Basic Biotechnology

Biotechnology is one of the major technologies of the twenty-first century. Its wide-ranging, multi-disciplinary activities include recombinant DNA techniques, cloning and the application of microbiology and other cell culture technologies to the production of a wide range of goods from bread to antibiotics. It continues to revolutionise treatments of many diseases, and is used to provide clean technologies and to deal with environmental problems.

Basic Biotechnology uniquely combines biology and bioprocessing topics to provide a complete overview of biotechnology. It explains the fundamental principles that underpin all biotechnology and provides a full range of examples showing how these principles are applied; from starting substrate to final product. A distinctive feature of this text are the discussions of the public perception of biotechnology and the business of biotechnology, which set the science in a broader context. This comprehensive text is essential reading for all students and practitioners of biotechnology and for researchers in academia, research institutes and biotechnology industries.

COLIN RATLEDGE is Emeritus Professor in the Department of Biological Sciences at the University of Hull where he has been teaching and researching for nearly 40 years. He has served on almost all the major biotechnology committees in the UK, including Chairperson of the Food Research Grants Board of the Biotechnology and Biological Sciences Research Council. He also acts as a consultant to many industrial companies in the UK, Europe and the USA.

BJØRN KRISTIANSEN is the Chief Executive Officer of EU Biotech Consulting in Norway. He is an active member of the European Federation of Biotechnology (EFB), including co-founder and interim chairperson for the Section on Biological Engineering Science.

Basic Biotechnology

Third Edition

Edited by

Colin Ratledge
University of Hull, UK

Bjørn Kristiansen
EU Biotech Consulting, Norway

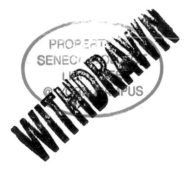

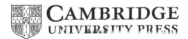
CAMBRIDGE
UNIVERSITY PRESS

CAMBRIDGE UNIVERSITY PRESS
Cambridge, New York, Melbourne, Madrid, Cape Town, Singapore, São Paulo

Cambridge University Press
The Edinburgh Building, Cambridge CB2 2RU, UK

Published in the United States of America by Cambridge University Press, New York

www.cambridge.org
Information on this title: www.cambridge.org/9780521840316

First published 2006

Printed in the United Kingdom at the University Press, Cambridge

A catalogue record for this publication is available from the British Library

ISBN-13 978-0-521-84031-6 hardback
ISBN-10 0-521-84031-7 hardback

ISBN-13 978-0-521-54958-5 paperback
ISBN-10 0-521-54958-2 paperback

Contents

Part I   Fundamentals and principles

Contributors

Allstair J. Anderson
Department of Biological Sciences, University of Hull, Hull, HU6
7RX, UK

David B. Archer
School of Biology, University of Nottingham, University Park,
Nottingham, NG7 2RD, UK

Frank Baganz
The Advanced Centre for Biochemical Engineering, Department of
Biochemical Engineering, University College London, Torrington
Place, London, WC1E 7JE, UK

Randy M. Berka
Research Fellow, Core Technology Department, Novozymes Biotech,
Inc., 1445 Drew Avenue, Davis, CA 95616, USA

Joaquim M.S. Cabral
Centro de Engenharia, Bioquimica e Quimica, Av Rovisco Pais,
Instituto Superior Technico, 1049–001 Lisboa, Portugal

Joel R. Cherry
Novozymes Biotech, Inc., 1445 Drew Avenue, Davis, CA 95616, USA

Yusuf Chisti
Institute of Technology and Engineering, Massey University, Private
Bag 11 222, Palmerston North, New Zealand

Mike Clark
Division of Immunology, Department of Pathology, University of
Cambridge, Tennis Court Road, Cambridge, CB2 1QP, UK

Steven D. Doig
The Advanced Centre for Biochemical Engineering, Department of
Biochemical Engineering, University College London, Torrington
Place, London, WC1E 7JE, UK

L. Eggeling
Research Centre Jülich, Biotechnologie 1, 52425 Jülich, Germany

Sven-Olof Enfors
Department of Biochemistry and Biotechnology, Riayl Institute of
Technology, S-100 44 Stockholm, Sweden

Sir Christopher Evans
Merlin Biosciences Ltd, 33 King Street, St James, London, SW1Y
6RJ, UK

Pedro Fernandes
Centro de Engenharia, Bioquimica e Quimica, Av Rovisco Pais,
Instituto Superior Technico, 1049–001 Lisboa, Portugal

Colin R. Harwood
Department of Microbiology and Immunology, The Medical School, University of Newcastle, Framlington Place, Newcastle upon Tyne, NE2 4HH, UK

J. J. Heijnen
TU Delft, Julianalaan 67, 2628 BC Delft, The Netherlands

C. J. Hewitt
Department of Chemical Engineering (Biochemical Engineering), The University of Birmingham, Edgbaston, B15 2TT, UK

Derek J. Hook
Senior Research Specialist, 3M Pharmaceuticals, Pharmacology, Building 0270-03-A10, 3M Center, St Paul, MN 55144-1000, USA

B. Isailovic
Department of Chemical Engineering (Biochemical Engineering), The University of Birmingham, Edgbaston, B15 2TT, UK

David J. Jeenes
Institute of Food Research, Norwich Research Park, Colney, Norwich, NR4 7UA, UK

Levente Karaffa
Department of Microbiology and Biotechnology, Faculty of Sciences, University of Debrecen, H-4010, PO Box 63, Debrecen, Hungary

Georg-B. Kresse, Head of Protein Discovery, Pharma Research, Roche Diagnostics GmbH, D-82372 Penzberg, Germany

Bjørn Kristiansen
EU Biotech Consulting, Gluppeveien 15, 1614 Fredrikstad, Norway

Christian P. Kubicek
Division of Gene Technology, Institut fur Verfahrenstechnik, Umwelttechnik und Techn, Biowissenschaften, Getreidemarkt 9/166, A-Vienna 1060, Austria

Gary J. Lye
The Advanced Centre for Biochemical Engineering, Department of Biochemical Engineering, University College London, Torrington Place, London, WC1E 7JE, UK

Donald A. MacKenzie
Institute of Food Research, Norwich Research Park, Colney, Norwich, NR4 7UA, UK

N. T. Mukwena
Department of Chemical Engineering (Biochemical Engineering), The University of Birmingham, Edgbaston, B15 2TT, UK

Jens Nielsen
Center for Process Biotechnology, Building 223, BioCentrum-DTU, Technical University of Denmark, DK-2800 Lyngby, Denmark

A. W. Nienow
Department of Chemical Engineering (Biochemical Engineering),
The University of Birmingham, Edgbaston, B15 2TT, UK

Henk J. Noorman
DSM Anti-Infectives, PO Box 425, 2600 AK Delft, The Netherlands

Marcel Ottens
Department of Biotechnology, Delft University of Technology,
Julianalaan 67, 2628 BC Delft, The Netherlands

W. Pfefferle
Degussa AG, Feed Additives Division, R&D, Kantstraese 2, 33790
Halle-Kuensebeck, Germany

Colin Ratledge
Department of Biological Sciences, University of Hull, Hull, HU6
7RX, UK

Jason Rushton
Merlin Biosciences Ltd, 33 King Street, St James, London,
SW1Y 6RJ, UK

H. Sahm
Research Centre Jülich, Biotechnologie 1, D-52425 Jülich, Germany

J. E. Smith
Department of Bioscience and Biotechnology, University of
Strathclyde, 204 George Street, Glasgow, G1 1XW, UK

Bernhard Sonnleitner
Zürich University of Applied Sciences, Winterthur, Institute for
Chemistry and Biotechnology, Postfach 805, 8401 Winterthur,
Switzerland

Hens J. G. ten Hoopen
Department of Biotechnology, Delft University of Technology, Delft,
The Netherlands

Luuk A. M. van der Wielen
Department of Biotechnology, Delft University of Technology,
Julianalaan 67, 2628 BC Delft, The Netherlands

Philippe Vandevivere
The Seawater Foundation, 4230E. Whittier Street,
Tucson, AZ 85711, USA

Robert Verpoorte
Department of Pharmacognosy, Section Metabolomics, IBL, Leiden
University, Leiden, The Netherlands

Willy Verstraete
Laboratory for Microbial Ecology and Technology, Ghent University,
Coupure L653, Belgium

Johannes A. Wesselingh
University of Groningen, Department of Chemical Engineering,
Nijenborgh 4, Groningen, NL-9747 AG, The Netherlands

Anil Wipat
Department of Microbiology and Immunology, The Medical School,
University of Newcastle, Framlington Place, Newcastle upon Tyne,
NE2 4HH, UK

James P. Wynn
Martek Biosciences Corp., 6480 Dobbin Road, Columbia, Maryland,
MD 21045, USA

Preface to the second edition

It is some 14 years since the first edition of this book appeared. Much has happened to biotechnology in these intervening years. Recombinant DNA technology, which was just beginning in the mid 1980s, is now one of the major cornerstones of modern biotechnology. Developments in this area have radically altered our concepts of healthcare with the arrival of numerous products that were unthinkable 20 years ago. Such is the pace of biotechnology that it can be anticipated in the next 14 years that even greater developments will occur thanks to such programmes as the Human Genome Project which will open up opportunities for treatment of diseases at the individual level. All such advances though rely on the application of basic knowledge and the appreciation of how to translate that knowledge into products that can be produced safely and as cheaply as possible. The fundamentals of biotechnology remain, as always, production of goods and services that are needed and can be provided with safety and reasonable cost.

Biotechnology is not just about recombinant DNA, of cloning and genetics; it is equally about producing more prosaic materials, like citric acid, beer, wine, bread, fermented foods such as cheese and yoghurts, antibiotics and the like. It is also about providing clean technology for a new millennium; of providing means of waste disposal, of dealing with environmental problems. It is, in short, one of the two major technologies of the twenty-first century that will sustain growth and development in countries throughout the world for several decades to come. It will continue to improve the standard of all our lives, from improved medical treatments, through its effects on foods and food supply and into the environment. No aspect of our lives will be unaffected by biotechnology.

This book has been written to provide an overview of many of the fundamental aspects that underpin all biotechnology and to provide examples of how these principles are put into operation: from the starting substrate or feedstock through to the final product. Because biotechnology is now such a huge, multi-everything activity we have not been able to include every single topic, every single product or process: for that an encyclopedia would have been needed. Instead we have attempted to provide a mainstream account of the current state of biotechnology that, we hope, will provide the reader with insight, inspiration and instruction in the skills and arts of the subject.

Since the first edition of this book, we sadly have to record the death of our colleague and friend, John Bu'Lock, whose perspicacity had led to the first edition of this book being written. John, at the time of his death in 1996, was already beginning to plan this second edition and it has been a privilege for us to have been able to continue in his footsteps to see it through into print. John was an inspiring figure in biotechnology for many of us and it is to the memory of a fine scientist, dedicated biotechnologist and a remarkable man that we dedicate this book to JDB.

Preface to the third edition

From antibiotics and production of other health care products to waste treatment and disposal, biotechnology continues to hold our attention. The breadth and scope of biotechnology continues to increase: each decade sees significant new advances across a wide range of topics. From the first edition of this book to the second edition took 14 years; from the second edition to this one has taken only five. The rapid pace of developments in molecular biology and genetics, and in their applications to biotechnology, ensures that progress in microbiology, animal and plant cell technology for the furtherance of our well-being never slackens. Biotechnology continues to be a world-driving force for the production of a whole range of products as well as being vitally important as a process technology for the care of the environment. The expectations are that biotechnology will remain as one of the leading scientific and industrially linked endeavours for at least the first half of this present century. Its contribution to our health, welfare, food and drink will, in fact, continue for as long as civilisation continues, such is the importance of biotechnology.

This new edition of *Basic Biotechnology* reflects these key developments in our subject but, at the same time, this new edition consolidates our knowledge of those fundamental principles of science and engineering that are vital to an understanding of the subject at its basic level. New chapters have been included on several topics both in the fundamentals and principles section as well as in the practical applications section; most of the other chapters have been extensively revised and all have been up-dated.

All our authors are internationally known for their contributions to biotechnology; all are exceptionally busy people and we therefore thank them most sincerely for taking time out to write their various chapters – both new and revised. Our task as editors has therefore been a rather easy one: curtailing a little too much detail here, or asking for clarification of a point, is about all we have had to do. Equally important is the enthusiasm of the publishers for this new edition. Their input in helping to produce a highly improved format, for what is already a highly regarded and popular book, is to be applauded. Obviously our publishers, like the purchasers of this book, know a good book when they see one.

We trust that this new edition adequately reflects the current status and trends in mainstream biotechnology. Given the diversity of biotechnology it will be an impossible task to cover every aspect of the field in one volume. Nevertheless, we feel that the major aspects of the subject are covered herein.

Part I

Fundamentals and principles

Chapter 1

Public perception of biotechnology

J. E. Smith

University of Strathclyde, UK

1.1   Introduction

Public perception of new technologies can have pronounced effects on the timing and direction of innovation, and on rates of uptake or discrimination of the technology, its products and services. Public perception can be area- or region-specific (e.g. North America, Southeast Asia, etc.) and will be dependent on several variables, namely

- economic affluence,
- level of education,
- cultural and religious values and traditions, and
- social and institutional ways of participation.

At the present time, public perception of biotechnology is generating much debate, especially in the EU.

Before entering into an examination of how the general public are believed to perceive modern biotechnology, especially genomics and proteomics, it is pertinent to highlight how biotechnology evolved historically to its present-day profound and positive impact on industry, medicine, agriculture, commerce and the environment. Historically, the microbial aspects of biotechnology evolved over many centuries

Basic Biotechnology, third edition, eds. Colin Ratledge and Bjørn Kristiansen.
Published by Cambridge University Press. © Cambridge University Press 2006.

as an artisan skill rather than as a science exemplified in the ancient manufacturing of beer, wine, cheese, yoghurts, fermented meats, such as salami, etc., where the methods of production were well understood but the actual microbial and biochemical mechanisms went unknown. Indeed, it was well into the seventeenth and eighteenth centuries before the causal microorganisms could be identified and their positive role confirmed. Consequently, with the advances in microbiology and biochemistry, all of the previously empirically driven processes became better understood and controlled. To these traditional and long-established products were added, more recently, antibiotics, vaccines, therapeutic proteins and countless others. *In all of these product examples, the industries involved with their manufacture contribute to national prosperity and the well-being of the population.*

Why, then, has there been such public awareness and concern for biotechnology in recent years? Without doubt, the main reasons can be attributed to the rapid advances in molecular biology, in particular recombinant DNA (rDNA) technology (gene technology), which is now allowing bioscientists a remarkable insight, understanding and control of biological processes. Using gene technologies, it is now increasingly possible to manipulate the heritable components of particular cells directly (that is, sections of DNA in which the desired gene is located) between different types of organisms (that is, between microbe and plant or animal, or from plant to animal, animal to microbe, etc.).

Developments in the domain of genomics and, more recently, proteomics, can be expected (and indeed have already been applied in some instances) to make important scientific advances in the field of human health, namely

- the use of genetically modified organisms for the production of biopharmaceuticals (i.e. insulin) and vaccines;
- elucidation of the molecular basis of many diseases;
- genome sequence obtention of more human pathogens, allowing better treatment for diseases;
- development of more successful gene therapy techniques for genetic diseases and cancer;
- more rapid and easily used disease diagnosis making use of molecular, biological and immunological techniques;
- improved nutrition by selected application of GM technology of food plants;
- the development of biosensors, such as DNA probes, for monitoring metabolites in the body.

Plant gene technology involves manipulating the genetic constitution of the plant (that is, by modifying a very small part of its DNA) so that it now has a more useful or better property; for example, a plant may now be resistant to insect or fungal attack; be more resistant to drought, or can produce higher quantities of a useful protein or compound (see Table 1.1). In some cases, an unwanted activity can be removed; for example, the enzyme responsible for tomatoes

Table 1.1	Important crop characteristics undergoing genetic modification

Pest resistance

Resistance to viral, bacterial and fungal diseases

Oil, starch and protein modification to provide sustainable supplies of raw materials for biodegradable plastics, detergents, lubricants, paper making and packaging; also, improvements in baking and brewing qualities

Herbicide tolerance to enable certain crop varieties to tolerate specific herbicides and, in many instances, reduce the number of herbicide applications to achieve effective weed control

Plant architecture and flowering, including plant height, flowering time and flower colour

Reduction in seed losses through shedding at harvest time

Modifications in fruit and tuber ripening and storage; research on potatoes is likely to reduce dependence on the use of antisprouting compounds applied to stored tubers

Increased tolerance to environmental stresses, including cold, heat, water and saline soils

Increase in the ability of certain plants to remove toxic metals from soils (bioremediation), e.g. from mining wastes

The elimination of allergens from certain crops, e.g. rice

The enhancement of vitamins, minerals and anticancer substances

The production of pharmaceutical substances, e.g. anticoagulant compounds, edible vaccines

Source: Dale, P. J. (2000). The GM debate: science or scaremongering? *Biologist* **47**: 7–10. Reproduced with permission.

overripening and splitting can be silenced so that tomatoes stay firm and in good condition for several weeks. All such plants are then known as 'genetically modified' or GM plants. The technology being used involves the direct application of molecular biology techniques and is, therefore, completely different from plant breeding, which seeks to improve the characteristics of plants by just using selective interbreeding between plants to bring out the desirable traits. GM techniques, because they are precise and are carried out in laboratories, can be a 100 times faster than plant breeding and their outcome is more certain (for an extended current report on GM crops see www.apec.umn.edu/faculty/frunge/globalbiotech04.pdf).

The focus of agriculture must be to use all scientific approaches, including GM technology, to improve human and animal nutrition so that it becomes possible to feed the growing world population at a time of decreasing availability of arable land. Worldwide acceptance and use of plant GM technology is clearly progressing rapidly in the Americas and Asia but is experiencing organised opposition in Europe!

The release of live GM microorganisms into various ecosystems when used as biopesticides or in bioremediation has raised concerns in some quarters. DNA probe analysis is now widely used in microorganism identification in complex ecosystems, while GM microorganisms are now increasingly used in pollution control for specific targeted compounds. While most innovations in modern biotechnology have not caused any noticeable public concern, three areas continue to generate levels of dissension, namely the potential, or imagined, health risks of GM foods and biopharmaceuticals; the advances in molecular genetics that relate to human reproduction; and ethical and moral issues arising from compiling human genetic information (relating to individuals).

1.2 | Public awareness of genetic engineering

Public perception of biotechnology is not only important, but also complex. In recent years, public policy makers on biotechnology have strived to balance the concerted interests of governments, industries, academia and environmental groups, often in a climate of tension and conflicting agenda. In gene technology, the central most important issue revolves around the question *'should regulation be dependent on the characteristics of the products produced by rDNA technology or on the use of rDNA technology per se?'* The 'product versus process' debate has lasted for many years and exposed conflicting views on what should represent public policies on new technology development. Should these important decisions be left to the scientists and technologists alone to decide or should the public also become part of the decision-making process? It is now apparent that many aspects of new biotechnology are matters for public deliberation and argument. *When arriving at important policy advice and moral judgements, there should be clearly defined reasons, criticisms, rebuttals, qualifications and careful analysis of scientific facts.* Social policy making should always be in the public, political realm and, in democratic countries, science policy must always be a matter for the people even though just a small minority of the population will understand the relevant science.

It is now well documented that gene technology provokes a variety of views within the general public that have not been so apparent with most other new technologies. In societies that include many different cultural, religious and political traditions, there will be a plurality of views that must be accommodated if democratic decisions are to be made. Public education in such complex areas of science as gene technology is paramount. Furthermore, *for many people there is an increasing concern about the ever-growing influence of technology, in general, in their lives and, in some instances, an unjustified mistrust of scientists.*

Over the last decade there have been many efforts made to gauge the public awareness of modern biotechnology by questionnaires, Eurobarometers and consensus conferences. Early EU studies highlighted public attitudes to the application of genetic engineering to a wide range of scenarios (Table 1.2). What then must be done to advance public understanding of genetic technology in the context of biotechnology? What does the public need to know and how can

Table 1.2 Public attitudes to applications of genetic manipulation

	Comfortable (%)	Neutral (%)	Uncomfortable (%)
Microbial production of bioplastics	91	6	3
Cell fusion to improve crops	81	10	10
Curing diseases such as cancer	71	17	9.5
Extension of the shelf life of tomatoes	71	11	19
Cleaning up oil slicks	65	20	13
Detoxifying industrial waste	65	20	13
Use of antiblood clotting enzymes produced by rats	65	14	22
Medical research	59	23	15
Making medicines	57	26	13
Making crops to grow in the Third World	54	25	19
Developing mastitis-resistant cows by genetic modification	52	16	31
Producing disease-resistant crops	46	29	23
Chymosin production by microorganisms	43	30	27
Improving crop yields	39	31	29
Using viruses to attack crop pests	23	26	49
Improving milk yields	22	30	47
Cloning prize cattle	7.2	18	72
Changing human physical appearance	4.5	9.5	84
Producing hybrid animals	4.5	12	82
Biological warfare	1.9	2.7	95

this be achieved to ensure that the many undoubted benefits that this technology can bring to humankind do not suffer the same fate as the food irradiation debacle in the UK in the early 1990s? While gamma irradiation of foods was demonstrated to be a safe and efficient method to kill pathogenic bacteria, it was not accepted by the lay public following the Chernobyl disaster, since most were unable to differentiate between the process of irradiation and radioactivity. Effective communication about the benefits and risks of genetic engineering will depend on understanding the underlying concerns of the public together with any foreseeable technical risks.

Eurobarometer surveys revealed a broad spectrum of opinions that were influenced by nationality, religion, knowledge of the subject and how the technology will be applied (Box 1.1). *A major contributory factor is the plurality of beliefs and viewpoints that are held explicitly or implicitly about the moral and religious status of Nature and what our relationship with it should be. Do we view Nature, in the context of human's dependency on plants and animals, as perfect and complete derived by natural means of reproduction and therefore should not be tampered with by 'unnatural' methods, or do we see it as a source of raw material for the benefit of humankind?* For centuries now, humans have been indirectly manipulating the genomes of plants and animals by guided matings primarily to enhance desired characteristics

> **Box 1.1** | **Eurobarometer (1997) on Public Perception of Biotechnology**
>
> - The majority of Europeans consider the various applications of modern biotechnology useful for society. The development of detection methods and the production of medicines are seen to be most useful and considered the least dangerous.
> - The use of modern biotechnology in the production of foodstuffs and the insertion of human genes into animals to obtain organs for humans were judged least useful and potentially dangerous.
> - Europeans believe that it is unlikely that biotechnology will lead to a significant reduction of hunger in the developing world.
> - The vast majority of Europeans feel genetically modified products should be clearly labelled.
> - The majority of Europeans tend to believe that we should continue with traditional breeding methods rather than changing the hereditary characteristics of plants and animals through modern biotechnology.
> - Less than one in four Europeans think that current regulations are sufficient to protect people from any risk linked to modern biotechnology.
> - Only two out of ten Europeans think that regulations of modern biotechnology should be primarily left to industry.
> - A third of Europeans think that international organisations such as the United Nations and the World Health Organisation are better placed to regulate modern biotechnology, followed by scientific organisations.

or minimise unwanted traits. In this way, present-day food plants and animals bear little resemblance to their predecessors. In essence, such changes have been driven by the needs and demands of the public or consumer, and have readily been accepted by them; almost invariably this has led to food becoming progressively less expensive. Indeed, the highest price ever paid for wheat was in the thirteenth century and the cheapest price was in 2005. *In the traditional methods used, the changes are made at the level of the whole organism, selection is made for a desired phenotype and the genetic changes are often poorly characterised and occur, together with other, possibly undesired, genetic changes. The new methods, in contrast, enable genetic material to be modified at the cellular and molecular level, are more precise and accurate, and consequently produce better characteristics and more predictable results while still retaining the aims of the classical breeder.* A great number of such changes can and will be done within species giving better and faster results than by traditional breeding methods.

Public responses must be properly gauged because the public itself is not a single entity and, consequently, cannot be considered as a homogeneous collection of attitudes, interests, values and level of education. A 2003 UK government-based public consultation has found that a majority of the 35 000 interviewees were opposed to genetically modified (GM) crops and distrusted both the agri-biotech industry and the government's ability to regulate such products. This

Table 1.3	Questions to be considered during safety assessment

- What is the function of the gene in the donor organism?
- What is the effect of the introduced gene(s) in the modified plant?
- Is there evidence of a change in allergenicity or toxicity?
- Will there be non-target effects on friendly organisms within the environment?
- Is there a change in the plant's ability to persist in agricultural habitat (weediness) or to invade natural habitats?
- Can the introduced gene be transferred to other plants (e.g. by pollination) or organisms, and what would be the likely consequences?

Source. Dale, P. J. (2000). The GM debate: science or scaremongering? *Biologist* **47**: 7–10. Reproduced with permission.

consultation 'GM Nation Public Debate' was designed as a comprehensive empirical study of public attitudes towards GM food and crops and of general public levels of awareness, understanding and perceived value of public debate on the commercialisation of agricultural biotechnology. The report has produced an interesting data set that will allow for a detailed exploration of public attitudes to this controversial issue. In reply, the pro-industry Agricultural Biotechnology Council (London) expressed some scepticism towards the findings claiming that the interviewees were unrepresentative and further implying that many responses had been orchestrated by anti-GM campaigning groups. *A worrying feature of public perception of genetic engineering is the extraordinary low and naïve public understanding of the genetic basis of life systems.* As a consequence various organisations have sought to generate public alarm and fear, especially of GM foods, while failing to set out a single piece of scientific data to support their claims. So-called Friends of the Earth activists trample and destroy legitimate field crop experiments that are designed to yield controlled scientific research into the safety and potential of GM plants. Such activists and provocative press articles (usually written by non-scientists) are, to a large extent, responsible for the wholly artificial sense of risk that has been ascribed, in particular, to GM foods. In the USA, the public acceptance of GM technology has continued with only minor disturbances and there is increased utilisation on farm of several GM crops. It is increasingly apparent that the worldwide acceptance and use of GM technology is progressing rapidly.

1.3 | Regulatory requirements

1.3.1 Safety of genetically engineered foods

There is now worldwide debate on the safety aspects of GM crop plants and derived products destined for public consumption. Some of the main questions on safety are presented in Table 1.3.

The Organisation for Economic Cooperation and Development (OECD), Paris, has included in its definition of food safety the passage 'reasonable certainty that no harm will result from intended uses under anticipated conditions of consumption'. When foods or food ingredients are derived from GM plants they must be seen to be as safe as, or safer than, their traditional counterparts. The concept of *substantial equivalence* is widely applied in the science-based determination of safety by comparing GM foods with analogous conventional food products, together with intended use and exposure. The concept of substantial equivalence can also be utilised as the premise for work based on the Codex Alimentarius Commusion (www.codexalimentarius.net/web/index_en.jsp or www.who.int/entity/foodsafety/codex/an. elaborate food standards and codes of practice for questions related to food), which has become the seminal global reference point for consumers, food producers and processors, national food control agencies and international food trade. The data used in establishing substantial equivalence will be largely derived from molecular and protein characterisation, which would involve tests to determine:

• gene expression patterns,
• protein profiling,
• changes in protein expression,
• differences in metabolite capabilities.

Such sophisticated testing protocols could make it difficult for many developing countries to comply with international food safety regulations. When novel products are moving into the marketplace, the consumer must be assured of their quality and safety. Thus, there must be toxicological and nutritional guidance in the evolution of novel foods and ingredients to highlight any potential risks which can then be dealt with appropriately. The approach should be in line with accepted scientific considerations, the results of the safety assessment must be reproducible and acceptable to the responsible health authorities, and the outcome must satisfy *and* convince the consumer!

A comprehensive regulatory framework is now in place within the EU with the aim of protecting human health and the environment from adverse activities involving genetically modified organisms (GMOs). There are two directives providing horizontal controls, i.e:

(1) contained use,
(2) deliberate release of GMOs.

The contained use of GMOs is regulated in Europe under the Health and Safety at Work Act through the Genetically Modified Organisms (Contained Use) Regulations, which are administered by the Health and Safety Executive (HSE) in the UK. The HSE receive advice from the Advisory Committee on Genetic Modification. These Regulations (which implement Directive 90/219/EEC), cover the use of all GMOs in containment and will incorporate GMOs used to produce food additives or processing aids. All programmes must carry out detailed risk assessments with special emphasis on the organism that is being modified and the effect of the modification.

Any deliberate release of GMOs into the environment is regulated in the UK by the Genetically Modified Organisms (Deliberate Release) Regulations, which are made under the Environmental Protection Act (and implement EC Directive 90/220/EC). Such regulations will cover the release into the environment of GMOs for experimental purposes (i.e. field trials) and the marketing of GMOs. Current examples could include the growing of GM food crop plants or the marketing of GM soya beans for food processing.

All experimental release trials must have government approval and the applicant must provide detailed assessment of the risk of harm to human health and/or the environment. All applications and the risk assessments are scrutinised by the Advisory Committee on Releases into the Environment, which is largely made up of independent experts who then advise the ministers.

The EC Novel Foods Regulation (258/97) came into effect on May 1997 and represents a mandatory EU-wide pre-market approval process for all novel foods. The regulation defines a novel food as one that has not previously been consumed to a significant degree within the EU. A part of their regulations will include food containing or consisting of GMOs as defined in Directive 90/220/EEC and food produced by GMOs but not containing GMOs in the final product.

In the UK the safety of all novel foods including genetically modified foods is assessed by the independent Advisory Committee on Novel Foods and Processes (ACNFP: now advises the UK, Food Standards Agency, www.foodstandards.gov.uk), which has largely followed the approach developed by the WHO and OECD in assessing the safety of novel foods. The ACNFP has encouraged openness in all of its dealings, publishing agenda, reports of assessments and annual reports, a newsletter and a committee website. By such means it hopes to dispel any misgivings that may be harboured by members of the public. The ultimate decisions are not influenced by industrial pressure and are based entirely on safety factors.

In all of the foregoing, the risk assessments of GMO products, etc., have been made by experts and judged on the basis of safety to the consumer. However, it must be recognised that subject experts define risk in a narrow technical way, whereas the public or consumer without sufficient knowledge generally displays a wider, more complex, view of risk that incorporates value-laden considerations such as unfamiliarity, catastrophic potential and controllability. Furthermore, the public, in general, will almost always overestimate risks associated with technological hazards such as genetic engineering and underestimate risks associated with 'lifestyle' hazards such as driving cars, smoking, drinking, fatty foods, etc. Perception of the risks inherent in genetic engineering may be moderated by recognition of the tangible benefits of specific products of genetic engineering that could be shown to have health or environmental benefits.

How do you achieve effective communication with the public about benefits and risks of genetic engineering? Trust in the information source is of major importance in communication about risk and this is associated with perceptions of accuracy, responsibility and concern with public welfare. In contrast, distrust may be generated when it is assumed that the facts are distorted or the information misused or biased.

1.3.2   Labelling: how far should it go?

Perhaps the most conscientious issue related to foods derived from genetic engineering is to what extent should they be labelled. The purpose of labelling a food product is to provide sufficient information and advice, accurately and clearly, to allow consumers to select products according to their needs, to store and prepare them correctly, and to consume them with safety. *Labelling of a product will only be relevant if the consumer is able to understand the information printed on the labels.* The US Food and Drug Administration (FDA) consider that labelling should not be based on the way a particular product is obtained. Their assumption is that this is, or should be, a part of normal approval for agricultural practice or industrial processes and, if approved, then labelling should be unnecessary, which is the common practice for most food products. It can be argued that certain consumers are, in principle, against a certain technique (such as genetic engineering) and such consumers should have the right to know if this technology has been used to produce the particular product.

At least within the EU there is considerable evidence that there is strong support for the clear labelling of genetically engineered foods. It can be argued that labelling is all about consumer choice and has nothing to do with health and safety. Where there is concern about the specific safety of products labelling will not solve the problem (note tobacco products are already labelled as injurious to health but are still bought by the public). The novel food regulations in the EU introduced specific labelling requirements over and above those already required for food. These stated that labelling would be required where there are special ethical concerns such as copies of animal or human genes or if the food product contained live GMOs. However, the EU has pressed for all foods that contain genetically modified material to be labelled clearly to enable consumers to have a real choice. Plant breeders are increasingly turning to the new genetic technologies to improve their plants and animals in order to produce the *cheap* food now demanded by the consumer. *If consumers insist that they want to choose whether or not to buy GM or non-GM products then there must be an adequate supply of non-GM foodstuffs.*

For over five years the EU banned GM foods on the specious grounds that they were unsafe. This has now been amended and GM foods will be allowed as long as the amount of GM material is labelled. The new EU labelling legislations will cover all foods and ingredients produced from GMOs, including animal feed and pet foods, irrespective of whether they contain detectable GM material. Since over 70% of processed foods, between them containing over 30 ingredients derived from maize and soya (current main GM food plants in the USA), will be required to be labelled unless manufacturers and suppliers take the necessary, but highly expensive and difficult, steps to avoid their use. While this legislation appears reasonable, it is, in reality, impractible. The financial consequences of these regulations will be vast, not only to industry but also to the consumer, with an anticipated 3–5% increase in the cost of processed foods. The EU is now clearly out of step with most other developed countries purely to satisfy the 'precautionary principle' propagated by the anti-GM lobby. The Royal Society of Canada concluded in 2002 that mandatory labelling of GM products cannot be justified on a scientific basis unless *there are clear, scientifically-established health risks or significant nutritional changes posed by the product itself*. There is no such evidence at this time! The Royal Society (UK) concluded also that there is no evidence to imply GM foods are a health risk. *GM modified foods have undergone more rigorous testing than any other foods and are safe. Why, then, the continued EU obstruction to their meaningful role in world food supply?* GM technology has predominantly been developed in North American and commercially marketed by North-America-located companies. Most European countries have been slow to develop this cutting-edge technology for agriculture and it has been strongly promulgated in the USA and Canada that these mandatory labelling requirements by the EU are simply old-fashioned trade protectionism. The USA and Canada have already filed legal challenges at the World Trade Organisation alleging unfair trade practices. Many European governments are projecting 'consumer protection' considerations purely for vote-gaining reasons. Many believe that these new regulations are ill-thought out, have serious practical limitations, will involve increased bureaucratic involvement and will be costly to industry and the consumer.

The whole aspect of labelling of GMO-derived foods is undergoing a fierce and often bitter and ill-informed debate. It can only be expected that in the near future all major food organisms, especially plants, will have had some level of genetic engineering in their breeding programmes. This will be necessitated by the need to produce food for an ever-increasing world population. *Let us not delude ourselves; without the addition of this technology to the armoury of the plant breeder there will be serious and indeed calamitous food shortages, especially in the developing world.*

If all aspects of genetic modification must be recognised and recorded, it can only lead to unacceptably complex labelling criteria.

Consumer rights, now recognised by all member states in the EU, involve a right to information and, its corollary, a duty to inform. As a consequence, labelling should be meaningful, but appropriate.

A recent US Institute of Food Technologists' Expert Panel concluded that continued development and use of food rDNA biotechnology could provide many important benefits to society:

- a more abundant and economical food supply for the world;
- continued improvements in nutritional quality, including foods of unique composition, for populations whose diets lack essential nutrients;
- fresh fruit and vegetables with improved shelf-life;
- further improvements in production agriculture through more efficient production practices and increased yields;
- the conversion of non-productive toxic soils, in developing countries, to productive arable land;
- more environmentally friendly agricultural practices through improved pesticides and pesticide-usage practices, less hazardous animal wastes, improved utilisation of land and reduced need for ecologically sensitive areas such as rainforests.

With respect to a range of environmental and economic concerns about rDNA-biotechnology-derived food products, the panel also reached the following conclusions:

- new rDNA-derived foods and food products do not inherently present any more serious environmental concerns or unintended toxic properties than those already present by conventional breeding practices;
- appropriate testing by technology developers, producers and processors, regulatory agencies and others should be continued for new foods and food products derived from all technologies, including rDNA technology;
- programmes should be developed to provide the benefits of safe and economical rDNA-technology-derived food products worldwide, including less-developed countries.

1.4 | Policy making

Policy making on genetic engineering throughout the industrial world is strongly influenced by the interests of governments, industry, academics and environmental groups. *After almost two decades of discussions, the dominant issue still is whether government regulations should depend on the characteristics of the products modified by rDNA technique or on the technique of rDNA employed.* As with other techniques, the genetic engineering debate could also prove to be a critical testing ground for efforts to insert into governmental policies, socio-economic and socio-cultural measures – the so-called 'fourth criterion'. The advocates of this approach consider that measures of efficacy, quality and safety are, alone, insufficient to judge the potential risks associated with such new techniques and their products, and to these they would add social and moral considerations.

These new approaches are having a significant impact on the pace of agricultural and environmental applications of genetic engineering. In contrast, biomedical applications have progressed relatively rapidly. *Millions of people throughout the world have accepted and benefited from medical diagnostics and drugs provided by the new biotechnology companies.* Examples include the GM products erthropoietin, for kidney dialysis patients, and insulin, for diabetics, while diagnostics developed by genetic engineering, in particular, keep dangerous pathogens, such as HIV and hepatitis viruses, out of the blood supplies. In agriculture there has been concerted opposition by activists against GM bovine somatotropin (BST, also known as bovine growth hormone) but almost total silence on the engineered chymosin enzyme used to clot milk in cheese production, which now claims about 40–45% of the US market. Millions of calves are now no longer required for this process.

How much of a role the fourth criterion will play in relation to genetic engineering in agriculture and environmental policy making is at an important cross-roads. While there is great need to increase the science literacy of the public, in general; a well-informed public must still rely heavily on experts on sophisticated technical issues.

1.5 | Areas of significant public concern

1.5.1 Antibiotic-resistance marker genes

Current plant DNA-delivery technology normally results in only a very small number of the targeted cells stably integrating the recombinant DNA with the designated gene. The difficulty in identifying these few transformed cells leads to the concept of selectable marker genes. Such genes are linked to the trait-conferring gene before transformation and their presence allows growth of the cell in a special medium while not allowing growth in the absence of the marker gene. The marker gene is incidental and has no function in the transformed crop. The most widely used marker genes confer to plant cells resistance to compounds such as antibiotics and herbicides. The most widely functional plant marker gene worldwide is *npt11*, which confers resistance to the antibiotics kanamycin and neomycin. In hindsight, this relatively simple laboratory system should not have been used in conjunction with commercial crops.

Could such antibiotic-resistance genes be transferred from a GM plant or microorganism into the human gut microflora and so increase antibiotic resistance in the human population? Bacterial resistance to commonly used antibiotics is now occurring worldwide and it is most probable that this incidence is the result of the transfer of antibiotic-resistance genes between bacteria followed by the selective pressures imposed by the use of antibiotics. *To date it has not been possible to demonstrate the transfer of antibiotic resistance from a selectable marker gene in a consumed GM plant to microorganisms normally present in the gut of humans and other animals.* However, the potential does exist and should not be ignored. European regulations have required a phasing out by 2006 of the use of markers conferring resistance to antibiotics used clinically. Methods are now being developed for the removal of antibiotic-resistance marker genes from transgenic crops. In theory, these methods should permit the phasing out of antibiotic-resistance markers and also reduce the amount of introduced recombinant DNA sequences.

1.5.2   Transfer of allergens

Food allergies arise when the immune system responds to specific allergens, which are usually proteins or glycoproteins in the food. This is now a major concern especially with respect to peanut and other tree nuts and severe anaphylactic reactions are not uncommon. Consequently, labelling of food products with respect to the presence of nuts, and especially peanuts, is now widely practised. With GM crop plants having wider access to diversity, crossing species barriers and introducing additional proteins into GM foods could potentially create allergic reactions in consumers. Thus, it becomes essential with GM foods to ensure that transfer of allergens does not occur from donor species to recipient species. Clearly, this is a complex process and one that all producers of GMOs are now fully alerted to and to which due consideration is being given. There have been no recorded examples of new allergies by the process of recombinant DNA technology.

Many databases that can identify proteins that could be problematic if inserted into food materials are now increasingly available. A GM corn called StarLink™ was approved for use in animal feed but not for human consumption, because the Cry9c protein in the transformed corn did not disappear as quickly as other proteins in test assays. When small amounts of StarLink™ corn appeared in taco shells it created a major GM controversy. In retrospect, the producer company, Aventis, should not have brought to market a corn product not approved for both food and feed use, since it is now obvious that segregation of the crops cannot be reliably achieved. The US FDA later developed an antibody assay to determine sensitivity to the Cry9c protein and, when compared to control samples, there were no allergenic reactions associated with Cry9c protein. The StarLink™ episode was hugely damaging to the public image of GM foods highlighting a wide range of significant issues, namely:

- the inadequacy of the US regulatory system for marketing GM products,
- the high-handed and irresponsible attitude of certain seed companies and farmers towards the use of GM crops,
- the problem of developing marketing systems to segregate GM products not approved for use in US food channels,
- the role of government to ensure the integrity of grain supply,
- the manner in which research and marketing decisions are achieved by the biotech industry,
- the negative impact on GM technology.

It is to be hoped that this relatively minor episode in GM food mismanagement will have alerted the biotech companies, seed companies, farmers and regulatory authorities to ensure that the correct procedures prevail throughout the entire food system. If such an event was to be repeated, it could have disastrous effects on the whole future of a well-regulated GM food market.

1.5.3 Pollen transfer from GM plants

While there have been many potential concerns expressed on the safety of GM foods, possible environmental hazards have also been considered. *The possibility of gene transfer from transgenic crop plants to compatible wild relatives has been subject to serious experimental examination. When all traditional commercial crop plants are considered, there are vanishingly few examples where this has happened since such crops require special cultivation practices and are unable to compete with the indigenous wild plant populations.* Could pest or herbicide resistance incorporated into transgenic plants be transferred into other closely related plants and increase their 'weediness'? Under normal conditions gene transfer by way of pollen between close relatives is exceptionally rare and there is little confirmed evidence that this will be different with transgenic plants. While, in theory, such occurrences are possible, they would be at such a low frequency that, in practice, the results are of virtually no consequence or concern. However, all commercially grown (released) transgenic plants are regularly monitored to confirm these conclusions.

1.5.4 Pharming

There are increasing efforts to produce human regulatory proteins, which normally occur (in humans) in very small concentrations and have mostly defied modern methods of extraction or synthesis, e.g. insulin. Previously, small quantities of such molecules were derived from organs of cadavers and from blood banks. Genetic engineering is now increasingly being used to produce these molecules in unrestricted quantities. This entails inserting the acquired human-derived gene constructs into suitable host microorganisms, which produce the therapeutic protein in quantities related to the scale of operation. Such products will be free of dangerous contaminants that could arise from extraction from cadavers.

Perhaps one of the most exciting and controversial issues in agricultural biotechnology at the present time is the concept of **'pharming'** – the production of genetically modified crops engineered to express some form of pharmaceutically useful product. *There is an anticipated short-fall in the production of therapeutic proteins by current-day technologies and, consequently, the acceptance of plants for this form of farming is now widely proposed.* However, from a legal aspect, the development of pharming raises a whole novel range of legitimate concerns about food safety risks related to using food crops to produce pharmaceutical products and the liability issues this will create.

The potential of pharming is enormous, but at the present time attention is being given to the choice of plants and how production can be contained without contamination of crops destined for the food product system.

1.5.5 Social, moral and ethical issues with plant and animal GMOs

Initial concerns about GMOs were perceived basically on safety issues; but more recently social, moral and ethical issues have become part of the decision-making process. The control of GM crop plants and their seeds by multi-national agrochemical companies and their need to recover the high investment costs could imply that only farmers making use of advanced technologies will be able to meet the full costs. *GM seeds are normally made sterile to prevent further propagation by farmers. However, this is normal practice by seed companies where the seeds used commercially are F1 hybrids that do not breed truly so that a constant supply of seed is needed for farmers to grow the right crops.* This ensures a fair return from the investment to produce them originally. The development of herbicide-resistant GM crops could well result in dependence by farmers on the specific herbicides and their producing companies. It is hoped that poor Third World farmers will benefit in the near future from these developments.

The concept of 'sustainability' would also have dramatic social impact on some developing countries. For example, several novel sweeteners have been developed, many times sweeter than sucrose, which could ultimately lead to a reduction in the traditional markets for sugar cane and sugar beet. In this way, these economies, predominantly in developing countries, could experience severe financial and employment disruption with alternatives difficult to find. Similarly, increased milk production from fewer cows by regular injection of genetically engineered bovine growth hormones (such as BST) may well cause severe difficulty for small farmers in the USA and EU. While this development has gone through quite successfully in the USA, there is a moratorium currently in operation in the EU to prevent its application in Europe.

It must be expected that many aspects of this new genetic technology, particularly when applied to agriculture and food production, could well lead to decreases in employment with an ensuing increase in poverty in developing economies. Different value judgements come into operation to reconcile the advantages to society against the disadvantages. *The developed nations must endeavour to assist the developing nations both technically and financially to be part of this agriculture revolution. To what extent this is now happening is variable and questionable. It is sad that public awareness of such issues is seldom voiced by the western activists against genetic engineering.*

It is in the area of animal transgenics that public awareness and concern is now being expressed. Transgenic animals are those incorporating foreign or modified genetic information resulting from genetic engineering. Genetic modification of animals with ensuing transgenesis may be considered by some on a religious basis as a fundamental breach in natural breeding barriers that nature developed through evolution to prevent genetic interplay between unlike species. Such viewpoints consider the species as 'sacred'. In contrast, in the reductional philosophy of most molecular biologists, the gene has become the ultimate unit of life and is merely a unique aggregation of organic molecules (largely common to all types of living cells) available for manipulation. In this way, most molecular biologists argue that there is no ethical problem created in transferring genes between species and genera. What are the foreseen reasons or benefits for pursuing animal transgenesis?

(1) There have been extensive animal studies aimed at understanding developmental pathways with a view to understanding gene action. The development of the Oncomouse for cancer studies could have significant values in developing anticancer drug treatment for humans. However, the fact that the mouse will suffer the development of cancer and die does raise issue of animal morality.

(2) Improved growth rates in animals and fish have been achieved by selected gene transfer, but will these GM organisms be fully accepted into the food chain?

(3) The insertion of human genes into lactating animals, e.g. sheep, has had dramatic and generally acclaimed results. There appears to be little effect on the animal and valuable human health proteins can be extracted from the milk of the transgenic animal and there is general public acceptance of such products. This is not seen as a contentious issue since the transgenic animal does not enter the food chain.

(4) Xenotransplantation, especially from pigs, is seen as an excellent source of organs for human transplants. Human complement-inactivating factors to prevent acute hyper-immune rejection of the transplant have been successfully transferred into the pig. This programme has obvious attraction and could overcome the acute shortage of human organs for essential transplants. The main concerns have been possible transfer of pig viruses to humans in the light of the BSE scare. Also the question of breeding pigs for this purpose, as opposed to the accepted current practice for eating purposes, does generate ethical concerns for some people!

(5) Biomarkers for detecting environmental pollution using transgenic nematodes would appear to be a worthwhile activity.

(6) As models for human genetic diseases with the ultimate aim to develop new drugs or gene-therapy treatments.

While many people see the aims of these studies to be of significant value to humankind, others express genuine concerns for animal welfare and whether we have the right to indulge in modifying an animal genome to human advantage. Central to public concern is a strong feeling of 'unnaturalness' in transferring human genes into animals with the new transgenic animal containing copies of the original human gene. *It is difficult for the average layperson to comprehend that while the transgene has human origin and structure, it is not its immediate source.* In the process of genetic manipulation, genes cannot be directly transported from the donor to the recipient but must progress through a complicated series of *in-vitro* clonings. In this manner a series of amplification steps are carried out in which the original gene is copied many times during the whole process – usually in a bacterium – such that the original genetic material is diluted 10^{55} times. Thus, the original DNA is not directly used; but, rather, similar DNA is synthesised artificially.

The issue of animal rights is highly contentious: do they have intrinsic rights or not? Some would assign equal moral worth to sentient animals as to humans, but where do you draw the line? The Advisory Committee on Novel Foods and Processes (ACNFP) some years ago considered some of the main ethical concerns arising from the food use of certain transgenic organs and prepared the following exclusions:

(1) Transfer of genes from animals whose flesh is forbidden for use as food by certain religious groups to animals that they normally consume (e.g. pig genes into sheep) would offend most Jews and Muslims.
(2) While transfer of human genes to food animals (e.g. transfer of the human gene for Factor IX, a protein involved in blood clotting, into sheep) is acceptable for pharmaceutical and medical purposes, the animals should not, upon slaughter, enter the food chain.
(3) Transfer of animal genes into food plants (e.g. for vaccine production), is acceptable for pharmaceutical and medical purposes, but plant remains should not then enter the animal and human food chain as they would be an anathema to vegetarians and, especially, vegans.
(4) Use of organisms containing human genes as animal feed (e.g. microorganisms modified to produce pharmaceutical human proteins such as insulin) should not be considered.

Close consultation with a wide range of religious faiths strongly suggested that there were no overwhelming objections to require an absolute ban on the use of food products containing copy genes of human origin. (This was particularly noticeable when the concept of the copy gene was understood). The report, however, strongly advocated that the insertion of ethically sensitive genes into food organisms be discouraged especially when alternative approaches were available. If transgenic organisms containing copy genes that are unacceptable to specific groups of the population subject to religious dietary restrictions were to be present in some foods, such foods should be compulsory and clearly labelled.

1.5.6 Genethics

Since the early days of the Human Genome Project there has been a growing apprehension of the anticipated ethical, social, legal and psychological issues that must emanate from research studies related to genetic testing, genetic databases, genetic screening, germ-line gene therapy, cloning, xenotransplantation and the use of embryonic stem cells (Table 1.4). Collectively, such studies will all fall into the area

Table 1.4	Areas of public concern in human genome research

Confidentiality of testing and screening results
Scope of genetic testing and screening
Discrimination and stigmatisation
Commercial exploitation of human genome data
Eugenic pressures
Effects of germ-line gene therapies on later generations

of 'genethics'. While the fundamental research on the analysis of the human genome will long continue to be essential, the potential repercussions could be considerable and will generate many questions concerned with confidentiality, privacy, community consent, stigmatism, access to genetic testing and screening, and how should financial resources be allocated.

Soon it may be possible to have a much fuller awareness of an individual's 'genetic portfolio' and possibly to diagnose future medical problems, e.g. potential to develop heart disease, cancer, etc., and advise treatment well in advance of the onset of the disease. It has been suggested that genetic testing and screening should only be carried out with disorders where treatment is presently available. Where genetic disorders have already been diagnosed and observed in families, it is now possible in limited cases to perform pre-natal testing to discover whether the foetus carries the defect. The parents may then be able to sanction a termination or be better prepared for the needs of the full-term baby.

The most sinister aspect of genetic testing is the use for which such information could be used by employers, and insurance and mortgage institutions. While, undoubtedly, genetic information of an individual could well reduce the financial risk to the business concern, the effects on the unfortunate individual would be disastrous, particularly when the potential genetic problem or risk identified may well never materialise in later years. Ethics committees are increasingly proposing that insurance companies and other related financial organisations should not require, or be allowed access to, an individual's genetic information as a pre-requisite for insurance or mortgage. However, this may well prove to be beyond the individual's control and, if permitted, could have catastrophic implications.

Medication based on the transfer of genes, gene therapy, could become important in combating inherited genetic diseases. Limited practice of somatic (non-sexual cells) gene therapy has been tried with little success and will remain under close supervision to satisfy medical safety, legal implications and public concerns. Germ-line (sexual cells, i.e. sperm cells) gene therapy is not allowed because it is ethically and socially unacceptable and would create major problems of eugenics.

The potential utilisation of human stem cells, undifferentiated primordial cells derived in most cases from a single fertilised egg, for regenerative medicine could have the potential to develop cures for many diseases, e.g. diabetes, Alzheimer's, etc. Stem cells could also lead the way to therapeutic cloning of organs (kidney, heart, etc.) for transplantation purposes. For those who could well benefit from such developments there is enthusiastic support, while others oppose on ethical and moral grounds! There will undoubtedly be major re-appraisals of stem cell research as this offers such potential gains to sick individuals.

A cautionary word must be said of those overzealous enthusi-asts who create unrealistic expectations concerning the capacity of biomedicine to control illness and aging. The all-too-often press state-ments on the imminent arrival of radically innovative biotechnologi-cally derived therapies more often create false expectations for those with illnesses and signs of aging. Much will be achieved in medicine by biotechnology, but it is essential not to turn biotechnology into an absolute belief system.

1.6 | Conclusions

The safety and impact of genetically modified organisms continues to be addressed by scientific research. Basic research into the nature of genes, how they work and how they can be transferred between organisms has served to underpin the development of the technol-ogy of genetic modification. In this way, basic information about the behaviour of genes and of GMOs will be built up and used to address the concerns about the overall safety of GMOs and their impact on the environment.

1.7 | Further reading

The following references should be consulted to achieve a fuller understand-ing of the many viewpoints related to the safety and impact of genetically modified organisms on society.

Atherton, K. T. *Genetically Modified Crops*: *Assessing Safety*. London: Taylor and Francis, 2002.

Dale, P. J. The GM debate: science or scaremongering? *Biologist*, **47**: 7–10, 2000.

Frewer, L. K. and Shepherd, R. Ethical concerns and risk perceptions associated with different applications of genetic engineering: interrelationship with the perceived need for regulation of the technology. *Agriculture and Human Values*, **12**: 48–57, 1995.

Horlick-Jones, T., Walls, J., Rower, G. *et al. A Deliberative Future? Public Debate about Possible Commercialisation of Transgenic Crops in Britain, 2003*, Understanding Risk Working Paper 04.02. Norwich: Centre for Environmental Risk, 2004.

Konig, A. A framework for designing transgenic crops: science, safety and citizen's concerns. *Nature Biotechnology* **21**: 1274–1279, 2002.

Lawrence, S. Agbio keeps on growing. *Nature Biotechnology* **23**: 281, 2005.

Miller, H. Cat and mouse in regulating genetic 'enhancement'. *Nature Biotechnology* **23**: 171–172, 2005.

Moore, P. A profile. *Nature Biotechnology* **23**: 280, 2005.

OECD. *Safety Evaluation of Food Derived by Modern Biotechnology*: Concepts and Principles. Paris: Organisation for Economic Cooperation and Development, 1993.

Poortinga, W. and Pidgeon, N. F. *Public Perceptions of Genetically Modified Food and Crops, and the GM Nation? Public Debate on the Commercialisation of Agricultural Biotechnology in the UK*, Understanding Risk Working Paper 04.01. Norwich: Centre for Environmental Risk, 2004.

Smith, J. E. *Biotechnology*, fourth edition. Studies in Biology. Cambridge: Cambridge University Press, 2004.

The Royal Society. *Genetically Modified Plants for Food Use*. London: The Royal Society, 1998, pp. 1–16.

The Royal Society. *Genetically Modified Plants for Food Use* and *Human Health: An Update*. London: The Royal Society, 2002.

Chapter 2

Biochemistry and physiology of growth and metabolism

Colin Ratledge

University of Hull, UK

2.1   Introduction

The First Law of Biology (if there was one) could be: the purpose of a microorganism is to make another microorganism.

In some cases biotechnologists, who seek to exploit the microorganism, may wish this to happen as frequently and as quickly as possible; in other words they wish to have as many microorganisms available at the end of the process as possible. In other cases, where the product is not the organism itself, the biotechnologist must manipulate it in such a way that the primary goal of the microbe is diverted. As the microorganism then strives to overcome these restraints on its reproductive capacity, it produces the product which the biotechnologist desires. The growth of the organism and its various products are therefore intimately linked by virtue of its metabolism.

In writing this chapter, I have not attempted to explain the structure of the main microbial cells: the bacteria, the yeasts, the fungi

Basic Biotechnology, third edition, eds. Colin Ratledge and Bjørn Kristiansen.
Published by Cambridge University Press. © Cambridge University Press 2006.

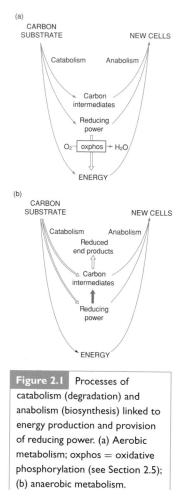

Figure 2.1 Processes of catabolism (degradation) and anabolism (biosynthesis) linked to energy production and provision of reducing power. (a) Aerobic metabolism; oxphos = oxidative phosphorylation (see Section 2.5); (b) anaerobic metabolism.

and the microalgae. These are available in most biology textbooks and these should be consulted if there are uncertainties about cell structures. However, biology textbooks rarely explain the chemistry that goes on in the living cell (i.e. their biochemistry) in simple terms but, as the biochemistry of the cell is fundamental to the exploitation of the organism, it is important to be acquainted with the basic systems that microbial cells use to achieve their multiplication.

The biochemistry of the cell is therefore described as an account of the chemical changes that occur within a cell as it grows and multiplies to become two cells. The physiology of the cell, however, goes beyond the biochemistry of the cell as this term extends the simple account of the flow of carbon, and the changes which occur to other elements, by describing how these processes relate to the whole growth process itself. The biochemical changes therefore are to be seen occurring in the three-dimensional array, which is the cell, with a fourth dimension of time being added. Not all reactions that are capable of happening will occur; some may occur during the period of its fastest growth while others may occur only as the growth rate of the organism is slowing down and entering a period of stasis. Physiology therefore is a complete understanding of the chemical changes within a cell related to its development, growth and life cycle.

2.2 | Metabolism

2.2.1 Some definitions

Metabolism is a matrix of two closely interlinked but divergent activities (see Fig. 2.1).

Anabolic processes are concerned with the building up of cell materials, not only the major cell constituents (protein, nucleic acids, lipids, carbohydrates, etc.) but also the intermediate precursors of these materials – amino acids, purine and pyrimidines, fatty acids, various sugars and sugar phosphates. Anabolism concerns processes that are endothermic overall (they 'require energy'). They also invariably require a source of reducing power which must come by the degradation of the substrate (or feedstock).

The compensating exothermicity is provided by various *catabolic (energy-yielding) processes* (see also Chapter 3). The degradation of carbohydrates, such as sucrose or glucose, ultimately to give CO_2 and water, is the principal exothermic process whereby 'energy generation' is accomplished. During this process reducing power needed for the subsequent anabolic processes is also generated. The same considerations, however, apply to all substances that are used by microorganisms: their degradation must yield not only carbon for new cells but also the necessary energy and reducing power to convert the metabolites into the macromolecules of the cell.

The combined processes of catabolism and anabolism are thus known as *metabolism*.

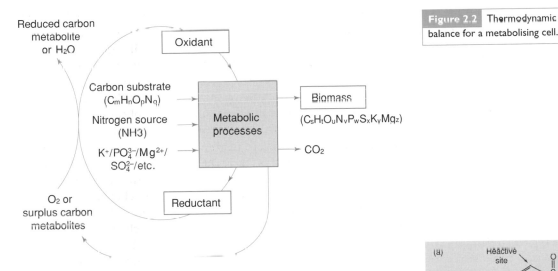

Figure 2.2 Thermodynamic balance for a metabolising cell.

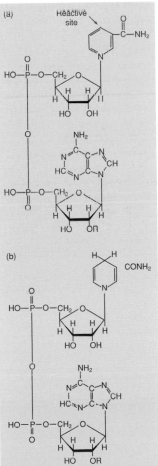

We can also distinguish between organisms that carry out their metabolism *aerobically*, using O_2 from the air, and those that are able to do this *anaerobically*, that is, without O_2. The overall reaction of reduced carbon compounds with O_2, to give water and CO_2, is a highly exothermic process; an aerobic organism can therefore balance a relatively smaller use of its substrates for catabolism to sustain a given level of anabolism, that is, of growth (see Fig. 2.1a), than can an anaerobic organism. Substrate transformations for anaerobic organisms are essentially *disproportionations*, with a relatively low 'energy yield', so that a larger proportion of the substrate has to be used catabolically to sustain a given level of anabolism (Fig. 2.1b).

The difference can be illustrated with an organism such as yeast, *Saccharomyces cerevisiae*, which is a facultative anaerobe – that is, it can exist either aerobically or anaerobically. Transforming glucose at the same rate, aerobic yeast gives CO_2, water and a relatively high yield of new yeast cells, whereas the yeast grown anaerobically has a lower yield of energy and reducing power. Consequently, fewer cells can be made than under aerobic conditions. Also it is not possible for the cells, in the absence of O_2, to oxidise all the reducing power that is generated during catabolism. Consequently, surplus carbon intermediates (in the case of yeast it is pyruvic acid) are reduced in order to recycle the reductants (see Fig. 2.2) and, in the case of yeast, ethanol is the product.

Overall, this process can be described by the simple reaction:

$$X + NADH \rightarrow XH_2 + NAD^+$$

where X is a metabolite and NADH is the reductant, and NAD^+ is its oxidised form (see Fig. 2.3a, b). NAD stands for nicotinamide adenine dinucleotide; NADH is therefore reduced NAD. There is also the phosphorylated form of NAD^+; NAD phosphate designated as $NADP^+$. This can also be reduced to NADPH and it can also function as a reductant but usually in anabolic reactions of the cell, whereas NADH is

Figure 2.3 (a) NAD^+NADP^+ (oxidised); (b) NADH/NADPH (reduced). In NAD^+ and NADH, R = H; in $NADP^+$ and NADPH, $R = PO_3^2$.

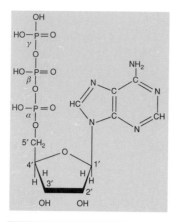

Figure 2.4 Adenosine triphosphate (ATP). When donating energy, the γ-bond is hydrolysed and the available energy is used to make a new bond in a molecule. Adenosine diphosphate (ADP) is without the last phospho group and adenosine monophosphate is without the last two phospho groups.

usually involved in the degradative reactions. All four forms (NAD$^+$, NADP$^+$, NADH and NADPH) occur in both aerobic as well as anaerobic cells: in the former cells re-oxidation of NADH and NADPH can occur by being linked to O_2, but this cannot take place in the anaerobe, hence the need for the alternative re-oxidation strategy (see Section 2.6).

A cell that grows obviously uses carbon, but many other elements are needed to make up the final composition of the cell. These will include nitrogen, oxygen, which may come from the air if the organism is growing aerobically (otherwise the O_2 must come from a rearrangement of the molecules in which the organism is growing, or even water itself), together with other elements such as K^+, Mg^{2+}, S (as SO_4^{2+}), P (as PO_4^{3+}) and an array of minor ions such as Fe^{2+}, Zn^{2+}, Mn^{2+}, etc. The dynamics of the system are set out in Fig. 2.2.

2.2.2 Catabolism and energy

The necessary linkage between catabolism and anabolism depends upon making the catabolic processes 'drive' the synthesis of reactive reagents, few in number, which in turn are used to 'drive' the full range of anabolic reactions. These key intermediates, of which the most important is adenosine triphosphate, ATP (Fig. 2.4), have, what biologists term, a 'high-energy bond'; in ATP it is the anhydride linkage in the pyrophosphate residue. Directly or indirectly the potential energy released by splitting this bond is used for the bond-forming steps in anabolic syntheses. Molecules such as ATP then provide the 'energy currency' of the cell. When ATP is used in a biosynthetic reaction it generates ADP (adenosine diphosphate) or occasionally AMP (adenosine monophosphate) as the hydrolysis product:

$$A + B + ATP \rightarrow AB + ADP + P_i \quad \text{or} \quad A + B + ATP \rightarrow AB + AMP + PP_i$$

(where A and B are both carbon metabolites of the cell, P_i = inorganic phosphate and PP_i = inorganic pyrophosphate).

ADP, which still possesses a 'high-energy bond', can also be used to produce ATP by the adenylate kinase reaction:

$$ADP + ADP \rightarrow ATP + AMP$$

Phosphorylation reactions, which are very common in living cells, usually occur through the mediation of ATP:

$$
\begin{array}{c}
\quad\quad\quad\quad\quad\quad\quad\quad\quad\quad\quad\quad O \\
| \quad\quad\quad\quad\quad\quad\quad\quad | \quad\quad || \\
- C - OH + ATP \rightarrow - C - O - P - OH + ADP \\
| \quad\quad\quad\quad\quad\quad\quad\quad | \quad\quad | \\
\quad\quad\quad\quad\quad\quad\quad\quad\quad\quad\quad\quad OH
\end{array}
$$

The phosphorylated product is usually more reactive (in one of several ways) than the original compound.

2.3 | Catabolic pathways

2.3.1 General considerations of glucose degradation

The purpose of breaking down a substrate is to provide the microorganisms with:

- building units for the synthesis of new cells;
- energy, principally in the form of ATP, by which to synthesise new bonds and new compounds;
- reducing power, which is mainly as reduced NAD (i.e. NADH) or reduced NADP (NADPH).

Both the ATP and the NAD(P)H (which can be used to denote both NADH and NADPH) act in conjunction with various enzymes in the conversion of one compound to another.

Although the microbial cell may be considered to be a vast collection of compounds, it can be simplified as being composed of:

- *proteins*, which can be either functional (such as enzymes) or structural as in some proteins associated with the cell wall or intracellular structures;
- *nucleic acids*, DNA and RNA;
- *lipids*, which are often based on fatty acids and are used in the formation of membranous structures surrounding either the whole cell or an organelle (a 'micro-organ') within the cell;
- *polysaccharides*, which are used mainly in the construction of cell walls, and cell capsules.

These, in turn, are made from simple precursors:

- proteins from amino acids;
- nucleic acids from nucleotide bases (plus ribose and phosphate);
- lipids from fatty acids, which are, in turn, produced from acetate (C_2) units;
- polysaccharides from sugars.

It is therefore possible to identify a mere nine precursors from which the cell can make all its molecules and, indeed, replicate itself (see Fig. 2.5). Thus, as long as the cell can produce these basic nine molecules from any substrate, or combination of substrates, it will be able to resynthesise itself (provided of course that in the formation of these precursors, ATP and NAD(P)H are also produced).

If we consider glucose as the usual growth substrate of a microbial cell, we can show how it is degraded into these nine key precursors (Fig. 2.5). Their formations are linked through the process of glycolysis, which is sometimes called the *Embden–Meyerhof–Parnas (EMP) pathway*, which is given in more detail in Fig. 2.6, and then by the further oxidation of pyruvate, as the end-product of glycolysis, through the reactions of the tricarboxylic acid cycle (see Fig. 2.9 below).

In addition to the glycolytic sequence, there is also an important adjunct to this that is responsible for forming pentose (C_5) phosphates

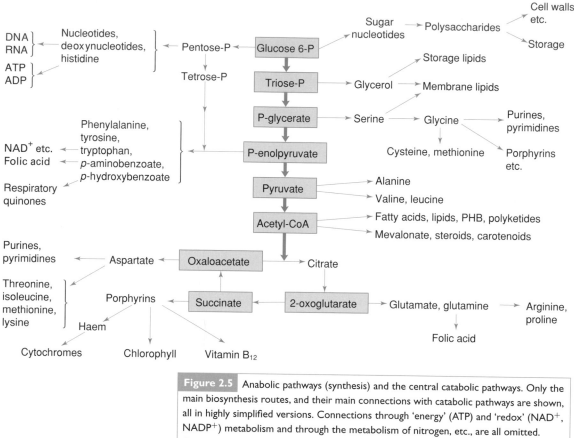

Figure 2.5 Anabolic pathways (synthesis) and the central catabolic pathways. Only the main biosynthesis routes, and their main connections with catabolic pathways are shown, all in highly simplified versions. Connections through 'energy' (ATP) and 'redox' (NAD$^+$, NADP$^+$) metabolism and through the metabolism of nitrogen, etc., are all omitted. (PHB, poly-β-hydroxybutyrate; P, phospho group). The nine principal precursors are in the shaded boxes.

and tetrose (C_4) phosphates. This is the *pentose phosphate pathway*, sometimes referred to as the pentose phosphate 'shunt' (see Fig. 2.7). The purpose of this pathway is two-fold: to provide C_5 and C_4 units for biosynthesis (see Fig. 2.5) and also to provide NADPH for biosynthesis.

Although the EMP pathway and the pentose phosphate (PP) pathway both use glucose 6-phosphate, the extent to which each route operates depends largely on what the cell is doing. During the most active stage of cell growth, both pathways operate in the approximate ratio 2 : 1 for the EMP pathway over the PP pathway. However, as growth slows down, the biosynthetic capacity of the cell also slows down and less NADPH and C_5 and C_4 sugar phosphates are needed so that the ratio between the pathways now moves to 10 : 1 or even to 20 : 1.

It is therefore apparent that metabolic pathways are controllable systems capable of considerable refinement to meet the changing needs of the cell. This is discussed later (see Section 2.8).

Although the EMP and PP pathways are found in most microorganisms, a few bacteria have an alternative pathway to the former

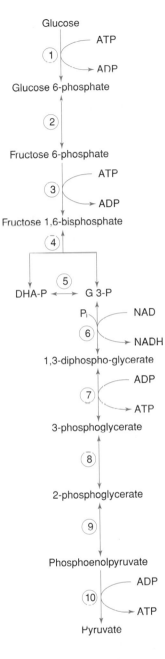

Glucose

Glucose 6-phosphate

Fructose 6-phosphate

Fructose 1,6-bisphosphate

DHA-P ⇌ G 3-P

1,3-diphospho-glycerate

3-phosphoglycerate

2-phosphoglycerate

Phosphoenolpyruvate

Pyruvate

Figure 2.6 The Embden–Meyerhof–Parnas pathway of glycolysis. Overall:

$$\text{Glucose} + 2NAD^+ + 2ADP + 2P_i$$
$$\rightarrow 2\text{pyruvate} + 2NADH$$
$$+ 2ATP$$

The reactions are catalysed by: (1) hexokinase, (2) glucose-6-phosphate isomerase, (3) phosphofructokinase, (4) aldolase, (5) triose phosphate isomerase, (6) glyceraldehyde-3-phosphate dehydrogenase, (7) 3-phosphoglycerate kinase, (8) phosphoglyceromutase, (9) phosphoenolpyruvate dehydratase, (10) pyruvate kinase. DHA-P dihydroxyacetone phosphate and G3-P = glyceraldehyde 3-phosphate. P_i represents an inorganic phosphate group.

pathway. This is the Entner–Doudoroff pathway (see Fig. 2.8), which occurs in pseudomonads and related bacteria. The pentose phosphate pathway, though, still operates in these bacteria as the Entner–Doudoroff pathway does not generate C_5 and C_4 phosphates.

2.3.2 The tricarboxylic acid cycle

The degradation of glucose, by whatever route or routes, invariably leads to the formation of pyruvic acid: $CH_3.CO.COOH$. The fate of pyruvate is different in aerobic organisms and anaerobic ones. In

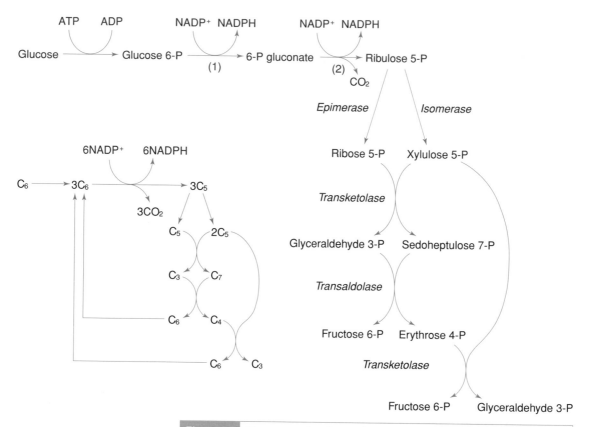

Figure 2.7 The pentose phosphate cycle (hexose monophosphate shunt). The numbered enzymes are: (1) glucose-6-phosphate dehydrogenase, (2) phosphogluconate dehydrogenase. Inset: summary showing stoichiometry when fructose 6-phosphate is recycled to glucose 6-phosphate by an isomerase; glyceraldehyde 3-phosphate can also be recycled by reverse glycolysis (Fig. 2.6). With full recycling the pathway functions as a generator of NADPH, but the transaldolase and transketolase reactions also permit sugar interconversions which are used in other ways.

Net reaction:

$$\text{Glucose} + \text{ATP} + 6\text{NADP}^+ \rightarrow \text{glyceraldehyde 3-P} + \text{ADP} + 6\text{NADPH} + 3\text{CO}_2$$

(Any removal of C_5 and C_4 sugars for biosynthesis will diminish the recycling process and thus the yield of NADPH will decrease.)

aerobic systems, pyruvate is decarboxylated (i.e. loses CO_2) and is simultaneously activated in the chemical sense, to acetyl coenzyme A (abbreviated as acetyl-CoA) in a complex reaction also involving NAD^+:

$$\text{pyruvate} + \text{CoA} + \text{NAD}^+ \rightarrow \text{acetyl-CoA} + \text{CO}_2 + \text{NADH}$$

This reaction is catalysed by *pyruvate dehydrogenase*. (The fate of pyruvate in anaerobic cells is described later.)

Acetyl-CoA, by virtue of it being a thioester, is highly reactive. It is capable of generating a large number of intermediates but its principal, though not sole, fate is to be progressively oxidised

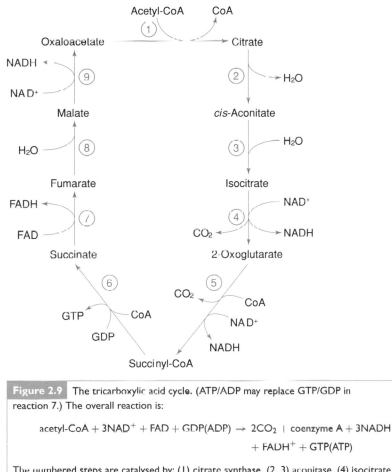

Figure 2.9 The tricarboxylic acid cycle. (ATP/ADP may replace GTP/GDP in reaction 7.) The overall reaction is:

$$\text{acetyl-CoA} + 3\text{NAD}^+ + \text{FAD} + \text{GDP(ADP)} \rightarrow 2\text{CO}_2 + \text{coenzyme A} + 3\text{NADH}$$
$$+ \text{FADH}^+ + \text{GTP(ATP)}$$

The numbered steps are catalysed by: (1) citrate synthase, (2, 3) aconitase, (4) isocitrate dehydrogenase, (5) 2-oxogluconate dehydrogenase, (6) succinate thiokinase, (7) succinate dehydrogenase, (8) fumarase, (9) malate dehydrogenase.

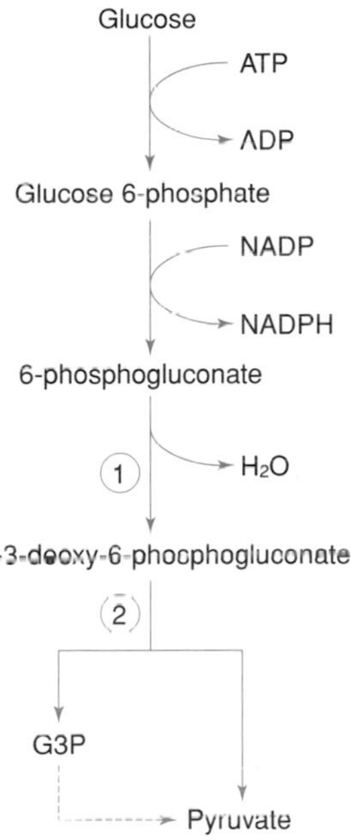

Figure 2.8 Entner–Doudoroff pathway. This sometimes replaces the Embden–Meyerhof–Parnas pathway (see Fig. 2.6) in some pseudomonads and related bacteria. Numbered enzymes are: (1) phosphogluconate dehydratase, (2) a specific aldolase. Glyceraldehyde 3-phosphate (G3P) is converted to pyruvate by the relevant enzymes given in Fig. 2.6.

through a cyclic series of reactions known as the *citric acid cycle*. This is also known as the *tricarboxylic acid cycle* or the *Krebs cycle* after its discoverer.

The reactions of the citric acid cycle are shown in Fig. 2.9. This cycle fulfils two essential functions:

- It provides key intermediates for biosynthetic reactions (see Fig. 2.5), principal of which are 2-oxoglutarate (to make glutamate and thence glutamine, arginine and proline), succinate (to make porphyrins) and oxaloacetate (to make aspartate and the aspartate family of amino acids – see Chapter 14);
- It produces energy from the complete oxidation of acetyl-CoA to CO_2 and H_2O. (This process is described in detail in Section 2.5.)

However the citric acid cycle cannot fulfil either function exclusively: if intermediates are removed for biosynthesis, then some energy production must be sacrificed; if all the acetyl CoA is oxidised

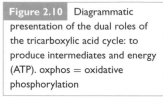

Figure 2.10 Diagrammatic presentation of the dual roles of the tricarboxylic acid cycle: to produce intermediates and energy (ATP). oxphos = oxidative phosphorylation

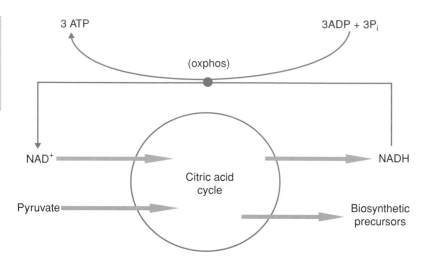

to CO_2 and H_2O there will be no intermediates left for biosynthesis. Consequently, the cycle runs as a balance between the two objectives. Pyruvate, coming from glucose, provides the input and the cycle provides the output in the way of energy *and* biosynthetic precursors (see Fig. 2.10). In meeting its twin objectives, the cycle cannot entirely replenish the initial oxaloacetate that is needed as a priming reactant to make citrate, as some of the intermediates must inevitably be used for biosynthetic purposes. (If they were not used for biosynthesis, there would be no point in the cycle just producing energy as this could not then be used in any sensible manner as there can be no biosynthesis without precursors.) It is therefore essential for there to be a second pathway by which oxaloacetate can be formed and this arises principally by the carboxylation of pyruvate:

$$\text{pyruvate} + CO_2 + ATP \rightarrow \text{oxaloacetate} + ADP + P_i$$

This reaction is carried out by *pyruvate carboxylase*. However, insofar as oxaloacetate is also produced from the activity of the cycle, the carboxylation of pyruvate must be regulated so that acetyl-CoA and oxaloacetate are always produced in equal amounts. This is usually achieved by the pyruvate carboxylase being dependent upon acetyl-CoA as a *positive effector* (see Section 2.8) for its activity; i.e. acetyl-CoA increases its activity but is not part of the enzyme reaction. The more acetyl-CoA that is present, the faster becomes the production of oxaloacetate. As oxaloacetate and acetyl-CoA are removed equally (to form citrate), the concentration of acetyl-CoA will fall; pyruvate carboxylase will then slow down but, as pyruvate dehydrogenase still operates as before, more acetyl-CoA will be produced. In this way not only will citric acid synthesis always continue, but the two reactions leading to the precursors of citrate will always be balanced (see Fig. 2.11). This type of reaction catalysed by pyruvate carboxylase is referred to as an *anaplerotic reaction*, meaning 'replenishing'.

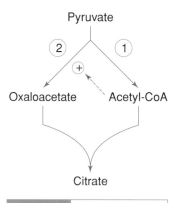

Figure 2.11 How the cell ensures equal supplies of oxaloacetate (OAA) and acetyl-CoA (AcCoA) for citric acid biosynthesis. The activity of pyruvate carboxylase (2) is stimulated by acetyl-CoA formed by pyruvate dehydrogenase (1).

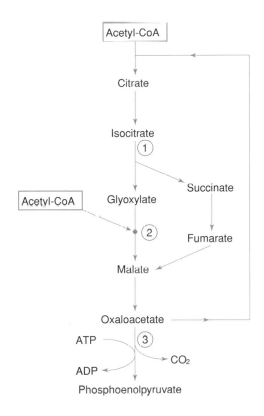

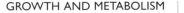

Figure 2.12 The glyoxylate by-pass. The additional reactions, beyond those of the tricarboxylic acid cycle (see Fig. 2.10), are (1) isocitrate lyase and (2) malate synthase. The scheme also shows how the by-pass functions to permit sugar formation from acetyl-CoA, with the added reaction (3) phosphoenolpyruvate carboxykinase, followed by reversed glycolysis (cf. Fig. 2.14). **NB** This by-pass only occurs in microbial and plant cells (the latter is in germinating plant seeds using stored triacylglycerols as sole carbon source) but not in animal cells.

2.3.3   The glyoxylate by-pass for growth on C_2 compounds

If a micro-organism grows on a C_2 compound, or on a fatty acid, hydrocarbon or any substrate that is degraded primarily into C_2 units (see Section 2.3.4), the tricarboxylic acid cycle is insufficient to account for its metabolism. Acetyl-CoA can be generated directly from acetate, if this is being used as a carbon source, or from a C_2 compound more reduced than acetate, i.e. acetaldehyde or ethanol:

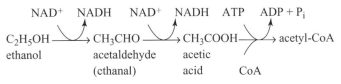

The manner in which acetate units are converted to C_4 compounds is known as the *glyoxylate by-pass* (see Fig. 2.12) for which two enzymes additional to those of the tricarboxylic acid cycle are needed: *isocitrate lyase* and *malate synthase*. The former enzyme cleaves isocitrate into succinate and glyoxylate. The latter enzyme then uses a second acetyl-CoA to add to the glyoxylate to give malate. Both these enzymes are 'induced' (i.e. they are synthesised only when the specific signal is given – see Section 2.8.4) when microorganisms are grown on C_2 compounds. The activity of both enzymes increases by some 20 to 50 times under such growth conditions. The glyoxylate by-pass does not supplant the operation of the tricarboxylic acid cycle; for example,

2-oxoglutarate will still have to be produced (from isocitrate) in order to supply glutamate for protein synthesis, etc. Succinate, the other product from isocitrate lyase, will be metabolised as before to yield malate and, thence, oxaloacetate. Thus, through the reactions of the glyoxalate cycle, C_4 compounds can now be produced from C_2 units and are then available for synthesis of all cell metabolites (see Fig. 2.5). Their conversion into sugars through the process of gluconeogenesis is detailed in Section 2.4.

2.3.4 Carbon sources other than glucose

Any compound that is used by a microorganism and can feed into any of the intermediates of glycolysis, or even into the citric acid cycle, can be handled by the organism with its existing complement of enzymes. However, a great many other substrates can be handled by microorganisms. In other words, all natural compounds are capable of degradation and the majority of this degradative capacity is found in microbial systems. The application of microorganisms as 'waste disposal units' is therefore paramount and this activity forms an intrinsic part of environmental biotechnology, which is explained in detail in Chapter 17.

To illustrate this diversity, the example of microbial degradation of fatty acids will be considered. The ability of microorganisms to grow on oils and fats is widespread. The difference between an oil and a fat is whether one is liquid or solid at ambient temperatures: they are both chemically the same, i.e they are fatty acyl triesters of glycerol:

$$
\begin{array}{ll}
CH_2OH & CH_2O.OC\text{-}(CH_2)_n\text{-}CH_3 \\
| & | \\
CHOH & CHO.OC\text{-}(CH_2)_m\text{-}CH_3 \\
| & | \\
CH_2OH & CH_2O.OC\text{-}(CH_2)_p\text{-}CH_3 \\
\textit{glycerol} & \textit{triacylglycerol}
\end{array}
$$

where n, m and p are typically 14 or 16; the long alkyl chain may be saturated as indicated or may have one or more double bonds giving unsaturated, or polyunsaturated, fatty acyl groups.

The oils, when added to microbial cultures, are initially hydrolysed by a *lipase* enzyme into its constituent fatty acids and glycerol. The latter is then metabolised by conversion to glyceraldehyde 3-phosphate (see Fig. 2.6). The fatty acids are taken into the cell and immediately converted into their coenzyme A thioesters. The fatty acyl-CoA esters are degraded in a cyclic sequence of reactions (see Fig. 2.13) in which the fatty acyl chain is progressively shortened by loss of C_2 units (as acetyl-CoA). This is known as the *β-oxidation cycle* as the initial attack on the fatty acyl chain is at the *β*- (or 3-) position. Each turn of the cycle produces a shorter fatty acyl-CoA ester, which then repeats the sequence of the four reactions until, finally, a C_4 fatty acyl group (butyryl-CoA) is produced which then gives rise to two acetyl-CoA units.

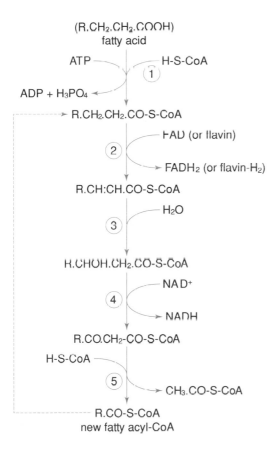

(R.CH$_2$.CH$_2$.COOH)
fatty acid

Figure 2.13 β-Oxidation cycle of fatty acyl-CoA esters. Enzymes are: (1) fatty acyl-CoA synthetase; (2) fatty acyl-CoA oxidase (in yeast and fungi) linked to flavin, or fatty acyl-CoA dehydrogenase in bacteria linked to FAD; (3) 2,3-enoyl-CoA hydratase (also known as crotonase); (4) 3-hydroxyacyl-CoA dehydrogenase; (5) 3-oxoacyl-CoA thiolase. The new fatty acyl-CoA then recommences the cycle at reaction (2).

For unsaturated fatty acids (see also Chapter 16), some adjustment in the position of the double bond may be needed to ensure that it is in the right position and configuration for it to be attacked by the second enzyme of the cycle, the hydratase (see Fig. 2.13).

The degradation of fatty acids liberates the energy as heat rather than metabolically usable energy in the form of ATP. This is by coupling the reoxidation of FADH$_2$ (see Fig. 2.13) to O$_2$, which produces H$_2$O$_2$. This is then cleaved by an enzyme, catalase, to give H$_2$O and 1/2O$_2$ with the liberation of considerable heat. Thus microorganisms growing on fatty acids and related materials, such as long chain alkanes, invariably generate considerable amounts of heat. As is explained in greater detail in Chapter 3, fatty acids and similar materials are energy-rich, carbon-low compounds, as opposed to glucose and other sugars being energy-low, carbon-rich compounds. Consequently, in the former case, degradative metabolism (i.e. catabolism) is geared so as to 'waste' energy that is surplus to requirements – which is then released as heat – and to conserve as much carbon as possible. The metabolism of the latter substrates, on the other hand, leads to a conservation of energy and 'wastage' of surplus carbon (as CO$_2$).

2.4 | Gluconeogenesis

When an organism grows on a C_2 or C_3 compound, or a material whose metabolism will produce such compounds at or below the metabolic level of pyruvate (e.g. acetate, ethanol, lactate or fatty acids), it is necessary for the organism to synthesise various sugars to fulfil its metabolic needs. This is termed *gluconeogenesis* (see Fig. 2.14). Though most of the reactions in the glycolytic pathways (see Figs. 2.5 and 2.6) are reversible, those catalysed by *pyruvate kinase* and *phosphofructokinase* are not and it is therefore necessary for the cell to circumvent them.

As phosphoenolpyruvate cannot be formed from pyruvate (there are, though, a few exceptions), oxaloacetate is used as the precursor:

$$oxaloacetate + ATP \rightarrow phosphoenolpyruvate + CO_2 + ATP$$

This reaction is catalysed by *phosphoenolpyruvate carboxykinase*, which is the key enzyme of gluconeogenesis. (The formation of oxaloacetate has already been discussed in relation to acetate metabolism, in Section 2.3.3.) For growth on lactate, or pyruvate itself, the lactate would be oxidised to pyruvate:

$$CH_3CH(OH).COOH + NAD^+ \rightarrow CH_3.CO.COOH + NADH$$

The pyruvate will be carboxylated to oxaloacetate using pyruvate carboxylase:

$$CH_3.CO.COOH + CO_2 + ATP \rightarrow COOH.CH_2.CO.COOH + ADP + P_i$$

The oxaloacetate is then converted to phosphoenolpyruvate (see above).

The net reaction for growth in lactate is therefore:

$$lactate + NAD^+ + 2ATP \rightarrow phosphoenolpyruvate + NADH$$
$$+ 2ADP + 2P_i$$

The irreversibility of the second glycolytic enzyme, phosphofructokinase (producing fructose 1,6-bisphosphate), is circumvented by the action of *fructose bisphosphatase*:

$$fructose\ 1,6\text{-}bisphosphate + H_2O \rightarrow fructose\ 6\text{-}phosphate + P_i$$

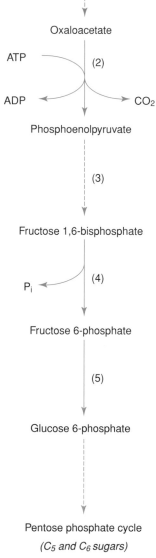

Figure 2.14 Gluconeogenesis sequence. From a substrate such as acetyl-CoA this is converted (1) by the reactions of the glyoxylate by-pass (see Fig. 2.12) to oxaloacetate and thence to phosphoenolpyruvate by phosphoenolpyruvate carboxykinase (2). This is converted by the reversed glycolytic sequence of enzymes (3) into fructose 1,6-bisphosphate (see also Fig. 2.6), which is then hydrolysed with the release of inorganic phosphate (P_i) by fructose 1,6-bisphosphatase (4). The product is then isomerised to glucose 6-phosphate (5), which can then be fed into the reactions of the pentose phosphate pathway (Fig. 2.7) or used for the biosynthesis of cell envelope polysaccharides.

Acetyl-CoA

(1)

Oxaloacetate

ATP

(2)

ADP — CO₂

Phosphoenolpyruvate

(3)

Fructose 1,6-bisphosphate

P_i (4)

Fructose 6-phosphate

(5)

Glucose 6-phosphate

Pentose phosphate cycle

(C₅ and C₆ sugars)

polysaccharides etc.

From this point, hexose sugars can be formed by the reversal of glycolysis and C_5 and C_4 sugars can now be formed via the pentose phosphate pathway (Fig. 2.7). Glucose itself is not an end-product of 'gluconeogenesis,' but glucose 6-phosphate is used for the synthesis of cell wall constituents and a large variety of extracellular and storage polysaccharides (see also Chapter 16).

2.5 | Energy production in aerobic microorganisms

It has already been explained how, in the metabolism of glucose (Figs. 2.6 and 2.7) and in the tricarboxylic acid cycle (Fig. 2.9), oxidation of the various metabolic intermediates is linked to the reduction of a limited number of co factors (NAD^+, $NADP^+$, FAD) producing the corresponding reduced forms (NADH, NADPH and $FADH_2$). The reducing power of these products is released by a complex reaction sequence that, in aerobic systems, is linked eventually to reduction of atmospheric O_2. This process is known as *oxidative phosphorylation* and the sequence of carriers that are used to convey the hydrogen ions and electrons, eventually to be coupled to O_2 to form H_2O, is referred to as the *electron transport chain*. The function of the electron-transport-coupled phosphorylation (ETP) system is the synthesis of ATP. The electron transport chain, together with ATP synthase, forms a multi-component system that is integrated into a membrane, which is either the cytosolic membrane of a bacterial cell or, in eukaryotic cells, is the mitochondrial membrane.

During the electron transport sequence, ATP is generated from ADP and inorganic phosphate (P_i) at two, or more usually three, specific points, depending on the nature of the original reductant. This is shown in Fig. 2.15. Although there are many variations in the respiratory chains [the principal systems for mitochondria (in eukaryotic organisms) and for bacteria as typified by *Escherichia coli* are shown in Fig. 2.15], the mechanism by which ATP is produced is similar in all cases. ATP synthase is a complex protein that sits across the membrane on one side of which are the reductants and on the other are protons (H^1; see Fig. 2.16). As the reductants become linked into the electron transport chain, further protons move back across the membrane and they literally drive the ATP synthase to revolve physically in its socket, which has the effect of coupling ADP with inorganic phosphate to give ATP. The system is referred to as having a *proton motive force* (PMF). Without a membrane creating two, otherwise unlinked, sides there could be no PMF, no ETP and, therefore, no energy production.

In the case of the three reductants, the overall reactions may be written as:

$$NADPH + 3ADP + 3P_i + \tfrac{1}{2}O_2 \rightarrow NADP^+ + 3ATP + H_2O$$
$$NADH + 3ADP + 3P_i + \tfrac{1}{2}O_2 \rightarrow NAD^+ + 3ATP + H_2O$$
$$FADH + 2ADP + 2P_i + \tfrac{1}{2}O_2 \rightarrow FAD + 2ATP + H_2O$$

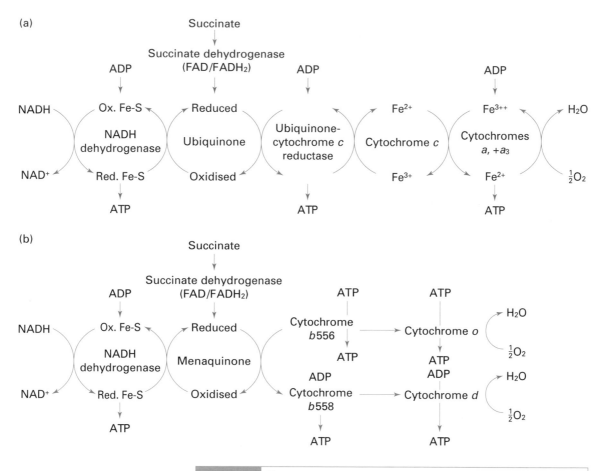

(a)

(b)

Figure 2.15 Electron-transport-coupled phosphorylation (ETP) system of: (a) mitochondria and (b) *E. coli*. Not all the electron carriers are shown, there being at least 16 proteins involved in each case. There are also considerable variations in the electron transport carriers. In the *E. coli* system, the electron transport chain divides and electrons and protons can flow through both the systems as described. The sites of phosphorylation of ADP to ATP are only indications as the actual formation of ATP is carried out by ATP synthases that are driven by the physical movement of proteins through the membrane (see also Fig. 2.16).

One can, therefore, describe the ATP yield, in each case, as being 3, 3 and 2, respectively. These are sometimes referred to as the *P/O ratios*, which is the amount of ATP gained from the reduction of $1/2 O_2$ to H_2O, and involves the transport of two electrons.

The yields of ATP per mole of glucose metabolised by the Embden–Meyerhof pathway (Fig. 2.6) and from the resulting pyruvate, metabolised by the reactions of the tricarboxylic acid cycle (Fig. 2.9) are summarised in Table 2.1. As can be seen, the vast majority of ATP is generated with the reactions of the electron transport chain coupled to the reactions of the citric acid cycle.

Table 2.1 ATP yields for glucose metabolism

	Moles ATP produced per mole hexose
Glycolysis (glucose to pyruvate):	
Net yield of ATP − 2 mol	2^a
NADH = 2 mol × 3	6
Pyruvate to acetyl-CoA:	
NADH = 1 mol × 3 (× 2 for 2 pyruvate)	6
Tricarboxylic acid cycle:	
NADH = 3 mol × 3 (× 2 for 2 acetyl-CoA)	18
FADH$_2$ = 1 mol × 2 (× 2 for 2 acetyl-CoA)	4
ATP = 1 mol (× 2 for acetyl-CoA)	2
Total	38

[a] Under anaerobic conditions these two moles of ATP represent the maximum attainable yield ('substrate-level phosphorylation', see Section 2.6.1).
[b] Produced from GTP (see Fig. 2.9) by nucleotide diphosphate kinase.

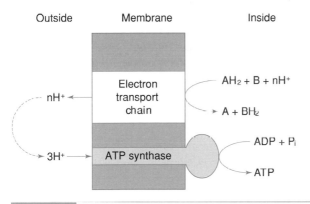

Figure 2.16 The coupling mechanism of ETP. The electron transport carriers (see Fig. 2.15) are located within a membrane. As the reductant (AH$_2$) is oxidised, this sets up a movement of protons through the membrane. These protons are then pumped back across the membrane driving the ATP synthase into coupling ADP with P$_i$ to give ATP.

2.6 | Anaerobic metabolism

2.6.1 General concepts

Under anaerobic conditions, the process of oxidative phosphorylation cannot occur, and the cell is deprived of its principal way of generating energy. Under such circumstances energy must be provided from the very process of degrading the original substrate. This process, known as *substrate-level phosphorylation*, yields only about 5--10% of the energy that can be produced under aerobic conditions (see Tables 2.1 and 2.2). This means that to produce a given weight of

Table 2.2 Substrate-level phosphorylation reaction in anaerobes

Enzyme	Reaction catalysed	Occurrence
1. Phosphoglycerol kinase	1, 3-bisphosphoglycerate + ADP → 3-phosphoglycerate + ATP	Widespread, see Fig. 2.6
2. Pyruvate kinase	phosphoenolpyruvate + ADP → pyruvate + ATP	Widespread, see Fig. 2.6
3. Acetate kinase	acetyl phosphate + ADP → acetate + ATP	Widespread
4. Butyrate kinase	butyryl phosphate + ADP → butyrate + ATP	E.g. enterobacteria on allantoin
5. Carbamate kinase	carbamoyl phosphate + ADP → carbamate + ATP	E.g. clostridia on arginine
6. Formyl-tetrahydrofolate synthetase	N^{10}-formyl-H_4 folate + ADP + P_i → formate + H_4 folate + ATP	E.g. clostridia on xanthine

cells, much more substrate must be degraded than under aerobic conditions. Or to put this another way, for a given amount of substrate (say, glucose), much fewer cells will be produced anaerobically than aerobically. Under anaerobic conditions, the cell is trying its utmost to maximise the formation of energy; the reducing power that is produced during the degradation of the substrate (see Figs. 2.1 and 2.2) has to be re-circulated for the process to continue as its supply is not limitless. The oxidation of the reducing equivalents therefore must be linked to the reduction of some of the carbon intermediates that are accumulating under these conditions:

$$X + NADH \rightarrow XH_2 + NAD^+$$

Only a little of the reducing power *per se* is needed for synthesis of new cells. Consequently, the reducing equivalents react with the accumulated carbon intermediates to reduce them in their turn (Fig. 2.1b). The only energy that is then available to the cell is that which comes from ATP formed during the anaerobic degradation of the substrate. Examples of substrate-level phosphorylation are given in Table 2.2. The energy yield from substrate-level phosphorylation will vary from organism to organism depending on the growth substrate being used and on whether acetate is accumulating as a final product, which will arise when acetyl kinase is in operation (see Table 2.2).

This process of anaerobic catabolism occurs not only in microorganisms, but may occur in higher animals too: an example would be the accumulation of lactic acid in muscle tissue during hyperactivity of an athlete. In microorganisms we can see a whole range of reduced carbon compounds being accumulated by organisms growing anaerobically. Examples may also include lactic acid itself (produced by lactic bacteria), but would include short chain fatty acids such as butyric or propionic acids, and alcohols such as butanol, propanol and ethanol (see Fig. 2.17). Some organisms, such as the *methanogenic*

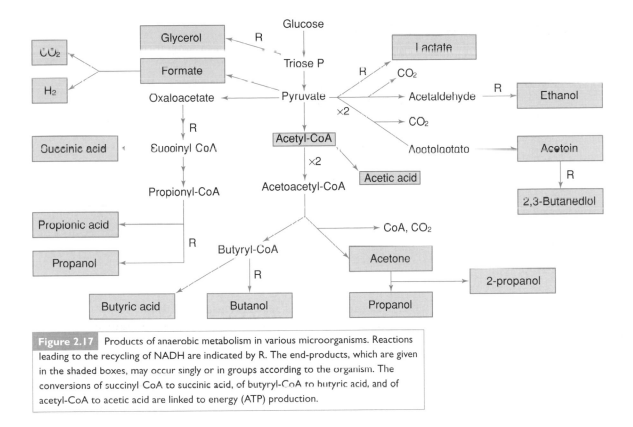

Figure 2.17 Products of anaerobic metabolism in various microorganisms. Reactions leading to the recycling of NADH are indicated by R. The end-products, which are given in the shaded boxes, may occur singly or in groups according to the organism. The conversions of succinyl CoA to succinic acid, of butyryl-CoA to butyric acid, and of acetyl-CoA to acetic acid are linked to energy (ATP) production.

bacteria, may go even further and produce, as the completely reduced end-product, methane (not shown in Fig. 2.17).

It is important to point out that pyruvate, produced by the glycolytic pathway (Fig. 2.6), will still enter the tricarboxylic acid cycle, which must continue, at least in part, to provide essential precursors for biosynthesis, principally 2-oxoglutarate, and oxaloacetate, but not to produce energy. The NADH produced in the cycle cannot be converted into ATP as the cells have no supply of O_2 to drive oxidative phosphorylation; however, in certain bacteria there are terminal electron acceptors other than O_2 that are capable of being coupled into the ETP system (Fig. 2.15) and that will allow the formation of ATP to take place. This includes microbes that can use nitrate (which is reduced to nitrite), nitrite (reduced to NH_4 or in some cases N_2 in a process known as *denitrification* – see also Chapter 17), CO_2 (reduced to methane by methanogens) or sulphate (reduced to H_2S by *sulphate-reducing bacteria*) as alternatives to O_2. In all cases, although the yield of ATP is less than occurs in aerobic systems, it is much greater than obtained by substrate-level phosphorylation alone.

2.6.2 Products of anaerobic metabolism
Figure 2.17 summarises some of the main reactions leading to the formation of reduced end-products in anaerobic microorganisms.

The major products are:

- *glycerol*, produced by yeasts when the conversion of pyruvate to ethanol is blocked;
- *lactic acid*, formed by lactic acid bacteria;
- *formic acid*, formed by enterobacteria via pyruvate-formate lyase and the formate can be converted to CO_2 and H_2 by formate dehydrogenase;
- *ethanol*, formed by yeasts (e.g. *Saccharomyces cerevisiae*), bacteria (e.g. *Zymomonas*) and by some fungi;
- *2,3-butanediol*, produced by various bacteria including *Serratia marcescens* and various *Bacillus* spp.;
- *butanol* with *acetone* and some *propanol* and/or 2-propanol, produced by *Clostridium* spp., some of which also produce butyric acid;
- *propionic acid*, produced by *Propionibacterium*.

Other products may arise from the anaerobic metabolism of compounds other than glucose, for example organic acids, such as citric acid, or amino acids and sometimes purines.

Methane (not shown in Fig. 2.17) is perhaps the ultimate reduced carbon compound and is produced by highly specialised Archaea (previously known as the Archaebacteria) by cleavage of acetate to CO_2 and CH_4 or in some cases by reduction of CO_2, methanol (CH_3OH), ethanol (CH_3CH_2OH) or formic acid (HCOOH) all in the presence of H_2.

2.7 | Biosynthesis

The provision of energy (ATP), reducing power (NADH and NADPH) and a variety of monomeric precursors (see Fig. 2.5) from the degradation of a substrate provides the cell with the necessary means of regenerating itself. The cell undertakes the biosynthesis of the macromolecules of the cell: nucleic acids (DNA and RNA), proteins (for enzymes and other functions), lipids for membranes and polysaccharides as components of the cell envelope, from these simple building blocks. As many of the biosynthetic pathways are covered elsewhere in this book (e.g. Chapters 14, 15 and 18) these need not be detailed here. However, a distinction needs to be drawn between primary metabolism and secondary metabolism as these have considerable importance for formation of biotechnological products.

2.7.1 | Primary metabolism

Primary metabolism occurs during *balanced growth*, sometimes known as the *tropophase*, of the organism in which all nutrients needed by the cell are provided in excess in the medium (see Fig. 2.18). Under such conditions the cells grow at an exponential rate in keeping with their mode of reproduction. The cells will have optimum contents of all the various macromolecules of the cell – DNA, RNA, proteins, lipids,

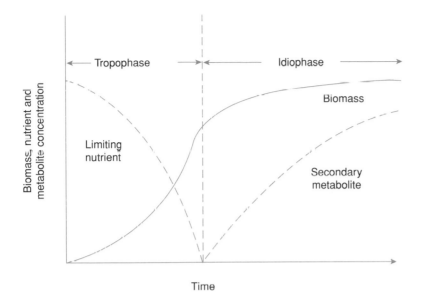

Figure 2.18 Microbial growth: primary and secondary metabolic phases. In the initial phase (balanced growth = tropophase) all nutrients are in excess. When one nutrient (not carbon) is consumed cell growth (——) slows down and secondary metabolite(s) are formed in the idiophase.

etc. – but their proportions will change as growth progresses and then slows down.

Eventually, though, the cell must run out of some nutrient, even if this is only O_2, and consequently the growth rate slows and eventually ceases. However, metabolism does not cease. The only time that metabolism completely ceases is when the cell dies; thus as long as the cell retains viability it is able to carry out some metabolic processes and, conversely and most importantly, if the cell wishes to remain alive it must carry out a modicum of metabolism.

2.7.2 Secondary metabolism

The need for the cell to keep a flux (or flow) of carbon going through it when active multiplication has ceased requires that the cell diverts its core metabolites into products other than the primary ones which are not needed in the same abundance. Some maintenance of vital components, though, must be carried out: key proteins must be replaced as all proteins undergo turnover; DNA must be repaired, RNA maintained, etc. Consequently, some primary metabolism must continue but the cell now switches into a secondary mode of metabolism (see Fig. 2.18). These secondary products then begin to arise sometimes as storage products within the cell (e.g. various polysaccharides or triacylglycerols – see Chapter 16), sometimes as increased amounts of primary metabolites (such as amino acids and organic acids, see Chapters 14 and 15), but sometimes new products are synthesised that are not normally present in any great abundance during the balanced phase of growth (e.g. numerous bioactive compounds including antibiotics – see Chapter 18) and these are, of consequence, of considerable biotechnological importance.

As the range of secondary metabolites varies almost with the species of organism being studied, this phase of unbalanced

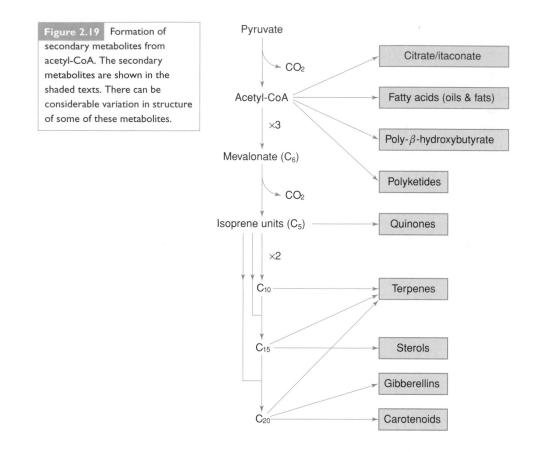

Figure 2.19 Formation of secondary metabolites from acetyl-CoA. The secondary metabolites are shown in the shaded texts. There can be considerable variation in structure of some of these metabolites.

metabolism has been referred to as the *idiophase*, in contrast to the tropophase phase of balanced growth. The secondary metabolites are usually synthesised from unwanted monomers that are still produced from glucose or fatty acid catabolism. Not surprisingly, acetyl-CoA is often used as a key starting point (Fig. 2.19).

The function of the secondary metabolites is uncertain. As they are not produced during balanced growth, they are evidentally not essential for growth and multiplication. As their type and occurrence varies enormously their roles may be equally diverse. Two schools of thought have been advanced:

- The secondary metabolites fulfil a functional role that probably has some benefit to the cell for its survival in a natural environment or they produce a response in the cell that is difficult to mimic in laboratory cultivation.
- Secondary metabolites per se have no value to the cell that produces them; it is the process of their formation that is important and not what the final product may be.

Whatever is the reason for the profusion of secondary metabolites, their properties make them some of the most exploited biotechnological products of all time.

2.8 | Control of metabolic processes

2.8.1 Metabolic flux

The concept of metabolic flux (or flow) has been developed that attempts to describe in mathematical terms the rate at which metabolic intermediates are moved along the various pathways. As this movement is invariably achieved by the action of the associated enzymes, then measurement of the individual enzyme reaction rates may, if one is extremely lucky, identify a single rate-controlling step. If this reaction can be de-regulated or its rate increased (or if a geneticist can change or amplify the appropriate gene coding for the enzyme to increase its activity – see Fig. 2.20 and also Chapters 4 and 5) then the rate-limiting step will be removed and increased product formation should result. Unfortunately, this rarely gives the required result as usually all the enzymes involved in a pathway are operating at similar rates and removal of one rate-limiting step merely identifies the next one. Entire pathways need to be 'engineered' (which can only be done at the genetic level) if a de-regulated pathway is needed for a particular product. Examples of removing some metabolic 'bottle-necks' are given in various chapters later in this book: overproduction of organic acids (Chapter 15), overproduction of amino acids (Chapter 14) and overproduction of antibiotics (Chapter 18).

Identification of the key enzymes that control the flux of carbon to various products is important for increasing the productivity of any process. The flux of carbon can be controlled in various ways and these are briefly described below. It should, however, be stated that many products have been increased by mutating microorganisms in a random manner and then picking out the one or two improved cells from the myriad of others that have an increased capacity to produce the desired product. However, with our considerably increased knowledge of biochemistry, of genetics and genetic manipulations, the current trend is to alter specific enzymes, or groups of enzymes, in order to effect improvements in a precise manner. This rational approach means that the key enzyme must be identified with great care otherwise considerable effort will be expended for little or no return. This understanding of how enzymes may be regulated, there-fore, is of considerable importance to the biotechnologist.

2.8.2 Nutrient uptake

Control of cell metabolism begins by the cell regulating its uptake of nutrients. Most nutrients, apart from O_2 and a very few carbon compounds, are taken up by specific transport mechanisms so that they may be concentrated within the cell from dilute solutions outside. Such 'active' transport systems require an input of energy. The processes are controllable so that once the amount of nutrient taken into the cell has reached a given concentration, further unnecessary (or even detrimental) uptake can be stopped. (This is also discussed in Section 2.8.5 on catabolite repression.) In some cases the rate at which

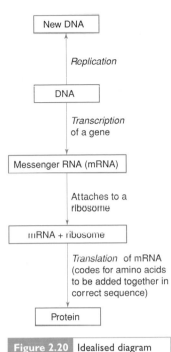

Figure 2.20 Idealised diagram showing how DNA can either be replicated to give new DNA (for new cell synthesis) or be transcribed into messenger RNA (mRNA) that is decoded (or translated) by it becoming attached to a ribosome which then makes a protein molecule by sequential addition of amino acids. Thus the original sequence of bases along the DNA (the gene) is first converted to a corresponding sequence of bases (mRNA) that gives rise to a new protein; see also Chapter 4, Fig. 4.1.

a carbon source, such as glucose, is taken up into the cell may be the limiting process for growth of the whole cell and, therefore, should receive particular attention when evaluating potential bottle-necks to increased productivity of a bioprocess.

2.8.3 Compartmentalisation

A simple form of metabolic control is the use of compartments, or organelles, within the cell, wherein separate pools of metabolites can be maintained. An obvious example is the mitochondrion of the eukaryotic cell which separates the tricarboxylic acid cycle reactions from reactions in the cytoplasm. Another would be the biosynthesis of fatty acids, which occurs in the cytoplasm of eukaryotic cells, whereas the degradation of fatty acids (see Fig. 2.13) occurs in a specialised organelle known as the *peroxisome* (which as its name suggests has a high activity of peroxidase/catalase enzymes that are involved in various degradative reactions). Separating the two sets of enzymes prevents any common intermediate being recycled in a futile manner. Other organelles (vacuoles, the nucleus, peroxisomes, etc.) are similarly used to control other reactions of the cell. Bacteria, however, do not have such compartments within their cells and, therefore, must rely on other means of metabolic control.

2.8.4 Control of enzyme synthesis

Many enzymes within a cell are present constitutively; i.e they are there under all growth conditions. Other enzymes only 'appear' when needed; e.g. isocitrate lyase of the glyoxylate by-pass (see Fig. 2.12) when the cell grows on a C_2 substrate. This is termed *induction of enzyme synthesis*. Conversely, enzymes can 'disappear' when they are no longer required; e.g. enzymes for histidine biosynthesis stop being produced if there is sufficient external histidine available to satisfy the needs of the cell. This is termed *repression* (of enzyme synthesis); when the gratuitous supply of the compound has gone, the enzymes for synthesis of the material 'reappear', i.e. their synthesis is *de-repressed*. The key to both induction and repression is that the genes coding for the synthesis of the proteins by the processes of transcription (see Fig. 2.20) are either switched on (induction) or off (repression) according to the metabolites present (or absent) in the cell. These processes are shown diagrammatically in Fig. 2.21.

2.8.5 Catabolic repression

This type of metabolic control is an extension of the ideas already set out with respect to enzyme induction and repression, being brought about by external nutrients added to the microbial culture. The term *catabolite repression* refers to several general phenomena seen, for example, when a microorganism is able to select, from two or more different carbon sources simultaneously presented to it, that substrate which it prefers to utilise. For example, a microorganism presented with both glucose and lactose may ignore the lactose until it has consumed all the glucose. This sequential utilisation of two

(a)

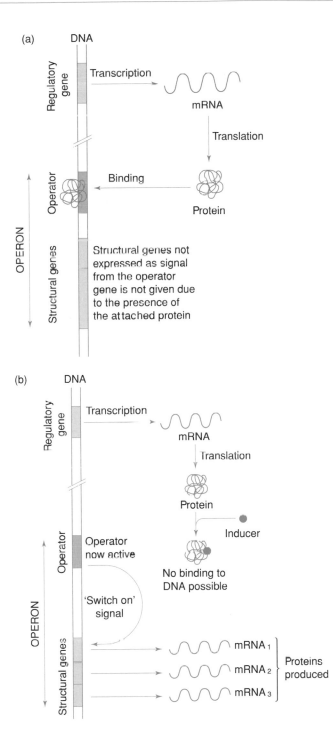

Figure 2.21 Control of enzyme synthesis through regulation of DNA expression. (a) Repression: in the absence of any inducing molecule the messenger RNA (mRNA) from the regulatory gene produces a protein that binds to an 'operator' gene further down the DNA molecule. As a result of this binding, the operator gene is inactivated and no signal is given to allow the structural genes (that would make active enzymes) to be expressed. (b) Induction: in the presence of an inducing molecule, the protein arising from the regulatory gene is now no longer able to bind to the operator gene. Consequently, the operator 'switches on' the structural genes and active proteins (enzymes) are now made.

(b)

substrates is referred to as *diauxic growth*. Similar selection may occur for the choice of a nitrogen source if more than one is available. The advantage to the cell is that it can use the compound that provides it with the most useful substrate for production of energy and provision of metabolites.

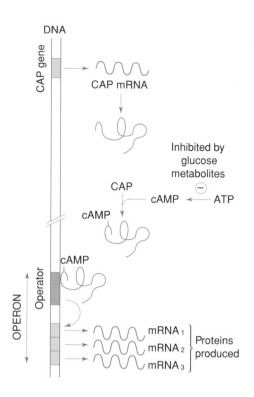

Figure 2.22 Catabolite repression. The mechanism shown is mediated by cyclic AMP (cAMP). An operon is controlled by the operator gene being activated by a complex found between a protein (the *catabolite activator protein*, *CAP*) and cyclic AMP *(cAMP)*. cAMP is only formed when glucose is absent. The structural genes are therefore 'switched off' (i.e. repressed) as long as glucose or its catabolites are present. Several operons may respond to the cAMP–CAP signal.

The mechanisms by which catabolite repression is achieved varies from organism to organism. A simple case is with *E. coli* where control is exerted via an effector molecule, cyclic AMP (cAMP). (In cAMP the single phospho group of AMP – see Fig. 2.4 – bridges across from the 3'-hydroxy group of ribose to the 5'-hydroxy group, thereby forming a cyclic diphosphoester.) cAMP interacts with a specific protein, *catabolite activator protein (CAP*; also known as the *CRP = catabolite receptor protein*), and the cAMP–CAP complex binds to DNA causing the genes that follow after (also referred to as being 'downstream' of) the binding site to be transcribed (see Fig. 2.22). These genes may then be used to synthesise new proteins for uptake and metabolism of the next substrate (e.g. lactose if the cells are growing on a glucose/lactose mixture). This positive system of genetic control is the reverse of the negative control system described in Fig. 2.21.

The key molecule is therefore cAMP. As long as glucose or its catabolites are present, cAMP is not formed as its synthesising enzyme (adenylate cyclase) is inhibited by these catabolites and thus lactose uptake and metabolism cannot occur. The catabolites therefore repress the synthesis of new enzymes. The repression is removed when the catabolites disappear, i.e. all the glucose has been consumed.

2.8.6 Modification of enzyme activity

Once an enzyme has been synthesised, its activity can be modulated by a variety of means.

Post-transcriptional modifications

This process is so-called because it occurs after the enzyme has been synthesised, i.e. after its formation by transcription (see Fig. 2.20).

Enzymes may be modified from one form to another, one form being active and the other inactive or less active:

$$E_{(active)} \leftrightarrow E_{(inactive)}$$

This process of activating or inactivating an enzyme is carried out by an entirely separate enzyme which has nothing to do with catalysing the reaction that the original enzyme will be involved with.

A common way of achieving this conversion is by phosphorylation of the enzyme using a new enzyme – a protein kinase. These protein kinases, of which there can be many, usually react with only one enzyme and thus are highly specific. They add a phospho group (from ATP) to a specific hydroxyl group (normally a serine residue) on the enzyme. The activated enzyme may be either the phosphorylated form or its dephosphorylated form. The dephosphorylation will be carried out by a specific phosphatase enzyme. The activities of the protein kinase and the phosphatase will be obviously controlled by other factors within the cell and will work according to the metabolic status of the cell.

There are other mechanisms of altering the activities of specific proteins by the attachment (or removal) of a simple molecule to a particular amino acid residue in an enzyme, but the addition of a phospho group is by far the most common.

Action of effectors

The second way in which an enzyme's activity can be controlled is by its response to various effectors. (Effectors can act positively, i.e. are *promoters*, or negatively, i.e. are *inhibitors*.) An example is the process known as *feedback inhibition*. Here, in a sequence of biosynthesis

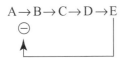

the end product, E, may be able to inhibit the first enzyme of the sequence (converting A to B). This will only occur when sufficient E has been produced by the cell for its immediate requirements and, therefore, no further carbon need be channelled down this pathway. As the cell continues to grow it will consume the accumulated E and thus diminish the amount of it in circulation. Thus, as E is withdrawn for the cell's own needs, the inhibitory effect will be withdrawn and the conversion of A to B will recommence, with the further synthesis of E then occurring to match the cell's requirements. This process will also occur if the end-product, E, is added to the growth medium of the organism. Here, as the product is now supplied gratuitously, the cell has no need to 'waste' its resources synthesising E, so the pathway is now inhibited. In addition to feedback inhibition, a high concentration of the end-product can also lead to the repression of the enzymes for the entire pathway; thus there is a 'quick' response mode to a high concentration of the end-product arising: the initial enzyme of the pathway is inhibited and there is no flux of carbon along the pathway; and then there is a longer-term response whereby all the enzymes needed for the pathway stop being synthesised by repression (see above) at the DNA level as they are surplus to requirement and their continued synthesis would be a waste of valuable amino acid precursors.

This process can, of course, be quite complicated should the pathway not be linear as depicted above but be a branching pathway with multiple end–products. This is of particular importance in the biosynthesis of amino acids several of which (such as phenylalanine, tyrosine and tryptophan) share a common initial pathway. This is discussed in greater detail in Chapter 14.

2.8.7 Degradation of enzymes

Enzymes are not particularly stable molecules and may be quickly and irreversibly destroyed. Their half-lives are very variable; they may be as short as a few minutes or as long as several days. Although the syntheses of enzymes can be regulated at the genetic level (see Section 2.8.4), once an enzyme has been synthesised it can remain functional for some time. If the environmental conditions change abruptly, it may not suffice for the synthesis of the enzyme to be 'switched off', i.e. repressed; the cell may need to inactivate the enzyme so as to avoid needless, or even perhaps deleterious, metabolic activity. This may be by feedback inhibition (Section 2.8.6). Additionally, under nitrogen-limited growth conditions, i.e. when a cell becomes depleted of nitrogen and cannot grow further (as N is needed for the synthesis of nucleic acids and proteins), proteases, that are proteolytic enzymes, may become activated. These enzymes then degrade surplus copies of proteins (e.g. enzymes) so that amino acids are released and can be used for the biosynthesis of new enzymes that may be still essential. Thus, enzymes may be 'turned over' more rapidly than may occur by simple denaturation.

2.9 | Efficiency of microbial growth

The overall efficiency of microbial growth is discussed in strict thermodynamic terms in Chapter 3. It is usually expressed in terms of the yield of cells formed per unit weight of carbon substrate consumed. The *molar growth yield, Y_S*, is the cell yield (dry weight) per mole of substrate, while the *carbon conversion coefficient*, which allows more meaningful comparisons between substrates of different molecular sizes, is the cell yield per gram of substrate carbon.

A particular feature in Table 2.3 is the lower growth yields attained when facultative organisms are transferred from aerobic to

Table 2.3 Growth yields of microorganisms growing on different substrates

Substrate	Organism	Molar growth yield (g organism dry wt g mol^{-1} substrate)	Carbon conversion coefficient (g organism dry wt g^{-1} substrate carbon)
Methane	*Methylomonas* sp.	17.5	1.46
Methanol	*Methylomonas* sp.	16.6	1.38
Ethanol	*Candida utilis*	31.2	1.30
Glycerol	*Klebsiella pneumoniae*	50.4	1.40
Glucose	*Escherichia coli:*		
	aerobic	95.0	1.32
	anaerobic	25.8	0.36
	Saccharomyces cerevisiae:		
	aerobic	90	1.26
	anaerobic	21	0.29
	Penicillium chrysogenum	81	1.13
Sucrose	*Klebsiella pneumoniae*	173	1.20
Xylose	*Klebsiella pneumoniae*	52.2	0.87
Acetic acid	*Pseudomonas* sp.	23.5	0.98
	Candida utilis	21.6	0.90
Hexadecane	*Yarrowia (Candida) lipolytica*	203	1.06

anaerobic conditions, a phenomenon which is obviously connected with decreased energy production under these conditions.

Empirically, the growth yield of a microorganism will depend on many factors:

(1) The nature of the carbon source.
(2) The pathways of substrate catabolism.
(3) Any supplementary provision of complex substrates (obviating the need for some anabolic pathways to operate).
(4) Energy requirements for assimilating other nutrients especially nitrogen.
(5) Varying efficiencies of ATP-generating reactions.
(6) Presence of inhibitory substrates, adverse ionic balance, or other medium components imposing extra demands on transport systems.
(7) The physiological state of the organism: nearly all microorganisms modify their development according to the external environment, and the different processes (e.g. primary and secondary metabolism) will entail different mass and energy balances.

In continuous culture systems, in which the growth rate and nutritional status of the cells are controlled (see Chapters 3 and 6), further factors can be identified:

(8) The nature of the limiting substrate: carbon-limited growth is often more 'efficient' than, for example, nitrogen-limited growth, in which catabolism of excess carbon substrate may follow routes

that are energetically 'wasteful' (however useful they may be to the biotechnologist!).

(9) The permitted growth rate: whereas the growth rate is decreased, the proportion of the substrate going towards maintaining the cells increases, thereby diminishing the amount of substrate that can go to other products.

As a final factor governing all aspects of microbial performances, one might usefully add:

(10) *The competence of the microbiologist.*

2.10 | Further reading

Hames, B. D. and Hooper, N. M. *Instant Notes: Biochemistry*, second edition. Oxford: Bios Scientific Publishers, 2000.

Holms, H. Flux analysis: a basic tool of microbial physiology. *Advances in Microbial Physiology* **45**: 271–340, 2001.

Horton, H. R., Moran, L. A., Scrimgeour, K. G., Perry, M. D. and Rawn, D. *Principles of Biochemistry* 4th edition. New Jersey, U. S. A: Pearson Education Inc., 2006.

Lengeler, J. W., Drews, G. and Schlegel, H., eds. *Biology of the Prokaryotes*. Oxford: Blackwell Science, 1999.

Moat, A. G., Foster, J. W. and Spector, M. P. eds. *Microbial Physiology*. New York: John Wiley & Sons, 2002.

White, D. *Physiology and Biochemistry of Prokaryotes*. Oxford: Oxford University Press, 1999.

Chapter 3

Stoichiometry and kinetics of microbial growth from a thermodynamic perspective

J. J. Heijnen

TU Delft, The Netherlands

Nomenclature

c_i	concentration	(mol i m^{-3})
$-\Delta G_{CAT}$	Gibbs energy produced in catabolism per mol organic electron donor or per mol of inorganic electron donor	(kJ mol^{-1})
$\Delta G_f^{\ominus}$	standard Gibbs energy of formation	(kJ mol^{-1})
$\Delta H_f^{\ominus}$	standard enthalpy of formation	(kJ mol^{-1})
K_s	affinity constant	(mol l^{-1})
m_i	maintenance coefficient of compound i	(C-mol i per C-mol x h^{-1})
q_i	biomass specific conversion rate of compound i	(mol i per C-mol x h^{-1})
r_i	specific conversion rate of compound i	(mol i m^{-3} h^{-1})
V	reactor liquid volume	(m^3)
X	biomass	(C-mol)

Basic Biotechnology, third edition, eds. Colin Ratledge and Bjørn Kristiansen.
Published by Cambridge University Press. © Cambridge University Press 2006.

Y_{ix}	yield of biomass (x) on compound i	(C-mol x per mol i)
Y_{sx}^{max}	maximal growth yield of biomass (x) on substrate (s) or electron donor (d)	(C-mol x per C-mol s)
μ	specific growth rate	(h^{-1})
μ_{max}	maximum specific growth rate	(h^{-1})
γ	degree of reduction	

3.1 | Introduction

Quantitative information on microbial growth is needed in many fermentation and biological waste treatment processes. Typically, growth is quantified using well-known parameters such as maximum biomass yield on substrate S (also called electron donor D) (Y_{sx}^{max} or Y_{dx}^{max}), maintenance requirements for substrate s or electron donor d (m_s or m_d), μ_{max} and K_s. A practical problem is that the values of these parameters vary by one to two orders of magnitude, depending on the growth systems being considered. Such growth systems are generally characterised (Fig. 3.1) by their catabolism using the available electron donor and electron acceptor, and the anabolism using the available C source and N source. In addition, HCO_3^-, H_2O and H^+ are involved in each growth system. A practical point is that many microorganisms have similar elemental compositions with one C-mol formula for biomass of $C_1H_{1.8}O_{0.5}N_{0.2}$. This permits the use of a standard biomass composition, in case this information is not specifically available. However, it is always preferable to determine the composition of the biomass, using elemental analysis. For practical purposes it is important to know the complete stoichiometry of growth. In fermentation processes information on the biomass yield from the substrate (Y_{sx} or Y_{dx}), the O_2 requirement, CO_2 production and heat production are important for the purpose of designing an optimal process. Therefore, methods of stoichiometric calculation are of fundamental value. In addition, the estimation of growth stoichiometry

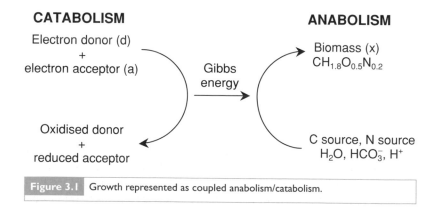

Figure 3.1 Growth represented as coupled anabolism/catabolism.

$$\frac{1}{Y_{dx}} \text{ electron donor} - \frac{1}{Y_{ax}} \text{ electron acceptor} + 1 \text{ C-mol biomass} + \frac{1}{Y_{hx}} \text{ kJ heat}$$

$$+ \frac{1}{Y_{Gx}} \text{ kJ Gibbs energy} + (\cdots) \text{ N source} + (\cdots) H_2O + (\cdots) HCO_3^- + (\cdots) H^+$$

Figure 3.2 General stoichiometric representation of the formation of one C-mol of biomass. Y_{ix} is the yield of one C-mol X on one mol or kJ of compound i; (. . .) are unknown stoichiometric coefficients.

for arbitrary growth systems is also relevant, for example, in biological waste treatment or in biogeological processes.

3.2 Stoichiometry calculations

3.2.1 Definition of the growth system

A microbial growth system is conveniently represented by an overall chemical reaction (Fig. 3.2) where one C-mol of biomass is formed and which takes into account the role of the N source, H_2O, HCO_3^-, H^+, electron donor and electron acceptor. In addition, heat and Gibbs energy are also involved. One C-mol of biomass is the amount of biomass that contains 12 grams of carbon. This usually amounts to about 25 grams of dry matter as the carbon content of biomass is typically about 45%. Energy must be generated for microbial growth to enable the construction of the complex biomass molecules from simple carbon compounds. This energy is generated in a redox reaction between the electron donor and electron acceptor. The proper measure of energy spent in growth processes is not the released heat but Gibbs energy, because Gibbs energy (ΔG) combines the heat related enthalpic (ΔH) and entropic (ΔS) contributions ($\Delta G = \Delta H - T\Delta S$). The stoichiometric coefficients in the reaction (Fig. 3.2) are related to well-known yield coefficients. Y_{dx}, Y_{ax}, Y_{hx} and Y_{gx} are the yields of biomass (in C-mol biomass) on electron donor (per C-mol for organic and per mol for inorganic compounds), on electron acceptor (per mol acceptor), on heat (per kJ) and Gibbs energy (per kJ), respectively. For biomass, the one C-mol composition is used. When a minus sign appears in any equation it signifies consumption.

3.2.2 Measuring yields

The biomass related yield coefficients Y_{ix} are ratios of conversion rates (r_x is given as C-mol biomass $m^{-3} h^{-1}$; r_i in mol i $m^{-3} h^{-1}$).

$$Y_{ix} = \frac{r_x}{r_i} \tag{3.1}$$

The rates are calculated from the correct mass balances using measurements from experiments, which may be either batch, continuous or fed-batch cultures. The most frequently measured growth stoichiometric coefficient is the biomass yield on substrate (or electron donor)

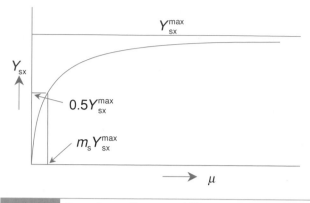

Figure 3.3 Dependence of biomass yield Y_{sx} on specific growth rate (maintenance effect), m_s is the substrate maintenance coefficient, Y_{sx}^{max} is the maximal biomass yield on substrate.

Y_{sx} (or Y_{dx}). In a constant volume batch culture (0 indicating time zero), Y_{sx} will be:

$$Y_{sx} = (c_x - c_{xo})/(c_{so} - c_s) \tag{3.2a}$$

In a chemostat, where input and outflow rates are equal, a similar equation holds, where $c_{xo} = 0$ and c_{so} is replaced by the concentration c_{si} of the incoming substrate. If volume variations occur, more complex relations can be derived from the mass balances. For batch reactors with initial volume V_o and variable volume V, we get:

$$Y_{sx} = (V c_x - V_o c_{xo})/(V_o c_{so} - V c_s) \tag{3.2b}$$

3.2.3 Maintenance effects

Initially Y_{sx} was introduced as a constant. However, after the introduction of the chemostat, cultivation of microorganisms under growth rates much lower than μ_{max} showed that Y_{sx} was dependent on the specific growth rate μ. This is explained in terms of the endogenous respiration, or maintenance, concept. In this concept it is assumed that maintenance of cellular functions requires the availability of a flow of Gibbs energy (for restoring leaky gradients, protein degradation, etc.). The Gibbs energy is produced by the catabolism of electron donor (= substrate) at a certain rate. This maintenance rate is called m_s or (m_d) C-mol substrate per C-mol biomass per hour and the following equation holds

$$\frac{1}{Y_{sx}} = \frac{1}{Y_{sx}^{max}} + \frac{m_s}{\mu} \tag{3.3}$$

Experimentally Y_{sx} is measured in a chemostat under different specific growth rates μ (see Chapter 6). From the obtained Y_{sx} and μ values, we can calculate, using Eq. 3.3, the model parameters Y_{sx}^{max} and m_s.

Figure 3.3 shows how Y_{sx} depends on μ:

- For high values of μ, Y_{sx} approaches the value of the model parameter Y_{sx}^{max}.
- For low μ-values, Y_{sx} drops significantly, becoming $\frac{1}{2} Y_{sx}^{max}$ when $\mu = m_s Y_{sx}^{max}$.

For most conventional processes, it can be shown that at normal growth temperatures the effect of maintenance on yield can be neglected for $\mu > 0.05$ h^{-1}. This means that in batch cultures during exponential growth (where $\mu \approx \mu_{max}$), $Y_{sx} \approx Y_{sx}^{max}$. However, in the fed-batch processes that are the norm in most industrial applications, where $\mu < 0.05$ h^{-1}, maintenance aspects dominate the biomass yield. In environmental applications of organisms, μ is also low and maintenance aspects are relevant.

3.2.4 Conservation principles to calculate the full stoichiometry of growth

Figure 3.2 shows that, besides Y_{sx} (or Y_{dx}), there are many more stoichiometric coefficients. Fortunately these need not be determined experimentally. The application of conservation principles often allows all other coefficients to be calculated if a single coefficient (Y_{sx}) is measured. This calculation and the use of the conservation principles are explained in the following example:

Use of conservation principles in the calculation of stoichiometric coefficients

An aerobic microorganism grows on oxalate using NH_4^+ as N source. The measured biomass yield is 1/5.815 C-mol X mol^{-1} oxalate. The standard biomass composition is used. The following overall reaction (according to Fig. 3.2) can be written based on one C-mol biomass being produced with a consumption of 5.815 mol oxalate:

$$-5.815 C_2O_4^{2-} + aNH_4^+ + bH^+ + cH_2O + dO_2 + eHCO_3^-$$
$$+ 1CH_{1.8}O_{0.5}N_{0.2}$$

There are five unknown stoichiometric coefficients (a to e) for which five conservation constraints can be formulated.

C conservation	$-11.63 + e + 1 = 0$
H conservation	$4a + b + 2c + 1e + 1.8 = 0$
O conservation	$-23.26 + c + 2d + 3e + 0.5 = 0$
N conservation	$a + 0.2 = 0$
Charge conservation	$+11.63 + a + b - e = 0$

Solving for a to e gives the full stoichiometry:

$$-5.815 C_2O_4^{2-} - 0.2NH_4^+ - 0.8H^+ - 1.8575O_2 - 5.415H_2O$$
$$+ 1CH_{1.8}O_{0.5}N_{0.2} + 10.63HCO_3^-$$

Thus we see that:

$$Y_{ax} = 1/1.8575 \text{ C-mol x mol}^{-1} O_2$$
$$Y_{cx} = 1/10.63 \text{ C-mol x mol}^{-1} HCO_3^-$$

For the overall reaction, using $\Delta H_f^\ominus$ and $\Delta G_f^\ominus 1$ values from thermodynamic tables (Table 3.1), we can also calculate $(-\Delta H_r)$ and $(-\Delta G_r)$ and thus we get values for $1/Y_{hx}$ and $1/Y_{gx}$.

3.2.5 Balance of degree of reduction

The application of the conservation constraints is straightforward. A useful short-cut of such calculations is to apply a degree of reduction balance. The degree of reduction (γ) is defined for each compound and is a stoichiometric quantity, defined in such a way that $\gamma = 0$ for the reference compounds H_2O, H^+, HCO_3^-, SO_4^{2-}, NO_3^-, Fe^{3+} and N source. The γ-value for each compound is found by calculating the redox half reaction, which converts the compound into the previous defined reference chemicals and a number of electrons. The γ-values will then be the number of produced electrons per mol for organic and inorganic compounds. For example, the degree of reduction of O_2 follows from the redox half reaction for oxygen:

$$O_2 + 4H^+ \rightarrow 2H_2O - 4e^-, \text{ giving } \gamma = -4.$$

For glucose, the redox half reaction is:

$$C_6H_{12}O_6 + 12H_2O \rightarrow 6HCO_3^- + 30H^+ + 24e^- \text{ and } \gamma$$
$$= 24 \text{ electrons mol}^{-1} \text{ glucose.}$$

It should be noted that for organic compounds one often defines γ per C-mol of carbon source, hence for glucose $\gamma = 24/6 = 4$.

Using the redox half reactions the γ-values for individual atoms and electric charge can also be calculated (Table 3.2). For example, for the carbon atom we obtain:

$$C + 3H_2O \rightarrow HCO_3^- + 5H^+ + 4e^-, \text{ giving a value of } \gamma = 4.$$

The γ-values for H, O, S, N, + and − charge are found in the same way (Table 3.1). It should be noted (Table 3.3) that the γ-value for the nitrogen atom present in the biomass and nitrogen present in the N source for growth depends on the N source used for growth. For example for NH_4^+ as N source using Table 3.3 (γ for H = 1, for + charge = −1) and Table 3.3 (γ for the N atom equals −3) the degree of reduction for NH_4^+ will be: $-3 + 4 - 1 = 0$. The degree of reduction of a molecule (Table 3.1) represents the amount of electrons becoming available from that molecule upon oxidation to the reference compounds. For organic molecules, the number of available electrons is usually normalised per C-mol, for inorganic molecules it is per mole. Table 3.1 shows that for organic molecules the γ-value ranges from 0 to 8. For biomass (standard composition) it follows that:

Table 3.1 Standard Gibbs energy and enthalpy (298 K, pH = 7, 1 bar, 1 mol l^{-1}), degree of reduction for relevant compounds in growth systems

Compound name	Composition	$\Delta G_f^{0'}$ (kJ mol^{-1})	ΔH_f^0 (kJ mol^{-1})	Degree of reduction (C-atom^{-1})
Biomass	$CH_{1.8}O_{0.5}N_{0.2}$	−67	−91	4.2 (N source NH_4^+)
Water	H_2O	−237.18	−286	−0
Bicarbonate	HCO_3^-	−586.85	−692	0
CO_2 (g)	CO_2	−394.359	−394.1	0
Proton	H^+	−39.87	0	0
O_2 (g)	O_2	0	0	−4
Oxalate^{2-}	$C_2O_4^{2-}$	674.04	−824	+1
Carbon monoxide	CO	−137.15	−111	+2
Formate$^-$	CHO_2^-	−335	−410	+2
Glyoxylate$^-$	$C_2O_3H^-$	−468.6	−	+2
Tartrate^{2-}	$C_4H_4O_6^{2-}$	−1010	−	+2.5
Malonate^{2-}	$C_3H_2O_4^{2-}$	−700	−	+2.67
Fumarate^{2-}	$C_4H_2O_4^{2-}$	−604.21	−777	+3
Malate^{2-}	$C_4H_4O_5^{2-}$	−845.08	−843	+3
Citrate^{3-}	$C_6H_5O_7^{3-}$	−1168.34	−1515	+3
Pyruvate$^-$	$C_3H_3O_3^-$	−474.63	−596	+3.33
Succinate^{2-}	$C_4H_4O_4^{2-}$	−690.23	−909	+3.50
Gluconate$^-$	$C_6H_{11}O_7^-$	−1154	−	+3.67
Formaldehyde	CH_2O	−130.54	−	+4
Acetate$^-$	$C_2H_3O_2^-$	−369.41	−486	+4
Dihydroxy acetone	$C_3H_6O_3$	−445.18	−	+5.33
Lactate$^-$	$C_3H_5O_3^-$	−517.18	−687	+4
Glucose	$C_6H_{12}O_6$	−917.22	−1264	+4
Mannitol	$C_6H_{14}O_6$	−942.61	−	+4.33
Glycerol	$C_3H_8O_3$	−488.52	−676	+4.67
Propionate$^-$	$C_3H_5O_2^-$	−361.08	−	+4.67
Ethylene glycol	$C_2H_6O_2$	−330.50	−	+5
Acetoine	$C_4H_8O_2$	−280	−	+5
Butyrate	$C_4H_7O_2^-$	−352.63	−535	+5
Propanediol	$C_3H_8O_2$	−327	−	+5.33
Butanediol	$C_4H_{10}O_2$	−322	−	+5.50
Methanol	CH_4O	−175.39	−246	+6
Ethanol	C_2H_6O	−181.75	−288	+6
Propanol	C_3H_8O	−175.81	−331	+6
n-Alkane (l)	$C_{15}H_{32}$	+60	−439	+6.13
Propane (g)	C_3H_8	−24	−104	+6.66
Ethane (g)	C_2H_6	−32.89	−85	+7
Methane (g)	CH_4	−50.75	−75	+8
H_2 (g)	H_2	0	0	+2
Ammonium	NH_4^+	−79.37	−133	+8
N_2 (g)	N_2	0	0	+10

(cont.)

Table 3.1 (cont.)

Compound name	Composition	$\Delta G_f^\circ kJ\,mol^{-1}$	$\Delta H_f^\circ kJ\,mol^{-1}$	Degree of reduction (C-atom^{-1})
Nitrite ion	NO_2^-	−37.2	−107	+2
Nitrate ion	NO_3^-	−111.34	−173	0
Iron II	Fe^{2+}	−78.87	−87	+1
Iron III	Fe^{3-}	−4.6	−4	0
Sulphur	S^0	0	0	+6
Hydrogen sulphide (g)	H_2S	−33.56	−20	+8
Sulphide ion	HS^-	+12.05	−17	+8
Sulphate ion	SO_4^{2-}	−744.63	−909	0
Thiosulphate ion	$S_2O_3^{2-}$	−513.2	−608	+8
Ammonium	NH_4^+	−79.37	−133	+8

- $\gamma_x = 4.2$ (from $1 \times 4 + 1.8 \times 1 + 0.5\,(-2) + 0.2\,(-3) = 4.2$) for NH_4^+ as a N source, and
- $\gamma_x = 5.8$ for NO_3^- as a N source.

Because electrons are conserved, it is possible to calculate the balance of degree of reduction as shown in the following example.

Application of the balance of degree of reduction

Consider the previous example of aerobic growth on oxalate and the overall chemical reaction, which contains $C_2O_4^{2-}$, NH_4^+, H^+, H_2O, O_2, HCO_3^- and biomass ($C_1H_{1.8}O_{0.5}N_{0.2}$) as reactants. Calculation of the degree of reduction (using the γ-values of atoms and charges in Table 3.3) of 1 molecule of oxalate ($C_2O_4^{2-}$) gives

$$\gamma = 2 \times 4 + 4 \times (-2) + (+2) = 2$$

The γ-value for biomass (NH_4^+ as a N source, therefore γ for the N atom $= -3$ according to Table 3.3 and using $C_1H_{1.8}O_{0.5}N_{0.2}$ as biomass

Table 3.2 Degree of reduction (γ) for atoms and charge

Atoms charge^{-1}	γ
H	1
O	−2
C	4
S	6
N	+5
Fe	+3
+ 1 charge	−1
− 1 charge	+1

Table 3.3 Degree of reduction for N present in N source and in biomass

N source used for growth	γ for N
NH_4^+	-3
N_2	0
NO_3^-	$+5$

composition) will be:

$$1 \times 4 + 1.8 \times 1 + 0.5(-2) + 0.2(-3) = 4.2$$

Similarly, the degree of reduction of O_2 will be -4. For HCO_3^- we obtain:

$$\gamma = 1 \times 1 + 1 \times 4 + 3 \times (-2) + 1 = 0$$

and for the N source NH_4^+ (using Tables 3.2 and 3.3) we get:

$$\gamma = -3 + 4 - 1 = 0$$

Also for the remaining compounds of the reaction (H_2O, H^+), $\gamma = 0$. This gives for the degree of reduction balance applied to the growth reaction:

$$-5.815 \times 2 - 4d + 4.2 = 0$$

It can be seen that in this balance, only the stoichiometric coefficients of substrate (or electron donor), the electron acceptor and biomass occur. This gives $d = -1.8575$, being identical to the full solution of conservation constraints obtained before. The other coefficients follow from application of the regular conservation constraints, i.e. the N source coefficient from the N balance, the HCO_3^- from the C balance, etc. From the example several points must be noted:

- The balance of degree of reduction always specifies a linear relation between the stoichiometric coefficients of electron donor, electron acceptor and biomass, making this relation extremely useful in practice.
- The balance of degree of reduction is not a new constraint: it is just a suitable combination of the C, H, N and charge conservation constraints.

Other useful applications of the conservation constraints can be found in the further reading list.

3.3 Stoichiometric predictions based on Gibbs energy dissipation

A number of methods have been proposed to estimate biomass yields (Y_{dx}) from correlations. A particularly simple, but useful and recent, method has been the thermodynamically based approach using Gibbs energy consumption per unit biomass $(1/Y_{gx})$ in kJ C-mol^{-1} X. This is a stoichiometric quantity that can be written as:

$$\frac{1}{Y_{gx}} = \frac{1}{Y_{gx}^{max}} + \frac{m_g}{\mu}$$ (3.4)

where m_g is the biomass specific rate of Gibbs energy consumption for maintenance purposes in kJ C-mol^{-1} X h^{-1} and Y_{gx}^{max} is the maximal biomass yield on Gibbs energy in C-mol X kJ^{-1}. Equation (3.4) shows that the Gibbs energy consumption contains a growth- and a maintenance-related term. Simple correlations have been proposed for $1/Y_{gx}^{max}$ and for m_g. These correlations cover a wide range of microbial growth systems and temperatures (heterotrophic, autotrophic, aerobic, anaerobic, denitrifying growth systems on a wide range of C sources, growth systems with and without Reversed Electron Transport, RET).

3.3.1 Correlation for maintenance Gibbs energy

The following correlation has been found to be valid for the maintenance Gibbs energy:

$$m_g = 4.5 \exp\left[-\frac{69\,000}{8.314}\left(\frac{1}{T} - \frac{1}{298}\right)\right]$$ (3.5)

This correlation holds for a temperature range of 278 to 348 K, for aerobic and anaerobic conditions. It is clear that m_g does not depend on the C source or electron donor or acceptor being applied and only shows a significant temperature dependency. This seems logical because maintenance processes only require Gibbs energy, irrespective of the electron donor/acceptor combination that provides the Gibbs energy.

3.3.2 Correlation for Gibbs energy needed for growth

For the growth-related Gibbs energy requirement $1/Y_{gx}^{max}$, in kJ Gibbs energy C-mol^{-1} X produced, the following correlations can be used.

For heterotrophic or autotrophic growth without RET:

$$\frac{1}{Y_{gx}^{max}} = 200 + 18(6 - c)^{1.8} + \exp\{[(3.8 - \gamma_s)^2]^{0.16}(3.6 + 0.4c)\}$$ (3.6a)

For autotrophic growth requiring RET:

$$\frac{1}{Y_{gx}^{max}} = 3500$$ (3.6b)

Equation (3.6a) shows that $1/Y_{gx}^{max}$ for heterotrophic growth is mainly determined by the nature of the C source used. The C source is characterised by its degree of reduction, γ_s, and the number of C atoms (parameter c) present in the C source (e.g. C = 6 and $\gamma_s = 4$ for glucose). Equation (3.6a) shows that $1/Y_{gx}^{max}$ ranges between about 200 and 1000 kJ of Gibbs energy required for the synthesis of one C-mol biomass, dependent on the C source used. For glucose as C source, the lower range is obtained; for CO, the higher value applies. Furthermore, it can be seen that $1/Y_{gx}$ increases for C sources that have fewer carbon atoms and for which the degree of reduction is higher or lower than about 3.8. This is because a C source with a low number of C atoms requires numerous biochemical reactions to produce the required C_4 to C_6 compounds needed in biomass synthesis. In addition, with the degree of reduction of biomass being about 4, it is clear that C sources, which are more reduced or more oxidised than biomass, require additional biochemical reactions for oxidation or reduction, respectively. Hence, increased values of $1/Y_{gx}^{max}$ reflect the increased requirement for additional biochemical reactions, which leads to a greater need for Gibbs energy. For example, making biomass from CO_2 ($\gamma_s = 0$, $c = 1$) requires, according to Eq. (3.6a), an amount of Gibbs energy of 986 kJ C-mol^{-1} X, whereas use of glucose ($\gamma_s = 4$, $C = 6$) only requires 236 kJ C-mol^{-1} X. This reflects the much higher energy requirement due to the larger number of biochemical reactions needed for growth using CO_2 as a C source.

To estimate the value of $1/Y_{gx}^{max}$ for autotrophic growth we need to know whether RET is required or not. This follows after establishing the biomass formation reaction from CO_2 using the available electron donor as the electron source. If $\Delta G_r \gg 0$ for this reaction, it is clear that the energy level of the electron donor electrons is insufficient to reduce CO_2 to biomass. The microorganism must then convert part of the donor electrons to a higher energy level, using a process called RET. Examples of such low-energy electron donor couples are:

- Fe^{2+}/Fe^{3+}
- NO_2^-/NO_3^-

For RET requiring electron donors, $1/Y_{gx}^{max}$ values are 3500 kJ C-mol^{-1} X (3.6b). This shows that RET requires many additional biochemical reactions leading to a much higher need for Gibbs energy.

Autotrophic electron donor couples such as H_2/H^+ or CO/CO_2 do not need RET. For these electron donors, $1/Y_{gx}^{max} \approx 1000$ kJ C-mol^{-1} X, as found from Eq. (3.6a), where $\gamma_s = 0$ and $c = 1$ (CO_2 is the C source).

Occurrence of Reversed Electron Transport (RET) in autotrophic growth

Consider the autotrophic aerobic microbial growth using Fe^{2+}/Fe^{3+} as the electron donor. HCO_3^- is the C source. This allows the following biomass formation (anabolic) reaction to be drawn up, where HCO_3^- is reduced using the donor electrons:

$$HCO_3^- + 4.2Fe^{2+} + 0.2NH_4^+ + 5H^+ \rightarrow 1CH_{1.8}O_{0.5}N_{0.2}$$
$$+ 4.2Fe^{3+} + 2.5H_2O$$

Using Table 3.1 one can calculate that $\Delta G_r^{\ominus 1} = +454$ kJ. Clearly, for the electron donor Fe^{2+}/Fe^{3+} RET is needed and Eq. (3.6b) applies.

3.3.3 Stoichiometric predictions using the Gibbs energy correlations

The correlations found for m_g and $1/Y_{gx}^{max}$ in Eqs. (3.5), (3.6a) and (3.6b) can be used to estimate, for each microbial growth system, the complete stoichiometry of the growth equation as a function of:

- applied C source,
- electron donor/acceptor combination,
- growth rate, and
- temperature.

It has been shown that for a wide range of microbial growth systems the estimation of Y_{dx} is possible in a range of 0.01 to 1 C-mol X mol^{-1} donor with a relative accuracy of about 10–15%. The calculation of the complete stoichiometry is best shown using an example.

Estimation of growth stoichiometry using the Gibbs energy correlations

Consider the aerobic autotrophic growth of a microorganism using Fe^{2+} to Fe^{3+} as electron donor at 50 °C, growing at a rate of 0.01 h^{-1} at a pH value of 1.5 and using NH_4^+ as N source. The following growth reaction can be specified for the production of one C-mol X, using seven unknown stoichiometric coefficients a to g:

$$+ a HCO_3^- + b NH_4^+ + c H_2O + d O_2 + e Fe^{2+} + 1 CH_{1.8}O_{0.5}N_{0.2} + f Fe^{3+}$$
$$+ g H^+ + 1/Y_{gx} \text{ kJ of Gibbs energy}$$

We can specify six conservation constraints and one Gibbs energy balance to calculate the seven (a to g) unknown stoichiometric coefficients. Using Eq. (3.4), $1/Y_{gx}$ follows from the correlations (knowing that RET is involved, that $\mu = 0.01$ h^{-1} and that T = 323 K) as:

$$1/Y_{gx} = 3500 + 38.84/0.01 = 7384 \text{ kJ C-mol}^{-1} \text{ X}$$

The six conservation constraints and the Gibbs energy balance (using $\Delta G_f^\circ 1$ values from Table 3.1) are as follows:

C conservation	$a + 1 = 0$
O conservation	$3a + c + 2d + 0.5 = 0$
Degree of reduction	$-4d + e + 4.2 = 0$
Iron conservation	$e + f = 0$
N conservation	$b + 0.2 = 0$
Charge conservation	$-a + b + 2e + 3f + g = 0$
Gibbs energy balance	$(-586.85)a + (-79.37)b + (-237.18)c$
	$+ (-78.87)e + (-67)d + (-4.6)f$
	$+ (-8.54)g + 7384 = 0$

Note that, for H$^+$, ΔG_f is recalculated from pH = 7 (in Table 3.2) to pH = 1.5 (which changes ΔG_{H^+} from -38.87 to -8.54 kJ mol H$^+$). Also the balance of degree of reduction has been used as a constraint (replacing the H constraint). After solving the six linear equations one obtains the complete stoichiometry as follows:

$$-1HCO_3^- \quad 0.2NH_4^+ - 218.88\,Fe^{2+} - 53.67O_2 - 219.68H^+$$
$$+ 1C_1H_{1.8}O_{0.5}N_{0.2} + 218.88Fe^{3+} + 109.84H_2O + 7384\,kJ\,Gibbs\,energy$$

From this obtained stoichiometry we can also calculate the heat of growth using the values of ΔH_f° in Table 3.1 and find that there is a production of heat of 12 620 kJ.

3.3.4 Algebraic relations to calculate stoichiometry

Because all the stoichiometric coefficients are, through the conservation constraints, related to $1/Y_{gx}$, one can also derive algebraic relations, between $1/Y_{ix}$ and $1/Y_{gx}$ using certain simplifying assumptions. For the biomass yield on electron donor Y_{dx} the following relation is obtained as an example:

$$Y_{dx} = \frac{(-\Delta G_{CAT})}{1/Y_{gx} + \gamma x/\gamma_d\,(-\Delta G_{CAT})} \tag{3.7}$$

where ΔG_{CAT} is the Gibbs energy of the catabolic reaction of one mol organic electron donor or of one mol inorganic electron donor in kJ (C) mol^{-1} donor, γ_x and γ_d are the degree of reduction for biomass and electron donor mol^{-1}. For the previous example the catabolic reaction of one mol electron donor is:

$$Fe^{2+} + \tfrac{1}{4}O_2 + H^+ \rightarrow Fe^{3+} + \tfrac{1}{2}H_2O$$

Using the values of $\Delta G_f^{\circ 1}$ from Table 3.1 with a ΔG_f value at pH = 1.5 of -8.54 kJ mol^{-1} for H$^+$, we will get $\Delta G_{CAT} = -35.78$ kJ mol^{-1} Fe^{2+}. In addition $\gamma_x = 4.2$, $\gamma_d = 1$ and $1/Y_{gx} = 7384$ kJ C-mol^{-1} X, resulting in $Y_{dx} = 0.0047$ C-mol X mol^{-1} Fe^{2+}. This shows that the stoichiometric coefficient e in the previous example equals 215 mol Fe^{2+} C-mol^{-1} X, which is very close to the calculated value of 218.9 mol Fe^{2+} -mol^{-1} X. Equation (3.7) shows that:

- Y_{dx} increases hyperbolically with increasing Gibbs energy production in catabolism $(-\Delta G_{CAT})$. This explains why anaerobic growth systems (with low $-\Delta G_{CAT}$ values) have lower Y_{dx} values as aerobic systems.
- Y_{dx} is higher for situations that need less Gibbs energy for synthesis of biomass. This means lower $1/Y_{gx}$ values found for high specific growth rate μ, low temperature, favourable C source and the absence of RET.
- Y_{dx} depends hyperbolically on μ substitute $1/Y_{gx}$ using Eq. (3.4) due to maintenance effects in agreement with Eq. (3.3).
- Y_{dx} has a theoretical maximal limit from the second law of thermodynamics of γ_d/γ_x C-mol X per mol^{-1} electron donor (according to the second law $1/Y_{gx}$ has a theoretical minimal value of 0 kJ C-mol^{-1} X).

3.3.5 Estimation of growth yields for non-conventional substrates and catabolic reactions

The correlations for $1/Y_{gx}^{max}$ are based on microbial growth on conventional substrates containing less than six carbon atoms per molecule, and which are directly connected to primary metabolism. In environmental biotechnology, many substrates, e.g. aromatics (benzene), polycyclic aromatic hydrocarbons (PAH), chelators as nitrilo triacetic acid (NTA), occur that are not funnelled immediately into primary metabolism. Special pathways are required, which involve mono- and dioxygenases consuming O_2, and which convert the non-conventional substrate into an intracellular primary metabolite (pyruvate, etc.). The consumed O_2 in these special pathways does not lead to metabolic energy, but to heat only. Methods for yield predictions for such situations have been presented, but are rather complex. A simpler approach would be to use the metabolic knowledge about the oxidative conversion of the non-conventional compound into primary metabolites. This reaction only produces heat. The produced primary metabolites are subsequently used as carbon and energy sources for growth and their stoichiometry can be calculated using (3.5), (3.6a) and (3.6b), as illustrated in the example in Section 3.3.3. The following two examples illustrate the procedure.

Growth stoichiometry on benzene

Benzene (C_6H_6) is converted by organisms into hydroxymuconic semi aldehyde $(C_6H_5O_4^-)$ according to the reaction:

$$C_6H_6 + 2O_2 \rightarrow C_6H_5O_4^- + H^+$$

This reaction provides no useful Gibbs energy due to oxygenation reactions. The metabolic intermediate (hydroxymuconic semialdehyde) serves as the 'real' carbon and energy source for growth and $\Delta G_{CAT} = 2516$ kJ mol^{-1} hydroxymuconic semialdehyde. Equation (3.6a), with $c = 6$ and $\gamma = 22/6 = 3.666$, gives $1/Y_{gx}^{max} = 233$ kJ C-mol^{-1} X. Use of Eq. (3.7), with $\gamma_X = 4.2$, $\gamma_d = 22$ electrons mol^{-1} semialdehyde, leads to $Y_{dx} = 3.57$ C-mol^{-1} X mol^{-1} benzene. This value is close to the measured value of 1.20 g X^{-1} g^{-1} benzene (equivalent to 3.42 C-mol X mol^{-1} benzene, using 90% organic matter in biomass and 24.6 gram organic biomass C-mol^{-1} X).

Growth stoichiometry on phenanthrene

Phenanthrene is converted, using oxygenases, into pyruvate and formate according to:

$$-1 \text{ phenanthrene} (C_{14}H_{10}) - 6O_2 + 4 \text{ pyruvate} (C_3H_3O_3^-)$$
$$+ 1 \text{ formate} (CHO_2^-)$$

The consumed O_2 does only lead to heat. The biomass is formed on pyruvate and formate. The biomass yield on pyruvate is obtained from $\Delta G_{CAT} = 1048.74$ kJ mol^{-1} pyruvate and $1/Y_{gx}^{max} = 373$ kJ (using Eq. (3.6a) with $c = 3$ and $\gamma_s = 3.333$, and Eq. (3.7) with $\gamma_X = 4.2$ and

$\gamma_d = 10$ electrons mol^{-1} pyruvate) and is 1.29 C-mol X mol^{-1} pyruvate. The biomass yield on formate ($\Delta G_{CAT} = 251.85$ kJ mol^{-1} formate and $1/Y_{\mu X}^{max} = 651$ kJ C-mol^{-1} X $\gamma_d = 2$) will be 0.213 C-mol X mol^{-1} formate. The biomass yield on phenanthrene then follows as $4 \times 1.29 + 1 \times 0.213 = 5.3$ C-mol X mol^{-1} phenanthrene. The measured yield is 6.5 C-mol X mol^{-1} phenanthrene. The discrepancy of 18% is probably due to the fact that in the case of phenanthrene there is no energy needed to transport the pyruvate and formate across the cell membrane. This leads to a small underestimation of the biomass yield on pyruvate and formate.

From these examples it appears that the thermodynamic yield prediction can be readily extended to non-conventional substrates, provided that the oxidative oxygenase-based conversion into primary metabolites is known. In bio-geochemical fields of application and in extreme environments (alkalophilic, high salt levels) there occur a diversity of catabolic reactions involving, e.g. metals and extreme conditions. Thermodynamic methods to calculate the catabolic Gibbs energy then become more complex.

3.3.6 Limitation of the yield prediction using the thermodynamic approach

The presented method provides Y_{sx} estimates, where the biochemical details of metabolism of conventional substrates, characteristic for each microorganism, are neglected. This is the attractive aspect of the method, because this knowledge is often not available. Some metabolic knowledge is needed for non-conventional substrates only, as shown in Section 3.3.5. However, one should always realise that differences in biochemistry are relevant. For example, ethanol fermentation from glucose is performed by *Saccharomyces cerevisiae* with Y_{sx} measured to be around 0.15 C-mol X C-mol^{-1} glucose. A similar Y_{sx} value is also obtained using the above method. However, *Zymomonas mobilis* performs the ethanol fermentation with a $Y_{sx} = 0.07$. The difference is caused by a different biochemical pathway (glycolysis versus Entner–Doudoroff route, see Chapter 2). This example shows that if the value of the estimated Y_{sx} deviates strongly from a measured Y_{sx}, one might expect that an unusual, possibly new, biochemical pathway is being used in catabolism (or anabolism).

3.4 | Growth kinetics from a thermodynamic point of view

Growth kinetics are generally characterised by the two parameters μ_{max} and K_s. It is known that variations in K_s values can be experienced, depending on the occurrence of passive diffusion, facilitated transport or active transport for the transfer of electron donor (substrate) into the microorganism. A general thermodynamic correlation for K_s is therefore not possible. Also for μ_{max} a very wide range (0.001

to 1 h^{-1}) of values is found, depending on the microorganism and cultivation conditions. However, it would seem reasonable to expect that a low maximal specific rate of Gibbs energy production from catabolism leads to a lower maximal specific growth rate. Using this concept of energy limitation one can derive the following expressions for the maximal specific rate of Gibbs energy production q_G^{max} (kJ C-mol^{-1} biomass h).

$$q_G^{max} = 3[(-\Delta G_{CAT})/\gamma_d] \exp\left[\frac{-69\,000}{R}\left(\frac{1}{T} - \frac{1}{298}\right)\right] \tag{3.8}$$

This relation is based on:

- A maximal electron transport rate of 3 mol electrons C-mol^{-1} X h at 298 K leading to the coefficient 3 in Eq. (3.8).
- A temperature effect on this rate according to an Arrhenius relation with an energy of activation of 69 000 J mol^{-1} (equivalent to a rate doubling for every 10 °C increase in temperature). R is the gas constant (equal to 8.314 J mol^{-1} K).
- The maximum rate of catabolic Gibbs energy production q_G^{max} is then the rate of electron transport multiplied by $(-\Delta G_{CAT}/\gamma_d)$, which is the catabolic energy release per transferred mole of electrons in the electron donor/acceptor reaction.

Equating the maximal rate of catabolic Gibbs energy production, Eq. (3.8), to the Gibbs energy needed for growth under maximal growth rate condition (being equal to the sum of μ_{max}/Y_{gx}^{max} and maintenance, which equals 4.5 times the temperature correction, see Eq. (3.5), gives the μ_{max} value (in h^{-1}) according to Eq. (3.9):

$$\mu_{max} = \frac{[3(-\Delta G_{CAT})/\gamma_d - 4.5]}{1\Big/Y_{gx}^{max}} \exp\left[\frac{-69\,000}{R}\left(\frac{1}{T} - \frac{1}{298}\right)\right] \tag{3.9}$$

Equation (3.9) can be shown to provide reasonable estimates of μ_{max} values for a wide variety of microorganisms (e.g. nitrifiers, methanogens, heterotrophic aerobes).

3.5 | Further reading

Amend, J. P. and Shock, E. L. Energetics of overall metabolic reactions of thermophilic and hyperthermophilic Archaea and Bacteria. *FEMS Microbiology Reviews* **25**: 175–243, 2001.

Heijnen, J. J. Bioenergetics of microbial growth. In *Encyclopedia of Bioprocesstechnology, Fermentation, Biocatalysis and Bioseparation*, eds. M. C. Flickinger and S. W. Drew. New York: John Wiley & Sons, 1999.

Heijnen, J. J. and van Dijken, J. P. In search of a thermodynamic description of biomass yields for the chemotrophic growth of microorganisms. *Biotechnology and Bioengineering* **39**: 833–858, 1992.

Heijnen, J. J., van Loosdrecht, M. C. M. and Tijhuis, L. A black box mathematical model to calculate auto- and heterotrophic biomass yields based on Gibbs energy dissipation. *Biotechnology and Bioengineering* **40**. 1139–1154, 1992.

Tijhuis, L., van Loosdrecht, M. C. M. and Heijnen, J. J. A thermodynamically based correlation for maintenance Gibbs energy requirements in aerobic and anaerobic chemotrophic growth. *Biotechnology and Bioengineering* **42**: 509–519, 1993.

van Briesen, J. M. Thermodynamic yield predictions for biodegradation through oxygenase activation reactions. *Biodegradation* **12**: 265–281, 2001.

van dam Westerhoff, H. V. K. *Mosaic Non-equilibrium Thermodynamics and the Control of Biological Free Energy Transduction*. Amsterdam: Elsevier, 1987.

van der Heijden, R. T. J. M., Heijnen, J. J., Hellinga, C., Romein, B. and Luyben, K. Ch. A. M. Linear constraint relations in biochemical reaction systems: I. Classification of the calculability and the balanceability of conversion rate. *Biotechnology and Bioengineering* **43**: 3–10, 1994.

van der Heijden, R. T. J. M., Romein, B., Heijnen, J. J., Hellinga, C. and Luyben, K. Ch. A. M. Linear constraint relations in biochemical reaction systems; II diagnosis and estimation of gross errors. *Biotechnology and Bioengineering* **43**: 11–20, 1994.

van der Heijden, R. T. J. M., Romein, B., Heijnen, J. J., Hellinga, C. and Luyben, K. Ch. A. M. Linear constraint relations in biochemical reaction systems: III. Sequential application of data reconciliation for sensitive detection of systematic errors. *Biotechnology and Bioengineering* **44**: 781–791, 1994.

Chapter 4

Genome management and analysis: prokaryotes

Colin R. Harwood
University of Newcastle, UK

Anil Wipat
University of Newcastle, UK

4.1 Introduction

Gene manipulation is a core technology used for a wide variety of academic and industrial applications. In addition to representing an extremely powerful analytical tool, it can be used to: (i) increase the yield and quality of existing products (e.g. proteins, metabolites or even whole cells); (ii) improve the characteristics of existing products (e.g. via protein engineering); (iii) produce existing products by new routes (e.g. pathway engineering); and (iv) develop novel products not

---

[1] A glossary of most of the specialised terms used in molecular biology and genetics is provided at the beginning of Chapter 5.

Basic Biotechnology, third edition, eds. Colin Ratledge and Bjørn Kristiansen.
Published by Cambridge University Press. © Cambridge University Press 2006.

Table 4.1 The usual size range of the various classes of genetic element found in bacterial cells

Genetic element	Size range (bp)[a]
Transposons	800–30 000
Plasmids	1 000–150 000
Prophages	3 000–300 000
Bacterial chromosomes	600 000–9 450 000

[a] bp, number of base pairs in the DNA.

previously found in nature (e.g. directed or hybrid biosynthesis). This chapter assumes knowledge of the basic structure and properties of nucleic acids, the organisation of the genetic information into genes and operons, and the mechanisms by which bacteria transcribe and translate this encoded information to synthesise proteins (see also Chapter 2).

4.2 | Bacterial chromosomes and natural gene transfer

4.2.1 Bacterial chromosomes

Chromosomes are the principal repositories of the genetic information, the site of gene expression and the vehicle of inheritance. The term chromosome, meaning dark-staining body, was originally applied to the structures visualised in eukaryotic organisms by light microscopy. The use of this term has now been extended to describe the physical structures that encode the genetic (hereditary) information in all organisms. The term genome is used in the more abstract sense to refer to the sum total of the genetic information of an organism. The term nucleoid is applied to a physical entity that can be isolated from a bacterial cell and that contains the chromosome in association with other components including RNA and protein. In addition to the main chromosome, other discrete types of replicating genetic material have been identified in bacterial cells, including transposable genetic elements (transposons), plasmids and prophages. The usual size ranges of the various genetic elements found inside bacterial cells are shown in Table 4.1.

The genetic material of bacteria consists of double-stranded (ds) DNA. The nucleotide bases are usually unmodified excepting for the addition of methyl residues that function to: (i) identify the 'old' (conserved) DNA strand following replication; (ii) protect the DNA from the action of specific nucleases; and (iii) time certain cell cycle events. Many viruses also use dsDNA as the genetic information (e.g. T-phages and lambda), while others have single-stranded (ss) DNA (e.g. ϕX174 and M13), ssRNA (e.g. MS2), or dsRNA (e.g. rotoviruses). Microbial chromosomes range in size over an order of magnitude and vary in their number, composition and topology (Table 4.2). Genome sizes

Table 4.2 Comparative properties[a] of viral, bacterial and fungal chromosomes with respect to size, composition and topography

Organism	Type	Number	Size	Nucleic acid	Topology
M13	bacteriophage	1	3.6 knt	ssRNA	circular
φX174	bacteriophage	1	5.4 knt	ssDNA	linear
lambda	bacteriophage	1	48.5 kbp	dsDNA	linear
T4	bacteriophage	1	174 kbp	dsDNA	linear
Mycoplasma genetalium	eubacterium	1	580 kbp	dsDNA	circular
Borrelia burgdorferi	eubacterium	1	910 kbp	dsDNA	linear
Campylobacter jejuni	eubacterium	1	1.7 Mbp	dsDNA	circular
Rhodobacter sphaeroides	eubacterium	2	3.2 Mbp + 0.9 Mbp	dsDNA	2 × circular
Bacillus subtilis	eubacterium	1	4.2 Mbp	dsDNA	circular
Escherichia coli	eubacterium	1	4.6 Mbp	dsDNA	circular
Streptomyces coelicolor	eubacterium	1	8.6 Mbp	ds DNA	linear
Myxococcus xanthus	eubacterium	1	9.45 Mbp	dsDNA	ND
Methannococcus junnaschii	archaea	1	1.6 Mbp	dsDNA	circular
Archaeoglobus fulgidus	archaea	1	2.8 Mbp	dsDNA	circular
Schizosaccharomyces pombe	eukaryote	3	3.5 to 5.7 Mbp total 18.8 Mbp	dsDNA	linear
Saccharomyces cerevisiae	eukaryote	15	0.2 to 2.2 Mbp total 12.43 Mbp	dsDNA	linear

[a] ND, not determined; dsDNA, double-stranded DNA; ssDNA, single-stranded DNA; bp, base pair(s); M, million; nt, nucleotide(s); k, thousand.

tend to reflect the organism's structural complexity and lifestyle. Obligate bacterial parasites such as *Mycoplasma genetalium* (580 kbp) tend to have small genomes, while bacteria with complex life cycles such as *Streptomyces coelicolor* (8.6 Mbp, i.e. 8.6 million base pairs of nucleotide bases) and *Myxococcus xanthus* (9.45 Mbp) tend to have large genomes. The genomes of more than 250 eubacterial, archaeal and simple eukaryotic micro-organisms have now been sequenced in their entirety.

The chromosome of *Escherichia coli* is typical of many eubacteria. It weighs 5 femtograms (5×10^{-15} g), is 1100 μm in length and its 4.6 Mbp of DNA codes for about 4400 proteins. The chromosome has a single set of genes (excepting for those encoding ribosomal RNA). At least 90% of the DNA encodes proteins/polypeptides, while the remaining 10% is used either for controlling gene expression or has a purely structural function. Genes of related function are often, but not always, clustered together on the chromosome. Protein coding sequences can be on either strand of the DNA, although there is a preference for an orientation in the direction in which the DNA is replicated. Gene expression involves two distinct, highly coordinated processes. The DNA is first transcribed by the enzyme RNA polymerase into messenger (m)RNA, an unstable molecular species with half-lives (i.e. the time taken for half of the RNA to be degraded) that are measured in minutes. Even as they are being transcribed, ribosomes (large nucleoprotein complexes) attach to specific sites on the mRNA,

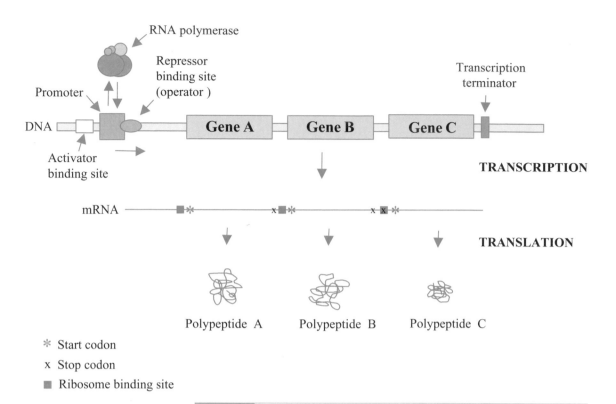

* Start codon

x Stop codon

■ Ribosome binding site

Figure 4.1 Schematic diagram illustrating the key components of a bacterial operon. The activator and repressor binding sites are control sites at which the frequency of transcription initiation are controlled. Although start and stop codons, and ribosome binding sites can be recognised in the DNA sequence, they are only functional in the mRNA.

the ribosome binding sites, and translate the encoded information into a linear polypeptide. To enable bacterial cells to regulate gene expression, the DNA is organised into transcriptional units or operons with distinct control sequences and transcriptional and translational start and stop points (Fig. 4.1).

The *E. coli* chromosome replicates by a bi-directional mode from the origin of replication (*oriC*) to the terminus (*terC*), primarily using the enzyme DNA polymerase III (Fig. 4.2). The rate of replication at 37 °C is about ~800 bases s^{-1} and, consequently, it takes approximately 40 minutes to replicate the entire chromosome. Since *E. coli* can divide by binary fission into two similarly sized cells every 20 minutes when growing on highly nutritious culture media, the chromosome of a single cell may have multiple sites of replication.

4.2.2 Mechanisms of gene transfer

The ability to engineer changes to the characteristics of a bacterium dates back to 1928 and the experiments of Fred Griffith who observed that of the two colonial morphologies exhibited by *Streptococcus pneumoniae*, namely rough and smooth, only the latter was able to infect mice. The rough and smooth characteristics (phenotypes) were due

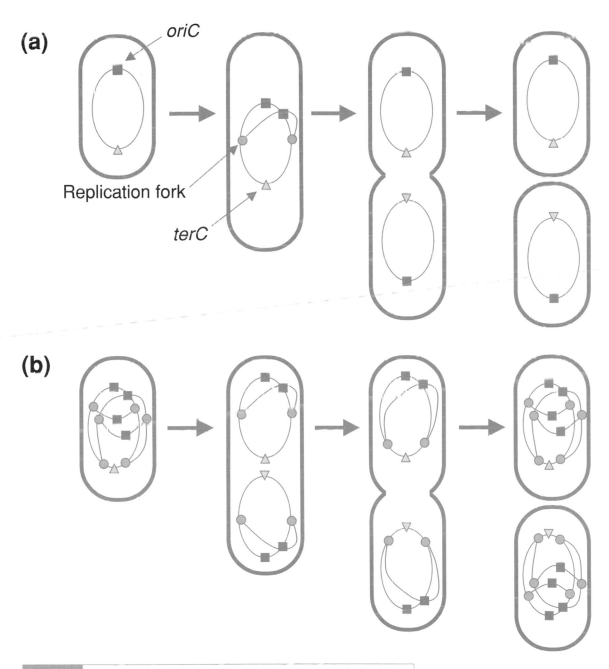

Figure 4.2 The bi-directional replication of the bacterial chromosome. Replication is initiated at the origin of replication (*oriC*) and is completed at the terminus (*terC*). (a) In slow growing cells (doubling time >60 min), each side of the chromosome has just one replication fork or site of DNA synthesis. (b) In rapidly growing cells (doubling time ~20 min), a new round of replication is initiated before the previous one has reached the terminus. Consequently, each side of the chromosome has more than one replication fork.

to the absence or presence, respectively, of a polysaccharide capsule that enables the bacterium to avoid the immune response. Griffith showed that if a rough (non-encapsulated) strain was injected into mice together with a heat-killed smooth strain, the rough strain could be transformed into a smooth strain to cause a fatal infection. It was some 16 years (1944) before the chemical responsible for transformation was identified as DNA, by Avery, MacLeod and McCarty, and another nine years (1953) before Watson and Crick determined its structure. The mechanism for transferring isolated DNA into a bacterium is still referred to as transformation, reflecting the rough to smooth transition of Griffith's pneumonococci. Cells that have received transforming DNA are referred to as *transformants*. Natural genetic transformation is exhibited by a wide variety of bacterial genera including *Azotobacter, Bacillus, Campylobacter, Clostridium, Haemophilus, Mycobacterium, Neisseria, Streptococcus* and *Streptomyces*. In addition, many strains that are not normally transformable can be induced to take up isolated DNA by chemical treatment or by the application of an electric field (see Section 4.4.5).

Two other mechanisms for transferring DNA between bacterial strains have been identified since the work of Griffith, namely *transduction* and *conjugation*. Transduction is the transfer of DNA from a donor cell to a recipient cell mediated by a bacterial virus (i.e. a bacteriophage, usually just referred to as a phage). It was first demonstrated in *Salmonella* by Zinder and Lederberg in 1952 using phage P22. During the replication of the phage in the donor, a small proportion of the phage particles (virions) encapsulate bacterial rather than phage DNA. These so-called transducing particles are still infective but, instead of injecting phage DNA, they infect the host cell with chromosomal DNA from the donor strain. The recipients of transduced DNA are referred to as *transductants*.

The third mechanism of gene transfer, *conjugation*, was discovered in 1946 by Lederberg and Tatum and involves cell-to-cell contact between the donor and recipient cells. Conjugation is usually mediated by a class of 'extrachromosomal, hereditary determinants' called plasmids. Plasmids are usually composed of covalently closed circular (*ccc*) molecules of double-stranded DNA that are able to replicate independently of the host chromosome, although occasionally they may integrate into the host chromosome. Plasmids are a common feature of bacterial strains where they confer a wide range of usually non-essential phenotypes, such as antibiotic resistance, toxin production, plant tumour formation, degradation of hydrocarbons and aromatic compounds (e.g. camphor, naphthalene, salicylate) and fertility. Plasmids tend to fall into the size range 1 to 150 kbp (kilo base pairs, i.e. gives the number of nucleotide bases in a particular piece of DNA) although mega-plasmids (>150 kb) have been found in representatives of a number of bacterial genera, including *Agrobacterium, Pseudomonas* and *Streptomyces*. Plasmids may account for between 0.1 and ~4% of their host's genotype, although in rare cases this may be as high as 20%. Plasmids such as the F plasmid of *E. coli* that confer fertility on their host cells are referred to as conjugative plasmids.

Bacterial conjugation involves the transfer of DNA from a donor to a recipient cell. Usually the DNA that is transferred to the recipient is plasmid DNA, and only rarely is it a part of the chromosomal DNA of the donor. The machinery involved is almost exclusively encoded by the conjugative plasmid, the main exception being the enzymes involved in DNA transfer replication. The transferred DNA is always in a single-stranded form and the complementary strand is synthesized in the recipient. The transfer of host chromosomal genes usually occurs at frequencies that are very much lower than that of plasmids, although some plasmids are exceptional in being able to mobilise host chromosomal genes at a frequency approaching 1, e.g. high frequency of recombination (Hfr) strains of E. coli.

Many small plasmids are capable of conjugal transfer even though they do not possess fertility functions of their own. These plasmids, which are referred to as *mobilisable plasmids*, exploit the fertility properties of co-existing conjugative plasmids. They have an active origin of transfer (*oriT*) and mobilisation (*mob*) genes encoding proteins required for their replicative transfer. When such plasmids are used as the basis of cloning vectors, the *mob* genes are usually omitted as a requirement of containment regulations designed to avoid the dissemination of the cloned genes to wild-type populations.

Although transfer between bacterial cells is the most common type of conjugation, transfer between bacteria and fungi and between bacteria and plants has also been demonstrated. In the latter case, strains of *Agrobacterium tumefaciens* with large (>200 kbp) tumour-inducing (Ti) plasmids can transfer part of their plasmid DNA – the so-called T-DNA (20–30 kbp) – into plant cells, where it interacts with the nuclear genome of the plant. This transfer is mediated by virulence (*vir*) genes, which show similarities to the components of bacterial conjugation systems. Agrobacterial Ti plasmids have been adapted to introduce new characteristics into plant species (transgenic plants), such as resistance to specific insect pests (see also Chapter 23).

Natural gene transfer methods have been used to generate genetic maps of many bacterial species that show the order and relative distances between the various genes. These classical genetic mapping techniques, highly developed in only a relatively small number of bacterial species, allowed detailed analysis of gene structure and the control of gene expression. These methods also allow strains with new characteristics to be constructed and have been adapted for use with more recently developed genetic engineering techniques.

4.3 | What is genetic engineering and what is it used for?

The ability to manipulate and analyse DNA using genetic engineering techniques (recombinant DNA technology) was foreseen in the mid 1960s and came to fruition in the early 1970s. The technology,

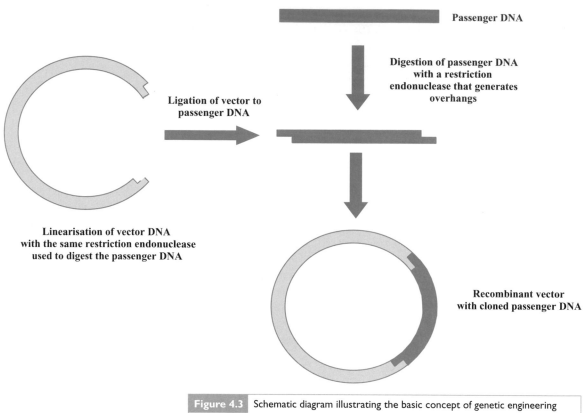

Passenger DNA

Digestion of passenger DNA with a restriction endonuclease that generates overhangs

Ligation of vector to passenger DNA

Linearisation of vector DNA with the same restriction endonuclease used to digest the passenger DNA

Recombinant vector with cloned passenger DNA

Figure 4.3 Schematic diagram illustrating the basic concept of genetic engineering using vector and passenger DNA.

which is still developing rapidly, evolved from a series of basic studies in the interrelated disciplines of biochemistry and microbial genetics. Key among these was the elucidation of the molecular basis of *bacterial restriction and modification* systems by Werner Arber that subsequently provided enzymes for cutting DNA at precise locations (target sites). These restriction endonucleases (*restriction enzymes*) were quickly exploited for the analysis and manipulation of DNA molecules from a variety of sources. From these relatively modest beginnings, techniques for manipulating and analysing both types of nucleic acid (DNA and RNA) have become remarkably powerful and sensitive, aided by the development of key technologies such as DNA sequencing, oligonucleotide synthesis and the polymerase chain reaction (PCR). At the same time, the provision of chemicals, reagents and equipment to facilitate this technology has become a multi-million dollar industry.

The advent of recombinant DNA technologies led to the realisation that DNA could be analysed to a resolution that was unimaginable only a few years before and consequently the genomes of almost any organism, prokaryote, archaea or eukaryote, could be manipulated to direct the synthesis of biological products that were normally only produced by their native hosts. This technology, illustrated in Fig. 4.3, has not only facilitated the production of certain proteins at a quantity and quality that was not previously achievable (see Chapter 21), but also opened up the possibility of developing highly modified or entirely new bioactive products. The technology has been applied to a wide range of industries particularly the pharmaceutical industry, where the main aims have been to produce natural compounds with proven or suspected therapeutic value and totally new products not found in Nature.

4.4 | The basic tools of genetic engineering

The techniques for isolating, cutting and joining molecules of DNA, developed in the early 1970s, have provided the foundations of our current technology for engineering and analysing nucleic acids. These allow fragments of DNA from virtually any organism to be cloned in a bacterium by inserting them into a vector (carrying) molecule that is stably maintained in the bacterial host.

4.4.1 Isolation and purification of nucleic acids

Biochemical techniques for preparing large quantities of relatively pure nucleic acids from microbial cells are an essential pre-requisite for in-vitro gene technology. The first step in the isolation of nucleic acids is the mechanical or enzymatic disruption of the cell to release the intracellular components that include the nucleic acids. Once released from the cell, the nucleic acids must be purified from other cellular components such as proteins and polysaccharides to provide a substrate of appropriate purity for nucleic acid modifying enzymes. The released nucleic acids are recovered using a combination of techniques including centrifugation, electrophoresis, adsorption to inert insoluble substrates or precipitation with non-aqueous solvents.

4.4.2 Cutting DNA molecules

The ability to cut molecules of DNA, either randomly or at specific target sites, is a requirement for many recombinant DNA techniques. DNA may be cleaved using mechanical or enzymatic methods. Mechanical shearing is non-specific and results in the production of random DNA fragments, which are often used to generate genomic libraries (see Section 4.4.5). When DNA molecules are mechanically sheared it is not possible to isolate a specific fragment containing, for example, a particular gene or operon. In contrast, when the DNA is cut using restriction endonucleases, which recognise and cleave specific target base sequences in double-stranded (ds)DNA, specific fragments can be isolated. Restriction endonucleases cut the phosphodiester backbone of both strands of the DNA to generate 3'OH and 5'PO$_4$ termini. Several hundred restriction endonucleases have been isolated from a wide variety of microbial species. Restriction endonucleases are classified into groups with distinct biochemical properties; type II enzymes are the main class used for genetic engineering purposes.

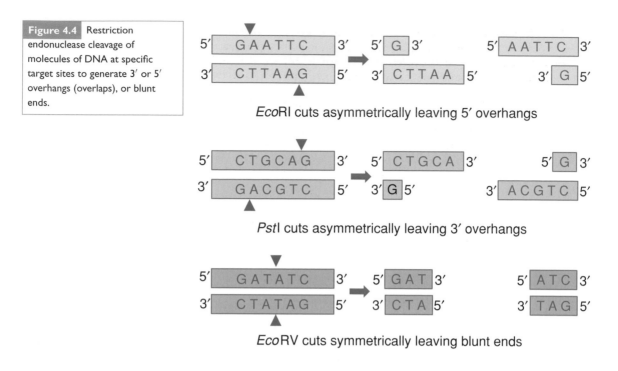

Figure 4.4 Restriction endonuclease cleavage of molecules of DNA at specific target sites to generate 3′ or 5′ overhangs (overlaps), or blunt ends.

*Eco*RI cuts asymmetrically leaving 5′ overhangs

*Pst*I cuts asymmetrically leaving 3′ overhangs

*Eco*RV cuts symmetrically leaving blunt ends

Restriction endonucleases are named according to the species from which they were originally isolated; enzymes isolated from *Haemophilus influenzae* are designated *Hin*, those from *Bacillus amyloliquefaciens*, *Bam*, etc. When more than one type of enzyme is isolated from a particular strain or species, the strain and isolation number (in roman numerals) are added to the name. Thus the three restriction endonucleases isolated from *H. influenzae* strain Rd are designated *Hin*I, *Hin*II and *Hin*III.

The target recognition sequences (restriction sites) of type II restriction enzymes are usually short, typically four to six bases in length. The length of the restriction sites and their nucleotide composition (i.e. the proportion of GC to AT bases) in relation to the rest of the target DNA, is important in determining the frequency at which the DNA is cut. For example, in DNA in which all four nucleotide bases occur randomly and with equal frequency, any given four base pair sequence will occur on average every 256 base pairs (4^4), while a six base pair recognition sequence will occur only once in every 4096 base pairs (4^6).

In most cases, restriction sites are palindromic, i.e. read the same on both strands with symmetry about a central point (Fig. 4.4). Cleavage usually occurs within the recognition sequence to generate either blunt ends or staggered ends with single-stranded overlaps. A list of commonly used restriction enzymes, their recognition sequences and cutting action is shown in Table 4.3.

4.4.3 Joining DNA fragments

DNA molecules with either blunt ends or with compatible (cohesive) overlapping ends may be joined together in vitro using specific

Table 4.3 Some common restriction endonucleases and their recognition sequences. Bases written in square brackets indicate variability of the bases in the recognition sequence. Sequences are written from 5' to 3' on one strand only. The point of enzymatic cleavage is indicated by an arrow

Enzyme	Source	Recognition site
BamHI	Bacillus amyloliquefaciens H	G↓GATCC
EcoRI	Escherichia coli RY13	G↓AATTC
EcoRII	Escherichia coli R245	↓CC[T/A]GG
HaeIII	Haemophilus aegyptius	GG↓CC
HindIII	Haemophilus influenzae Rd	A↓AGCTT
KpnI	Klebsiella pneumoniae	GGTAC↓C
NotI	Nocardia otitidis-caviarum	GC↓GGCCGC
PstI	Providencia stuartii	CTGCA↓G
Sau3A	Staphylococcus aureus 3A	↓GATC
SmaI	Serratia marcescens	CCC↓GGG

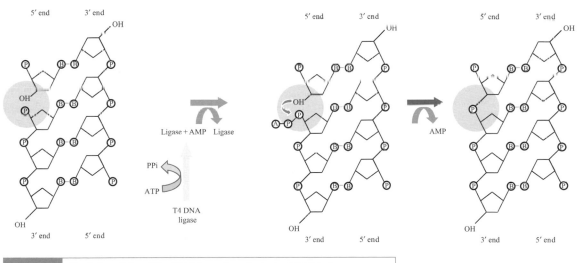

Figure 4.5 Catalytic activity of the DNA ligase from bacteriophage T4. An enzyme–AMP complex forms that binds to breaks in the phosphodiester backbone of the DNA and makes a covalent bond between the exposed 3'OH and 5'PO$_4$ groups on each side of the break.

'joining enzymes' called DNA ligases. These enzymes catalyse the formation of phosphodiester bonds between 3'OH groups at the terminus of one strand, with the 5'PO$_4$ terminus of another strand. The DNA ligase encoded by phage T4 is widely used for joining DNA molecules with both blunt-ended or cohesive ends. T4 DNA ligase activity requires ATP as a co-factor to form an enzyme–AMP intermediary complex. It then binds to the exposed 3'OH and 5'PO$_4$ ends of the interacting DNA molecules to create the covalent phosphodiester bond (Fig. 4.5).

Ligation reactions usually involve joining a fragment of passenger DNA (i.e. the piece of new DNA to be 'carried') to a vector molecule (Fig. 4.3). To increase the probability of the vector attaching to passenger DNA rather than to itself or another vector molecule, the molar ratio (i.e. number rather than mass of DNA) of passenger to vector DNA is usually about 10. An alternative strategy is to use a phosphatase (e.g. calf intestinal phosphatase, CIP) to remove phosphate groups from the $5'PO_4$ ends of the linearised vector DNA. Since this phosphate group is essential for joining the two ends of the vector together, recircularisation is impossible. However, when passenger DNA is present, it can provide the $5'PO_4$ ends for ligation to the $3'OH$ ends of the vector. This generates a circular molecule with single gaps in each of its nucleotide strands that are separated by the length of the passenger DNA. This structure is stable enough to be transformed into a cloning host where repair systems will seal the gaps.

Ligation reactions with T4 DNA ligase are relatively inefficient (~60%) and time consuming (2–12 hours) particularly when blunt-ended DNA is used as a substrate in the reaction. In recent years, various technologies have been introduced to improve the efficiency of ligation reactions. One such reaction uses the DNA topoisomerase I from *Vaccinia* virus, which functions both as a restriction endonuclease and a DNA ligase (Fig. 4.6). In nature, this enzyme relieves supercoiling in dsDNA by recognising the specific pentameric sequence, $5'$-(C/T)CCTT-$3'$, introducing a single-strand cleavage event immediately after the recognition sequence and allowing the DNA to unwind. The energy released during cleavage is conserved by the formation of a covalent interaction between tyrosine at position 274 on the enzyme and the resulting $3'PO_4$. The reaction can be reversed in the presence of $5'OH$ residues which can attack the phospho-tyrosyl bond on the vector, resulting in a highly efficient ligation reaction. Commercial systems, in which linearised vectors are supplied with *Vaccinia* topoisomerase I covalently attached to their 3-ends, facilitate the efficient ligation (95%) of either blunt-ended fragments or PCR products with $3'$ adenosine overlaps generated by non-proof-reading DNA polymerase such as *Taq*.

Novel approaches have also been developed to increase the efficiency with which target DNA sequences can be moved from one cloning vector to another. One such approach is based on the characteristics of the site-specific integration/excision mechanism of phage lambda. When lambda infects *E. coli*, it either enters the lytic cycle, generating approximately 200 copies of itself at the expense of the host cell, or the lysogenic state, in which case it integrates into the bacterial chromosome at a specific attachment (*att*) site. Integration, driven by a phage-encoded integrase (Int), involves a site-specific crossover recombination between the *attB* site on the bacterial chromosome and the *attP* site on the phage chromosome, to generate *attL* and *attR* sites at the junctions between the phage and bacterial genomes. The reaction is reversible, but it does require the combined actions of Int and a second phage-encoded excision enzyme, Xis. When this system is used to move DNA between different vectors, the target DNA is located between lambda '*att*' sequences (*attB* × *attP* ↔ *attL* × *attR*; see Fig. 4.7). The required directionality of the reaction is driven by the

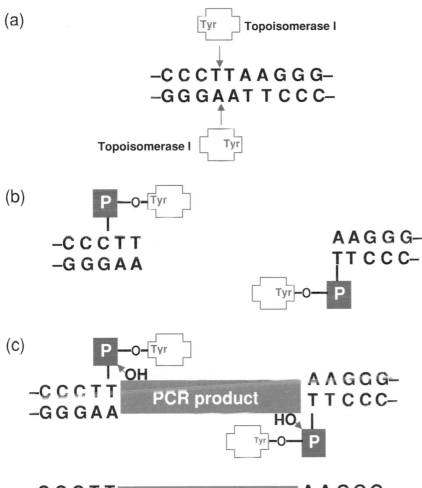

(a)

(b)

(c)

(d)

Figure 4.6 DNA topoisomerase I form *Vaccinia* virus has both restriction endonuclease and ligase activities that may be used for cloning DNA fragments. (a) DNA topoisomerase I recognises the sequence 5'-CCCTT-3'. (b) DNA topoisomerase I generates a single-strand nick immediately downstream of the recognition sequence – here there are recognition sequences on each strand resulting in two single-strand nicks opposite each other. The enzyme remains covalently attached to the nicked end via a tyrosine (Tyr) residue at position 274. (c) The phosphor-tyrosyl bond is attacked by the OH residue at the 5' terminus of a PRC product generated with non-phosphory primers. (d) The PRC product is ligated into the vector *via* a phosphodiester bond between the 3'PO$_4$ and 5'OH groups, respectively, at the ends of the vector and PCR product.

addition of either Int or Int + Xis, and the products transformed into a suitable *E. coli* cloning host. The destination plasmid containing the required target DNA is selected on the basis of its antibiotic-resistance gene. However, to avoid selection of the original destination plasmid, the sequences between the *att* sites encode a toxin that is lethal to *E. coli*.

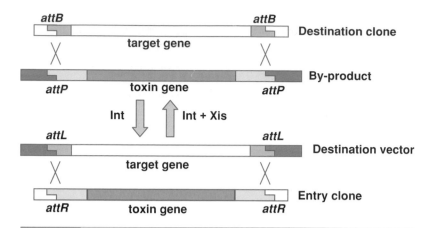

Figure 4.7 Cloned DNA can be moved between different vectors without the need for conventional sub-cloning. The system uses the site-specific recombination system of phage lambda. The target DNA is cloned initially into an entry vector to give the entry clone. Entry clone DNA is mixed with the destination vector and a mixture of Int and Xis recombinases added. Recombination is unidirectional, forming at high efficiency the destination clone and by-product. After transformation into a host that is sensitive to the toxin encoded by the toxin gene, destination clones are selected on the basis of their antibiotic-resistance phenotype. The reaction is reversible if Int alone is added to the reaction mixture, in which case the roles of the various vectors are reversed.

4.4.4 The polymerase chain reaction (PCR) and its uses

Since its introduction in the mid 1980s, the polymerase chain reaction (PCR) has had a major impact on recombinant DNA technology. PCR facilitates the amplification of virtually any fragment of DNA from about 0.2 to 40 kbp in size. Because the amplification reaction is cyclical and the concentration of DNA doubles at each cycle, the total amount of DNA in the reaction increases exponentially; the theoretical yield from each original template molecule is about 10^6 molecules after 20 cycles, and about 10^9 molecules after 30 cycles. PCR requires a thermostable DNA polymerase, template DNA, a pair of specific oligonucleotide primers and a complete set of deoxynucleotide triphosphates (i.e. dATP, dCTP, dGTP and dTTP) substrates.

Oligonucleotide primers for PCR are synthesised chemically to be complementary to sequences that flank the region to be amplified and are usually about 20 nucleotides in length. The primers are designed to bind (anneal) specifically to the opposite strands of the template molecule, in such a way that their 3′ ends face the region to be amplified. It is the specificity of the primer annealing reaction which ensures that the PCR amplifies the appropriate region of the template DNA. A key feature of the PCR is that the entire DNA amplification reaction is carried out in a single tube containing enzyme, template, primers and substrates. Each cycle of amplification therefore involves annealing, extension and denaturation reactions, each brought about at different temperatures (Fig. 4.8). Since the dissociation reaction may occur at temperatures as high as 95 °C, and there may be as

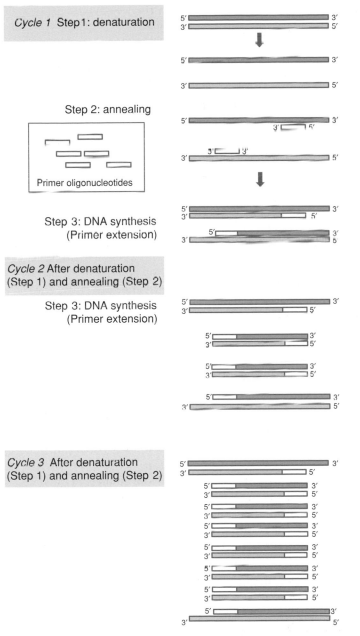

Cycle 1 Step 1: denaturation

Step 2: annealing

Primer oligonucleotides

Step 3: DNA synthesis
(Primer extension)

Cycle 2 After denaturation
(Step 1) and annealing (Step 2)

Step 3: DNA synthesis
(Primer extension)

Cycle 3 After denaturation
(Step 1) and annealing (Step 2)

Figure 4.8 The polymerase chain reaction, showing the cyclical nature of the annealing, synthesis and denaturation reactions which are carried out automatically in a dedicated thermocycler (PCR machine).

Cycles repeated 20–35 times, leading to exponential doubling of the target sequence

many as 35 cycles in a single PCR, a highly thermostable DNA polymerase is a basic requirement for PCR. *Taq* polymerase, was isolated from an archea bacterium, *Thermus aquaticus*, found growing in a hot Icelandic spring. It was the first thermostable DNA polymerase to be employed in PCR. *Taq* polymerase lacks a 3′ to 5′ exonuclease proofreading function and consequently has a high error rate for the incorporation of incorrect nucleotides. However, proof-reading thermostable DNA polymerases, such as *Pfu* polymerase from *Pyrococcus furiosus*, another archaea, have been recently introduced with considerably reduced mis-incorporation error rates.

The first step in the polymerase chain reaction (Fig. 4.8) is the denaturation of the double-stranded DNA template by heating to about 95 °C. The reaction mixture is then cooled to allow the oligonucleotide primers to anneal to the resulting single-stranded templates. The temperature at which annealing occurs is dependent on the length and G + C content of the primer sequences, but is usually designed to be in the range 50–65 °C. After the annealing step the temperature is raised to about 70 °C, the optimum temperature for the synthesis of the complementary strand by thermostable DNA polymerases. The cycle of denaturation, annealing and synthesis is repeated 20–35 times in a typical PCR. Although the maximum size of fragment that can be amplified with *Taq* polymerase is about 4 kbp, optimisation of the components in the reaction and the use of a mixture of thermostable polymerases means that it is now possible to amplify DNA fragments of up to 40 kbp in size.

PCR has been developed for a whole host of other applications, including DNA sequencing, the introduction of specific nucleotide changes (site-directed mutagenesis), DNA labelling and in the fusion of DNA fragments to generate chimeric genes. Additionally, by incorporating target sites for restriction endonucleases into the 5′ ends of the oligonucleotide primers, the amplified PCR products can be digested and subsequently ligated into a specific site on the cloning vector (Section 4.5). In addition, real-time (RT)-PCR is increasingly used to quantitate the expression of specific genes. mRNA is converted to DNA with reverse transcriptase (RNA-dependent DNA polymerase) and the resulting copy DNA quantified by RT-PCR. The real-time amplification reactions are carried out using fluorescently labelled primers in a thermocycler that detects the accumulated fluorescent signal. The fluorophore is positioned in the unincorporated primer so that it is quenched (i.e. emits very little fluorescence), but becomes unquenched when incorporated into double-stranded DNA. The reactions are carried out in a capillary tube and the accumulating unquenched fluorescent signal resulting from successive PCR cycles is measured in real-time by a micro volume fluorimeter incorporated into the thermocycler. The RT-PCR process is extremely sensitive, accurate and reproducible.

4.4.5 Transformation and other gene transfer methods

The ability to introduce foreign DNA into a bacterial cell host lies at the very heart of recombinant DNA technology. *Transformation*, in which the exogenous DNA is taken up by the host cell, is the most widely applied gene transfer technique for cloning purposes. While some bacteria possess natural transformation systems others, such as *E. coli*, require chemical pre-treatment to make them competent for the uptake of DNA.

Although transformation is efficient for most cloning purposes, there are some procedures, such as the generation of genomic libraries, for which transformation is not efficient enough. In these cases it is possible to circumvent the transformation procedure by packaging the recombinant DNA into virus particles in vitro (Section 4.5.2). More recently it has been shown that bacteria are able to take up DNA when given a high voltage pulse. In this process, called electroporation, mixtures of cells and exogenous DNA are subjected to a brief (typically of millisecond duration) electric pulse of up to 2500 volts. The high field strength induces pores to form in the cell membrane, permitting the entry of the negatively charged DNA that is itself mobilised by the electrical gradient. In many cases electroporation is more efficient than transformation and some types of bacteria may only be transformed by this procedure.

4.4.6 Selection and screening of recombinants

After most cloning procedures it is necessary to screen the resulting clones to isolate those carrying the required gene or fragment of DNA. At the simplest level this may be done by selecting bacterial transformants that contain a copy of the vector. This is achieved by incorporating an antibiotic-resistance marker gene into the vector so that only transformed bacteria that have received a copy of the vector are able to grow on media containing the appropriate antibiotic. More advanced systems have been developed to allow the discrimination of transformants containing a vector with or without a cloned insert. These systems include the use of gene disruption methods that result in the loss of a particular trait upon insertion of foreign DNA (Section 4.5.4).

Clones containing a specific gene or fragment can be identified directly by selection techniques or indirectly by restriction endonuclease mapping, PCR or hybridisation techniques. If the target gene is expressed, its presence may be selected by complementation of a defect in the cloning host (e.g. restoration of the ability to utilise a particular substrate or to grow in the absence of an otherwise essential nutrient). In the case of restriction mapping, plasmid DNA extracted from a number of representative clones is digested with specific restriction endonucleases. Only clones containing the required gene or DNA fragment will generate the correct pattern of bands after agarose gel electrophoresis. Restriction mapping is only feasible if the target clones are likely to occur at a high frequency among the population to be screened. Diagnostic PCR, using oligonucleotide primers specific to the target DNA sequence, may also be used to identify clones containing the required gene or DNA fragment. Since PCR may be used directly on unprocessed samples of colonies, it is feasible to test many more clones.

If the target DNA is likely to occur at a low frequency in a population of clones, as would be the case with a genomic library (Section 4.5.5), a large number of clones need to be screened. In this case the method of choice is hybridisation of the bacteria colony that grows from a single cell (or in the case of phage vectors, the viral plaque). Colony or plaque hybridisation makes use of labelled nucleic acid probes (DNA or RNA) that are able to detect the presence of specific DNA sequences within individual colonies or plaques. Biomass from individual transformant colonies or plaques is transferred to a membrane onto which denatured DNA, released by breaking the cells open, will bind. The membrane is then exposed to a labelled probe (Section 4.4.7) that binds specifically to the immobilised target DNA, revealing the identity of colonies or plaques containing the appropriate cloned DNA.

4.4.7 Nucleic acid probes and hybridisation

Nucleic acid probes are used to detect specific target DNA molecules. Traditionally, a soluble probe binds (i.e. hybridises) to the target DNA that is immobilised onto a solid matrix (e.g. nylon, nitrocellulose glass or silicon), although this situation is reversed in the case of DNA arrays (Section 4.4.8). Hybridisation is used for a variety of biotechnological applications including the detection of cloned DNA (Section 4.4.6), the analysis of genetic organisation and the diagnosis of genetic diseases. Although nucleic acid hybridisation techniques are used in a wide variety of contexts, the same basic principles apply. Nucleic acid hybridisation exploits the ability of single-stranded probe nucleic acid (DNA or RNA) to anneal to complementary single-stranded target sequences (DNA or RNA) within a population of non-complementary nucleic acid molecules.

The original technique, referred to as *Southern blotting* after its inventor, Ed Southern, involved the size separation of restriction endonuclease digested fragments of DNA by gel electrophoresis, and their transfer by blotting onto nitrocellulose membranes. The probe nucleic acid is applied as an aqueous solution and, under appropriate hybridisation conditions, binds to immobilised target DNA. The location of bound probe nucleic acid on the membrane is indicated by the presence of a readily and sensitively detected label. When the technique was extended to detect target RNA it was referred to as *Northern blotting* (Section 4.7.1).

Nucleic acid probes used in hybridisation reactions must be in the form of single-stranded (ss) RNA or DNA molecules; when double-stranded DNA is used it must be denatured prior to hybridisation. Since the function of the probe is to detect the specific target sequences, it means that the probe itself must be easily detected. Traditionally this is achieved by the incorporation of a radionuclide such as ^{32}P or ^{35}S and detection by exposure to photographic (e.g. X-ray) film.

In recent years, concerns over safety and pollution have led to the development of methods for labelling nucleic acids that avoid the need to use radionuclides, and nucleotide analogues containing biotin or digoxigenin are incorporated in their place. Ligand (i.e. binding) molecules with a high affinity for the incorporated nucleotide analogue (e.g. streptavidin for biotin), and which are cross-linked to enzymes such as peroxidases or alkaline phosphatases, are used to detect the probe after hybridisation to its target. Detection is based on the enzymatic cleavage of either a colourless chromogenic substrate, with release of a coloured product, or a chemiluminescent substrate, with the production of light. The latter is detected using photographic film in a similar manner to radionuclides.

RNA probes are preferred for hybridisation reactions in which the target molecule is RNA (e.g. Northern blotting) and these are synthesised in vitro using a phage RNA polymerase. A DNA fragment encoding all or parts of the target sequence is cloned behind the appropriate phage promoter. After extraction of the plasmid, the phage RNA polymerase is used to synthesise an RNA transcript that is complementary to the target nucleic acid. As with the labelling of DNA, radiolabelled nucleotides or nucleotide analogues are incorporated during the synthesis reaction.

4.4.8 DNA array technology

The availability of numerous complete microbial genome sequences, together with advances in microfabrication technology, has led to the development of a powerful technology that allows the transcription of every gene in a bacterium to be monitored in a single experiment. DNA array technology has revolutionised the analysis of gene expression profiling (Fig. 4.9). Microfabrication techniques are used to attach specific DNA probes at high density onto a glass or silicon substrate – the array or chip. Two types of probe are used: PCR products containing all or part of the target gene (ORFmer), or oligonucleotides of between 20 and 70 nucleotides in length. In most cases the probes are synthesised independently and then spotted onto the array using a robotic printer; however, more advanced systems use photolithography to synthesise the probes in situ. The probe density can vary from 10 000 to 500 000 spots per array, depending on the printing technology.

Target nucleic acid is usually labelled with a fluorescent dye. Messenger RNA is dye-labelled during the reverse transcription reaction that generates copy DNA. The use of complementary dyes, Cy3 (green) and Cy5 (red), facilitates the direct comparison of signals from independent sources on a single array. The signals are detected and quantified using a laser-scanning fluorimeter; Cy3 is excited at 532 nm and detected between 557 and 592 nm, while Cy5 is excited at 635 nm and detected between 650 and 690 nm.

4.4.9 DNA sequencing

DNA sequencing is one of the most powerful techniques available for the analysis and directed manipulation of DNA. Knowledge of the DNA sequences of target DNA molecules and cloning vectors is fundamental to the construction of advanced bacterial protein production systems. It also facilitates the design of specific probes or primers and the production of computer-generated transcription and restriction maps.

Control system
(e.g. wild-type or non-stressing
growth conditions)

Experimental system
(e.g. mutant or stress-inducing
growth conditions)

Extract RNA

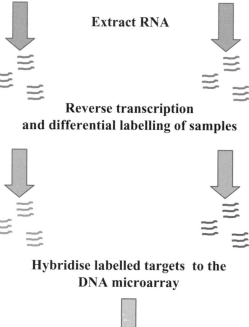

Reverse transcription
and differential labelling of samples

Hybridise labelled targets to the
DNA microarray

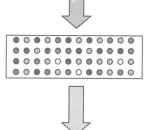

Quantitation by laser scanning fluorimetry

> Figure 4.9 The principle of a DNA array experiment to compare the expression profile of an experimental system with that of a control system.

The Maxam and Gilbert method for DNA sequencing uses chemical reagents to bring about the base-specific cleavage of the DNA. Although still used for a limited number of applications, this chemically based technique has generally been replaced by the elegant chain-terminator method developed by Sanger and colleagues. The *Sanger procedure* exploits the ability of a variant of *E. coli* DNA polymerase I (the so-called Klenow fragment) to synthesise a complementary strand of DNA from a single-stranded DNA template, incorporating both the natural deoxynucleotides and 2′,3′-dideoxynucleotide analogues. Dideoxynucleotides lack a hydroxyl group at the 3′ position and are therefore not able to act as a substrate for further chain

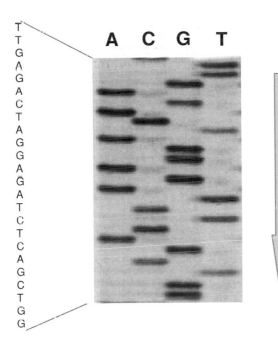

Direction
of electrophoresis

Figure 4.10 An autoradiograph of part of a DNA sequencing gel generated by the Sanger chain termination method. The lanes are labelled according to the nucleotides at which they are terminated, namely; A, adenine; C, cytosine; G, guanine; T, thymine. The sequence specified by the gel is shown to the left of the gel.

elongation. Their incorporation therefore terminates the synthesis of the DNA strand in question. A specific oligonucleotide primer, used to initiate the chain elongation process, determines the start point for all of the newly synthesised DNA molecules. DNA polymerase synthesises DNA from a single-stranded template in the presence of all four deoxynucleotide triphosphate substrates (dATP, dCTP, dGTP, dTTP), one of which is radiolabelled (e.g. $(\alpha\text{-}^{35}\text{S})$-dATP). Identical reactions are carried out in four tubes excepting that each tube also includes, at a lower concentration, one of the four possible dideoxynucleotide triphosphate analogues (ddATP, ddCTP, ddGTP, ddTTP). When the appropriate relative concentrations of normal and dideoxy nucleotides are used, newly synthesised DNA strands will be terminated at every possible base position and a set of fragments of all possible lengths will be generated. The products of the four reaction mixtures are separated by denaturing polyacrylamide gel electrophoresis and subjected to autoradiography. The resulting banding pattern allows the DNA sequence to be read directly (Fig. 4.10).

The demands of large-scale sequencing projects has led to the automation of DNA sequencing technology. This has been achieved by changing the format of the chain-termination technique to allow real-time detection of the DNA bands within capillary polyacrylamide gels, using fluorescent dye-labelled substrates. Up to 1000 bases may be read from a single reaction using this technology and the data are captured directly in electronic format.

4.4.10 Site-directed mutagenesis

Site-directed mutagenesis, the specific replacement of nucleotides in a sequence of DNA, is used to analyse or modify the activity of genes

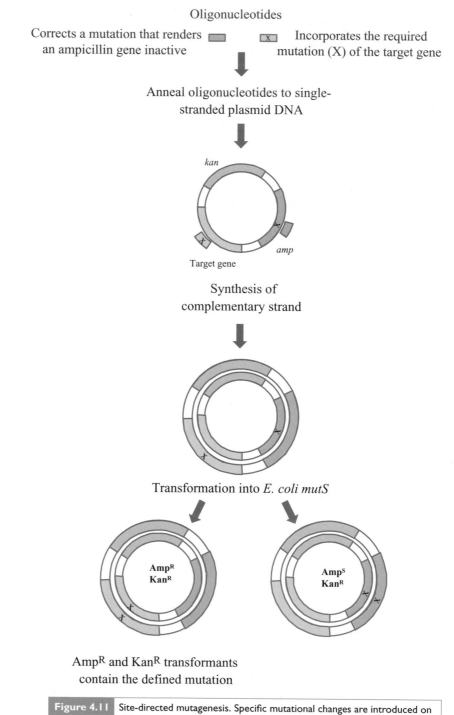

Figure 4.11 Site-directed mutagenesis. Specific mutational changes are introduced on oligonucleotide primers that reconstitute a double-stranded plasmid molecule from a single-stranded template containing the target gene. After transformation into *E. coli*, mutated and wild-type plasmids segregate among the progeny. Plasmids with the required mutation are selected on the basis of their newly acquired ampicillin resistance.

or gene products. For example, specific amino acid replacements have been use to improve the characteristics of many industrial enzymes. The mutational changes are introduced in the DNA using in vitro techniques; the DNA is then introduced back into the bacterium where the resulting phenotypes are observed. Oligonucleotide site-directed mutagenesis is an important tool for achieving this aim, since it permits the introduction of highly specific changes in the target DNA sequence. Although many methodologies have been developed for site-directed mutagenesis, the principles are generally similar to the example shown in Fig. 4.11. The target DNA is cloned into a plasmid vector, which is able to be replicated to form single-stranded DNA (Section 4.5.4). In addition to the target DNA, the vector also contains two antibiotic-resistance markers. One of the resistance genes, here the ampicillin-resistance gene, has been inactivated by the inclusion of a single base substitution. The single-stranded form of the plasmid is annealed with two oligonucleotide primers: one complementary to the target gene excepting for the inclusion of the desired base substitution(s), the other complementary to the mutated region of the ampicillin-resistance gene, but incorporating a base substitution that reverses the ampicillin-sensitive phenotype by restoring the wild-type gene sequence. The addition of DNA polymerase and DNA ligase leads to the synthesis of a complementary strand of DNA. The resulting double-stranded plasmid contains two deliberate mismatches, one that corrects the mutation in the ampicillin-resistance gene and the other generating the specific change(s) to the target gene. It is transformed into E. coli, where repair of the mismatches by the host's mismatch repair systems is avoided by use of a mutant (e.g. *mutS*) that is defective in this function. After replication, each strand will form a double-stranded molecule without mismatches and these will segregate into separate daughter cells. One molecule will contain the mutations introduced by the oligonucleotides, whilst the other will be identical to the original plasmid. Cells harbouring plasmids with the desired mutation are selected by virtue of their newly acquired ampicillin-resistance phenotype.

4.5 | Cloning vectors and libraries

A cloning vector is a molecule of DNA into which passenger DNA can be cloned to allow it to be replicated inside a bacterial host cell. The vector and passenger DNA are covalently joined by ligation (Section 4.4.3). Cloning vectors have four basic characteristics: (i) they must be easily introduced into the host bacterium by transformation or, after in vitro packaging, by phage infection; (ii) they must be able to replicate in the host bacterium, preferably so that the number of copies of the vector (copy number) exceeds that of the host chromosome by between 50 and 200; (iii) they should contain unique sites for the action of a variety of restriction endonucleases; and (iv) they should encode a means for selecting or screening host cells that contain a copy of the vector. Cloning vectors are derived from naturally occurring DNA molecules, such as plasmids and phages, which are capable of replicating independently of the host chromosome. A wide variety of cloning vectors has been developed for specific applications and these are briefly described below.

4.5.1 General purpose plasmid vectors

General purpose plasmid vectors are designed for cloning relatively small (<10 kbp) fragments of DNA, usually into E. coli. The vectors are usually introduced into their bacterial host by transformation, and transformants that have received a copy of the vector are selected using a vector-based antibiotic-resistance gene. Modern general purpose vectors have purpose-designed fragments (multiple-cloning site or MCS) incorporating a variety of unique restriction sites.

General purpose vectors usually include a system for detecting the presence of a cloned DNA fragment, based on the loss of an easily scored phenotype. The most widely used system involves the *lacZ'* gene encoding the α-peptide from the N terminus of E. coli β-galactosidase. The synthesis of this peptide, from a gene located on the vector, complements an otherwise inactive version of this enzyme, encoded by the host's chromosome. The result is an active β-galactosidase enzyme that can be detected by its ability to liberate a blue chromophore from the colourless chromogenic substrate 5-bromo-4-chloro-3-indolyl-β-D-galactoside, referred to as X-gal. Cloning a fragment of DNA within the vector-based gene encoding the α-peptide prevents the formation of an active β-galactosidase. If X-gal is included in the selective agar plates, transformant colonies are blue in the case of a vector with no inserted DNA and white in the case of a vector containing a fragment of cloned DNA. The same detection system is used in a variety of modern vectors, including phage vectors that consequently generate blue or white plaques. The most widely used general-purpose plasmid vectors are those of the pUC series (Fig. 4.12).

4.5.2 Bacteriophage and cosmid vectors

Bacteriophage lambda (λ), which infects E. coli, has provided the basis for the most commonly used phage vectors. Lambda has been of greatest value for cloning relatively large fragments (>10 kbp) that are not easily cloned by general-purpose plasmid vectors. Lambda has a linear dsDNA genome of approximately 48.5 kbp in size with short 12-base pair single-stranded 5′ projections at each end to facilitate its circularisation in E. coli. The site generated by the circularisation reaction is known as the *cos* site (cohesive ends). In the development of lambda cloning vectors, non-essential genes have been removed to provide space for the insertion of DNA fragments of up to 23 kbp in size. Additionally, because the phage genome is only circularised upon infection of the host, lambda vectors can be supplied as separate 'left' and 'right' arms. Each arm has an appropriate restriction endonuclease site at one of its ends and the recombinant DNA is

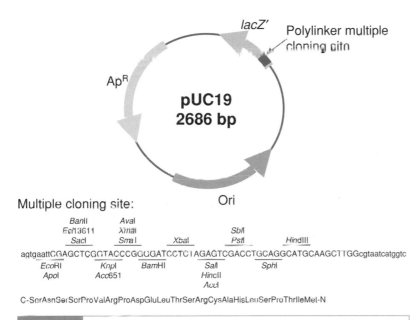

Multiple cloning site:

C-SerAsnSerSerProValArgProAspGluLeuThrSerArgCysAlaHisLeuSerProThrIleMet-N

Figure 4.12 The general purpose plasmid cloning vector pUC19 is a member of the pUC series of plasmid vectors. The pUC vectors have been generated in pairs that differ only with respect to their multiple cloning site which are located in opposite orientation, allowing the passenger DNA to be located in either the same direction or apposed to the transcription of the *lacZ'* gene. The arrows on the *lacZ'*, ampicillin-resistance (Ap^R) and replication protein (Ori) genes indicate the direction of transcription. The sequence of the multiple-cloning site (capitals) and adjacent (lower case) sequences are shown together with restriction endonuclease target site and translated amino acids.

cloned between the arms (Fig. 4.13). The transformation of lambda molecules into *E. coli* is relatively inefficient and this has led to the development of in vitro phage packaging systems for the efficient delivery of recombinant lambda genomes into their bacterial hosts.

Cosmid vectors combine the advantages of a plasmid cloning vector (e.g. ease of cloning and propagation) with the high efficiency of delivery and cloning capacity of a phage vector. Cosmids are plasmids that have a copy of the *cos* site normally found on the lambda genome. The presence of the *cos* site enables these plasmids to be

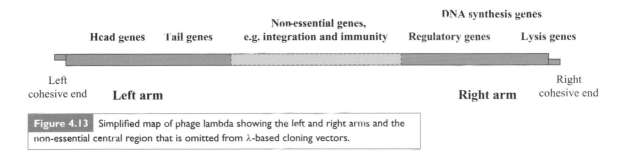

Figure 4.13 Simplified map of phage lambda showing the left and right arms and the non-essential central region that is omitted from λ-based cloning vectors.

used in conjunction with a lambda *in-vitro* packaging system. This means that molecules of cosmid DNA with large insertions of passenger DNA can be introduced efficiently into an appropriate *E. coli* host. Since the cosmid vector itself is typically only about 5 kbp in size, inserts of about 32–47 kbp can be accommodated in the phage. The packaged cosmid DNA is injected into the bacterial cell as if it was lambda DNA where it circularises and starts to replicate using its plasmid replication functions.

4.5.3 Bacterial artificial chromosomes

Bacterial artificial chromosomes (pBACs, where 'p' refers to 'plasmid') have been developed for cloning very large (>50 kbp) sequences of DNA. BAC vectors are usually based on the F plasmid of *E. coli* and are able to accept DNA inserts as large as 300 kbp. pBACs are maintained as single copy plasmids in *E. coli*, excluding the replication of more than one pBAC in the same host cell. Ordered pBAC libraries of bacterial genomes may be constructed in which the entire genome sequence is represented by a series of clones with overlapping inserts.

4.5.4 Special purpose vectors

In addition to the vectors described above, a range of special purpose vectors have been developed and are described briefly below.

Expression vectors

Expression vectors are designed to achieve high level, controlled expression of a target gene with resulting production of a protein product at concentrations as high as 40% total cellular protein. Expression vectors often incorporate a system that adds an affinity tag to the protein to facilitate its purification by affinity chromatography. Expression vectors are mostly plasmid based and often use the tightly controlled and highly efficient phage T7 RNA polymerase gene expression system. The target gene is cloned downstream of the transcriptional (promoter) and translational (ribosome binding site) control signals derived from T7. The vector is transformed into an *E. coli* host with a chromosomally located gene encoding the T7 RNA polymerase. Switching the polymerase gene on leads to high-level synthesis of the target gene.

If the target gene is not fused to an affinity tag, the protein must be purified using expensive methodologies. However, a number of affinity tag systems have been developed in recent years that provide for highly specific purification protocols. A variety of tags have been used, including a tag of six adjacent histidine residues ($6 \times$ His) that binds to nickel and glutathione-S-transferase that binds to glutathione. The ligand is attached to an insoluble resin and the tagged fusion protein recovered by passing through a chromatographic column containing the resin-bound ligand (Fig. 4.14). The bound fusion protein is eluted as a virtually pure protein and the affinity tag removed by treatment with a chemical or by digestion with a protease.

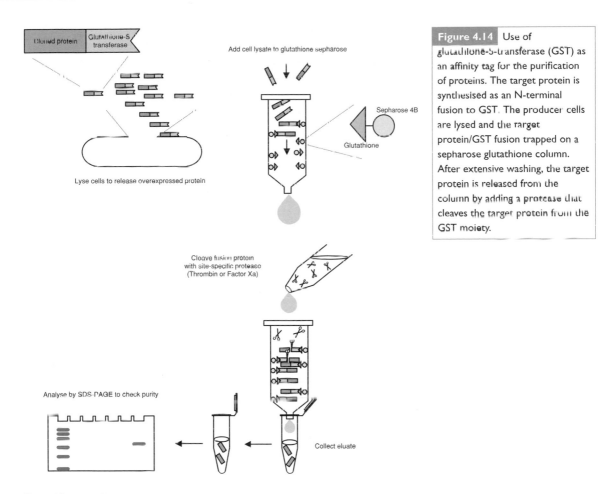

Add cell lysate to glutathione sepharose

Sepharose 4B

Glutathione

Lyse cells to release overexpressed protein

Cleave fusion protein
with site-specific protease
(Thrombin or Factor Xa)

Analyse by SDS-PAGE to check purity

Collect eluate

Figure 4.14 Use of glutathione-S-transferase (GST) as an affinity tag for the purification of proteins. The target protein is synthesised as an N-terminal fusion to GST. The producer cells are lysed and the target protein/GST fusion trapped on a sepharose glutathione column. After extensive washing, the target protein is released from the column by adding a protease that cleaves the target protein from the GST moiety.

Secretion vectors

Currently, most systems for the production of recombinant proteins lead to the intracellular accumulation of the product. However, intracellular accumulation can lead to lower production levels, protein aggregation, proteolysis and permanent loss of biological activity (Section 4.9.4). This can sometimes be overcome by secreting the target protein directly into the culture medium since secreted proteins can potentially be accumulated to higher concentrations and are usually correctly folded. For a protein to be secreted into the culture medium it needs to be directed to the secretion apparatus located in the cytoplasmic membrane. This requires the use of a secretion vector (Fig. 4.15) in which the target protein is synthesised as a fusion protein with an N-terminal signal peptide. The signal peptide directs the protein to a secretory translocase located in the membrane. Once translocated, the signal peptide is removed by cleavage with a signal peptidase located on the outer surface of the cell membrane.

Shuttle or bifunctional vectors

Rapid advances in microbial genetics and the development of cloning vectors mean that it is now possible to manipulate the genomes of

(a) Signal peptide structure (~25 residues):

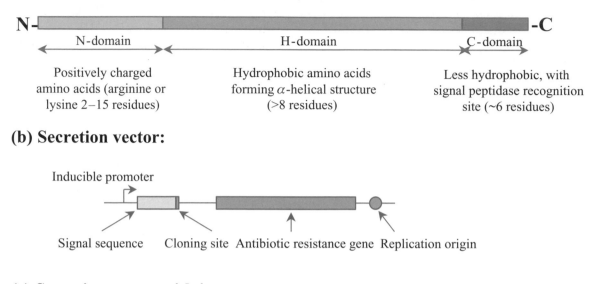

Positively charged amino acids (arginine or lysine 2–15 residues)

Hydrophobic amino acids forming α-helical structure (>8 residues)

Less hydrophobic, with signal peptidase recognition site (~6 residues)

(b) Secretion vector:

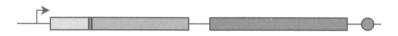

Inducible promoter

Signal sequence   Cloning site   Antibiotic resistance gene   Replication origin

(c) Secretion vector with insert:

Target gene sequence fused in-frame with the signal sequence

Figure 4.15 Properties of a secretion vector. (a) Structure of a typical *E. coli* signal (or leader) peptide required to target a protein across the cytoplasmic membrane. (b) Organisation of a secretion vector with cloning site immediately downstream of the signal sequence. (c) Secretion vector with the DNA sequence of the target protein fused in-frame downstream of the signal sequence.

a broad range of micro-organisms. However, in many cases transformation efficiency remains stubbornly low and it is often expedient to use *E. coli* as an intermediate cloning host. This can be achieved by using a shuttle or bifunctional vector that has replication origins that are functional in *E. coli* and the target micro-organism. More recently certain plasmids have been found to have broad host range replication functions and these have been used for the development of a new generation of shuttle plasmids.

Single-stranded phage and phagemid vectors
It is sometimes necessary to generate single-stranded DNA, particularly for DNA sequencing and oligonucleotide-directed mutagenesis. Messing developed a series of vectors based on phage M13, a filamentous ssDNA phage of *E. coli*. The mp series of M13 vectors incorporates

a multiple cloning site within a gene encoding the α-peptide fragment of β-galactosidase. They are therefore amenable to blue/white plaque selection (Section 4.3.1) for the detection of cloned inserts. M13-based vectors infect F$^+$ strains of *E. coli* via the F pilus. It is the double-stranded replicative form of the phage genome that is used for cloning purposes.

Phagemids are plasmids that contain the origin of replication for a ssDNA phage (Fig. 4.16), usually that of phage f1 which is closely related to M13. *Escherichia coli* is able to maintain a phagemid as dsDNA by virtue of a plasmid origin of replication. However, if the cell is infected with a so-called helper f1 phage, the f1 replication origin is activated and the vector switches to a mode of replication that generates ssDNA that is packaged into phage particles as they are extruded from the host cell.

Integration vectors

Integration vectors are designed to integrate all or part of themselves into the chromosome of a host bacterium. They are used in a variety of specific contexts including cloning genes at low copy numbers, the generation of insertion mutations, gene replacements and the generation of gene fusions. Integration vectors are usually based on plasmids that are either unable to replicate in the target host, or which have temperature-sensitive replication functions. Integration can occur by either single or double cross-over recombination events, using homologous DNA sequences on the plasmid and the host.

In single *cross-over recombination*, also referred to as 'Campbell-type integration', the vector integrates into the host chromosome in its entirety. Integration takes place by a cross-over event between homologous regions on the host and the vector. The frequency of integration is host dependent and it may be necessary to grow the host in the presence of the vector for several generations – this can be achieved by growing transformants for several generations at a temperature that permits the replication of the vector. Selection for integrants is achieved by raising the temperature to the non-permissive level and selecting for an antibiotic-resistance phenotype encoded by the vector. The specificity of the integration event can be confirmed by a diagnostic PCR using primer pairs in which a primer specific to adjacent chromosomal DNA is orientated towards the insert and the other, specific for the insert, is orientated towards the adjacent DNA. The outcome of a single cross-over event with respect to the functionality of the target gene is dependent on the homologous fragment cloned into the vector. If the fragment carries an intact gene, two functional copies will be present on the chromosome (Fig. 4.17a). If the fragment contains one or other of the ends of the target gene, then one functional and one deleted copy will be present on the chromosome (Fig. 4.17b). However, if the fragment contains sequences that are internal to the target gene, no functional copies will be present on the chromosome after integration (Fig. 4.17c).

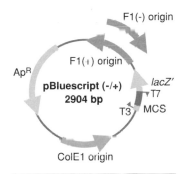

Figure 4.16 The phagemid pBluescript, is a plasmid vector used for the generation of single-stranded DNA molecules. Cells containing the phagemid are infected with an f1 'helper' phage that stimulates the f1 replication origin to generate ssDNA that is assembled into phage particles and released from the bacterium. Two versions of pBluescript, the (+) or (−) derivatives, allow for replication of either the positive or negative strand as required. T3 and T7 promoters either side of the multiple-cloning site allow the single-stranded DNA to be used as a substrate from in vitro RNA synthesis using the cognate RNA polymerase and NTP substrates. An ampicillin-resistance gene (Ap^R) is used to select for and to maintain the phagemid in *E. coli*.

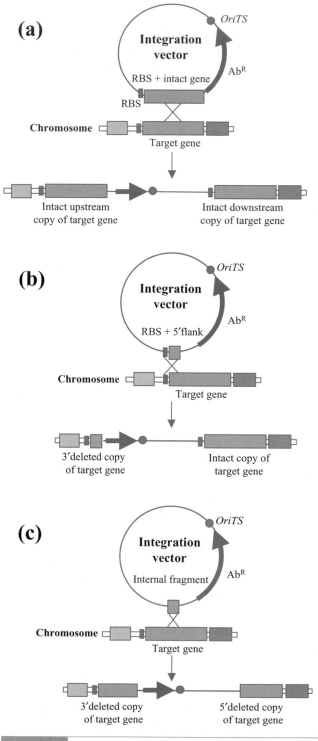

(a)

(b)

(c)

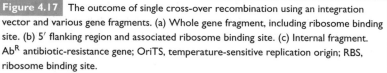

Figure 4.17 The outcome of single cross-over recombination using an integration vector and various gene fragments. (a) Whole gene fragment, including ribosome binding site. (b) 5′ flanking region and associated ribosome binding site. (c) Internal fragment. Ab^R antibiotic-resistance gene; OriTS, temperature-sensitive replication origin; RBS, ribosome binding site.

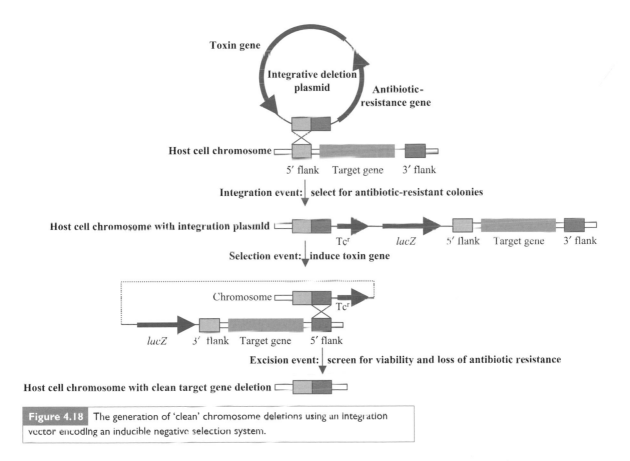

Figure 4.18 The generation of 'clean' chromosome deletions using an integration vector encoding an inducible negative selection system.

A specialised use of single cross-over recombination is the generation of 'clean' deletions (Fig. 4.18), in which target sequences are removed from the chromosome without their replacement with a marker gene. Sequences flanking the target gene are cloned into the integration vector. After transformation, integrants resulting from a single cross-over recombination event are selected. Although Fig. 4.18 shows a cross-over between the 5' flanking ends, it can occur with equal frequency between the 3' flanking ends. The final step is to screen for an excision event between the flanking ends not involved in the original cross-over recombination – in the example shown in Fig. 4.18, between the 3' flanking ends. The required deletion event can be selected if the vector encodes an inducible toxic gene product that kills cells still containing the inserted vector sequences.

In contrast to single cross-over recombination, double cross-over recombination (also known as *allele replacement*) results in only one copy of the target DNA fragment. Typically, a region of chromosomal DNA is replaced by sequences containing either mutationally altered homologous DNA or heterologous DNA. Sequences either side of the chromosome target are incorporated into the integration vector and all or part of the target gene sequence is replaced with a selectable marker gene and, if required, additional gene sequences. A double

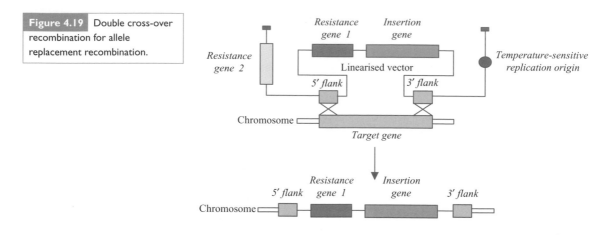

Figure 4.19 Double cross-over recombination for allele replacement recombination.

cross-over recombination between the vector and target sequence on the chromosome leads to the integration only of the sequences between the flanking regions (Fig. 4.19). Linearising the vector before transformation forces the selection of integrants that have resulted from a double rather than single cross-over recombination, since the latter would be lethal to the host. The absence of the original vector can be tested by confirming the absence of the antibiotic-resistance phenotype encoded by a resistance gene outside the integrating fragment.

4.5.5 Genomic and gene libraries

A *genomic library* is a collection of recombinant clones containing, at a theoretical level, representatives of all of the genes encoded by the genome of a particular organism. In practice, the best that can be achieved is a library with a high probability (usually >95%) that a particular gene will be represented. Libraries are produced by 'shotgun cloning' randomly generated DNA fragments into a suitable cloning vector. These fragments may be generated by mechanical shearing or by enzymatic digestion. Libraries may also be generated using copy DNA that has been synthesised from the mRNA of a particular tissue or organism using the enzyme reverse transcriptase.

4.6 | Analysis of genomes/proteomes

The genetic information of a bacterial cell is physically located on its chromosome(s). The physical organisation of bacterial chromosomes is much more variable than was previously supposed, and both linear and circular chromosomes have been recognised as a result of the application of physical mapping techniques such as *pulsed-field gel electrophoresis* (PFGE) and DNA sequencing.

4.6.1 DNA fingerprinting/physical mapping/pulsed-field gel electrophoresis

Prior to whole genome sequencing, various physical mapping methods were developed to determine the physical structure of bacterial genomes and determine relatedness between individual bacterial strains. The latter are particularly useful for strain identification and epidemiological studies.

Physical maps of the chromosome can be constructed by use of PFGE, a method developed specifically to resolve very large (30–2000 kbp) fragments of DNA. To avoid mechanical shearing, the DNA is extracted directly from bacterial cells in agarose blocks and, when required, digested *in situ* with restriction endonucleases that cleave the genome sequences infrequently (e.g. 10–30 times). The agarose block is then incorporated into a slab of agarose and subjected to an oscillating electric field. Separation is based on the time taken for the individual molecules of DNA to re-orientate in the modulating electric field; larger molecules taking longer than smaller molecules. The various fragments are aligned using a variety of strategies that include digesting the DNA with two rare-cutting enzymes, hybridisation between fragments isolated from separate digests and transformation of purified fragments into mutants with specific lesions.

Genome fingerprinting methods have been developed for examining the relationships between strains for epidemiological studies (e.g. monitoring outbreaks of disease) or heterogeneity in natural populations. The banding patterns generated by restriction endonucleases (e.g. *restriction fragment-length polymorphism* or RFLP) or PCR-based techniques using specific (e.g. *amplified fragment length polymorphism* or AFLP) or *random oligonucleotide primers* (e.g. *random amplified polymorphic DNA* or RAPD) can either be used diagnostically or for revealing relationships between strains.

4.6.2 Analysis of the proteome

The term *proteome* is used to define the proteins specified by the genome of an organism. Characterisation of the proteome provides a link between an organism's genetics and physiology. It helps to validate the genome sequence, aids the identification of *regulons* (genes or operons controlled by the same regulatory proteins) and *stimulons* (genes or operons controlled by the same inducing signal) and allows the response of the organism to its environment to be evaluated. *Escherichia coli*, with a genome size of 4.6 Mbp, encodes about 4400 proteins. A combination of experimental evidence and homology with proteins in other organisms has led to an identification of the functions of about 60% of these proteins. The biological roles of the remaining proteins (about 1800) are unknown but are under active investigation. A similar proportion of proteins of unknown function are observed even for a bacterium such as *Mycoplasma genitalium* which has a very much smaller genome (0.58 Mbp).

The expression of individual proteins for which antisera are available can be detected by Western blotting. Released cellular proteins are separated by sodium dodecyl sulphate-polyacrylamide gel electrophoresis (SDS-PAGE), and are then transferred and bound to a nitrocellulose or nylon membrane. Specific proteins are revealed by reacting (probing) with an antiserum which is then detected using a secondary antibody or probe.

The current system of choice for analysing the proteome involves a combination of two-dimensional polyacrylamide gel (2-DPAG) electrophoresis and their identification by mass spectrometry. Two-dimensional PAG electrophoresis facilitates the separation of hundreds of polypeptides extracted from whole cells. Polypeptides are initially separated in the first dimension on immobilised pH gradient gels on the basis of their pI. These gels are then separated in a second direction by SDS-PAGE in which the rate of migration is primarily based on their size. The migration of individual polypeptides in the two dimensions is extremely reproducible. Individual polypeptides can be detected by staining techniques or by radiography, using radio-labelled amino acids. Independent gels can be overlaid using warping software and compared directly to reveal, for example, the polypeptides that are induced in response to a particular growth phase, stress or change of substrate. Moreover, individual protein spots can be excised from the gel and, after digestion with trypsin, identified by high-resolution mass spectrometry [e.g. matrix-assisted laser desorption/ionisation – time of flight (MALDI-TOF) or electro-spray mass spectrometry].

4.7 | Analysis of gene expression

Promoters influence the frequency of initiation rather than the rate of transcription, and strong promoters have a high affinity for RNA polymerase binding. A comparison of a number of *E. coli* promoters has led to the recognition of a consensus promoter sequence: 5′--TATAAT–3′, centred around 10 nucleotides upstream of (prior to) the transcription initiation site (−10 region) and 5′–TTGACA–3′, located about 35 nucleotides upstream (−35 region). The strongest promoters are those that show the closest identities to this sequence. Additionally, the spacing between the −10 and −35 regions is important, the optimal being 17 nucleotides. The ability to analyse gene expression is an important pre-requisite for optimising the biotechnological potential of bacteria and many highly sensitive and precise techniques have been developed for this purpose.

4.7.1 Analysis of messenger RNA (mRNA) transcripts

Three methods are used for the analysis of mRNA transcripts: Northern blotting (see p. 90), S1-nuclease mapping and primer extension analysis. The last two techniques have the potential to identify the transcription initiation sites.

Northern blotting involves the separation of mRNA species by electrophoresis through agarose or polyacrylamide. Formamide, urea or other denaturants are included to avoid the single-stranded molecules forming secondary structures (e.g. duplexes, loops) that would affect their mobility. The separated mRNA species are transferred to

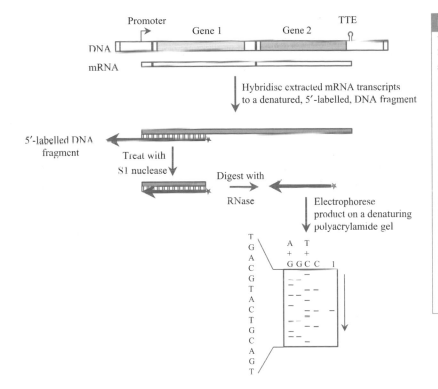

Figure 4.20 Mapping of transcription initiation points using S1 nuclease. RNA is hybridized to a denatured DNA fragment that has been labelled at its 5′ end. The DNA fragment is chosen so that its 5′ end is internal to the target mRNA, while the 3′ end extends beyond the putative mRNA start point. The RNA/DNA hybrid molecule has single-stranded extensions that are degraded by the single-strand-specific activity of S1 nuclease. The 3′ end of the DNA fragment is determined by running it on a denaturing gel against a DNA sequencing of the original fragment generated by the Maxam and Gilbert chemical cleavage method.

activated nylon membranes by blotting and then covalently cross-linked. Specific mRNA species are detected by hybridisation (Section 4.4.7), using labelled oligonucleotide, DNA or RNA probes. The use of markers with different molecular sizes allows the sizes of specific transcripts to be estimated which provides clues as to the organisation of the transcriptional unit from which the transcript was synthesised.

S1-Nuclease and primer extension analyses facilitate the identification of the 5′-prime ends of mRNA transcripts or the processed products of primary transcripts. In the case of S1-mapping (Fig. 4.20), mRNA is hybridised to a specific species of ssDNA that overlaps the start of the target transcript. The resulting RNA/DNA hybrid molecule has an overlap of DNA at the 3′ end that is digested by the single-strand-specific S1 nuclease. The size of the processed ssDNA molecule, which is labelled at its unmodified 5′ end, is determined by denaturing polyacrylamide gel electrophoresis using a DNA sequence ladder as a molecular-size marker.

In the case of primer extension analysis (Fig. 4.21), a 5′ end labelled oligonucleotide, hybridising about 60–100 nucleotides downstream of the predicted transcription initiation site, is used to prime the synthesis of a DNA copy of the mRNA transcript, using the enzyme reverse transcriptase. Synthesis of the complementary DNA strand terminates at the 5′ end of the transcript, to generate a product of defined length. Again this can be sized using a DNA sequence ladder, generated using the same primer oligonucleotide, as a molecular-size marker.

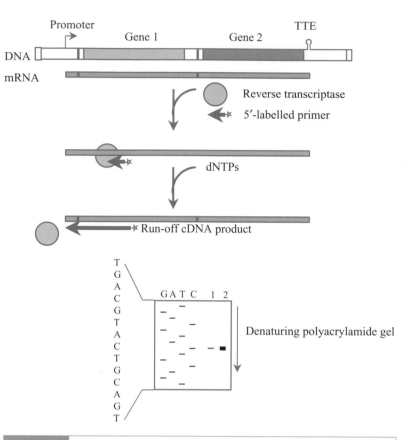

Figure 4.21 Primer extension analysis of a specific mRNA transcript. An oligonucleotide primer, radiolabelled at its 5′ end, is annealed to extracted mRNA about 60–100 nucleotides downstream of the putative transcript start point. Reverse transcriptase (an RNA-dependent DNA polymerase) and deoxyribonucleotide triphosphate (dNTP) substrates are added, and copy (c) DNA synthesis intitiated. cDNA synthesis terminates at the 5′ end of the mRNA transcript and the size of the run-off cDNA product is determined on a sequencing gel (lanes 1 and 2 on the gel) using a DNA sequence ladder generated with the same primer as a molecular-size marker. This allows the precise nucleotide at which the transcript was initiated to be identified. Primer extension analysis is semi-quantitative, and the strength of the signal from each primer extension reaction reflects the amount of the specific mRNA. The reactions can also be used to compare the strength of adjacent promoters.

4.7.2 Gene fusion technology

One of the most powerful and widely used techniques for analysing gene expression is *reporter gene technology*. Reporter genes are generally used when the gene or operon under investigation does not encode an easily assayed product. Fusion to a reporter gene therefore allows the factors controlling gene expression to be identified. In recent years, gene fusion technology has been developed to facilitate the study of target gene expression at the single-cell level, allowing visualisation of population heterogeneity and the location of specific proteins within the cell.

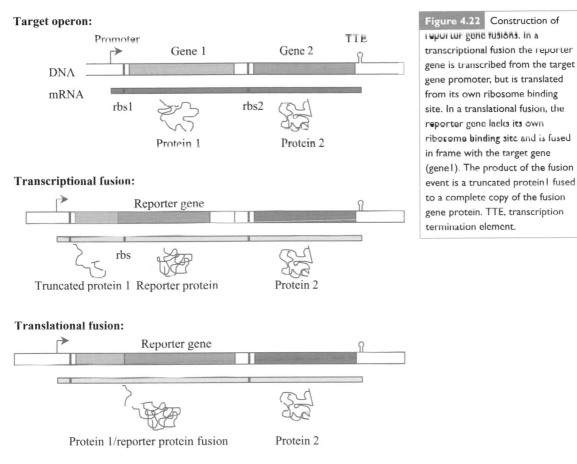

Target operon:

Transcriptional fusion:

Translational fusion:

Figure 4.22 Construction of reporter gene fusions. In a transcriptional fusion the reporter gene is transcribed from the target gene promoter, but is translated from its own ribosome binding site. In a translational fusion, the reporter gene lacks its own ribosome binding site and is fused in frame with the target gene (gene1). The product of the fusion event is a truncated protein1 fused to a complete copy of the fusion gene protein. TTE, transcription termination element.

The use of reporter gene technology involves three main variables: (i) the type of fusion constructed (i.e. transcriptional or translational); (ii) the type of reporter gene used; and (iii) the method of detection (e.g. enzyme, immuno- or cytochemical assay).

Types of gene fusion

Reporter genes can be fused as either transcriptional or translational fusions (Fig. 4.22). In the case of a *transcriptional fusion*, the reporter gene is cloned downstream of the promoter controlling the transcription of the target gene or operon and must include a ribosome binding site for translation initiation that is functional in the host bacterium. Transcriptional reporters can only be used for monitoring the activities of the target promoter and associated control sequences; post-transcriptional control cannot be detected with such a fusion.

In the case of a *translational fusion* (Fig. 4.22), the reporter gene is fused in the same codon reading frame as the target gene so that when the target gene is transcribed and translated, the product is a hybrid protein consisting, for example, of a portion of the target protein at the N terminus and the entire reporter at the C terminus. The length of the target protein depends on the type of analysis. If the purpose is simply to understand mechanisms controlling synthesis, the portion of target may be as few as 10 amino acid residues. However, if the purpose is to identify the cellular location of the target protein, virtually all of the target protein may be required to be fused to the reporter protein.

Reporter genes

A variety of reporter genes have been developed for particular applications and most can be adapted for use in a wide range of bacterial species. These include chromogenic reporters (e.g. *E. coli lacZ*, encoding β-galactosidase) that are detected on the basis of colour change, enzyme assay or immuno-detection techniques; antibiotic-resistance gene reporters (e.g. *cat*, encoding chloramphenicol acetyl transferase that confers resistance to chloramphenicol) that are detected using selective techniques or enzyme assay; or fluorescent and luminescent reporters (e.g. *luxAB*, encoding luciferase which catalyses a light-emitting reaction or *gfp*, encoding a green fluorescent protein) that are detected by spectrometry, luminometry or video/photo-microscopy.

Genome-wide expression profiling

The genes transcribed by a bacterium at any particular time are referred to as the *transcriptome*. DNA arrays (Section 4.4.8) are now widely used to monitor the expression of all of the genes in the genome in a single experiment. They can be used to compare changes in the expression profile in response to stresses (e.g. oxidative stress, nutrient deprivation), macrophage engulfment or specific mutations. They can also be used to monitor gene expression during fermentation.

4.8 | Engineering genes and optimising products

Many commercially important biotechnological processes have been developed using micro-organisms found in the environment. These include traditional processes such as the production of milk products (e.g. yoghurt production by *Lactococcus casei*), the synthesis of organic solvents (e.g. acetone production by *Clostridium acetobutylicum*), and the production of enzymes for domestic and industrial catalysis (e.g. α-amylases, proteases and penicillin acylases from *Bacillus* species). These processes are usually distinct from those found in nature and may place particular requirements on the catalyst, be it a whole organism or an industrial enzyme, that are not encountered in natural environments. The organism or enzyme may therefore have to be engineered as part of the process optimisation.

4.8.1 Protein and pathway engineering

A well-studied example of enzyme optimisation is that of subtilisin, an alkaline protease isolated from *Bacillus subtilis* and close relatives (e.g. *B. licheniformis*, *B. stearothermophilus*) and used as a stain remover in the detergent industry. Subtilisin is used in 95% of washing detergent formulations and allows protein stains to be removed more effectively and at lower temperatures than are usually needed for laundry processing. The ideal requirements for such an enzyme are stability up to 70 °C and within the pH range 8–11, resistance to non-ionic detergents and oxidising reagents such as hydrogen peroxide, and the absence of metal ion requirements. Based on an extensive knowledge of its catalytic activity and three-dimensional structure, subtilisin was engineered by site-directed mutagenesis (Section 4.4.10) to produce variant enzymes with combinations of these improved characteristics.

An alternative approach has been used to improve the enzymatic characteristics of *Bacillus* α-amylases. In this case natural recombination was used to generate functional hybrid amylases from genes encoding closely related enzymes from *B. amyloliquefaciens*, *B. licheniformis* and *B. stearothermophilus*. The genes for these enzymes were cloned in pair-wise combinations and then allowed to undergo rounds of reciprocal recombination. This generated a population of cells with a large number of hybrid α-amylases, which were then screened for cells producing amylases with improved catalytic or structural characteristics. More recently, knowledge of the three-dimensional structure of these amylases, together with information on the relationship between structure and functional characteristics such as thermostability, has enabled more directed approaches to be used. These have included the use of PCR gene splicing techniques for the construction of specific hybrid α-amylases.

Comparative DNA and protein sequence studies have demonstrated the importance of recombination of blocks of sequence rather than point mutation alone in the evolution of protein structure. These studies have led to the development of molecular techniques, such as *DNA shuffling* or *sexual PCR*, to facilitate the rapid evolution of proteins. The principle involves mixing randomly fragmented DNA encoding closely related genes and then using PCR (Section 4.4.4) to re-assemble them into full length fragments, with the individual fragments acting as primers. The PCR products are used to generate a library (Section 4.4.5) of chimaeric genes for the selection of proteins with modified or improved characteristics. This system has been used to generate a variant of an *E. coli* β-galactosidase with a 60-fold increase in specific activity for sugar that is normally a poor substrate for this enzyme and a variant of the green fluorescent protein (Section 4.7.2) with a 45-fold increase in fluorescent signal.

Bacteria produce a number of compounds that, if synthesised at suitable concentrations, represent commercially viable products. Traditionally, bacteria that make a significant amount of a potentially commercial product can be directed to synthesise larger amounts. This may be achieved by randomly mutagenising a population of the target organism, and screening for mutants producing higher concentrations of the product, or by cloning the synthetic genes together and placing them under the control of efficient transcription and translation signals. While there are examples that testify to the success of such approaches (e.g. antibiotic production, synthesis of amino acids), recently more rational approaches have been made by engineering metabolic pathways, either to increase productivity or to direct synthesis towards specific products.

4.9 Production of heterologous products

Traditionally, genetic techniques have been applied by industry to increase the production of natural products such as enzymes, antibiotics and vitamins (see Chapters 14, 15, 18, 20 and 21 for examples). Only a limited number of protein products were produced commercially, and these were produced using existing technologies from their natural hosts (e.g. proteases from *Bacillus* species). Specific genes can now be isolated from virtually any biological material and cloned into a bacterium or other host system. However, cloning a gene does not, per se, ensure its expression, nor does expression ensure the biological activity of its product. Many factors need to be considered to ensure commercially viable levels of production and biological activity. For example, the choice of host/vector systems determines both the strategy used for the cloning and expression, and these in turn can affect the quantity and fidelity of the product. In some cases, it is not possible to use a bacterial system to produce a biologically active product or one that is acceptable for pharmaceutical purposes. Instead host/vector systems based on higher organisms, for example mammalian or insect cell culture systems, may be used.

4.9.1 Host systems and their relative advantages

Prior to the 1970s, the only methods for obtaining proteins or polypeptides for analysis or for therapeutic purposes were to isolate them from natural sources or, in a limited number of cases (e.g. bioactive peptides), to synthesise them chemically. Recombinant DNA technology opened up the possibility to clone the gene responsible for a particular product and to produce it in unlimited amounts in a bacterium such as *E. coli*. Initially, the only eukaryotic genes that could be cloned were those encoding products that were already available in relatively large amounts and that had very sensitive assays (e.g. insulin, human growth hormone, interferon). This was because it was necessary to have extensive information about their amino acid sequence, and protein sequencing techniques available at that time required relatively large amounts of the purified protein. Current technical improvements permit almost any characterised protein to be cloned, either directly via copy DNA synthesis from mRNA extracted from biological material, or indirectly by gene synthesis.

Although recombinant technology was developed in bacterial systems, it has been increasingly expanded into a range of eukaryotic organisms, using a wide variety of interesting and novel technologies (see Chapter 5). However, from an economic point of view, bacteria are still the organisms of choice because of the ease with which they can be genetically manipulated, their rapid growth rate and relatively simple nutritional requirements.

Proteins derived from recombinant technology are expected to meet the same exacting standards as conventionally produced drugs; particularly with respect to product potency, purity and identity. Sensitive analytical techniques are used to characterise the products, with particular attention being paid to undesirable biological activities, such as adverse immunogenic and allergenic reactions. These exacting requirements, laid down by various regulatory authorities [such as the US Food and Drug Administration (FDA)] to increase the authenticity (and supposed safety) of pharmacological products, have led producers to switch from bacterial to eukaryotic systems for the production of certain products. These requirements have been driven by the increasing sensitivity of analytical techniques such as high-performance liquid chromatography (HPLC), mass spectrometry, nuclear magnetic resonance (NMR) and circular dichroism that are able to reveal subtle differences in the structures of natural and recombinant proteins.

Often, a great deal of effort can be put into devising a cloning strategy only to discover that the level of production of a particular protein is much lower than is anticipated. In many cases, the reasons for these failures are not easily determined. Some of the causes of low recombinant protein productivity are given below.

4.9.2 Transcription

The cloning of a DNA fragment encoding a protein of interest is not in itself sufficient to ensure its expression. Instead, the cloning strategy has to include sequences designed to express the DNA at an appropriate time and level in the host bacterium. Transcription is facilitated by cloning the target gene downstream of a promoter sequence and associated translation signals. Promoter strength is a key factor affecting the level of expression of a cloned gene and a wide range of promoters is currently available, including those that are tightly regulated and others whose expression is constitutive. In *E. coli*, expression from a strong promoter can lead to the production of a recombinant protein at levels that are equivalent to about 50% of the total cell protein.

A number of naturally occurring promoters have been used to direct high-level expression of recombinant genes. However, with an increased knowledge of the factors required to generate strong promoters, hybrid and even totally synthetic promoters have been constructed. Promoters that are induced by expensive and potentially toxic chemicals are not suitable for large-scale fermentations and, consequently, promoters have been designed in which induction is mediated simply by increasing the temperature of the culture medium. Other promoters have been developed that are induced at low oxygen tension or with cheap, readily available sugars.

Expression from strong promoters imposes a high metabolic load on the host cell and consequently their transcriptional activity must be tightly controlled. One aspect of this control is the incorporation of *efficient transcription termination elements* (TTE). The failure to include such TTEs can lead to diminished levels of expression of the target gene, since energy is unnecessarily diverted into the synthesis of non-productive mRNA species. This is especially important when the target gene is expressed from a multi-copy plasmid vector since highly active transcriptional activity over regions necessary for plasmid replication and/or segregation can lead to greatly increased vector instability.

4.9.3 Translation

The efficient translation of mRNA transcripts requires the incorporation of an efficient *ribosome binding site* (RBS), located about 5 bp upstream of (prior to) the translational start codon. The structure of the RBS tends to vary from bacterium to bacterium according to the sequences at the 3′OH end of the 16S ribosomal (r)RNA that interact with the mRNA.

The genetic code is degenerate and many amino acids are specified by more than one codon (triplet of nucleotide bases). Codons that specify the same amino acid are said to be synonymous but are not necessarily used with similar frequencies. In fact, most bacterial species exhibit preferences in their use of codons, particularly for highly expressed genes. Variations in codon usage are, in part, a reflection of the %GC content of the organism's DNA, with favoured codons corresponding to the organism's most abundant transfer (t)RNA species. Since most codons are recognised by specific aminoacyl tRNA molecules, the use of non-favoured codons results in a reduction in the rate of translation and an increase in the misincorporation of amino acids above that of the normal error rate of about 1 in 3000 amino acids. Codon bias can be determined by calculating the *relative synonymous codon usage* (RSCU) of individual codons:

$$RSCU = \frac{\text{observed number of times a particular codon is used}}{\text{expected number if all codons are used with equal frequency}}$$

therefore:

if RSCU equals 1, the codon is used without bias
if RSCU is less than 1, the codon is 'non-favoured'
if RSCU is more than 1 the codon is 'favoured'.

Gene synthesis technology allows genes to be constructed so as to optimise the codon usage of the host producer strain. The significance of codon usage was demonstrated in studies on the production of interleukin-2 (IL-2) by *E. coli*. When the native IL-2 gene (399 bp) was analysed for its codon usage only 43% of the codons were 'favoured' by *E. coli*. When an alternative copy of the IL-2 gene was generated by gene synthesis, it was possible to adjust the codon usage such that 85% of the codons corresponded to those favoured by *E. coli*. When the two versions were cloned and expressed in *E. coli* on identical vectors, despite their producing identical amounts of mRNA, eight times more biologically active IL-2 was produced from the synthetic gene as compared with the native gene

4.9.4 Formation of inclusion bodies

Many recombinant proteins, particularly when produced at high concentrations, are unable to fold properly within the producing cell and instead associate with each other to form large protein aggregates referred to as inclusion bodies. Inclusion bodies are particularly common in bacteria expressing mammalian proteins. The proteins in inclusion bodies can vary from a native-like state that is easily dissociated, to completely mis-folded molecules that are dissociated only under highly denaturing conditions. The size, state and aggregation density of inclusions are affected by the characteristics of the recombinant protein itself and factors that affect cell physiology (e.g. growth rate, temperature, culture medium, etc.). In some cases aggregation can be prevented or reduced by modulating the fermentation conditions.

Inclusion body formation can lead to: (i) the production of biologically inactive proteins, (ii) sub optimal yields, (iii) extraction and purification problems. However, in some cases, inclusion body formation can be advantageous since a body is composed of relatively pure protein that is insoluble under mild extraction conditions. It is therefore possible to devise protocols that recover the target protein in this insoluble state and re-fold it under conditions that favour the biologically active conformation. In some cases problems associated with inclusion body formation can be overcome by use of a secretion vector system (Section 4.5.4) in which the target protein is directed into the periplasm or culture medium.

4.10 | In silico analysis of bacterial genomes

The availability of entire genome sequences for a significant number of micro-organisms opens up new approaches for the analysis of bacteria, and the rapidly expanding field of bioinformatics has the potential to reveal relevant and novel insights on bacterial evolution and gene function. It has the potential to provide answers to long standing questions relating to evolutionary mechanisms and to the relationships between gene order and function.

One of the most significant advances in methods for studying and analysing micro-organisms has come about through the availability of powerful personal computers that, together with the development of the internet, grid and parallel processing technologies, provide researchers with access to immensely powerful bioinformatical tools. The combination of bioinformatics and in vivo and in vitro methodologies has led to the emergence of systems biology, which attempts to integrate data from a variety of high-throughput technologies.

The ultimate goal is to model the behaviour of whole organisms, including aspects of their evolution. Although not currently a substitute for in vivo and in vitro experimentation, such models are beginning to show their potential to direct the focus of more traditional approaches.

Several types of computer program are available for analysing bacterial genome sequences. These include programs that attempt to identify protein-encoding genes, sequence signals such as ribosome binding sites, promoters and protein binding sites, and relationships to previously sequenced DNA of whatever source. Programs that attempt to identify protein-encoding genes translate the DNA sequence in all six reading frames (i.e. the three possible reading frames on each of the two strands of the DNA duplex) and then analyse the resulting data for the presence of long stretches of amino-acid-encoding codons, uninterrupted by termination codons. These so-called *open reading frames* (ORF) can range from tens to several thousand amino acids in length. The more advanced programs for predicting protein coding genes are able to search for the presence of ribosome binding sites located immediately upstream of a putative start codon and even to identify potential DNA sequencing errors that generate frame-shift mutations.

Once putative proteins have been identified, other bioinformatical tools can be used to determine their relationships to previously identified proteins or putative proteins. A pre-requisite for this type of analysis is the availability of data libraries, which act as repositories of currently available DNA and protein sequences. The databases can be routinely accessed via the internet, using programs such as FASTA and BLAST that provide a list of DNA sequences and proteins, respectively, showing homology to all or part of the query sequence. The internet is also a source of molecular biological tools that facilitate a wide range of analyses including the identification of putative transmembrane domains, secondary structures and the signal peptides of secretory proteins. Finally graphical approaches have been used to model regulatory networks, protein : protein interaction networks and metabolic pathways.

4.11 | Further reading

Davies, J. E. and Demain, A. L. *Manual of Industrial Microbiology and Biotechnology*, second edition. Washington, DC: American Society for Microbiology, 1999.

Glazer, A. N. and Nikaido, H. *Microbial Biotechnology: Fundamentals of Applied Microbiology*. New York: W. H. Freeman & Company, 1995.

Lewin, B. *Genes VIII*. Oxford: Oxford University Press, 2004.

Primrose, S. B., Twyman, R. M. and Old, R. W. *Principles of Gene Manipulation: An Introduction to Genetic Engineering*, sixth edition. Oxford: Blackwell, 2001.

Snyder, L. and Champness, W. *Molecular Genetics of Bacteria*. Washington, DC: American Society for Microbiology, 1997.

Streips, U. N. and Yasbin, R. E. *Modern Microbial Genetics*, second edition, New York: Wiley-Liss, 2002.

Wren, B. and Dorrell, N. *Functional Microbial Genomics*. London: Academic Press, 2002.

Zhou, J., Thompson, D. K., Xu, Y. and Tiedje, J. M. *Microbial Functional Genomics*. New York: Wiley-Liss, 2004.

Chapter 5

Genetic engineering: yeasts and filamentous fungi

David B. Archer
University of Nottingham, UK

Donald A. MacKenzie
Institute of Food Research, UK

David J. Jeenes
Institute of Food Research, UK

Glossary

Auxotrophic mutation A mutation in a gene that confers the requirement for a growth factor to be supplied rather than synthesised by the organism. A gene that **complements** this auxotrophic mutation is one that can return the organism to its normal **phenotype** (i.e. not requiring the growth factor).

cDNA Single-stranded DNA with a *complementary* sequence to messenger RNA (mRNA), synthesised in vitro. Double-stranded cDNA can then be made. cDNA libraries contain double-stranded cDNA molecules, each of which forms part of a **vector** (q.v.). The collection of cDNA molecules, each in a separate vector, forms the cDNA **library**.

Chaperone A protein that assists the folding of another protein.

Chromatin A highly organised complex of protein and DNA.

Chromosome A discrete unit of DNA (containing many genes) and protein. Different species have different numbers of chromosomes (see Table 5.1).

Basic Biotechnology, third edition, eds. Colin Ratledge and Bjørn Kristiansen.
Published by Cambridge University Press. © Cambridge University Press 2006.

Circular DNA molecule See **plasmid**.

Complementation The ability of a gene to convert a mutant **phenotype** (q.v.) to the **wild-type**.

Cosmid Plasmid (q.v.) containing sequences (phage lambda cos sites) that permit packaging of the **plasmid** into the proteinaceous phage coat.

Cross-over See **homologous recombination**.

Dimorphism Ability to exist as two structurally distinct forms.

Endoplasmic reticulum (ER) Intracellular membrane structure in eukaryotes forming the early part of the protein secretory pathway.

Exons The coding regions of a gene (excluding the **introns**).

Expressed sequence tag (EST) A portion of a cDNA, usually of sufficient length to provide useful sequence information to enable identification or cloning of a full-length gene.

Expression cloning A term used to describe the process of protein synthesis from a gene.

Expression cassette An arrangement of DNA which permits the **transcription** of a gene for protein production, i.e. includes a **promoter**, the **open reading frame** and a **transcriptional terminator**.

Gene A region of DNA which is transcribed into RNA.

Genome The entire DNA in an organism.

Genotype/genotypic The information contained in the DNA of an organism.

Heterologous Pertaining to a gene or protein which is foreign in relation to the system being studied.

Homologous recombination The breakage and re-joining of two double strands of DNA that have closely related sequences. The process of homologous recombination, also called crossing-over, permits the integration of genes into specific genomic loci (see Fig. 5.4) but the term is used more widely, for example in exchange of genetic material between chromosomes during meiosis. In **transformations** using circular **plasmids**, a single **cross-over** leads to incorporation of the entire plasmid into a **chromosome**. A double cross-over employs a linearised DNA molecule and leads to the replacement of a chromosomal gene by a gene with sequence similarity to the chromosomal gene at the cross-over regions.

Intron A segment of RNA which is excised before the mRNA is translated into protein. Introns are common in eukaryotic genes but very rare in prokaryotes.

Library A collection of cloned genomic DNA fragments or cDNA molecules.

Linkage The tendency of genes that are physically close to be inherited together.

Linkage group A group of genes that is inherited or transferred as a single unit and represents an entire **chromosome**.

Metabolome The complement of metabolites produced by an organism at any one time.

Microarray Miniaturised solid support (typically a glass slide) containing a grid of single-stranded DNA fragments that can represent all, or a sub-population of, the genes from an organism.

Mycelium Typical vegetative growth form of filamentous fungi, consisting of branched filaments.

Nucleotide Building block for DNA and RNA, a base-(deoxy)ribose-phosphate molecule. The nucleotides are referred to by base. Purines: A (adenine), G (guanine). Pyrimidines: C (cytosine), T (thymine), U (uracil). DNA has AGCT, RNA has AGCU.

Open reading frame (ORF) Stretch of **codons** uninterrupted by stop codons and therefore presumed to be coding for a functional protein.

Origin (*ori*) The site of initiation of DNA replication

Phenotype Properties (e.g. biochemical or physiological) of an organism which are determined by the **genotype**.

Plasmid DNA molecule that replicates independently of the **chromosomes**.

Ploidy The number of complete sets of **chromosomes** in a cell, e.g. haploid (1), diploid (2), polyploid (>2).

Polymerase chain reaction (PCR) A procedure for exponential amplification of DNA fragments (see Fig. 4.8).

Promoter The region of DNA upstream (i.e. 5′) of a gene which contains signals for initiating and regulating **transcription** of the **gene**.

Proteome The complement of proteins produced by an organism at any one time.

Protoplasts Cells from which the cell wall has been removed by the action of carbohydrase enzymes. These cells are bounded by the plasma membrane and are osmotically fragile.

Recombination The exchange of DNA between two DNA molecules or the incorporation of one DNA molecule into another, e.g. between the **chromosome** and introduced DNA.

Restriction enzyme Enzyme that cleaves at or near a specific, short DNA sequence (restriction site).

Shuttle vector A vector that can replicate independently in more than one type of organism, e.g. can 'shuttle' between a bacterium and a yeast.

Southern blotting Process by which DNA fragments are separated according to size by electrophoresis, transferred to a membrane and probed with a labelled DNA segment to detect complementary sequences (named after Ed Southern).

Splicing The excision of introns from RNA molecules which is followed by re-joining of the **exons**. This normally occurs in the nucleus.

Synteny Gene order in a **chromosome** being physically the same in different organisms.

Transcription The synthesis of RNA coded by the DNA sequence.

Transcription factor A protein that binds to DNA in the **promoter** region, or binds to other protein factors, and regulates the **transcription** of one or more genes.

Transcription terminator A DNA sequence that causes the RNA polymerase to stop synthesis of RNA.

Transcriptional start point (tsp) The site at which RNA synthesis is initiated.

Transcriptome The complement of mRNA molecules produced by an organism at any one time.

Transformation (genetic) The uptake and stable incorporation of exogenous DNA into a cell.

Vector A DNA molecule (usually a plasmid) used for transferring DNA into an organism.

Wild-type Strain of an organism not deliberately mutated or modified by genetic manipulation. The term can also be used to describe the **phenotype** of such a strain.

Figure 5.1 Phase contrast micrograph of (a) the yeast *Saccharomyces cerevisiae*, (b) the yeast (above right) and hyphal (below right) forms of *Yarrowia lipolytica*, (c) bright field micrograph of the filamentous fungus *Aspergillus niger* grown on a cellophane sheet, (d) differential interference contrast micrograph of protoplast formation from *Aspergillus nidulans*. Note the branching of hyphae. Barmarkers = 10 μm. Cs, conidiospores (asexual); H, hypha; P, protoplast. Micrographs (a)–(c) are courtesy of Linda and James Barnett.

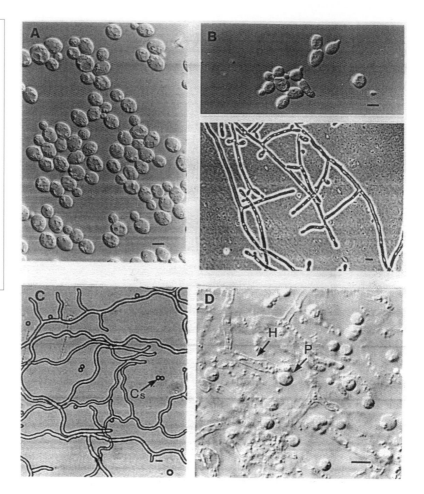

5.1 | Introduction

Fungi are eukaryotes classified as either yeasts or filamentous fungi primarily by their predominant form of growth in culture. Those species that are normally unicellular are the yeasts and thus superficially distinguished from their filamentous relatives. This distinction is not always adhered to by the organisms themselves as several are able to grow in both forms and are called **dimorphic** (Fig. 5.1). More discriminatory **genotypic** methods are now enabling a more soundly based classification of the fungi, but the substantial similarities between yeasts and filamentous fungi enable us to treat them together in one chapter. Despite the similarities, their differences have given rise to a wide diversity of biotechnological applications, which is increasing as the number of different species examined rises and as their exploitation is extended by genetic engineering.

In this chapter, we focus on the molecular biology involved in genetic engineering of fungi and describe applications of the fungi as hosts for the production of proteins encoded by introduced

Table 5.1 | Some fungal genome sequences

	Number of chromosomes	Genome size (Mb)[a]	Website[b]
Ashbya gossypii	7	9.2	http://agd.unibas.ch/
Saccharomyces cerevisiae	16	12	http://genome-www.stanford.edu/saccharomyces/
Schizosaccharomyces pombe	3	14	http://www.sanger.ac.uk/Projects/S_pombe/
Candida albicans	8	16	http://sequence-www.stanford.edu/group/candida/
Neurospora crassa	7	40	http://www.broad.mit.edu/annotation/fungi/neurospora/
Aspergillus nidulans	8	30	http://www.broad.mit.edu/annotation/fungi/aspergillus/

[a] Approximate haploid genome size excluding the mitochondrial genome.

[b] Suggested websites for genome information. Note that websites can change and there is a larger and increasing number of fungal genomes available. There are also some general fungal sites that provide links to other relevant sites: http://www.fgsc.net, http://www.eurofung.net/frameset.php, http://www.aspergillus.man.ac.uk/.

foreign **genes**. Many of the experimental approaches adopted in this work have been described in the preceding chapter (Chapter 4) with prokaryotes and are essentially the same with fungi. Their descriptions are not repeated here except where differences between bacteria and fungi require alterations to the protocols. Differences arise primarily because fungi are larger in both size and **genome** than bacteria and the organising principles for many of their cellular functions are typical of complex higher organisms rather than simple bacterial cells. Thus, fungi have defined membrane-bound nuclei containing several **chromosomes** and other membrane-bound organelles, including a membranous intracellular system called the **endoplasmic reticulum (ER)** into which proteins are transported for targeting either to the cell exterior or to other sub-cellular organelles. Fungal cell walls do not contain peptidoglycan, which is found only in bacteria. Rather, their walls are composed primarily of various polysaccharides (e.g. glucans, mannans, chitin, chitosan) and glycoproteins depending on the species. Fungi can have complex life cycles, exhibiting normal (vegetative) cell growth as a **mycelium** followed by morphogenesis (change in form) with the formation of either sexual (resulting from the mating of two strains) or asexual spores. For most biotechnological purposes, fungi are grown vegetatively with associated mitotic nuclear division. Meiosis will not concern us here. For the interested reader reference to information on the fungal cell cycle can be found in general texts cited at the end of the chapter.

Fungal genes are organised within chromosomes, which can be separated by electrophoresis. The number of chromosomes varies with species and equates to the number of **linkage groups** where the **linkage** of genetic markers has been studied. Some examples are given in Table 5.1 together with examples of fungal genome sizes. The amount of DNA in fungi is much larger than that in prokaryotes (cf. 4.7 Mb, 4.7 million nucleotide bases in length, for *Escherichia coli*). This is due to fungi having more genes and more DNA which does not code for proteins, either within genes (as **introns**) or as 'spacer' DNA between genes. Bacteria economise on non-coding DNA in comparison with fungi. For example, some bacterial genes can be physically adjacent to each other with **transcription** directed and regulated by a single **promoter**, to form an *operon* (see Fig. 4.1). Operons are not found in fungi and even where genes encoding functionally related enzymes are clustered (i.e. grouped together), the transcription of each gene is regulated by an independent promoter. Knowledge of the regulatory mechanisms of transcription is necessary to design rational approaches for genetic modification of an organism in order to achieve the desired **phenotype**. We therefore discuss in this chapter examples of wide-domain (multi-pathway) and pathway-specific transcriptional regulatory mechanisms.

Chromosomes from eukaryotes are composed of **chromatin**, which is an approximately equal weight of DNA and protein (mainly histones). Histones bind to DNA and help to package it into complex structures. For example, DNA associates with particular histones to form nucleosomes, which can be visualised by electron microscopy as 'beads on a string'. Nucleosome arrangements can control access of proteins (**transcription factors**) that are required to initiate transcription at a promoter, a level of regulation not seen in prokaryotes. Discussion of the regulation of transcription at the level of chromatin is beyond the scope of this chapter, but its mention is a reminder of the level of complexity in eukaryotes. Fortunately, many important fungi are amenable to investigation of their biology at the molecular level and we are able to modify these species genetically in order to alter either the types or amounts of product formed.

5.2 | Introducing DNA into fungi (fungal transformation)

5.2.1 Background

The first fungal **transformation** experiments in the early 1970s were performed by transferring chromosomal DNA fragments from **wild-type** strains into mutant hosts that had a specific growth requirement for an amino acid or **nucleotide** base (examples of **auxotrophic mutants**). Successful transformation relied on converting the fungal cells into **protoplasts** (Fig. 5.1d) by digesting away the cell wall (a major barrier to DNA uptake) with carbohydrase enzyme mixtures before introducing the transforming DNA. Transformants could then be selected by their ability to grow without supplementation for the auxotrophic requirement due to the activity of the wild-type gene, a process known as genetic **complementation**. The fate of the transforming DNA in the cell could not be studied in great detail until the advent of more sophisticated molecular techniques in the late 1970s and early 1980s when it was subsequently shown that the DNA in these early experiments had integrated by genetic **recombination** into the fungal chromosomes.

Subsequently, transformation methods were developed for the yeast *Saccharomyces cerevisiae*, using **shuttle vectors**, which could be propagated as intact **plasmids**, without chromosomal integration, in both *E. coli* and yeast. Manipulation of these plasmids and 'bulking up' the amount of vector DNA were more effectively performed in *E. coli* prior to their introduction into yeast. Similar vectors have been designed for the transformation of filamentous fungi, but in most cases the introduced DNA integrates into the fungal chromosomes rather than replicating as a plasmid. Transformation was accomplished first in genetically well characterised organisms such as *S. cerevisiae*, *Neurospora crassa* and *Aspergillus nidulans* because these fungi had been studied extensively in the laboratory and a number of suitable auxotrophic mutants and their corresponding wild-type genes were available. Methods are now continually being modified or adapted for more biotechnologically important fungi in which genetic systems may be less well defined. In cases where auxotrophic complementation of industrial strains is not feasible, other selection markers, such as resistance to an antibiotic, can be used in the transformation.

5.2.2 Transformation protocols

For the transformation of many filamentous fungi, the method of choice still relies on converting the fungal mycelium into protoplasts, which are prepared in a buffer containing an osmotic stabiliser to prevent cells from bursting (Fig. 5.2). Vector DNA is then added to the protoplast suspension in the presence of Ca^{2+} and DNA uptake is induced by the addition of polyethylene glycol (PEG). Not all protoplasts can regenerate into viable fungal cells by producing new cell walls and only a proportion of these will contain the transforming DNA. Thus, there is a need to have effective selection methods to obtain those cells containing the introduced DNA. Transformation frequencies, in terms of the number of transformants obtained per microgramme of vector DNA added, can vary significantly depending on the organism and transformation protocol used. Since the first reports of fungal transformation, various modifications to this basic method have been described that improve transformation frequencies by orders of magnitude. Alternative methods that obviate the need for protoplast formation, such as the lithium acetate/yeast whole cell method, electroporation of germinating spores or biolistic transformation of fungal mycelia, have had varied success but these suffer from the limitations of suitable host range and the need for specialised equipment in some cases. A list of transformation methods is given in Table 5.2.

Figure 5.2 Typical transformation protocol using protoplasts derived from a filamentous fungus. Following harvesting, the filtered mycelium is resuspended in a buffer containing an osmotic stabiliser such as sorbitol or KCl to prevent protoplasts from bursting. The selective agar can either be a minimal medium (lacking the required growth supplement which is now supplied by the activity of the introduced gene) or it can contain an antibiotic. For antibiotic selection, the transformants are normally allowed to regenerate their cell walls and express the antibiotic-resistance protein before being challenged with the antibiotic. PEG, polyethylene glycol.

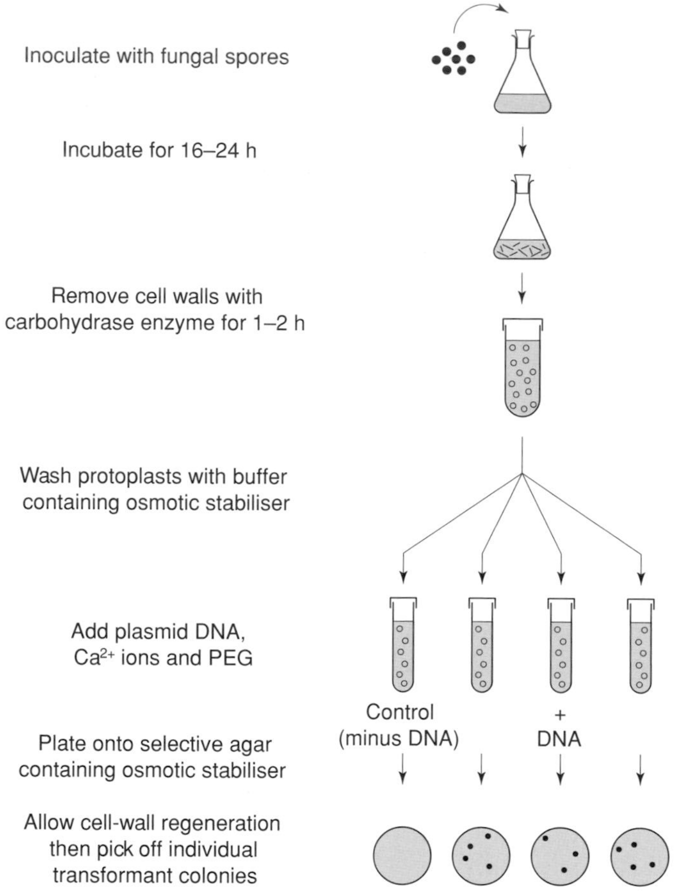

Inoculate with fungal spores

Incubate for 16–24 h

Remove cell walls with carbohydrase enzyme for 1–2 h

Wash protoplasts with buffer containing osmotic stabiliser

Add plasmid DNA, Ca^{2+} ions and PEG

Control (minus DNA)   + DNA

Plate onto selective agar containing osmotic stabiliser

Allow cell-wall regeneration then pick off individual transformant colonies

5.2.3 Transformation vectors

Transformation vectors can be designed to introduce DNA that either integrates into the recipient organism's genome (integrative transformation) or can be maintained as a plasmid. Integrative transformation is used to insert DNA either at site(s) in the chromosome that show significant sequence similarity to a region on the plasmid (integration by **homologous recombination**) or randomly at one or more locations (ectopic integration). Yeast **shuttle vectors** contain genes that allow for their selection in both bacterial and yeast cells. They also contain bacterial and yeast **origins of replication** (*ori*), sequences that are essential for the initiation of plasmid DNA replication in both organisms. A stylised yeast shuttle vector that is capable of replication without integration into the yeast chromosomes (extrachromosomal vector) or that can be specifically targeted into a region of a chromosome (integrative vector) is illustrated in Fig. 5.3.

In order to find those cells that are 'transformed', i.e. contain the introduced DNA, the transformation vector is designed to contain a gene that confers a selectable characteristic on the transformed cells. These 'selection markers' fall into three main groups. First, a number of genes from wild-type fungi have been cloned which complement

Table 5.2 Fungal transformation methods

Method or treatment		Examples of fungi transformed	Transformation frequency[a]	Remarks
Protoplasts PEG[b]/CaCl$_2$		Saccharomyces cerevisiae, Pichia pastoris	10^2–10^5	Most widely used method but frequencies generally lower with filamentous fungi
		Aspergillus nidulans, A. niger, Trichoderma reesei, Mucor circinelloides	10^0–10^3	
Protoplasts	Electroporation[c]	S. cerevisiae, A. niger, T. reesei	10^0–10^3	Can be as efficient as the PEG/CaCl$_2$ method
Whole cells	Electroporation	S. cerevisiae, A. niger, A. oryzae, Neurospora crassa	10^0–10^3	For filamentous fungi, best results are obtained using germinating conidiospores with weakened cell walls
Whole cells	LiAc[d]/PEG	S. cerevisiae, Yarrowia lipolytica	10^3–10^7	Only applicable to a few yeast species and not effective with filamentous fungi
Whole cells	Biolistics[e]	S. cerevisiae, A. nidulans, N. crassa, Trichoderma harzianum	10^0–10^3	Most effective with intact yeast cells or conidiospores, but mycelium can also be used
Protoplasts or whole cells	Agrobacterium tumefaciens[f]	S. cerevisiae, Aspergillus awamori, T. reesei, N. crassa	10^2–10^4[g]	Equally effective with protoplasts or conidiospores, but transformation frequency is species dependent

[a] Expressed as the number of transformants obtained per microgramme of vector DNA added. Values depend on the organism, type of vector and method used.

[b] Polyethylene glycol.

[c] Introduction of DNA into cells by applying a short-pulse, high-voltage electric field.

[d] Lithium acetate.

[e] Shooting DNA-coated metal particles (normally gold or tungsten) at high velocity into cells under vacuum.

[f] DNA is transferred to the fungus from the bacterium A. tumefaciens in a manner similar to plant transformations.

[g] Transformation frequency in this case is expressed as number of transformants obtained per 10^7 recipient cells.

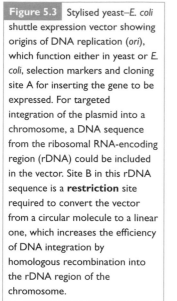

Figure 5.3 Stylised yeast–*E. coli* shuttle expression vector showing origins of DNA replication (*ori*), which function either in yeast or *E. coli*, selection markers and cloning site A for inserting the gene to be expressed. For targeted integration of the plasmid into a chromosome, a DNA sequence from the ribosomal RNA-encoding region (rDNA) could be included in the vector. Site B in this rDNA sequence is a **restriction** site required to convert the vector from a circular molecule to a linear one, which increases the efficiency of DNA integration by homologous recombination into the rDNA region of the chromosome.

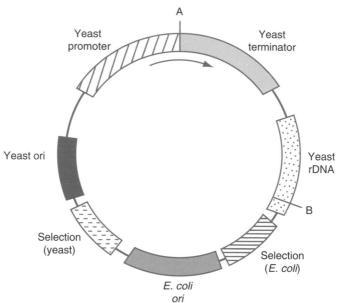

auxotrophic growth requirements, as already explained. In many cases, genes from one fungus are able to complement the appropriate mutations in a different fungus (**heterologous** transformation). However, for some fungi, only their own genes are able to complement mutations (homologous transformation). If the required auxotrophic mutant is not available, a second class of selection marker, based on resistance to antibiotics, such as hygromycin B, phleomycin, kanamycin or benomyl, can be used. One drawback with this type of marker is that the fungus must be reasonably sensitive to the antibiotic in question. For example, a bacterial gene that encodes resistance to kanamycin can be expressed weakly from its own promoter in yeast. Higher levels of drug resistance can be achieved, however, if a yeast promoter is used instead for expression. For filamentous fungi too, optimisation of antibiotic-resistance systems normally requires the use of a fungal promoter. Finally, a third group of vectors exploit genes that confer the ability to grow on carbon or nitrogen sources which the host strain would not normally be able to use. A good example is the acetamidase gene (*amdS*) of *A. nidulans*, which allows growth of the recipient strain on acetamide or acrylamide as the sole nitrogen source. This marker has been introduced into a number of *Aspergillus* and *Trichoderma* spp. and is particularly useful in generating transformants that contain multiple copies of the integrated vector.

In yeast, plasmid vectors are maintained within the cell provided the transformants are grown under selective conditions, e.g. in the presence of an antibiotic. When the selective pressure is removed, plasmids can be lost relatively rapidly from the cells because there is no advantage to the cells in maintaining a plasmid. All plasmids must contain an *ori*, which can be derived either from naturally occurring plasmids or from chromosomal DNA sequences. Vectors with an *ori* from one yeast can normally function in a variety of different yeast hosts, albeit not always with the same degree of efficiency. Plasmid vectors can be present at up to 200 copies per cell and thus provide a simple system for increasing the number of copies of the introduced genes. This often leads to higher yields of the protein encoded by the introduced gene. The disadvantage is that selective pressure is normally required to avoid significant plasmid loss, i.e. maintaining the desired characteristic can be a problem, particularly in *S. cerevisiae*. Conversely, in other yeasts, such as *Kluyveromyces lactis*, some extrachromosomal vectors are comparatively stable without the need for continuous selection.

Integration of the plasmid into the yeast genome brings enhanced stability but lower numbers of the introduced gene. One way of achieving this in *S. cerevisiae* has been to target the plasmid to *ribosomal DNA sequences* (rDNA), which can be present at about 150 tandemly repeated copies per genome. Incorporation of rDNA sequences into a vector (Fig. 5.3) enhances integration of that plasmid into the chromosomal rDNA region by recombination of homologous sequences, especially when the vector has been linearised in the rDNA region. The number of gene copies can be increased by placing the gene used for selection under the transcriptional control of weak, or deliberately weakened, promoters. This approach encourages the selection of multiple gene copies through selection pressure for a critical level of gene product. This approach is used together with rDNA targeting to obtain high numbers of integrated gene copies.

Vectors that integrate into the chromosomes have several important uses in the molecular manipulation of fungi. In addition to increasing the number of copies of a particular gene in a chromosome, they can also be used to disrupt or replace a desired gene. In *S. cerevisiae*, the use of 'replacement cassette' vectors has permitted the deletion of each of the 6000 or so genes identified by the Yeast Genome Sequencing Project to test the function of each gene in the cell. Each cassette, which consists of a kanamycin (G418) selection gene flanked at each end by short regions of gene-specific sequence, is released from the vector by cutting with a **restriction enzyme**. **Homologous recombination** between the ends of the cassette and the target gene in the chromosome leads to the specific deletion of that gene (Fig. 5.4). In these studies, individual genes, or groups of genes, were deleted from the yeast and changes in phenotype were then looked for. In this way, a particular gene might be associated with a particular function although, in practice, the deletion of a gene does not always give a detectable phenotype. The systematic deletion of individual genes within the *S. cerevisiae* genome has, in that way, been achieved by exploiting homologous recombination with introduced PCR-derived sequences. This is easier in yeast than filamentous fungi where the efficiency of homologous recombination appears to be lower and much longer regions of homologous DNA sequences are often necessary. In yeast, each deletion was tagged with a unique DNA sequence that served as a bar-code for that mutant.

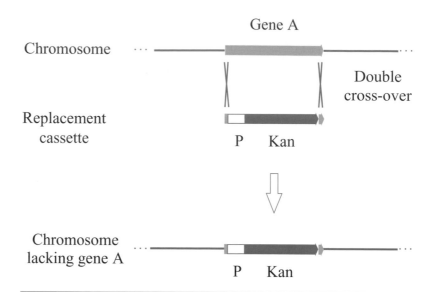

Figure 5.4 Gene deletion in *S. cerevisiae* using the kanamycin (G418) 'replacement cassette'. The cassette consists of the kanamycin-(G418)-resistance gene (Kan) under the control of a fungal promoter (P) and short flanking sequences of only about 40 bp (■), which correspond to the ends of the gene to be deleted. A double **cross-over** by homologous recombination between these ends and the chromosome leads to the deletion of the gene. At the cross-over sites, chromosomal DNA molecules are broken enzymically and DNA strands exchanged with that of the incoming cassette DNA via a DNA repair mechanism which re-joins the DNA molecules. Because many genes are essential for survival, gene deletion is first carried out in diploid cells where only one of the two copies of the gene is deleted. Yeast diploid transformants containing the deleted gene are selected on medium containing the antibiotic G418, which is more effective against yeast cells than kanamycin, and these are then forced to undergo sporulation (involving meiosis) to produce haploid spores, 50% of which contain the deleted gene. Growth tests can then be carried out to determine if the gene is essential and to discover the gene's function in the cell.

The majority of vectors used for transforming filamentous fungi rely on random, integration events, which occur at a relatively low frequency in most cases. One approach to increase transformation frequencies has been the use of *restriction enzyme-mediated integration* (REMI). In this method, the plasmid DNA is added to the cells along with a **restriction enzyme** (see Chapter 4) which cuts once in the vector. Under these conditions, the DNA is targeted to the corresponding restriction sites in the genome. With standard integrative transformation in filamentous fungi, the vector is found predominantly as multiple copies at one or more sites in the genome, but with REMI the proportion of single copies at several different sites is increased (Fig. 5.5).

The extent to which an introduced gene is able to lead to production of the protein it encodes is affected by its site of integration in the host's genome. Therefore, methods have been developed to target genes to specific chromosomal locations that ensure good **expression**.

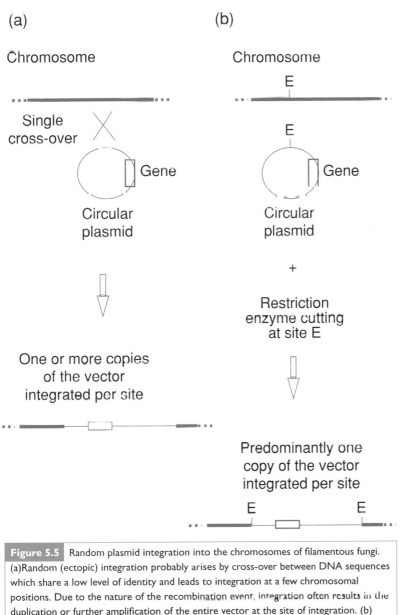

Figure 5.5 Random plasmid integration into the chromosomes of filamentous fungi. (a)Random (ectopic) integration probably arises by cross-over between DNA sequences which share a low level of identity and leads to integration at a few chromosomal positions. Due to the nature of the recombination event, integration often results in the duplication or further amplification of the entire vector at the site of integration. (b) Restriction enzyme-modified integration (REMI) involves the addition of a vast excess of a particular restriction enzyme which cuts the plasmid only at one site (E), along with the plasmid DNA during the transformation procedure. It is thought that the enzyme enters the cell's nucleus and cuts genomic DNA randomly at several sites in the chromosomes. Conversion of the circular vector molecule to a linear one by cutting at the same restriction site allows integration of the entire plasmid at several chromosomal sites. This process results in a higher proportion of vector molecules integrated as single copies at many more sites in the fungal genome but, due to its random nature, not all chromosomal sites contain the vector.

(a)

Chromosome

Vector

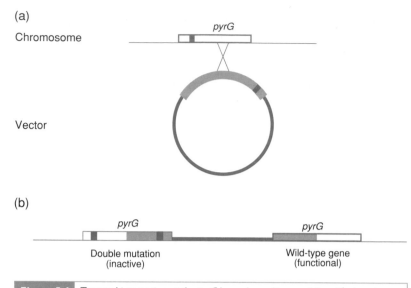

(b)

Figure 5.6 Targeted integration at the *pyrG* locus (encoding orotidine- 5′-phosphate decarboxylase) in *Aspergillus awamori*. The host strain of *A. awamori* contains a mutant (non-functional) *pyrG* gene conferring a growth requirement for uridine. The transformation vector contains a non-functional *pyrG* with a mutation in a different part of the gene. By a single homologous recombination (a single cross-over) event (a), the entire vector is integrated at the *pyrG* locus and a functional *pyrG* gene is created (b). The cross-over event involves breakage and re-joining of DNA molecules both in the vector and chromosome by a DNA repair mechanism similar to that outlined in Fig. 5.4. Fungal transformants are selected by their ability to grow without the need for added uridine in the growth medium.

(a)

Chromosome

Linearised vector

(b)

Chromosome

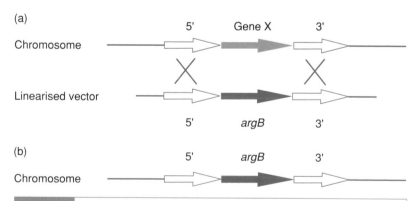

Figure 5.7 Specific gene deletion in filamentous fungi. Upstream (5′) and downstream (3′) regions of at least 1 kb in size, immediately adjacent to the chromosomal gene to be deleted (gene X), are incorporated into a vector containing a suitable selection marker, e.g. the *argB* gene of *A. nidulans* which encodes ornithine carbamoyl transferase, an enzyme involved in arginine biosynthesis. The plasmid which is normally a circular molecule of DNA is converted to a linear one by cutting with a restriction enzyme that cuts the plasmid once. This linearised vector is then transformed into an *argB* mutant strain. A double homologous recombination event (double cross-over, as outlined in Fig. 5.4) in the 5′ and 3′ regions (a) replaces gene X in the chromosome with the *argB* selection marker (b). Fungal transformants are selected by their ability to grow without the need for added arginine in the growth medium.

One method for gene targeting, developed in *Aspergillus* spp., relies on transforming a strain that has one mutation in a particular gene with an integrative plasmid that contains the same gene with a different mutation. A functional gene will only be formed if vector integration occurs at the site of the gene in question by a single cross-over event (Fig. 5.6). Up to 40% of transformants can contain the vector inserted as a single copy at the correct gene locus but transformation frequencies are normally quite low. Specific gene disruption in fungi, using circular plasmids with the appropriate marker, is quite a rare event. For gene deletion or replacement in filamentous fungi, regions adjacent to the gene in question, usually larger than 1 kilobase (kb) in size, have to be incorporated into the vector, which is linearised with a restriction enzyme prior to transformation. Gene replacement by a double cross-over event occurs at a frequency of anything from 1 to 50% but is species and gene dependent (Fig. 5.7).

5.3 | Gene cloning

The success with which fungal genes are isolated and characterised is still heavily dependent on the species being studied. Several different approaches have been adopted to overcome problems presented by genetically poorly characterised, but biotechnologically useful, fungi. The use of mutant strains has been the cornerstone of fungal gene cloning. In this approach, mutant strains are transformed to the wild-type phenotype by introduction of DNA and, when that DNA contains only one gene, it identifies the function of the gene. Other options are now available that exploit the rapidly expanding amount of gene sequence information available in gene databases although a functional assessment of a cloned gene must always be made. For some genes, 'expression cloning' is a convenient and efficient approach that is based on the introduction into yeast of a new metabolic activity detectable by a simple plate assay. We describe the basic principles involved in these and other strategies below.

5.3.1 Mutant isolation

The complementation of defined mutants remains the most effective means for isolating genes of known function although the generation of such mutants remains a problem for many fungi of interest. Physico-chemical mutagens, e.g. ultraviolet or nitrosoguanidine, are still the most common means for generating fungal mutants which may, on occasion, be characterised quickly when simple growth tests are available. Because mutations in other genes in a biosynthetic pathway can confer the same growth requirement, the mutant is tested for its ability to metabolise different substrates to confirm the precise step that has been affected.

A disadvantage of physico-chemical mutagenic methods is that treatment may induce more than one mutation per cell. This may then obscure the real factors underlying an observed property of the mutant. Thus, alternative methods for obtaining mutants have been developed in model organisms such as *S. cerevisiae, A. nidulans* and *N. crassa*, which have provided useful systems applicable to less genetically well-characterised species. Mutagenesis by means of inserting a piece of DNA into a gene so that the normal DNA sequence is altered (*insertional inactivation*) or by complete gene deletion are preferred methods where the need for a defined genetic background is paramount. Fragments of DNA, termed *transposons*, with the ability to move from one site to another within the host genome, occur naturally in many species and can be used for this purpose. The transposon, Ty, is used in this way in *S. cerevisiae* and similar elements have been identified in *Schizosaccharomyces pombe, Candida albicans* and other yeasts. As already discussed, the genome sequences of several fungal species have been determined so the next steps are to predict the positions of genes within the genome and, then, to characterise the gene products functionally. This has been achieved on a genome-wide scale in yeast species using transposon (e.g. the bacterial transposon Tn7) mutagenesis. Although less well developed in filamentous fungi, large-scale gene disruptions using transposons are showing promise. Other insertional inactivation systems are available and include restriction enzyme-mediated integration (REMI), as already described in Section 5.2.3.

Of necessity, mutants must provide an easily assayed phenotype so that large numbers of colonies can be quickly tested. Screening for the production of extracellular products provides a simple and rapid means to do this. Agar plates containing substrates which, for example, allow the detection of clearing zones or colour changes are frequently used to isolate genes encoding those extracellular enzymes associated with the saprophytic lifestyle of many filamentous fungi. Thus, agar plates containing starch as the sole carbon source can be used to test for the production of amylases. Often, specific strategies can be employed to isolate particular classes of mutant. For example, the location of a protein within a cell can be exploited: if an essential protein is normally located in the cytoplasm but has been genetically engineered to contain signals that will divert it through the secretory pathway to the outside of the cell, then mutants in the secretory pathway that prevent this occurring can be selected for.

5.3.2 Mutant complementation

DNA fragments that collectively represent the entire genome of an organism can be cloned into a vector to produce a population of DNA molecules termed a **library**. Complementation of defined fungal mutants by transformation with a library of fungal DNA is a well-established procedure only for those fungi, e.g. *S. cerevisiae* and *A. nidulans*, that can be transformed at high frequency (Fig. 5.8). Alternatively, some gene products are sufficiently well conserved across species boundaries that they will function in a bacterial background. Thus,

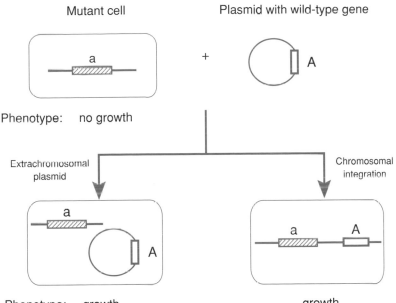

Mutant cell

Plasmid with wild-type gene

a

+

A

Phenotype: no growth

Extrachromosomal plasmid

Chromosomal integration

a

A

a   A

Phenotype: growth

growth

Figure 5.8 Complementation of a mutant gene 'a' in a cell with the corresponding wild-type gene 'A' on a plasmid. ▨ represents the mutant gene 'a' and □ represents the wild-type gene 'A'. The presence of gene A within the cell, either as a plasmid or integrated into the chromosome, allows growth.

a number of fungal genes have been isolated via complementation of *E. coli* mutants although transformation of fungal hosts remains the norm. The surest route to assess gene function relies on the integration of a single copy of the gene in question into the fungal host DNA. Many yeasts, such as *S. cerevisiae*, and some filamentous fungi allow the introduction of a gene on a **circular DNA molecule (plasmid)**, which can be present at several copies per cell. In some cases, this allows closely related (but not identical) genes to complement the mutation and can therefore provide a misleading picture of the gene's function.

Plasmids that replicate extrachromosomally are much less common in filamentous fungi than in yeasts. Despite this, such vectors can still be exploited to identify fungal genes that are able to complement specific mutations (Fig. 5.9). For example, if an *A. nidulans* mutant is transformed with a mixture of a plasmid, containing only a bacterial selection marker and a fungal *ori*, and linear genomic DNA isolated from the fungus under study, two distinct classes of transformant are obtained. The first shows a stable, wild-type phenotype on plates resulting from direct integration of the complementing DNA into the *A. nidulans* chromosomes. The second class of transformant shows uneven growth within colonies on plates where certain sectors of each colony appear wild-type whilst other sectors display the mutant phenotype. This 'sectored' morphology results from recombination between the two source DNAs producing plasmids that carry the complementing gene but which can be lost during the process of cell division. Extraction of the total DNA from such unstable *A. nidulans* colonies, and transformation into *E. coli*, permits the isolation of the plasmids containing the fungal DNA fragment that complemented the original *A. nidulans* mutation.

Figure 5.9 Isolation of a gene by complementation of a defined mutant in a filamentous fungus. ▨ represents the mutant gene 'a' and ☐ represents the wild-type gene 'A' found in genomic DNA (–). ■ represents the fungal origin of replication (*ori*) on the plasmid. Recombination between the genomic DNA and the plasmid results in an unstable inheritance of the wild-type gene 'A' which causes a sectored colony morphology, i.e. growth occurs where the plasmid is present but is prevented when parts of the colony lose the plasmid. The plasmid containing gene 'A' can be recovered from the colonies showing sectored growth.

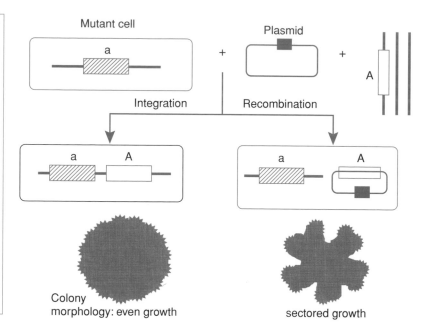

Advantages of the method are that it is rapid and it is not necessary to construct a library of individual genes from the total DNA of the fungus.

5.3.3 Gene isolation by the polymerase chain reaction

Extensive use of the **polymerase chain reaction** (PCR; see Fig. 4.8) is now made to isolate many specific genes. This approach requires proteins with the same function to have been identified in other organisms and for the gene sequences to be available in a DNA sequence database (e.g. on the Internet). Fortunately, there is an available resource of fungal genome sequences and the number of fungal species with a sequenced genome is increasing. Annotation of the genomes (into putative genes with assigned function) is also often available. Alignment of the protein sequences encoded by these genes against one another can then be used to identify highly conserved regions and allows short sequences of single-stranded DNA (PCR primers) corresponding to these regions to be designed. Because the genetic code is redundant, i.e. more than one triplet of nucleotide bases (codon) can encode the same amino acid, these primers are often mixtures of different DNA sequences which nevertheless encode the same amino acid sequence. Ideally, those conserved regions would contain amino acids which are encoded by a low number of codons to avoid the generation of many different PCR fragment species. If this is not possible, a number of strategies may be used to overcome this problem. The most obvious example is to employ 'nested' primers, i.e. a second set of primers, which are internal to the first set, and are designed from additional conserved regions, in a second round of PCR

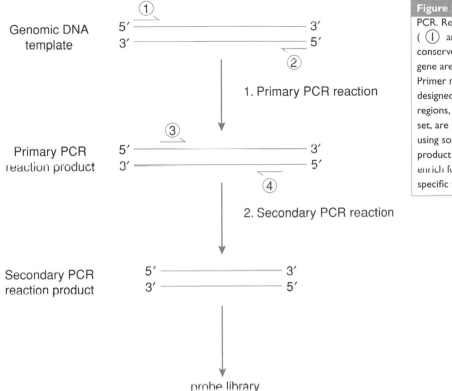

Genomic DNA
template

Primary PCR
reaction product

Secondary PCR
reaction product

1. Primary PCR reaction

2. Secondary PCR reaction

probe library

Figure 5.10 'Nested primer' PCR. Redundant primer mixes ((1) and (2)) designed against conserved regions of the target gene are used in the initial PCR. Primer mixes ((3) and (4)) designed against further conserved regions, internal to the first primer set, are used in a second PCR using some of the first PCR product as template. This should enrich for PCR-amplified products specific to the target gene.

(Fig. 5.10). These can be successful in amplifying fragments of a specific size from a first round reaction, which gives a smeared appearance when the PCR products are electrophoresed through an agarose gel. The temperature at which a single-stranded primer binds to its complementary sequence in the template DNA is termed the annealing temperature and depends upon the DNA base composition; therefore, there may only be a narrow range of possible annealing temperatures when a mixture of primers is used. Also, in practice, several temperatures and buffer component concentrations should be examined in order to optimise yields of fragments specific only to those reactions containing both sets of primers. Potential candidate fragments should be cloned, if necessary, then sequenced to verify identity to the desired gene and used as probes to isolate clones containing the complete gene sequence from a library.

The major disadvantage of any approach to isolate a gene, other than complementation of a known mutation, is that information on the functionality of the gene is missing. Identifying a gene by a comparison of its DNA sequence with sequences of genes from other organisms rarely provides a conclusive answer, especially when dealing with novel or poorly characterised organisms. Gene deletion experiments should be done to ascertain whether the gene is essential for growth. However, if no clear phenotype emerges from this

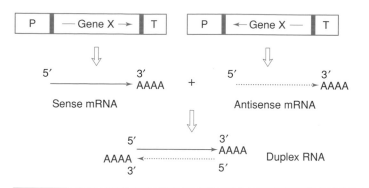

Figure 5.11 Possible mechanism for the down-regulation of protein production by 'antisense' RNA transcripts. Open boxes represent the target gene X cloned in either of two orientations and flanked by promoter (P) and terminator (T) sequences. Transcription provides sense and antisense mRNA molecules (both with polyA tails) depending on the orientation of the gene relative to the promoter. These two complementary RNA molecules bind together to form a duplex RNA. Formation of duplex RNA in the nucleus reduces the amount of mature mRNA available for translation in the cytoplasm.

type of experiment, complementation of a defined mutant should be used. An additional strategy, which is especially useful when the gene in question is essential for growth, is to decrease the amount of a protein produced within cells. This uses a process known as *antisense* in which a messenger RNA (mRNA) sequence complementary to the sense mRNA interferes with the production of the protein encoded by the target gene (Fig. 5.11). This approach is becoming more commonly used for the functional assessment of cloned genes in yeasts and filamentous fungi although it has not always proved successful.

5.3.4   PCR and fungi

In addition to its use in the isolation of genes, PCR is also commonly used in screening for the outcome of specific DNA manipulations in many systems. For some filamentous fungi, however, the cell wall has proved a substantial barrier to obtaining DNA of sufficient quantity or purity for large-scale screening by PCR. A protocol has now been developed in which fungal colonies are grown in liquid culture in microtitre plates and their cell walls removed by enzymic digestion to release protoplasts. The 'hot' denaturing step of the PCR cycle lyses the protoplasts providing DNA which can be used to screen for the presence of specific DNA fragments (Fig. 5.12). Other protocols, which use mycelia, spores or cells and incorporate a short heating step to burst the cells prior to PCR amplification, work well with many fungal species.

5.3.5   Heterologous gene probes

A third strategy for the isolation of specific genes involves the use of radioactively labelled DNA fragments (probes) from other organisms

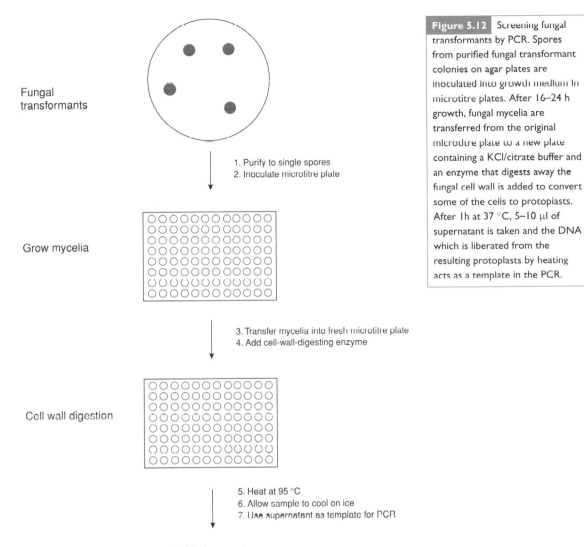

Fungal transformants

1. Purify to single spores
2. Inoculate microtitre plate

Grow mycelia

3. Transfer mycelia into fresh microtitre plate
4. Add cell-wall-digesting enzyme

Cell wall digestion

5. Heat at 95 °C
6. Allow sample to cool on ice
7. Use supernatant as template for PCR

PCR fragments

Figure 5.12 Screening fungal transformants by PCR. Spores from purified fungal transformant colonies on agar plates are inoculated into growth medium in microtitre plates. After 16–24 h growth, fungal mycelia are transferred from the original microtitre plate to a new plate containing a KCl/citrate buffer and an enzyme that digests away the fungal cell wall is added to convert some of the cells to protoplasts. After 1h at 37 °C, 5–10 μl of supernatant is taken and the DNA which is liberated from the resulting protoplasts by heating acts as a template in the PCR.

which encode the same protein as that of the fungal gene required. These are termed heterologous gene probes. Initial experiments in which single-stranded (denatured) fungal genomic DNA is transferred to a nylon membrane after agarose gel electrophoresis (**Southern blotting**) can be used to determine the efficacy of this approach and to determine optimal conditions for hybridisation. Because the sequence of the heterologous probe may be substantially different from the fungal gene due to its different origin, the temperature at which the radioactive probe is annealed to the fungal DNA (hybridisation) is a critical parameter. Improved specificity can be gained by altering the salt concentration of the washes used following hybridisation. Once hybridisation conditions have been optimised, a DNA library from the organism under study can be screened.

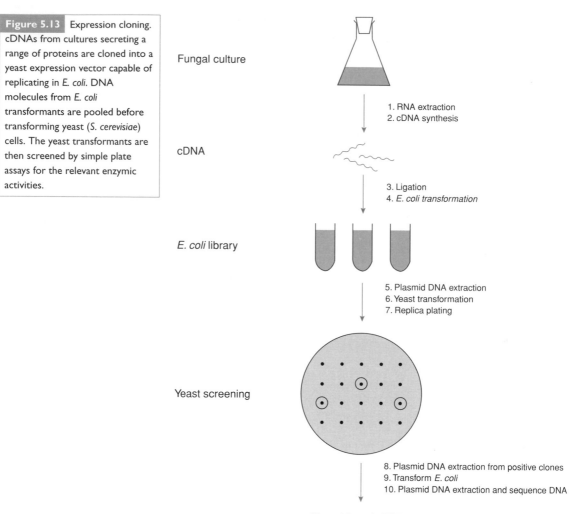

Figure 5.13 Expression cloning. cDNAs from cultures secreting a range of proteins are cloned into a yeast expression vector capable of replicating in *E. coli*. DNA molecules from *E. coli* transformants are pooled before transforming yeast (*S. cerevisiae*) cells. The yeast transformants are then screened by simple plate assays for the relevant enzymic activities.

Fungal culture

1. RNA extraction
2. cDNA synthesis

cDNA

3. Ligation
4. *E. coli transformation*

E. coli library

5. Plasmid DNA extraction
6. Yeast transformation
7. Replica plating

Yeast screening

8. Plasmid DNA extraction from positive clones
9. Transform *E. coli*
10. Plasmid DNA extraction and sequence DNA

Cloned fungal cDNA

5.3.6 Database and linkage-based methods for gene isolation

Finally, two other strategies may be used for gene isolation. The first, termed **synteny**, relies upon the fact that even where there are significant differences between the DNA sequences of genes from different species, gene linkages may be physically maintained. Thus, if in organism X, genes A and B are neighbours on the same chromosome then, if the same case pertains in the fungal system, screening for gene B may allow one to isolate gene A. The main requirement for such a method to work is a detailed genome map of the model organism (X). A number of genomes have been, or are currently being, sequenced and maps established which should provide a basis for this approach (see Table 5.1).

An alternative approach employs partial complementary DNA (cDNA) libraries, which can be made from fungal RNA samples using readily available cDNA synthesis kits. These cDNAs are termed expressed sequence tags (ESTs) since they comprise the ends of transcribed sequences. When allied to automated sequencing, this approach rapidly provides information that can be used to identify those genomic sequences in the gene sequence databases which are transcribed.

5.3.7 Expression cloning

The lifestyles of some fungi mean that they secrete high concentrations of protein, many of which have application in a variety of industries. A quick and effective method, termed **expression cloning**, has recently been developed to isolate genes encoding extracellular enzymes (Fig. 5.13). In this method, the fungus is grown under conditions expected to induce expression of the target gene(s), and the mRNA is extracted and used to construct a cDNA library in *E. coli*. This library is then used to transform *S. cerevisiae* and the transformants are grown on media that provide a simple assay for the newly acquired enzyme activity. Other yeast hosts, such as *Yarrowia lipolytica*, *K. lactis*, *Pichia angusta* (formerly *Hansenula polymorpha*) and *S. pombe*, may be preferred for the transformation step. The effectiveness of this system has been demonstrated by its use to clone genes encoding over 150 fungal enzymes including arabinanases, endoglucanases, galactanases, mannanases, pectinases, proteases and many others. This approach requires that the cDNA step synthesises full-length products to ensure the presence of a protein secretion signal which is also functional in the yeast host. Expression of the enzymes in the yeast host and an easily assayed phenotype are also pre-requisites.

5.4 | Gene structure, organisation and expression

In general, transcriptional signals in genes from higher organisms are more complex than those found in bacterial systems. Within fungi, gene organisation shares many common features across a wide number of genera. The three main organisational units in fungal genes can be split up into those signals that (a) control the switching on or off of gene transcription (*promoters*), (b) control the termination of transcription (*terminators*) and (c) control the necessary excision of introns from mRNA.

Unlike their bacterial counterparts, fungal promoters can extend a substantial distance (>1 kb) upstream of the **transcriptional start point (tsp)**. Early cloning experiments in *S. cerevisiae* suggested that native *S. cerevisiae* promoters were required for the expression of foreign genes although subsequent experiments have shown that some promoters from other yeasts, e.g. *K. lactis*, can also function in *S. cerevisiae*. In filamentous fungi, promoters tend to function well within their own genus but are less predictable in more distantly related species.

Promoters can generally be defined as either constitutive, i.e. they are switched on permanently, or inducible, i.e. contain elements that allow them to be switched on or off in a regulated fashion. In both types of promoter, one or more tsp can exist. Sequences in the promoter region define both the tsp and the binding sites for regulatory proteins. TA-rich regions, known as *TATA-boxes*, are often involved in determining the tsp and also maintaining a basal level of transcription. An illustration of their function is provided by the *S. cerevisiae* HIS4 promoter where transcription can occur either with or without a TATA-box (the HIS4 gene encodes histidinol dehydrogenase involved in histidine biosynthesis); high transcription levels are only observed from the HIS4 promoter containing a TATA-box. However, there are also strong yeast promoters that lack a TATA-box. Since many yeast and filamentous fungal promoters do not contain this sequence, other motifs, such as the pyrimidine-rich tracts (CT-boxes) found in filamentous fungal promoters, can perform the same function. These sequences can be used to describe what is essentially a 'core' promoter. A third sequence, CCAAT, is also often associated with core promoter function. However, most (~95%) *S. cerevisiae* genes appear not to require CCAAT-boxes for function although this motif is known to function in *A. nidulans*. It should be stressed that in the majority of fungal promoters that have been isolated, the functional significance of sequences identified in them has not been determined and therefore remains unclear.

With a constitutive promoter, the basal level of transcription is determined by the binding to the *core promoter* of a protein complex which contains RNA polymerase and the so-called general or upstream factors. In contrast, the expression of an inducible gene can change by orders of magnitude. The regulatory elements responsible for mediating this switch are usually found upstream of the core promoter sequences and are termed *upstream activation* or *upstream repression sequences* (UAS or URS). These UAS/URS sequences bind regulatory proteins that are thought to stabilise (or destabilise), either directly or indirectly, the transcriptional complex bound to the core promoter thus elevating/decreasing the rate of transcriptional initiation.

Regulatory sequences which control expression of an inducible promoter may often be found in promoters of several genes that encode proteins of unlinked function, all of which are controlled by a single regulatory protein. Such a network of co-regulated genes may respond to physiological parameters affecting the cell such as pH, carbon or nitrogen source. For example, in the filamentous fungus *A. nidulans*, a protein (termed PacC) that binds to a specific sequence in the promoters of genes encoding pH-responsive proteins has been identified (Fig. 5.14). When the ambient pH is alkaline, PacC is activated by a protease to a form that permits expression of a wide range of alkaline-expressed genes (e.g. isopenicillin N synthase) and represses many genes normally expressed under acid conditions (e.g. acid phosphatases). Similarly, in *S. cerevisiae* and some *Kluyveromyces* spp., the DNA-binding protein, Mig1p, binds in a glucose-dependent fashion to GC-rich regions (GC-boxes) of many promoters of genes

Alkaline pH

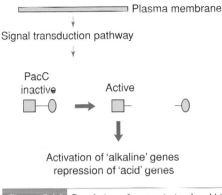

Activation of 'alkaline' genes
repression of 'acid' genes

Figure 5.14 Regulation of transcription by pH in filamentous fungi. The external pH is sensed by cells and leads to changes in gene expression. In fungi, the transcription of genes which encode proteins that are necessary for survival at alkaline pH is mediated by a transcription factor (PacC). Alkaline pH is sensed and leads, through a signal transduction pathway, to the cleavage of an inactive form of PacC to produce the active form. The activated PacC stimulates the transcription of genes leading to enzymes such as alkaline phosphatase that are active at alkaline pH ('alkaline' genes) and represses the transcription of 'acid' genes. The truncated form of PacC activates genes by binding to its target promoters at the sequence 5'-GCCARG-3' (where R = G or A).

involved in carbon source utilisation. Mig1p forms a complex with other proteins that represses transcription of genes required for the catabolism of carbon sources which are less efficient in producing energy than glucose and related sugars, a process known as carbon catabolite repression. In filamentous fungi, such as *A. nidulans* and *Trichoderma reesei*, a similar function is performed by the CreA and Cre-1 proteins, respectively, which bind to GC-boxes in the promoters of genes involved in carbon catabolism. Another network of genes, whose control is mediated by the regulatory protein AreA in *A. nidulans* (Nit2 in *N. crassa*), is that involved in the synthesis of enzymes for nitrogen catabolism. In the presence of the preferred simple nitrogen sources, ammonium and glutamine, genes responsible for breaking down complex nitrogen sources are switched off.

In addition to these regulatory systems of broad specificity covering networks of genes, there are also control mechanisms specific to a particular metabolic pathway. Thus, the positive regulatory protein, AflR, co-ordinates the expression of at least 25 different genes responsible for the synthesis of the fungal toxin, aflatoxin. All those genes examined so far contain a specific sequence in their promoters to which the AflR protein binds and activates transcription. Although in this instance the genes are clustered on a small region of one chromosome, there is no known requirement for genes which are co-ordinately regulated (either in a global or pathway-specific context) to be physically contiguous or even be on the same chromosome.

What knowledge there is regarding termination of transcription in fungi has derived mainly from studies with *S. cerevisiae* where it is tightly coupled to a process called *polyadenylation*, that is the addition of long stretches of adenine nucleotides to form polyA mRNA tails. A major function of polyadenylation is to increase the stability of mRNA; in mutants of *S. cerevisiae* where the rate of polyA removal is slowed down, mRNA stability is increased. Most yeast genes lack the sequence AATAAA associated with polyadenylation in higher eukaryotes although two other motifs have been associated with terminator function: a TTTTTAT motif, which functions only in one orientation, and a tripartite signal based on a TAG . . (T-rich) . . TA(T)GT . . (AT-rich) . . TTT sequence, which can function in either orientation. It seems likely that a number of signals are used to terminate transcription in *S. cerevisiae*.

The genes of higher organisms also differ from their bacterial counterparts through the presence of introns, which must be excised from the mRNA before it is translated into protein; a process known as **splicing**. *S. cerevisiae* and filamentous fungal genes show considerable differences with regard to the presence and nature of their **intron**s. The majority of *S. cerevisiae* genes lack introns altogether and those that do contain introns often contain only one. Genes from filamentous fungi, and those of *S. pombe*, often have several introns, usually between 50 and 100 bp in size. The fact that the introduction of filamentous fungal genes into *S. cerevisiae* results in incorrect splicing suggests that the splicing mechanisms differ significantly between some fungal species, although the *amdS* gene from *A. nidulans*, which has three introns, is spliced correctly in several filamentous fungal species. Intron position, though not sequence, is often conserved across filamentous species and introns need not necessarily be within the coding region but can be found in the region between the tsp and the point at which translation of the mRNA starts.

5.5 | Other methodologies

5.5.1 Yeast two-hybrid system

This genetic-based assay was developed in *S. cerevisiae* to test whether proteins of interest interact within the cell (Fig. 5.15a). The method can be used either to study two proteins whose genes have already been isolated or, more importantly, to identify genes from a cDNA library whose gene products will interact with a known protein of interest, termed the 'bait' protein. The two-hybrid assay relies on the fact that most eukaryotic transcription factors are single proteins which contain regions involved either in promoter DNA-binding or transcription initiation. A common system used is based on the Gal4p transcription activator protein which regulates galactose utilisation in *S. cerevisiae*. Typically, the 'reporter' gene, whose expression is measured in the yeast transformants, is the *lacZ* gene that encodes β-galactosidase, an easily measured enzyme activity. Positive interactions between the proteins under study result in an increased production of β-galactosidase compared with negative controls. This

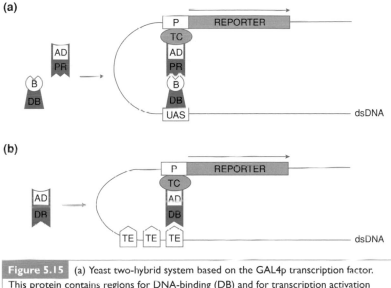

Figure 5.15 (a) Yeast two-hybrid system based on the GAL4p transcription factor. This protein contains regions for DNA-binding (DB) and for transcription activation (AD) and is involved in switching on galactose utilisation in *S. cerevisiae*. P, GAL4p-activated yeast promoter; TC, transcription complex including the RNA polymerase; DB, the GAL4p DNA-binding region fused to B, the 'bait' protein of known function; PR, the 'prey' protein under study or the products of a cDNA library fused to AD, the GAL4p activation region; UAS, upstream activation sequence required for initiation of transcription at the promoter; dsDNA, double-stranded DNA. Expression of the reporter gene, e.g. the *lacZ* gene encoding β-galactosidase, is switched on if the AD and DB regions of the GAL4p transcription activator are brought together through interaction of the 'bait' and 'prey' proteins. (b) Yeast one-hybrid system, which is also based on the GAL4p transcription factor. TE, target element (DNA sequence), normally constructed as at least three repeated copies; AD-DB, the GAL4p activation region fused to the DNA-binding protein of interest or to the products from a cDNA library; other labelling as in (a). Expression of the reporter gene (e.g. *lacZ*) is switched on if the putative DB region binds to the TEs.

flexible system can be used to investigate interactions between proteins from any organism but once a positive result has been obtained, the interaction in question must be verified biochemically. The two-hybrid system is now commercially available in a number of different kits.

5.5.2 Yeast one-hybrid system

The one-hybrid system was developed from the two-hybrid version to identify genes that encode proteins recognising known specific DNA sequences, such as transcription factors that regulate gene expression or proteins that bind to other sequences such as DNA replication origins (Fig. 5.15b). Positive clones that show increased 'reporter' gene activity are analysed by searches through DNA databases for sequence identity to known DNA-binding proteins and their functional activity verified by protein-DNA binding assays.

5.5.3 Cosmids and artificial chromosomes

With the development of **vectors** that can carry large fragments of chromosomal DNA, up to 50 kb in size, it is now possible to clone entire fungal pathways, provided all the genes are clustered in one region of the genome, and to transfer these into another organism. **Cosmid vectors** have been constructed that can be propagated in *E. coli* or in filamentous fungi. Like other vectors, these DNA molecules can be designed to either integrate into the chromosome or replicate extrachromosomally when introduced into the fungus. Cosmids with overlapping inserts have been used to clone the entire pathway for aflatoxin/sterigmatocystin biosynthesis, a total of at least 25 co-regulated genes, from a number of *Aspergillus* spp. In another case, a cosmid containing the three structural genes for penicillin biosynthesis from *Penicillium chrysogenum* has been integrated into the chromosomes of *Aspergillus niger* and *N. crassa*, both of which then gained the ability to synthesise penicillin.

Yeast artificial chromosomes (YACs) are now also available for cloning large DNA fragments. These are large linear molecules up to 620 kb in size and can be considered to behave as small chromosomes. Problems of YAC stability have led to the development of alternative bacterial artificial chromosome (BAC) systems, but YACs still prove useful in several applications. They have been used to analyse foreign gene expression in mammalian cell lines and also in whole animals. YACs have also been used to study chromosome damage in higher cells, to map ESTs in the genome and to clone large DNA fragments for genome sequencing projects.

5.5.4 Genomic and post-genomic technologies

The ability to sequence the entire genome of an organism has led to the development of some extremely powerful tools for studying fundamental cellular processes. The DNA sequence itself provides the data to construct microarrays (see Section 4.7.2) on glass slides suitable for a wide variety of applications; the sequence also provides the means to construct genome-wide deletion sets for functional analysis (see Section 5.2.3).

Arrays containing sequences considered to represent the majority of the transcribed DNA can be used to analyse the transcriptional profile (**transcriptome**) of an organism under any given set of conditions. Comparisons of data obtained under different conditions have defined genes associated with pathogenesis, signal transduction pathways, protein secretion and many other coordinated regulatory networks. In fungi, such an approach will prove powerful in unravelling the complexities associated with growth, differentiation and metabolism, the production of secondary metabolites, the stress response imposed by protein overproduction and many other biotechnologically significant processes. An important caveat to transcriptome analysis is that changes in transcript level do not necessarily translate into a similar change in the corresponding protein.

The increased amount of DNA sequence data has also driven the development of other technologies, the most well established of which is proteomic analysis. Here, proteins from total or fractionated cell extracts are separated in two dimensions (based on charge and size) on polyacrylamide gels (**proteome**). Protein spots are then extracted, digested with trypsin and analysed by mass spectrometry (MS). Comparison of the tryptic products generated with publicly available DNA/protein databases is then used to identify the protein. This process can be used to examine the changes in both protein level and modification status from cells grown under different conditions. Although transcriptomic approaches present an opportunity to examine all known genes, the available methods for proteome analysis can only cover a proportion of the cellular proteins. Improved methods for the extraction and separation of proteins (especially membrane proteins), not necessarily involving separation on polyacrylamide gels, will be important in the improvement of proteomic analyses. In the same way that transcript levels may not reflect those of translated protein, proteomic analysis may not always give an accurate picture of the activity of the cell's proteins, i.e. the cell's metabolism.

This has led to the development of **metabolomics**, which quantifies the metabolite levels in a cell by means of mass spectrometry (MS), usually coupled with separation by gas chromatography (GC-MS) or high-performance liquid chromatography (LC-MS). The metabolome generated in this way may be a truer measurement of the cell's metabolic activity. Recently, *metabolic footprinting* of yeast strains by MS directly from spent growth media has been developed for rapid high-throughput screening and has made use of the 6000 or so defined gene knock-out strains already described in Section 5.2.3 (see also Chapter 12).

Despite their power, none of these technologies, in themselves, provide a complete picture of the complex relationship between genome and phenotype and emphasises the need to use a combination of techniques to study a given process.

5.6 | Biotechnological applications of fungi

Genetic engineering of yeasts and filamentous fungi is now commonly used for investigating aspects of their biological function and also for constructing strains for particular biotechnological applications. Although genetic engineering is well developed for only a few species, the technology can normally be developed for most species provided sufficient effort is expended. Some of the commercially important products and species are shown in Table 5.3. Each product is a target for improved production using genetically modified strains: this is most advanced in the production of enzymes and antibiotics.

The use of yeasts and filamentous fungi to produce **heterologous** proteins, i.e. proteins not naturally produced from that species and encoded by a **gene** derived from another organism, serves as a

Table 5.3 | Useful products from yeasts and filamentous fungi. These products provide targets for genetic manipulation. GM strains are most advanced for the production of antibiotics and enzymes

Product	Uses	Yeast[a]	Filamentous fungus[a]
Biomass	Foods	Saccharomyces cerevisiae	Agaricus bisporus Fusarium venenatum
Ethanol	Beer, wine	Saccharomyces cerevisiae	
CO_2	Bread, wine	Saccharomyces cerevisiae	
Sulphite	Preservative (beer)	Saccharomyces cerevisiae	
Flavours (e.g. lactones, peptides, terpenoids)	Foods, beverages	Saccharomyces cerevisiae Pichia guilliermondii Sporobolomyces odorus	Trichoderma viride Gibberella fujikuroi Mucor circinelloides Phycomyces blakesleeanus
Polyunsaturated fatty acids	Foods	Cryptococcus curvatus	Mortierella alpina Mucor circinelloides
Organic acids (e.g. citric, gluconic, itaconic)	Preservatives, food ingredients, chemical synthesis	Yarrowia lipolytica	Aspergillus niger Aspergillus terreus
Antibiotics (e.g. penicillin, cephalosporin, polyketides)	Health		Penicillium chrysogenum, Acremonium chrysogenum Penicillium griseofulvum Aspergillus tamorii
Homologous enzymes (e.g. amylases, cellulases, proteases)	Food processing, paper production, detergents	Kluyveromyces lactis	Aspergillus spp. Rhizopus spp. Trichoderma spp.
Heterologous proteins	Foods, therapeutics	Saccharomyces cerevisiae Kluyveromyces lactis Pichia pastoris Pichia angusta Yarrowia lipolytica	Aspergillus niger Aspergillus oryzae Aspergillus nidulans Trichoderma reesei

Notes:
[a] Main species only

convenient topic for a comparative discussion. This is because both yeasts and filamentous fungi are used as hosts for heterologous protein production (see also Chapter 21), the technology has advanced sufficiently for commercial use and research is still active in order to improve the systems. To be effective, a production system must deliver sufficient yields (whether it be for commercial viability or to provide research material) of the target protein and the protein must be authentic in its properties, i.e. the same as, or close to, those of the protein from its natural source.

5.6.1 Protein production: the importance of secretion

Most of the commercially available enzymes are secreted from their source organisms although some important enzymes are extracted from cell biomass. The main advantage of producing secreted, as opposed to intracellular, enzymes to a commercial enterprise is the ease (and therefore relative cheapness) of purifying the enzyme. Secreted enzymes are normally correctly folded and active because this is a function of the quality control system within the secretory pathway. Enhanced production of intracellular proteins can lead to the accumulation of improperly folded and inactive protein; or the extraction process itself, which is expensive, may inactivate a proportion of the protein thus reducing recoverable yields. The secretory pathway is also the site of protein glycosylation, which may contribute to the function or stability of some proteins. Both N-linked (at asparagine) and O-linked (at serine or threonine) glycosylation of proteins occur, sometimes with both forms within the same protein. The composition of the glycan component of secreted glycoproteins varies according to species and the glycosylation of heterologous proteins will differ according to the production host. Whether this presents a difficulty in practice will depend upon the intended application of the enzyme. It is likely to be most acute if the heterologous protein is intended for therapeutic use in humans since the glycans of human and fungal proteins have different compositions and their antigenicity can lead to their rapid clearance from the bloodstream. Enzyme activity per se need not be affected by alterations in glycosylation.

A high secretion capacity in the producing organism is desirable although not essential. Those species that naturally secrete a range of enzymes as part of their lifestyles might therefore be expected to be systems of choice for use as hosts for the production of heterologous proteins. Many species of filamentous fungi secrete enzymes to degrade polymeric organic matter and, in laboratory and commercial-scale culture, secrete prodigious amounts of enzymes. It is not surprising that the filamentous fungi are the sources of about 10 times the number of commercial (homologous) enzymes that yeasts produce. For the production of heterologous proteins, however, both yeasts and filamentous fungi have been developed as hosts and each system has its attractions and adherents.

5.6.2 Heterologous proteins from yeasts

Saccharomyces cerevisiae is widely used in the production of bread and alcohol, and is regarded as safe. Gene transfer and gene regulation/expression have been extensively studied in S. cerevisiae and its widespread familiarity makes it a superficially attractive host organism for heterologous protein production. A large number of different heterologous proteins have been produced following gene transfer into *S. cerevisiae* and the proteins are produced at sufficient yields for commercialisation (e.g. human serum albumin and human insulin). Despite its advantages, there are two major difficulties. The first problem is that many target proteins are 'hyperglycosylated', i.e. the N-linked carbohydrate chains are often extremely long and of a high-mannose type, which is not characteristic of human glycans. Human serum albumin, on the other hand, is not naturally glycosylated and is not glycosylated when produced by yeast. The second problem is that secreted yields are often initially very low.

A number of alternative yeast expression systems have been developed for the utilisation of cheap, widely available substrates or for more efficient protein secretion. *Kluyveromyces lactis*, grown on lactose-containing whey, is used commercially for the production of lactase (β-galactosidase) and the strong, inducible promoter of the encoding gene is used to drive heterologous gene expression. Chymosin from *K. lactis* has been produced commercially and various other proteins have also been produced with yields of secreted proteins reported in the literature generally higher than those of *S. cerevisiae*. Two methanol-utilising yeasts, *Pichia angusta* and *P. pastoris*, possess the strong, methanol-inducible promoter from the methanol oxidase gene which is used to drive the expression of introduced genes. Impressive secreted yields of several heterologous proteins have been reported from both species particularly when high cell densities are obtained in bioreactors. Also, hyperglycosylation appears not to be a major problem in proteins secreted at high yields from *P. pastoris*. *Yarrowia lipolytica* (Fig. 5.1b) is unusual in being capable of growth on some hydrocarbons although this capacity has not yet been exploited through provision of promoters to drive heterologous gene expression. Rather, the regulated promoter of the gene encoding the major secreted alkaline protease has been used to drive expression but other promoters are also available. A wide range of proteins is naturally secreted by *Y. lipolytica*, unlike some other yeasts, which indicates a well-developed secretory capacity.

The **expression cassettes** used for heterologous protein production have several interesting features (see Fig. 5.4). The foreign gene (usually a cDNA gene to avoid the possibility of splicing introns incorrectly in a heterologous host organism) is flanked by a yeast promoter and transcriptional terminator. In general, a promoter derived from the host yeast is preferred, although some promoters operate effectively across species (e.g. the promoter from the *S. cerevisiae* PGK gene (coding for phosphoglycerol kinase) is used in *K. lactis*). A short (15–30 amino acids) peptide sequence, called a signal sequence, at the N-terminal end of the protein to be produced is a requirement for the secretion of proteins (see Fig. 4.15). Cleavage of the signal sequence is carried out in the cell by a specific intracellular endopeptidase upon entry of the protein to the endoplasmic reticulum (ER), which is the start of the secretory system in eukaryotes. The cleavage site is not sequence specific but is governed primarily by the size and charge distribution (usually a positively charged N-terminal region and a hydrophobic core) of the signal sequence. Several heterologous, homologous and synthetic signal sequences have been examined with many working effectively It has become more common to include a short 'pro-sequence' after the signal sequence and before the N-terminus of the target protein. Pro-sequences are naturally present in many secreted homologous proteins and can aid folding. In S. cerevisiae, the signal sequence and pro-sequence of the secreted a-mating factor protein is often employed. This pro-sequence ends in a di-basic pair of amino acids, lysine–arginine, and an endopeptidase that is located in the Golgi body (an organelle in the secretory pathway) cleaves after the lysine–arginine to release mature target protein with its correct N-terminal sequence. This endopeptidase is called Kex2p in S. cerevisiae and equivalent enzymes are found in other yeasts and filamentous fungi.

Many heterologous proteins are produced at yields that are too low (for commercial viability or for experimental purposes) or are structurally and functionally different from the authentic protein. Yeasts are no different in this regard to other expression systems and modifications to the standard procedures have been pursued in order to overcome the difficulties. The use of vectors that replicate at high copy number can titrate out the necessary transcription factors so that they become limiting. This occurs in S. cerevisiae with the galactose-inducible, GAL1, promoter. Increasing the expression of the associated regulatory protein (Gal4p) overcomes this titration effect.

Many of the limitations leading to low secreted yields are post-translational and relate to the secretory pathway or to proteolytic degradation. Thus, protease-deficient mutants have been examined and, conversely, enhancement of the specific proteolytic activities of the signal peptidase and Kex2 protease have also been examined. Each approach has shown some promise without wholly overcoming the bottle-necks to high yields. Folding of proteins during secretion occurs within the ER and is assisted by resident **chaperone** proteins. Other proteins, termed foldases, also catalyse folding by the formation of disulphide bonds within the ER. Up-regulated expression of foldases and chaperones has increased the secreted yield of some, but not all, heterologous proteins from S. cerevisiae. Mutagenesis of strains has been used to increase secreted protein yields and in a few cases mutations have been localised to particular genes. Mutations that affect all aspects, including transcription, proteolysis, secretion and glycosylation, have been recorded. Although mutagenesis will continue to be used as a tool for improving yields, many mutations are recessive and not easily incorporated into polyploid commercial strains that have multiple copies of each chromosome. Thus targeted gene manipulations provide a complementary and valuable approach.

5.6.3 Heterologous proteins from filamentous fungi

Typical fungal expression vectors are not dissimilar to those described already for yeast. As discussed in Section 5.2.3, the main difference

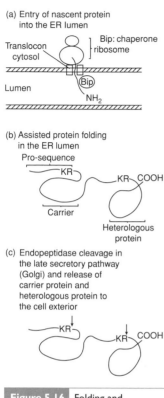

(a) Entry of nascent protein into the ER lumen

Translocon cytosol

Bip: chaperone ribosome

Lumen

Bip

NH₂

(b) Assisted protein folding in the ER lumen

Pro-sequence

KR

KR COOH

Carrier

Heterologous protein

(c) Endopeptidase cleavage in the late secretory pathway (Golgi) and release of carrier protein and heterologous protein to the cell exterior

KR

KR COOH

Figure 5.16 Folding and processing of secretory fusion proteins in filamentous fungi. (a) Entry of nascent polypeptide into the lumen of the endoplasmic reticulum (ER). The signal sequence that directs entry of the polypeptide is removed by signal peptidase so that the emerging polypeptide within the lumen lacks the signal sequence. BiP is an abundant chaperone within the lumen which is associated with early protein folding events. Other chaperones and foldases (see text) are also present. (b) Folding of the full-length fusion protein within the ER. (c) The fusion protein is cleaved within the Golgi body by a specific peptidase (Kex2p in *S. cerevisiae*) to release the heterologous protein to the cell exterior following transport of the protein by membrane-bound vesicles.

is that autonomous replication of nuclear plasmids is not normally an option with commercial filamentous fungi, and all vectors, with the exception of some used for research purposes, are designed to integrate into the fungal genome. As with yeast integration vectors, genomic integration of the transforming DNA brings added, though not necessarily complete, stability, but some uncertainty about the levels of gene expression expected and a limit to the number of gene copies that can be integrated. From a practical standpoint, a fungal transformation produces transformed strains that differ in their level of heterologous protein produced. One of the reasons for variation in gene expression upon genomic integration of the vector is that some parts of the genome are more transcriptionally active than others. Multiple copies of transforming DNA can be achieved through selection pressure and an elegant example in *A. niger* is the use of the *amdS* gene from *A. nidulans*, described earlier in Section 5.2.3. It is not, however, advantageous to increase the copies beyond a certain limit because there is no advantage in terms of protein yields. For example, beyond about 20 copies of the *A. niger glaA* promoter, essential transcription factors become limiting. Analogous observations were made in yeast (Section 5.6.2) and, there, the limitation was overcome by upregulating the expression of the transcription factor(s). This strategy may work also in filamentous fungi.

Aside from the gene dosage strategy just described, mutagenesis of protein-producing strains and screening the resulting mutants for improved protein production is another effective method for strain optimisation. Indeed, the combination of targeted *genetic modification* (GM) with conventional mutagenesis-based strain improvement provides a very powerful approach for improved production of heterologous proteins. Two further GM-based strategies are now routinely used (see also Chapter 21). The most commonly exploited fungi secrete proteases that might degrade the target heterologous protein. Therefore, one strategy is to use either protease-deficient mutant strains or strains in which specific protease genes have been eliminated by gene disruption or gene deletion. The second strategy is to employ gene fusions whereby the target gene is fused downstream of a gene encoding a naturally well-secreted 'carrier' protein such as glucoamylase in *A. niger* or cellobiohydrolase in *Trichoderma reesei*. When this tactic was used for production of calf chymosin, the chymosin (which is a protease) cleaved itself from the glucoamylase–prochymosin fusion at the pro-sequence boundary to release mature chymosin. For most heterologous proteins this approach is not possible and a cleavable protease site is included at the fusion junction. The site usually employed is the dibasic lysine–arginine sequence, which, in yeast, is the site for cleavage by the Kex2 protease. This works well too in filamentous fungi (Fig. 5.16). The fusion protein strategy appears to increase secreted protein yields by enhancing mRNA stability and by easing the passage of protein through the secretory pathway, although the underlying mechanisms are not known.

Recognition of bottle-necks in achieving high yields of secreted proteins that have the activities expected of the authentic proteins is the first step towards defining strategies to overcome the problems. It is already clear that, as with yeast expression, several factors can conspire to present a bottle-neck and that their relative importance depends on the heterologous protein. Foreign genes that use codons not common in fungi, the presence of sequences that destabilise mRNA, differences in the protein folding/secretory pathway and the abundance of proteases all contribute to the observed bottle-necks. In addition, although hyper-glycosylation of heterologous proteins is not such a problem with filamentous fungi as it is with *S. cerevisiae*, it can still be a difficulty. In addition, the patterns of glycosylation differ from those seen in mammalian cells, which could be important for therapeutic protein production. The glycan structures in fungal glycoproteins are being analysed and the genes that encode enzymes responsible for glycan assembly are being cloned, providing the possibility in the future of manipulating glycan synthesis.

The essential details of the secretory pathway in filamentous fungi appear to be qualitatively very similar to those in the yeast system, which has been studied more extensively. Some of the genes that encode chaperones and foldases have been cloned, as have genes that encode proteins involved in vesicular transport. Although successful manipulation of the protein secretory pathway using these genes has not yet been reported, the necessary tools to do so are becoming available.

5.7 | Further reading

Arora, D. K. (ed.) *Handbook of Fungal Biotechnology*, second edition. New York and Basel. Marcel Dekker, 2004.

Ausubel, F. M., Brent, R., Kingston, R. E. *et al. Short Protocols in Molecular Biology: A Compendium of Methods from Current Protocols in Molecular Biology*, fifth edition. New York: John Wiley & Sons, 2002.

Castrillo, J. O. and Oliver, S. G. Yeast as a touchstone in post-genomic research: strategies for integrative analysis in functional genomics. *Journal of Biochemical and Molecular Biology* **37**: 93–106, 2004.

Gellissen, G. and Hollenberg, C. P. Application of yeasts in gene expression studies: a comparison of *Saccharomyces cerevisiae, Hansenula polymorpha* and *Kluyveromyces lactis*. A review. *Gene* **190**: 87–97, 1997.

Gow, N. A. R. and Gadd, G. M. (eds.) *The Growing Fungus*. London: Chapman & Hall, 1995.

Gow, N. A. R., Robson, G. D. and Gadd, G. M. (eds.) *The Fungal Colony*. Cambridge: Cambridge University Press, 1999.

Luban, J. and Goff, S. P. The yeast two-hybrid system for studying protein–protein interactions. *Current Opinions in Biotechnology* **6**: 59–64, 1995.

MacKenzie, D. A., Jeenes, D. J. and Archer, D. B. Filamentous fungi as expression systems for heterologous proteins. In *Genetics and Biotechnology*, vol. 2, *The Mycota*, second edition, ed. U. Kuck. Berlin: Springer-Verlag, pp. 289–315, 2004.

Oliver, R. P. and Schweizer, M. (eds.) *Molecular Fungal Biology*. Cambridge: Cambridge University Press, 1999.

Talbot, N. (ed.) *Molecular and Cellular Biology of Filamentous Fungi: A Practical Approach*. Oxford: Oxford University Press, 2001.

Wolf, K. (ed.) *Non-Conventional Yeasts in Biotechnology*. Berlin: Springer-Verlag, 1996.

Chapter 6

Microbial process kinetics

Jens Nielsen

Technical University of Denmark

6.1 | Introduction

Quantitative description of cellular processes is an indispensable tool in the design of fermentation processes. Thus, the two most important quantitative design parameters, *yield* and *productivity*, are quantitative measures that specify how the cells convert the substrates to the product. The yield specifies the amount of product obtained from the substrate (or raw material) and the productivity specifies the rate of product formation. These two design parameters can easily be derived from experimental data, e.g. from measurement of the substrate consumption and the product formation. However, what is more difficult is to predict how they change with the operating conditions, e.g. if the medium composition changes or the temperature changes. In order to do this it is necessary to set up a mathematical model (see Box 6.1), which may be anything from a simple empirical correlation that specifies the product formation rate as a function of the medium composition, to a complex model that accounts for all the major cellular reactions involved in the conversion of the substrates to the product. Independent of the model structure, the process of defining a quantitative description of a fermentation process involves a number of steps (Fig. 6.1).

A key aspect in setting up a model is to specify the model's complexity. This depends much on the aim of the work, i.e. what the model is going to be used for, as discussed in Section 6.2.1. Specification of

Basic Biotechnology, third edition, eds. Colin Ratledge and Bjørn Kristiansen.
Published by Cambridge University Press. © Cambridge University Press 2006.

Figure 6.1 Different steps in quantitative description of fermentation processes.

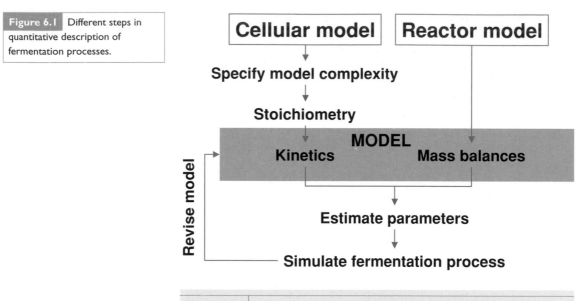

Figure 6.1 Different steps in quantitative description of fermentation processes.

Box 6.1 | Mathematical models

A mathematical model is a set of relationships between the variables in the system being studied. These relationships are normally expressed in the form of mathematical equations, but they may also be specified as logic expressions (or cause/effect relationships) that are used in the operation of a process. The variables include any properties that are of importance for the process, e.g. the agitation rate in the bioreactor, the feed rate to the bioreactor, pH and temperature of the medium, the concentration of substrates in the medium, the concentration of metabolic products, the biomass concentration, and the state of the biomass – often represented by the concentration of a set of key intracellular compounds. In order to set up a mathematical model it is necessary to specify a control volume wherein all the variables of interest are taken to be uniform, i.e. there are no variations in their values throughout the control volume. For fermentation processes the control volume is typically given by the volume of liquid in the whole bioreactor, but for large bioreactors the medium may be inhomogeneous due to mixing problems and here it is necessary to divide the bioreactor into several control volumes (see also Section 6.3). When the control volume is the whole bioreactor it may either be of constant volume or it may change with time, depending on the operation of the bioprocess. When the control volume has been defined, a set of balance equations can be specified for the variables of interest. These balance equations specify how material is flowing into and out of the control volume and how material is converted within the control volume. The conversion of material within the control volume is specified by so-called rate equations (or kinetic expressions), and together with the mass balances these two specify the complete model (see Fig. 6.1).

the model's complexity involves defining the number of reactions to be considered in the model, and specification of the stoichiometries for these reactions. When the model's complexity has been specified, rates of the cellular reactions considered in the model are described with mathematical expressions, i.e. the rates are specified as functions of the variables – namely the concentration of the substrates (and in some cases the metabolic products). These functions are normally referred to as *kinetic expressions*, since they specify the kinetics of the reactions considered in the model. This is an important step in the overall *modelling cycle* and in many cases different kinetic expressions have to be examined before a satisfactory model is obtained. The next step in the modelling process is to combine the kinetics of the cellular reactions with a model for the reactor in which the cellular process occurs. Such a model specifies how the concentrations of substrates, biomass and metabolic products change with time, and what flows in and out of the bioreactor. These *bioreactor models* are normally represented in terms of simple mass balances over the whole reactor, but more detailed reactor models may also be applied, if inhomogeneity of the medium is likely to play a role (see Section 6.3). The combination of the kinetic and the bioreactor model makes up a complete mathematical description of the fermentation process, and this model can be used to simulate the profile of the different variables of the process, e.g. the substrate and product concentrations. However, before this can be done it is necessary to assign values to the parameters of the model. Some of these parameters are operating parameters, which depend on how the process is operated, e.g. the volumetric flow in and out of the bioreactor, whereas others are kinetic parameters that are associated with the cellular system. In order to assign values to these parameters it is necessary to compare model simulations with experimental data, and hereby estimate a parameter set that gives the best fit of the model to the experimental data. This is referred to as parameter estimation. The evaluation of the fit of the model to the experimental data can be done by simple visual inspection of the fit, but generally it is preferred to use a more rational procedure, e.g. by minimising the sum of squared errors between the model and the experimental data. If the model simulations are considered to represent the experimental data sufficiently well the model is accepted, whereas if the fit is poor (for any set of parameters) it is necessary to revise the kinetic model and go through the modelling cycle again.

In the following we will consider the two different elements needed for setting up a bioprocess model, namely kinetic modelling and mass balances for bioreactors. This will lead to a description of different types of bioreactor operation, and hereby simple design problems can be illustrated.

6.2 | Kinetic modelling of cell growth

Models are used by all researchers in life sciences when results from individual experiments are interpreted and when results from several different experiments are compared with the aim of setting up a model that may explain the different observations. Thus biologists use models to interpret experiments on gene regulation and expression, and these models are very important when the message from often quite complicated experiments is to be presented. Most of these biological models are qualitative *only*, and they do not allow quantitative analysis. Often these *verbal models* can be relatively easy transferred to quantitative models, but a major obstacle in applying these quantitative models is estimation of the parameters of the model. In order to do this precise measurement of the different variables of the system is necessary and at different experimental conditions. Thus, quantitative description (or model simulations) goes hand-in-hand with experimental work, and quantitative modelling is often limited by the availability of reliable experimental data. During the last ten years there has been a revolution in experimental techniques applied in life sciences, and this has made possible far more detailed modelling of cellular processes. Furthermore, the availability of powerful computers has made it possible to solve even complex numerical problems within a reasonable computational time. At present, even complex mathematical models for biological processes can therefore be handled and experimentally verified. However, such detailed (or mechanistic) models are often of little use in the design of a bioprocess, whereas they mainly serve a purpose in fundamental research of biological phenomena. In this presentation we will focus on models that are useful for the design of bioprocesses, but in order to give an overview of the different mathematical models applied to describe biological processes we start the presentation of kinetic models with a discussion of model complexity.

6.2.1 Model structure and model complexity

Biological processes are extremely complex per se. Cell growth and metabolite formation are the result of a very large number of cellular reactions and events like gene expression, translation of mRNA into functional proteins, further processing of proteins into functional enzymes or structural proteins, and long sequences of biochemical reactions leading to building blocks needed for synthesis of cellular components. All these different reactions can roughly be divided into four groups as shown in Fig. 6.2. It is quite clear that a complete description of all the possible reactions and events cannot be included in a mathematical model. In fermentation processes, where there is a large population of cells, inhomogeneity of the cells with respect to activity and function may add further to the complexity. In setting up fermentation models, lumping of cellular reactions and events is therefore always done, but the detail level considered in the model, i.e. the degree of lumping, depends on the aim of the modelling.

Fermentation models can roughly be divided into four groups depending on the level of detail included in the model (Fig. 6.3). The simplest description is the so-called *unstructured models* where the biomass is described by a single variable (often the total biomass concentration) and where no segregation in the cell population is considered, *i.e.* all the cells in the population are assumed to have identical properties. These models can be combined with a *segregated*

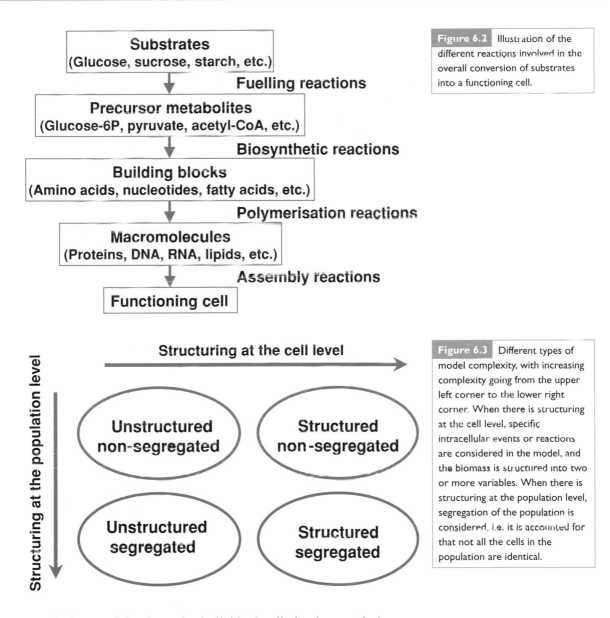

Figure 6.2 Illustration of the different reactions involved in the overall conversion of substrates into a functioning cell.

Figure 6.3 Different types of model complexity, with increasing complexity going from the upper left corner to the lower right corner. When there is structuring at the cell level, specific intracellular events or reactions are considered in the model, and the biomass is structured into two or more variables. When there is structuring at the population level, segregation of the population is considered, i.e. it is accounted for that not all the cells in the population are identical.

population model, where the individual cells in the population are described by a single variable, e.g. the cell mass or cell age, but often it is relevant to add further structure to the model when segregation in the cell population is considered. In the so-called *structured models* the biomass is described with more than one variable, i.e. structure in the biomass is considered. This structure may be anything from a simple structuring into a few compartments to a detailed structuring into individual enzymes and macromolecular pools.

From the above it is clear that a very important element in mathematical modelling of fermentation processes is defining the model structure (or specifying the complexity of the model), and for this a general rule can be stated as: *as simple as possible, but not simpler*. This rule implies that the basic mechanisms should always be included and that the model structure depends on the aim of the modelling exercise (see Box 6.2). Thus, if the aim is to simulate the biomass concentration in a fermentation process, a simple unstructured model (Sections 6.2.3 and 6.2.4) may be sufficient. However, if the aim is to analyse a given system in further detail it is necessary to include much more structure in the model and, in this case, one often describes only individual processes within the cell, e.g. a certain pathway or gene transcription from a certain promoter.

Box 6.2 | Model complexity

A simple illustration of difference in model complexity is the quantitative description of the fractional saturation y of a protein at a ligand concentration c_l. This may be described either by the Hill equation:

$$y = \frac{c_l^h}{c_l^h + K} \tag{1}$$

where h and K are empirical parameters, or the equation of Monod:

$$y = \frac{\left[L a \left(1 + \dfrac{a c_l}{K_R} \right)^3 + \left(1 + \dfrac{c_l}{K_R} \right)^3 \right] \dfrac{c_l}{K_R}}{L \left(1 + \dfrac{a c_l}{K_R} \right)^4 + \left(1 + \dfrac{c_l}{K_R} \right)^4} \tag{2}$$

where L, a and K_R are parameters. Both equations address the same experimental problem, but whereas Eq. (1) is completely empirical with h and K as fitted parameters, Eq. (2) is derived from a hypothesis for the mechanism and the parameters therefore have a direct physical interpretation. If the aim of the modelling is to understand the underlying mechanism of the process, Eq. (1) cannot obviously be applied since the kinetic parameters are completely empirical and give no (or little) information about the ligand binding to the protein. In this case, Eq. (2) should be applied, since by estimating the kinetic parameter the investigator is supplied with valuable information about the system and the parameters can be directly interpreted. If, on the other hand, the aim of the modelling is to simulate the ligand binding to the protein, Eq. (1) may be as good as Eq. (2) – one may even prefer Eq. (1) since it is more simple in structure and has fewer parameters and it actually often gives a better fit to experimental data than Eq. (2). Thus, the answer to which model one should prefer depends on the aim of the modelling exercise.

6.2.2 Definitions of rates and yield coefficients

Before we turn to description of different unstructured models a few definitions are needed. Figure 6.4 is a representation of the overall conversion of substrates into metabolic products and biomass components (or total biomass). The rates of substrate consumption can be determined during a fermentation process by measuring the concentration of these substrates in the medium. Similarly, the formation rates of metabolic products and biomass can be determined from measurements of the corresponding concentrations. It is therefore possible to determine what flows into the total pool of cells

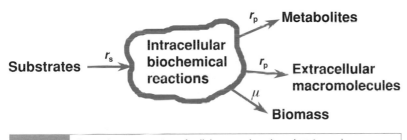

Figure 6.4 General representation of cellular growth and product formation. Substrates are converted, via the large number of intracellular biochemical reactions, into metabolic products, e.g. ethanol, lactate or penicillin (and other secondary metabolites), extracellular macromolecules, e.g. a secreted enzyme, a heterologous protein or a polysaccharide, and into biomass constituents, e.g. cellular protein, lipids, RNA, DNA and carbohydrates.

and what flows out of this pool. The inflow of a substrate is normally referred to as the substrate uptake rate and the outflow of a metabolic product is normally referred to as the product formation rate. From the direct measurements of the concentrations one obtains so-called *volumetric rates* [units: g (l h)$^{-1}$ or moles (l h)$^{-1}$]. Often it is convenient to normalise the rates with the amount of biomass (DW = dry wt) to obtain *specific rates*, and these are often represented as r_i [units: g (g DW h)$^{-1}$ or moles (g DW h)$^{-1}$], where the subscript, i, indicates whether it is a substrate (s) or a metabolic product (p). The *specific growth rate* of the total biomass is also an important variable, and it is generally designated μ [unit: g DW (g DW h)$^{-1}$ or simply h^{-1}]. The specific growth rate is related to the *doubling time* t_d(h) of the biomass through:

$$t_d = \frac{\ln 2}{\mu} \tag{6.1}$$

The doubling time t_d is equal to the generation time for a cell, *i.e.* the length of a cell cycle for unicellular organisms, which is frequently used by life scientists to quantify the rate of cell growth.

The specific rates – or the flow in and out of the cell – are very important design parameters, since they are related to the productivity of the cell. Thus, the specific productivity of a given metabolite directly indicates the rate at which the cells synthesise this metabolite. Furthermore, if the specific rate is multiplied by the biomass concentration in the bioreactor one obtains the volumetric productivity, or the synthesis rate of the biomass population per reactor volume. In simple kinetic models the specific rates are specified as functions of the variables in the system, e.g. the substrate concentrations. In more complex models where the rates of the intracellular reactions are specified as functions of the variables in the system, the substrate uptake rates and product formation rates are given as functions of the intracellular reactions rates.

Another class of very important design parameters are the yield coefficients, which quantify the amount of substrate recovered in

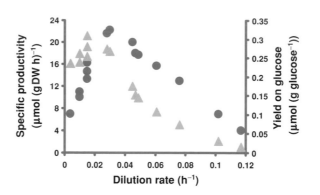

Figure 6.5 The specific penicillin productivity ● and the yield of penicillin ▲ on glucose for different specific growth rates (equal to the dilution rate in a chemostat, see Section 6.3.3).

biomass and the metabolic products. The yield coefficients are given as ratios of the specific rates, e.g. for the yield of biomass on a substrate:

$$Y_{sx} = \frac{\mu}{r_s} \tag{6.2}$$

and similarly for the yield of a metabolic product on a substrate:

$$Y_{sp} = \frac{r_p}{r_s} \tag{6.3}$$

The yield coefficients are determined by how the carbon in the substrate is distributed among the different cellular pathways towards the end-products of the catabolic and anabolic routes. These parameters can be considered as an overall determination of metabolic fluxes, a key aspect in modern physiological studies where methods to quantify intracellular, metabolic fluxes have become important tools. In the production of low-value-added products, e.g. ethanol, bulk antibiotics and amino acids, it is important to optimise the yield of product on the substrate, and the target is therefore to direct as much carbon as possible towards the product and minimise the carbon flow to other products (including biomass). For aerobic processes, the yield of carbon dioxide on oxygen is often used to characterise the metabolism of the cells. This yield coefficient is referred to as the *respiratory quotient* (RQ), and with pure respiration it is close to 1 whereas if a metabolite is formed it deviates from 1 (see also Section 6.2.4).

The yield coefficients are always given with a double index which indicates the direction of the conversion, i.e. the yield for the conversion of substrate to biomass ($s \rightarrow x$) has the index sx. With the definitions of the yield coefficients it is clear that:

$$Y_{ij} = \frac{1}{Y_{ji}} \tag{6.4}$$

Thus, the yield coefficient Y_{xs} specifies the amount of substrate used per unit biomass formed, and similarly the yield coefficient Y_{xp} specifies the amount of product formed per unit biomass formed. With the yield coefficient and the specific rate defining two very important design parameters in terms of optimisation of fermentation processes, it is unfortunately rarely possible to optimise both parameters

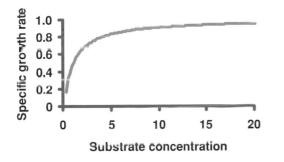

Figure 6.6 The specific growth rate as a function of the concentration of the limiting substrate when the Monod model is applied. Both parameters of the model are normalised to 1, i.e. $\mu_{max} = K_s = 1$.

at the same time. This is illustrated in Fig. 6.5, where the specific productivity of penicillin is shown together with the yield of penicillin on glucose for different specific growth rates. The data clearly show that the yield is optimum for a lower specific growth rate compared with the specific rate, and it is therefore important to weigh the relative importance of these two parameters in the overall optimisation of the process.

6.2.3 Black box models

The most simple mathematical presentation of cell growth is the so-called *black box* model, where all the cellular reactions are lumped into a single overall reaction. This implies that the yield of biomass on the substrate (as well as the yield of all other compounds consumed and produced by the cells) is constant. Consequently the specific substrate uptake rate can be specified as a function of the specific growth rate of the biomass, simply by rewriting Eq. (6.2):

$$r_s = Y_{xs}\mu \tag{6.5}$$

The specific uptake rate of other substrates, e.g. uptake of oxygen, and the formation rate of metabolic products is similarly proportional to the specific growth rate. In the black box model, the kinetics reduce to a description of the specific growth rate as a function of the variables in the system. In the most simple model description it is assumed that there is only one limiting substrate, typically the carbon source (which is often glucose), and the specific growth rate is therefore specified as a function of the concentration of this substrate only. A very general observation for cell growth on a single limiting substrate is that at low substrate concentrations (c_s) the specific growth rate μ is proportional to c_s, but for increasing values there is an upper value for the specific growth rate. This verbal presentation can be described with many different mathematical models, but the most often applied is the Monod model, which states that:

$$\mu = \mu_{max}\frac{c_s}{c_s + K_s} \tag{6.6}$$

where μ_{max} represents the maximum specific growth rate of the cells and K_s is numerically equal to the substrate concentration at which the specific growth rate is $0.5\mu_{max}$. The influence of the substrate concentration on the specific growth rate with the Monod model is

Table 6.1 Typical K_s values for different microbial cells growing on different sugars

Species	Substrate	$K_s(mg\ l^{-1})$
Aerobacter aerogenes	Glucose	8
Aspergillus oryzae	Glucose	5
Escherichia coli	Glucose	4
Klebsiella aerogenes	Glucose	9
	Glycerol	9
Klebsiella oxytoca	Glucose	10
	Arabinose	50
	Fructose	10
Penicillium chrysogenum	Glucose	4
Saccharomyces cerevisiae	Glucose	180

Table 6.2 Compilation of different unstructured, kinetic models

Model name	Kinetic expression
Tessier	$\mu = \mu_{max}\left(1 - e^{-c_s/K_s}\right)$
Moser	$\mu = \mu_{max}\dfrac{c_s^n}{c_s^n + K_s}$
Contois	$\mu = \mu_{max}\dfrac{c_s}{c_s + K_s x}$
Blackman	$\mu = \begin{cases} \mu_{max}\dfrac{c_s}{2K_s}; & c_s \le 2K_s \\ \mu_{max}; & c_s \ge 2K_s \end{cases}$
Logistic law	$\mu = \mu_{max}\left(1 - \dfrac{x}{K_x}\right)$

illustrated in Fig. 6.6. The parameter K_s is sometimes interpreted as the affinity of the cells towards the substrates. Since the substrate uptake often is involved in the control of substrate metabolism, the value of K_s is also often in the range of the K_m values of the substrate uptake system of the cells. However, K_s is an overall parameter for all the reactions involved in the conversion of the substrate to biomass, and it is therefore completely empirical and has no physical meaning. Table 6.1 summarizes the K_s value for different microbial systems.

The Monod model is not the only kinetic expression that has been proposed to describe the specific growth rate in the black box model. Many different kinetic expressions have been presented and Table 6.2 compiles some of the most frequently applied models. In the Contois kinetics, an influence of the biomass concentration x is included, i.e. at high biomass concentrations there is an inhibition on cell growth. It is unlikely that the biomass concentration as such inhibits cell growth, but there may well be an indirect effect, e.g. by the formation of an inhibitor compound by the biomass or high biomass concentrations may give a very viscous medium that results in mass transfer problems. These different expressions clearly demonstrate the empirical nature of these kinetic models, and it is therefore futile to discuss which model is to be preferred, since they are all simply data fitters, and one should simply choose the model that gives the best description of the system studied.

All the kinetic expressions presented above assume that there is only one limiting substrate, but often more than one substrate concentration influences the specific growth rate. In these situations complex interactions can occur which are difficult to model with unstructured models unless many adjustable parameters are admitted. Several different multi-parameter, unstructured models for growth on multiple substrates have been proposed, and here one often distinguishes between whether a second substrate is growth enhancing or also growth limiting. A general kinetic expression that accounts for both types of substrates is:

$$\mu = \left(1 + \sum_i \frac{c_{s_i,e}}{c_{s_i,e} + K_{e,i}}\right) \prod_j \frac{\mu_{max,j} c_{s,j}}{c_{s,j} + K_{s,j}} \tag{6.7}$$

where $c_{s,e}$ is the concentration of a growth-enhancing substrate and c_s is the concentration of a substrate essential for growth. The presence of growth-enhancing substrates results in an increased specific growth rate whereas the essential substrates are absolutely necessary for growth to take place. A special case of Eq. (6.7) is the growth in the presence of two essential substrates, i.e.

$$\mu = \frac{\mu_{max,1} \mu_{max,2} c_{s,1} c_{s,2}}{(c_{s,1} + K_1)(c_{s,2} + K_s)} \tag{6.8}$$

If the concentration of both substrates is at a level where the specific growth rate for each substrate reaches 90% of its maximum value, i.e. $c_{s,i} = 0.9\ K_i$, then the total rate of growth is limited to 81% of the maximum possible value. This is hardly reasonable and several alternatives to Eq. (6.8) have therefore been proposed, and one of these is

$$\frac{\mu}{\mu_{max}} = \min\left(\frac{c_{s,1}}{c_{s,1} + K_1}, \frac{c_{s,2}}{c_{s,2} + K_2}\right) \tag{6.9}$$

Growth on two or more substrates, which may substitute for each other, e.g. glucose and lactose, cannot be described by any of the unstructured models described above. Consider, for example, growth of *Escherichia coli* on glucose and lactose. Glucose is a more favourable substrate and will therefore be metabolised first. The metabolism of lactose will only begin when the glucose is exhausted. The bacterium needs one of the sugars to grow, but in the presence of glucose there is no growth-enhancing effect of lactose. To describe this so-called *diauxic* growth it is necessary to apply a structured model and, in general, it is advisable to consider a single limiting substrate in black box models only.

In some cases growth is inhibited either by high concentrations of the limiting substrate or by the presence of a metabolic product.

In order to account for these aspects the Monod kinetics is often extended with additional terms. Thus for inhibition by high concentrations of the limiting substrate we get:

$$\mu = \mu_{\max} \frac{c_s}{c_{s^2}/K_i + c_s + K_s} \tag{6.10}$$

and for inhibition by a metabolic product:

$$\mu = \mu_{\max} \frac{c_s}{c_s + K_s} \frac{1}{1 + p/K_i} \tag{6.11}$$

Equations (6.10) and (6.11) may be a useful way of including product or substrate inhibition in a simple model. Extension of the Monod model with additional terms or factors should, however, be done with some hesitation since the result may be a model with a large number of parameters but of little value outside the range in which the experiments were made.

6.2.4 Linear rate equations

In the black box model all the yield coefficients are taken to be constant. This implies that all the cellular reactions are lumped into a single overall growth reaction where substrate is converted to biomass. A requirement for this assumption is that there is a constant distribution of fluxes through all the different cellular pathways at different growth conditions. This assumption is not valid as the yield of biomass on substrate is not constant. To describe this observation the concept of *endogenous metabolism* was introduced, which specified substrate consumption for this process in addition to that for biomass synthesis, *i.e.* substrate consumption takes place in two different reactions. In a parallel development it was also established that lactic acid bacteria produce lactic acid under non-growth conditions, which was consistent with an endogenous metabolism of the cells. The result indicated a linear correlation between the specific lactic acid production rate and the specific growth rate:

$$r_p = a\mu + b \tag{6.12}$$

where a and b are two constants. Later, the term *maintenance*, a linear correlation between the specific substrate uptake rate and the specific growth rate, was introduced to replace the endogenous respiration concept (see Box 6.3). The linear correlation for maintenance takes the form

$$r_s = Y_{xs}^{true}\mu + m_s \tag{6.13}$$

where Y_{xs}^{true} is referred to as the true yield coefficient and m_s as the maintenance coefficient. The maintenance coefficients quantify the rate of substrate consumption for cellular maintenance, and it is normally given as a constant. In principle this gives rise to a conflict since this may result in substrate consumption even when the substrate concentration is zero ($c_s = 0$), and in some cases it may therefore be necessary to specify m_s as a function of c_s.

Box 6.3 | Maintenance

Substrate consumption for maintenance of cellular function is a result of many different processes in the cells. Common for all these processes is that they consume Gibbs free energy (typically in the form of ATP) without net formation of new cell mass. In order to supply this Gibbs free energy, the substrate needs to be catabolised and the overall result is therefore substrate consumption without net formation of cell mass. The three most important maintenance processes are:

- Maintenance of concentration and electrical gradients across cellular membranes. Across the cytoplasmic and other cellular membranes there are large concentration gradients of many different compounds, especially of protons, minerals and other ions. These gradients result in electrical gradients across the membranes, which are essential for cellular function.
- Futile cycles. In the cells there are pairs of reactions that result in the net consumption of Gibbs free energy only. An example is the phosphorylation of fructose 6-phosphate to fructose 1,6-bisphosphate with the consumption of ATP (catalysed by phosphofructokinase) and the reverse reaction, which does not lead to formation of ATP (catalysed by fructose 1,6-bisphosphatase). The hydrolysis of fructose 1,6-bisphosphate to fructose 6-phosphate is repressed by glucose, and is therefore not very active when there is a high glycolytic flux. However, there is always some activity of the hydrolysis reaction, and a futile cycle is therefore active.
- Turnover of macromolecules. A number of macromolecules are continuously synthesised and degraded, and this is a special group of futile cycles, since the net result is consumption of Gibbs free energy without formation of cell mass. Among the most prominent group of macromolecules that is continuously synthesised and degraded is mRNA, which has a very short half-life in the cell.

With the introduction of linear correlations, the yield coefficients obviously cannot be constants. Thus for the biomass yield on the substrate:

$$Y_{sx} = \frac{\mu}{Y_{xs}^{true}\mu + m_s} \tag{6.14}$$

which shows that Y_{sx} decreases at low specific growth rates where an increasing fraction of the substrate is used to meet the maintenance requirements of the cell. For large specific growth rates, the yield coefficient approaches the reciprocal of Y_{xs}^{true}. This corresponds to the situation where the maintenance substrate consumption becomes negligible compared with the substrate consumption for biomass growth, and Eq. (6.13) can be approximated to Eq. (6.5). Despite its simple structure the linear rate equation Eq. (6.13) has been found to be valid for many different species, and Table 6.3 compiles true yield coefficients and maintenance coefficients for various microbial species.

The empirically derived, linear correlations are very useful to correlate growth data, especially in steady-state continuous cultures where linear correlations similar to Eq. (6.13) are found for most of the important specific rates. The remarkable robustness and general

Table 6.3 True yield and maintenance coefficients for different microbial species and growth on glucose or glycerol

Organism	Substrate	Y_{xs}^{true} $(g(gDW)^{-1})$	m_s $(g(gDWh)^{-1})$
Aspergillus awamori	Glucose	1.92	0.016
Aspergillus nidulans		1.67	0.020
Aspergillus niger			
Aspergillus oryzae			
Candida utilis		2.00	0.031
Escherichia coli		2.27	0.057
Klebsiella aerogenes		2.27	0.063
Penicillium chrysogenum		2.17	0.021
Saccharomyces cerevisiae		1.85	0.015
Aerobacter aerogenes	Glycerol	1.79	0.089
Bacillus megatarium		1.67	–
Klebsiella aerogenes		2.13	0.074

validity of the linear correlations indicates that they have a fundamental basis, and this basis is likely to be the continuous supply and consumption of ATP, since these two processes are tightly coupled in all cells. Thus the role of the energy producing substrate is to provide ATP to drive both the biosynthetic and polymerisation reactions of the cell and the different maintenance processes according to the linear relationship

$$r_{ATP} = Y_{xATP}\mu + m_{ATP} \tag{6.15}$$

which is a formal analogue to the linear maintenance correlation. Equation (6.15) states that ATP produced balances the consumption for growth and for maintenance, and if the ATP yield on the energy producing substrate is constant, i.e. r_{ATP} is proportional to r_s, it is quite obvious that Eq. (6.15) can be used to derive the linear correlation Eq. (6.13). Notice that Y_{xATP} in Eq. (6.15) is not a real yield coefficient but a parameter.

6.2.5 Effect of temperature and pH

The reaction temperature and the pH of the growth medium are process conditions with a bearing on the growth kinetics. It is normally desired to keep both of these variables constant (and at their optimal values) throughout the cultivation process – hence they are often called *culture parameters* to distinguish them from other variables such as reactant concentrations, stirring rate, oxygen supply rate, etc., which can change dramatically from the start to the end of a cultivation. The influence of temperature and pH on individual cell processes can be very different, and since the growth process is the result of many enzymatic processes the influence of both variables (or culture parameters) on the over-all bioreaction is quite complex.

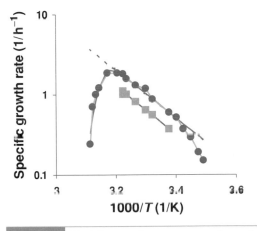

Figure 6.7 The influence of temperature on the maximum specific growth rate shown by a typical Arrhenius plot (reciprocal absolute temperature on the abscissa and log (μ) on the ordinate) for *E. coli*. (■) Growth on a glucose-rich medium, (•) growth on a glucose-poor medium. The linear portion of the curve between ~21.0 and 37.5 °C is well represented by Eq. (6.16), while the sharp bend and rapid decrease of μ for $T >$ 39 °C shows the influence of the denominator term in (6.17).

The influence of temperature on the maximum specific growth rate of a microorganism is similar to that observed for the activity of an enzyme: an increase with increasing temperature up to a certain point where protein denaturation starts, and a rapid decrease beyond this temperature. For temperatures below the onset of protein denaturation the maximum specific growth rate increases in much the same way as for a normal chemical rate constant:

$$\mu_{\max} = A \exp\left(-\frac{E_g}{RT}\right) \tag{6.16}$$

where A is a constant and E_g is the activation energy of the growth process.

Assuming that the proteins are temperature denatured by a reversible chemical reaction with free energy change ΔG_d and that denatured proteins are inactive one may propose an expression for $\mu_{\max}$:

$$\mu_{\max} = \frac{A \exp\left(-E_g/RT\right)}{1 + B \exp\left(-\Delta G_d/RT\right)} \tag{6.17}$$

The influence of pH on the cellular activity is determined by the sensitivity of the individual enzymes to changes in the pH. Enzymes are normally only active within a certain pH interval, and the total enzyme activity of the cell is therefore a complex function of the environmental pH. As an example we shall consider the influence of pH on a single enzyme, which is taken to represent the cell activity. The enzyme is assumed to exist in three forms:

$$e \leftrightarrow e^- + H^+ \leftrightarrow e^{2-} + 2H^+ \tag{6.18}$$

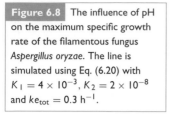

Figure 6.8 The influence of pH on the maximum specific growth rate of the filamentous fungus *Aspergillus oryzae*. The line is simulated using Eq. (6.20) with $K_1 = 4 \times 10^{-3}$, $K_2 = 2 \times 10^{-8}$ and $ke_{tot} = 0.3 \ h^{-1}$.

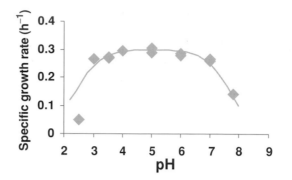

where e^- is taken to be the active form of the enzyme while the two other forms are assumed to be completely inactive. K_1 and K_2 are the dissociation constants for e and e^-, respectively. The fraction of active enzyme e^- is calculated to be:

$$\frac{e^-}{e_{tot}} = \frac{1}{1 + [H^+]/K_1 + K_2/[H^+]} \tag{6.19}$$

and the enzyme activity is taken to be $k = k_e e^-$. If the cell activity is determined by the activity of the enzyme considered above, the maximum specific growth rate will be:

$$\mu_{max} = \frac{ke_{tot}}{1 + [H^+]/K_1 + K_2/[H^+]} \tag{6.20}$$

Although the dependence of cell activity on pH cannot possibly be explained by this simple model it has been found that Eq. (6.20) gives an adequate fit for many microorganisms, and Fig. 6.8 shows fit of the model for some data of the filamentous fungus *Aspergillus oryzae*.

6.3 | Mass balances for ideal bioreactors

The last step in modelling of fermentation processes is to combine the kinetic model with a model for the bioreactor. A bioreactor model is normally represented by a set of dynamic mass balances for the substrates, the metabolic products and the biomass, which describes the change in time of the concentration of these state variables. The bioreactor may be any type of device ranging from a test tube or a shake flask to a well-instrumented bioreactor. Normally the bioreactor is assumed to be completely (or ideally) mixed, i.e. there is no spatial variation in the concentration of the different medium compounds. For small volume bioreactors (<50 litres), including shake flasks, this can generally be achieved through aeration and agitation. In larger bioreactors there may be significant concentration gradients through-out the bioreactor, and for simulation of fermentation processes at an industrial scale it may be necessary to consider concentration gradients in the bioreactor (see Chapter 8). This can be done by defining different control volumes in the bioreactor, and then by setting up mass balances for each control volume. Agitation and aeration in the bioreactor will ensure exchange of material between the different control volumes. Many different models have been proposed for description of such inhomogeneities in bioreactors, but we will only consider the simple case where the bioreactor volume is assumed to be completely mixed. Figure 6.9 is a general representation of a bioreactor.

The bioreactor may be operated in three different modes:

- **batch**, where $F = F_{out} = 0$, i.e. the volume is constant;
- **continuous**, where $F = F_{out} > 0$, i.e. the volume is constant; and
- **fed-batch** (or semi-batch), where $F > 0$ and $F_{out} = 0$, i.e. the volume increases.

In the following these three different operation modes are described in detail and Table 6.4 summarises their advantages and disadvantages. The mass balances for the different bioreactor modes can all be derived from a set of general mass balances, and we therefore start to consider these general balances.

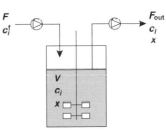

Figure 6.9 General representation of a bioreactor with addition of fresh, sterile medium at a flow rate F ($l\,h^{-1}$) and removal of spent medium at a flow rate of F_{out} ($l\,h^{-1}$), where c_i^f is the concentration of the ith compound (typically a substrate) in the feed and c_i is the concentration of the ith compound in the spent medium. The reactor has the volume V (l) and is assumed to be well mixed (or ideal), whereby the concentration of each compound in the spent medium becomes identical to its concentration in the bioreactor. The biomass concentration in the bioreactor is designated x.

6.3.1   General mass balance equations

The basis for derivation of the general dynamic mass balances is the mass balance equation:

$$\text{Accumulation} = \text{Net formation rate} + \text{Flow} - \text{Flow out} \quad (6.21)$$

The term *accumulation* specifies the rate of change of the compound in the bioreactor, e.g. the rate of increase in the biomass concentration during a batch fermentation. For substrates the term *net formation rate* for metabolic products and biomass is given by the formation rate of these variables (which will all be positive), whilst for a substrate it will be given by the substrate uptake, or consumption, rate (which will be negative). The term *flow in* is the flow of the compounds into the bioreactor and the term *flow out* is the flow of compounds out from the bioreactor. For the ith substrate, which is added to the bioreactor via the feed and is consumed by the cells present in the bioreactor the mass balance is:

$$\frac{d(c_{s,i}V)}{dt} = -r_{s,i}xV + F\,c_{s,i}^f - F_{out}c_{s,i} \quad (6.22)$$

were r_i is the specific substrate uptake rate [moles (g DW h)$^{-1}$], $c_{s,i}$ is the concentration in the bioreactor, which is assumed to be the same as the concentration in the outlet (moles or g l^{-1}), $c_{s,i}^f$ is the concentration in the feed (moles or g l^{-1}) and x is the biomass concentration in the bioreactor (g DW l^{-1}). The first term in Eq. (6.22) is the accumulation term, the second term accounts for substrate consumption (or net formation), the third term accounts for the inlet and the last term accounts for the outlet. Rearrangement of Eq. (6.22) gives:

$$\frac{dc_{s,i}}{dt} = -r_{s,i}x + \frac{F}{V}c_{s,i}^f - \left(\frac{F_{out}}{V} + \frac{1}{V}\frac{dV}{dt}\right)c_{s,i} \quad (6.23)$$

For a fed-batch reactor we have:

$$F = \frac{dV}{dt} \quad (6.24)$$

Table 6.4	Advantages and disadvantages of different modes of bioreactor operation	
Reactor	Advantages	Disadvantages
Batch	Versatile, since it can be used for many different processes Low risk of contamination Complete conversion of substrate possible	High labour cost Much idle time, due to cleaning and sterilisation after each fermentation
Continuous	High efficiency of the reactor capacity High productivity can be maintained for long periods of time Automation is simple Constant product quality	Problems with infection Possibility of the appearance of low levels of mutant production during long operation Inflexible since it can rarely be used for different processes without substantial retrofitting Downstream processing has to be adjusted to the flow through the bioreactor (or holding tanks are required)
Fed-batch	Allows operating at well-controlled conditions by controlling the feed addition Allows very high cell densities and thereby high final titres	Some of the same problems as for the batch and continuous reactor, but generally the disadvantages are less pronounced with this mode of operation

and $F_{out} = 0$, the term within the parenthesis becomes equal to the so-called *dilution rate* given by:

$$D = \frac{F}{V} \tag{6.25}$$

For a continuous and a batch reactor the volume is constant, i.e. $dV/dt = 0$, and $F = F_{out}$, and for these bioreactor modes the term within the parenthesis becomes equal to the dilution rate also. Equation (6.23) therefore reduces to the mass balance equation (6.26) for any type of operation:

$$\frac{dc_{s,i}}{dt} = -r_{s,i}x + D\left(c_{s,i}^f - c_{s,i}\right) \tag{6.26}$$

Dynamic mass balances for the metabolic products are derived in analogy with those for the substrates and take the form:

$$\frac{dc_{p,i}}{dt} = r_{p,i}x + D\left(c_{s,i}^f - c_{s,i}\right) \tag{6.27}$$

where the first term on the right-hand side is the volumetric formation rate of the ith metabolic product. Normally the metabolic products are not present in the sterile feed to the bioreactor and $c_{p,i}^f$ is therefore often zero. With sterile feed the mass balance for the total biomass is:

$$\frac{d(xV)}{dt} = \mu xV - F_{out}x \tag{6.28}$$

which, in analogy with the substrate balance, can be rewritten as:

$$\frac{dx}{dt} = (\mu - D)x \tag{6.29}$$

6.3.2 The batch reactor

This is the classical operation of the bioreactor, and it is used extensively. Batch experiments have the advantage of being easy to perform, and by using shake flasks a large number of parallel experiments can be carried out. The disadvantage in research is that the experimental data are difficult to interpret since there are dynamic conditions throughout the experiment, i.e. the environmental conditions experienced by the cells vary with time. In well-instrumented laboratory bioreactors many variables, e.g. pH and dissolved oxygen tension, may be kept constant, and this allows study of the effect of a single substrate on the biomass growth and product formation. The dilution rate is zero for a batch reactor and the mass balances for the biomass and the limiting substrate[1] therefore takes the form:

$$\frac{dx}{dt} = \mu x; \quad x(t = 0) = x_0 \tag{6.30}$$

$$\frac{dc_s}{dt} = -r_s x; \quad c_s(t = 0) = c_{s,0} \tag{6.31}$$

where x_0 indicates the initial biomass concentration, which is obtained right after inoculation, and $c_{s,0}$ is the initial concentration of the limiting substrate. According to these mass balances the biomass concentration will increase and the substrate concentration will decrease until its concentration reaches zero and growth stops. Assuming Monod kinetics, the mass balances for biomass and the limiting substrate can be rearranged into one first-order differential equation in the biomass concentration and an algebraic equation relating the substrate concentration to the biomass concentration. The algebraic equation is given by:

$$c_s = c_{s,0} - Y_{xs}(x - x_0) \tag{6.32}$$

and the solution to the differential equation for the biomass concentration is given by:

$$\mu_{max}t = \left(1 + \frac{K_s}{c_{s,0} + Y_{xs}x_0}\right)\ln\left(\frac{x}{x_0}\right)$$
$$- \frac{K_s}{c_{s,0} + Y_{xs}x_0}\ln\left(1 + \frac{x_0 - x}{Y_{xs}c_{s,0}}\right) \tag{6.33}$$

Using these equations the profiles of the biomass and the glucose concentrations during a typical batch culture are easily derived (see Fig. 6.10). Since the substrate concentration is zero at the end of the

---

[1] In a batch fermentation the limiting substrate is defined as the substrate that is first exhausted.

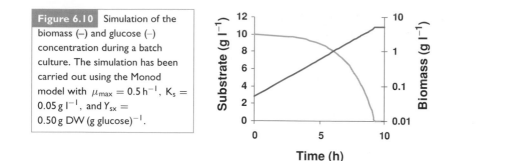

Figure 6.10 Simulation of the biomass (–) and glucose (–) concentration during a batch culture. The simulation has been carried out using the Monod model with $\mu_{max} = 0.5\,h^{-1}$, $K_s = 0.05\,g\,l^{-1}$, and $Y_{sx} = 0.50\,g$ DW (g glucose)$^{-1}$.

cultivation the overall yield of biomass on the substrate can be found from:

$$Y_{sx}^{overall} = \frac{x_{final} - x_0}{c_{s,0}} \tag{6.34}$$

where x_{final} is the biomass concentration at the end of the cultivation. Normally $x_0 \ll x_{final}$, and the overall yield coefficient can therefore be estimated from the final biomass concentration and the initial substrate concentration alone.

Notice that the yield coefficient determined from Eq. (6.34) is the overall yield coefficient and not Y_{sx} nor Y_{xs}^{true}. The yield coefficient Y_{sx} may well be time dependent since it is the ratio between the specific growth rate and the substrate uptake rate (see Eq. (6.2)). However, if there is little variation in these rates during the batch culture (e.g. if there is a long exponential growth phase and only a very short declining growth phase) the overall yield coefficient may be very similar to the yield coefficient. If there is maintenance metabolism the true yield coefficient is difficult to determine from a batch cultivation, since it requires information about the maintenance coefficients, which is difficult to estimate from a batch experiment. However, if the specific growth rate is close to its maximum throughout most of the growth phase, the substrate consumption due to maintenance will be negligible and, according to Eq. (6.14), the true yield coefficient is close to the observed yield coefficient determined from the final biomass concentration.

6.3.3 The chemostat

A typical operation of the continuous bioreactor is the so-called *chemostat*, where the added medium is designed such that one single substrate is limiting. This allows for controlled variation in the specific growth rate of the biomass. By varying the feed flow rate to the bioreactor the environmental conditions can be varied and thereby valuable information concerning the influence of the environmental conditions on the cellular physiology can be obtained. Other examples of continuous operation besides the chemostat are the *pH-stat*, where the feed flow is adjusted to maintain the pH constant in the bioreactor, and the *turbidostat*, where the feed flow is adjusted to maintain the biomass concentration at a constant level. From the biomass mass balance equation (6.29) it can be seen that in a steady-state continuous reactor the specific growth rate equals the dilution rate:

$$\mu = D \tag{6.35}$$

Thus, by varying the dilution rate (or the feed flow rate) in a continuous culture different specific growth rates can be obtained. This allows detailed physiological studies of the cells when they are grown at a specified specific growth rate (corresponding to a certain environment experienced by the cells). At steady state the substrate mass balance (6.36) gives:

$$0 = -r_s x + D \left(c_s^f - c_s \right) \tag{6.36}$$

which upon combination with Eq. (6.35) and the definition of the yield coefficient gives:

$$x = Y_{sx} \left(c_s^f - c_s \right) \tag{6.37}$$

Thus, the yield coefficient can be determined from measurement of the biomass and the substrate concentrations in the bioreactor (it is assumed that the substrate concentration in the feed flow is known).

If the Monod model applies the mass balance for the biomass gives:

$$D = \mu_{max} \frac{c_s}{c_s + K_s} \tag{6.38}$$

or

$$c_s = \frac{D K_s}{\mu_{max} - D} \tag{6.39}$$

Thus the concentration of the limiting substrate increases with the dilution rate. When substrate concentration becomes equal to the substrate concentration in the feed the dilution rate attains its maximum value, which is often called the *critical dilution rate*:

$$D_{crit} = \mu_{max} \frac{c_s^f}{c_s^f + K_s} \tag{6.40}$$

When the dilution rate becomes equal to or larger than this value the biomass is washed out of the bioreactor. Equation (6.39) clearly shows that the steady-state chemostat is well suited to study the influence of the substrate concentration on the cellular function, e.g. product formation, since by changing the dilution rate it is possible to change the substrate concentration as the only variable. Furthermore, it is possible to study the influence of different limiting substrates on the cellular physiology.

Besides quantification of the Monod parameters the chemostat is well suited to determine the maintenance coefficient. As the dilution rate equals the specific growth rate, a combination of Eqs. (6.14) and (6.37) gives:

$$x = \frac{D}{Y_{xs}^{true} D + m_s} \left(c_s^f - c_s \right) \tag{6.41}$$

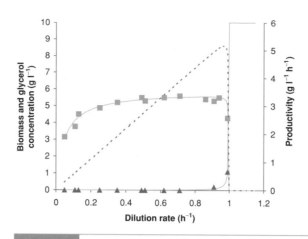

Equation (6.41) shows that the biomass concentration decreases at low specific growth rates, where the substrate consumption for maintenance is significant compared with that for growth. At high specific growth rates (high dilution rates) maintenance is negligible and the yield coefficient becomes equal to the true yield coefficient. Since $\mu = D$ at steady state Eq. (6.13) expresses that there is a linear relation between the specific substrate uptake rate and the dilution rate. In this linear relationship the true yield coefficient and the maintenance coefficient can easily be estimated using linear regression.

For production of biomass, e.g. baker's yeast or single cell protein, and growth-related products the chemostat is very well suited since it is possible to maintain a high productivity over very long periods of operation. The productivity of biomass is given by:

$$P_x = D x \tag{6.42}$$

and in Fig. 6.11 the productivity is shown as a function of the dilution rate.

By inserting the expression for the biomass concentration (6.41) into Eq. (6.42), with Eq. (6.39) inserted for the substrate concentration, it is possible to calculate the dilution rates that give maximum productivity. If there is no maintenance, i.e. $m_s = 0$, the optimal dilution rate is given by:

$$D_{opt} = \mu_{max} \left(1 - \sqrt{\frac{K_s}{c_s^f + K_s}}\right) \tag{6.43}$$

It is important to emphasise that this optimum only holds for Monod kinetics without maintenance. When maintenance is included, finding the optimum dilution rate will involve solving a third-degree polynomial. This polynomial will have one solution in the possible range of dilution rates. However, instead of solving the third-degree polynomial it is generally easier to find the solution numerically.

6.3.4 The fed-batch reactor

This operation is probably the most common operation in industrial processes, since it allows for control of the environmental conditions, e.g. maintaining the glucose concentration at a certain level, as well as enabling formation of very high titres (up to several hundred grams per litre for some metabolites), which is of importance for subsequent downstream processing. There is striking similarity between the fed-batch reactor and the chemostat, and for the fed-batch reactor the mass balance for biomass and substrate are given by the general mass balances (6.26) and (6.29). Normally the feed concentration c_s^f is very high, i.e. the feed is a very concentrated solution, and the feed flow is low giving a low dilution rate. The dilution rate is given by:

$$D = \frac{1}{V}\frac{dV}{dt} \tag{6.44}$$

and if D is to be kept constant there needs to be an exponentially increasing feed flow to the bioreactor. If the yield coefficient is constant, combining the mass balances for the biomass and the substrate gives:

$$\frac{d(x + Y_{sx}c_s)}{dt} = [(\mu - D)x - Y_{sx}r_s x + Y_{sx}D\left(c_s^f - c_s\right)] \tag{6.45}$$

or, since $\mu = Y_{sx}r_s$

$$\frac{d\left[x - Y_{sx}\left(c_s^f - c_s\right)\right]}{dt} = -D\left[x - Y_{sx}\left(c_s^f - c_s\right)\right] \tag{6.46}$$

Through combination with Eq. (6.44) this differential equation can easily be solved with the solution given by:

$$\frac{Y_{sx}\left(c_s^f - c_{s,0}\right) - x_0}{Y_{sx}\left(c_s^f - c_s\right) - x} = \frac{V}{V_0} \tag{6.47}$$

where x_0, $c_{s,0}$ and V_0 are the biomass concentration, the substrate concentration and the reactor volume at the start of the fed-batch process. The substrate concentration in the feed c_s^f is normally very high and much higher than both the initial substrate concentration and the substrate concentration during the process (c_s); this means that $Y_{sx}c_s^f$ is larger than the biomass concentration, both initially and during the process. Consequently the increase in volume can be kept low even when there is a very high increase in the biomass concentration.

If there is an exponential feed flow to the bioreactor there will be substantial biomass growth and, since the biomass concentration increases, this may lead to limitations in the oxygen supply. The feed flow is therefore typically increased until limitations in the oxygen supply set in, whereafter the feed flow is kept constant. This will give a decreasing specific growth rate. However, since the biomass concentration normally will increase, the volumetric uptake rate of substrates (including oxygen) may be kept approximately constant. From the above it is quite clear that there may be many different feeding strategies in a fed-batch process, and optimisation of the operation is a complex problem that is difficult to solve empirically. Even when a very good process model is available, calculation of the optimal feeding strategy is a complex optimisation problem. In an empirical search for the optimal feeding policy the two most obvious criteria are:

- keep the concentration of the limiting substrate constant;
- keep the volumetric growth rate of the biomass (or uptake of a given substrate) constant.

A constant volumetric growth rate (or uptake of a given substrate) is applied if there are limitations in the supply of oxygen or in heat removal, and this is often the case. A constant concentration of the limiting substrate is often applied if the substrate inhibits product formation, and the chosen concentration therefore depends on the degree of inhibition and the desire to maintain a certain growth of the cells. The required feeding profile to maintain a constant substrate concentration c_s corresponding to a constant specific growth rate μ_0 is quite simple to derive. From (6.28) with $F_{out} = 0$,

$$\frac{d(xV)}{dt} = \mu_0 xV \tag{6.48}$$

or

$$xV = x_0 V_0 e^{\mu_0 t} \tag{6.49}$$

Since the substrate concentration is constant the substrate balance gives:

$$-Y_{xs}\mu_0 x + D\left(c_s^f - c_s\right) = 0 \tag{6.50}$$

or

$$F(t) = \frac{Y_{xs}\mu_0}{c_s^f - c_s} xV = \frac{Y_{xs}\mu_0}{c_s^f - c_s} x_0 V_0 e^{\mu_0 t} \tag{6.51}$$

Finally, the biomass concentration $x(t)$ is obtained from Eq. (6.47) with $c_s = c_{s,0}$:

$$\frac{x(t)}{x_0} = \frac{e^{\mu_0 t}}{1 - ax_0 + ax_0 e^{\mu_0 t}} \tag{6.52}$$

where

$$a = \frac{Y_{xs}}{c_s^f - c_s} \tag{6.53}$$

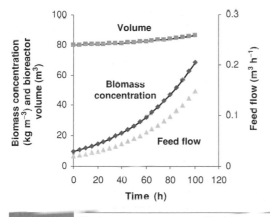

Figure 6.12 The biomass concentration (♦), the bioreactor volume (■) and the feed flow rate (∧) to a fed-batch reactor operated with a constant substrate concentration. The yield coefficient Y_{sx} is taken to be 0.5 g DW (g glucose)$^{-1}$, the constant specific growth rate μ_0 is taken to be 0.02 h^{-1} and the substrate concentration in the feed c_s^f is taken to be 400 kg m^{-3}. The substrate concentration is assumed to be much less than c_s^f. The initial biomass concentration x_0 and the initial bioreactor volume are taken to be 10 kg m^{-3} and 80 m^3, respectively.

The bioreactor volume is given by:

$$\frac{V}{V_0} = 1 - ax_0 + ax_0 e^{\mu_0 t} \tag{6.54}$$

Figure 6.12 specifies typical profiles for the biomass concentration, the bioreactor volume and the feed flow rate during a fed-batch process with constant substrate concentration.

Fed-batch cultures were used in the production of baker's yeast as early as 1915, where it was introduced by Dansk Gærindustri (and therefore sometimes referred to as the Danish method). In modern fed-batch processes for yeast production the feed of molasses is under strict control based on the automatic measurement of traces of ethanol in the exhaust gas of the bioreactor. Although such systems may result in low growth rates, the biomass yield is generally close to the maximum obtainable, and this is especially important in the production of baker's yeast where there is much focus on the yield. Besides its application in the production of baker's yeast, the fed-batch process is today applied in the production of secondary metabolites (where penicillins are the most prominent group of compounds), industrial enzymes and many other products derived from fermentation processes.

6.4 | Further reading

Herbert, D. Some principles of continuous culture. *Recent Progress in Microbiology* 7: 381–396, 1959. A reference paper on maintenance metabolism. Very clear in its presentation.

Monod, J. *Recherches sur la Croissance des Cultures Bacteriennes.* Paris: Hermann et Cie, 1942. A classic paper on kinetics of microbial growth. The original paper specifies the kinetics and gives a qualitative description of cellular growth kinetics.

Neidhardt, F. C., Ingraham, J. L. and Schaechter, M. *Physiology of the Bacterial Cell. A Molecular Approach.* Sunderland: Sinauer Associates, 1990. An excellent monograph on microbial physiology. The book gives a very comprehensive description of the growth physiology of bacteria. The description of microbial biochemistry is very well structured and excellent for both teaching and research.

Nielsen, J., Villadsen, J. and Lidén, G. *Bioreaction Engineering Principles*, second edition. New York: Kluwer Academic/Plenum Publishers, 2002. A comprehensive monograph on modelling of fermentation processes. The book treats both growth kinetics and design of bioreactor operation.

Pirt, S. J. The maintenance energy of bacteria in growing cultures. Proceedings of The Royal Society *London, Series B* **163**: 224–231, 1965. A classic paper on maintenance metabolism. The paper is very clear in its presentation.

Roels, J. A. *Energetics and Kinetics in Biotechnology.* Amsterdam: Elsevier Biomedical Press, 1983. An excellent monograph on thermodynamics and kinetics of cellular growth.

Stephanopoulos, G., Nielsen, J. and Aristodou, A. *Metabolic Engineering. Principles and Methodologies.* San Diego: Academic Press, 1998. A comprehensive monograph on modern theoretical methods applied in fermentation physiology and metabolic engineering. The book describes the theory behind metabolic flux analysis, metabolic control analysis, and thermodynamics of cellular reactions.

Chapter 7

Bioreactor design

Yusuf Chisti

Massey University, New Zealand

Nomenclature

A_d	cross-sectional area of the downcomer (m^2)
A_H	area for heat transfer (m^2)
A_r	cross-sectional area of the riser (m^2)
a	parameter in Eq. (7.8) (–)
C_p	specific heat capacity of the broth (J kg^{-1} °C^{-1})
c	dimensionless constant (–)
d	characteristic length dimension (m)
d_i	diameter of the impeller (m)
d_p	particle diameter (m)
d_T	diameter of bubble column or tank (m)
d_w	fermenter wall thickness (m)
E	energy dissipation rate per unit mass of fluid (J s^{-1} kg^{-1})
Gr	Grashof number (–)
g	gravitational acceleration (m s^{-2})
h_f	jacket side fouling film heat transfer coefficient (J s^{-1} m^{-2} °C^{-1})
h_i	film heat transfer coefficient for the cooling water on the jacket side (J s^{-1} m^{-2} °C^{-1})
h_L	height of gas-free liquid (m)
h_o	broth film heat transfer coefficient (J s^{-1} m^{-2} °C^{-1})

Basic Biotechnology, third edition, eds. Colin Ratledge and Bjørn Kristiansen.
Published by Cambridge University Press. © Cambridge University Press 2006.

k	parameter in Eq. (7.8) (m^{-1})
k_i	impeller-dependent constant (–)
k_T	thermal conductivity of the culture broth (J s^{-1} m^{-1} °C^{-1})
k_w	thermal conductivity of the fermenter wall (J s^{-1} m^{-1} °C^{-1})
ℓ	mean length of the energy dissipating fluid eddy (m)
N	rotational speed of the impeller (s^{-1})
Nu	Nusselt number (–)
n	flow behaviour index of a fluid (–)
P	power input in gas-free state (J s^{-1})
P_G	power input in presence of gas (J s^{-1})
Po	power number (–)
Pr	Prandtl number (–)
Q	volumetric gas flow rate (m^3 s^{-1})
Q_H	heat transfer rate (J s^{-1})
Re	Reynolds number (–)
Re$_i$	impeller Reynolds number (–)
SG	sight glass
ΔT	temperature difference (°C)
U_G	superficial gas velocity based on the total cross-sectional area of the vessel (m s^{-1})
U_{Gr}	superficial velocity of gas in riser (m s^{-1})
U_H	overall heat transfer coefficient (J s^{-1} m^{-2} °C^{-1})
U_L	superficial liquid velocity (m s^{-1})
V_L	volume of liquid in the reactor (m^3)
β	coefficient of volumetric expansion (m^3 kg^{-1} °C^{-1})
γ	average shear rate (s^{-1})
γ_{max}	maximum shear rate (s^{-1})
ε_L	volume fraction of liquid (–)
μ_L	viscosity of liquid (kg m^{-1} s^{-1})
μ_w	viscosity of water (kg m^{-1} s^{-1})
μ_{Lw}	viscosity of liquid at wall temperature (kg m^{-1} s^{-1})
ρ_L	density of liquid or slurry (kg m^{-3})
τ	shear stress (N m^{-2})

7.1 | Introduction

A bioreactor, or fermenter, is any device or vessel that is used to carry out one or more biochemical reactions to convert any substance (i.e. a substrate) to some product. Bioreactors are a necessary part of any biotechnology based production process whether it is for producing biomass or metabolites, biotransforming one compound into another or degrading unwanted wastes. The reactions occurring in a bioreactor are driven by biocatalysts – enzymes, micro-organisms, cells of animals and plants, or sub-cellular structures such as mitochondria and chloroplasts. The bioreactor provides an environment that is conducive to optimal functioning of the biocatalyst. A bioproduction facility typically has a train of bioreactors ranging from

20 litres to 250 m^3. Still larger vessels are encountered in certain processes. In a great majority of processes, the reactors are operated in a batch or fed-batch mode, under sterile or monoseptic conditions. The most common operational practice starts with culturing micro-organisms or cells in the smallest bioreactor. After a pre-determined batch time the content of this reactor is transferred to a larger, pre-sterilised, medium-filled reactor and this process is repeated until the production fermenter, the largest reactor in the train, is reached. Most commercial processing is carried out as submerged culture with the biocatalyst suspended in a nutrient medium in a suitable reactor.

This chapter focuses on the common types of bioreactors used in various industrial processes and the design considerations for such reactors. The major types of bioreactor configurations discussed include

- stirred tank reactors,
- bubble columns,
- airlift devices,
- packed beds,
- fluidised beds,
- photobioreactors.

Irrespective of the specific reactor configuration that may be demanded by a given application, designing a bioreactor requires attention to several other aspects:

(1) The need to maintain monoseptic operation.
(2) Mixing to ensure suspension of the biocatalyst and attain a relatively homogeneous environment in the bioreactor.
(3) Supply of oxygen and removal of carbon dioxide.
(4) Supply of various other nutrients in such a way that the rate of supply does not limit the performance of the biocatalyst.
(5) Heat transfer for temperature control.
(6) Control of the shear stress levels in the bioreactor so that the biocatalyst is not damaged by various hydrodynamic forces.

7.2 | Bioreactor configurations

7.2.1 Stirred tank reactors

Stirred tank bioreactors consist of a cylindrical vessel with a motor-driven central shaft that supports one or more agitators. The shaft may enter through the top or the bottom of the reactor vessel. A typical stirred tank reactor is shown in Fig. 7.1. Microbial culture vessels are generally provided with four baffles projecting into the vessel from the walls to prevent swirling and vortexing of the fluid. The baffle width is one-tenth or one-twelfth of the tank diameter. The aspect ratio (i.e. height to diameter ratio) of the vessel is 3 to 5, except in animal cell culture applications where aspect ratios do not

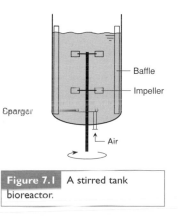

Figure 7.1 A stirred tank bioreactor.

Figure 7.2 Some commonly used impellers: (a) Rushton disc turbine, (b) a concave bladed turbine, (c) a hydrofoil impeller and (d) a marine propeller.

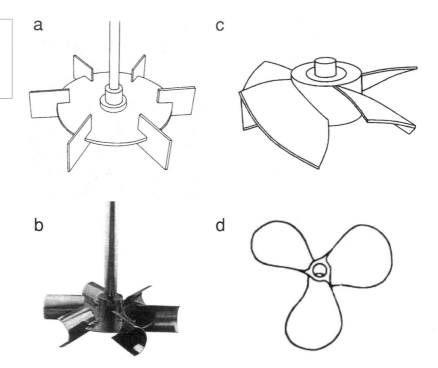

a

c

b

d

normally exceed 2. Often, the animal cell culture vessels are unbaffled (especially small-scale reactors) to reduce turbulence that may damage the cells. The number of impellers depends on the aspect ratio. The bottom impeller is located at a distance of about one-third of the tank diameter above the bottom of the tank. Additional impellers are spaced approximately one to two impeller diameter distances apart. The impeller diameter is about one-third of the vessel diameter for gas dispersion impellers such as Rushton disc turbines and concave bladed impellers (Fig. 7.2). Larger hydrofoil impellers (Fig. 7.2) with diameters of 0.5 to 0.6 times the tank diameter are especially effective bulk mixers and are used in fermenters for highly viscous mycelial broths. Animal cell culture vessels typically employ a single, large diameter, low-shear impeller such as a marine propeller (Fig. 7.2). Gas is sparged into the reactor liquid below the bottom impeller using a perforated pipe ring sparger with a ring diameter that is slightly smaller than that of the impeller. Alternatively, a single hole sparger may be used.

In animal or plant cell culture applications, the impeller speed generally does not exceed about 120 rpm in vessels larger than about 50 litres. Higher stirring rates are employed in microbial culture, except with mycelial and filamentous cultures where the impeller tip speed (i.e. $\pi \times$ impeller diameter $\times$ speed of rotation) does not in general exceed 7.6 m s^{-1}. Even lower speeds have been documented to damage certain mycelial fungi. The superficial aeration velocity (i.e. the volumetric gas flow rate divided by the cross-sectional area of the vessel) in stirred vessels must remain below the value needed to flood the impeller. (An impeller is flooded when it receives more gas than it can effectively disperse.) A flooded impeller is a poor mixer. Superficial aeration velocities do not generally exceed 0.05 m s^{-1}. Stirred tanks are among the most widely used types of bioreactors, especially in production of antibiotics and organic acids.

7.2.2 Bubble columns

A bubble column bioreactor is shown on Fig. 7.3. Usually, the column is cylindrical with an aspect ratio of 4 to 8. Gas is sparged at the base of the column through perforated pipes, perforated plates, or sintered glass or metal microporous spargers. Oxygen (O_2) transfer, mixing and other performance factors are influenced mainly by the gas flow rate and the rheological properties of the fluid. Internal devices such as horizontal perforated plates, vertical baffles and corrugated sheet packings may be placed in the vessel to improve mass transfer and modify the basic design. The column diameter does not affect reactor behaviour so long as the diameter exceeds 0.1 m. One exception is the axial mixing performance. For a given gas flow rate, the mixing improves with increasing vessel diameter. Mass and heat transfer and the prevailing shear rate increase as gas flow rate is increased. In bubble columns the maximum aeration velocity does not usually exceed 0.1 m s^{-1}. The liquid flow rate does not influence the gas–liquid mass transfer coefficient so long as the superficial liquid velocity remains below 0.1 m s^{-1} (see also Chapter 8). Bubble columns are particularly suited to use in the biological treatment of wastewater and other relatively less viscous aerobic fermentations.

7.2.3 Airlift bioreactors

In airlift bioreactors the fluid volume of the vessel is divided into two interconnected zones by means of a baffle or draft tube, as shown in Fig. 7.4. Only one of the two zones is sparged with air or other gas. The sparged zone is known as the riser; the zone that receives no gas is the downcomer. The bulk density of the gas–liquid dispersion in the gas-sparged riser tends to be lower than the bulk density in the downcomer, consequently the dispersion flows up in the riser zone and down in the downcomer. Sometimes the riser and the downcomer are two separate vertical pipes that are interconnected at the top and the bottom to form an external circulation loop. For optimal gas–liquid mass transfer performance, the riser to downcomer cross-sectional area ratio should be between 1.8 and 4.3. External-loop airlift reactors are less common in commercial processes compared to the internal-loop designs. The internal-loop configuration may be either a concentric draft-tube device or a split cylinder.

Airlift bioreactors are highly energy efficient relative to stirred fermenters, yet the productivities of both types are comparable. Being especially suited to shear-sensitive cultures, airlift devices are often employed in large-scale manufacture of biopharmaceutical proteins obtained from fragile animal cells. In addition, airlift devices are used in high-rate biotreatment of wastewater, production of insecticidal

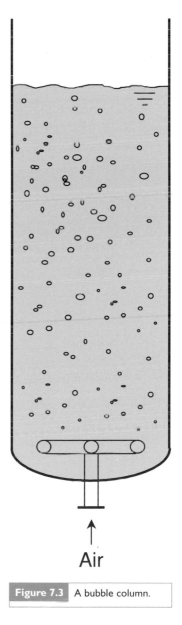

Air

Figure 7.3 A bubble column.

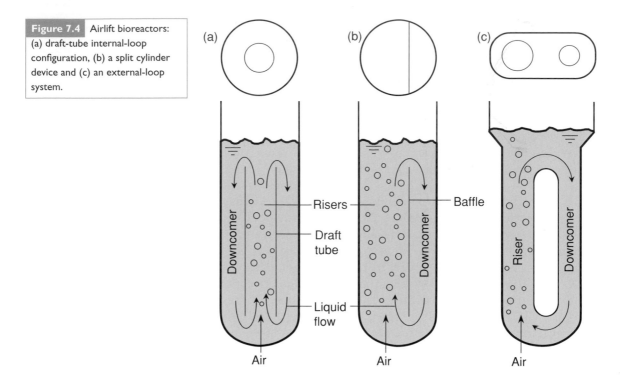

Figure 7.4 Airlift bioreactors: (a) draft-tube internal-loop configuration, (b) a split cylinder device and (c) an external-loop system.

nematode worms and other low-viscosity fermentations. Heat and mass transfer capabilities of airlift reactors are at least as good as those of other systems, and airlift reactors are more effective in suspending solids than are bubble columns. All performance characteristics of airlift bioreactors are linked ultimately to the gas injection rate and the resulting rate of liquid circulation. In general, the rate of liquid circulation increases with the square root of the height of the airlift device. Consequently, the reactors are designed with high aspect ratios. Because the liquid circulation is driven by the gas hold-up difference between the riser and the downcomer, circulation is enhanced if there is little or no gas in the downcomer. All the gas in the downcomer comes from being entrained with the liquid as it flows into the downcomer from the riser near the top of the reactor. Various designs of gas–liquid separators are sometimes used in the head zone to reduce or eliminate the gas carry-over to the downcomer. Relative to a reactor without a gas–liquid separator, installation of a suitably designed separator will always enhance liquid circulation, i.e. the increased driving force for circulation will more than compensate for any additional resistance to flow due to the separator.

7.2.4 Fluidised beds

Fluidised bed bioreactors are suited to reactions involving a fluid-suspended particulate biocatalyst such as the immobilised enzyme and cell particles or microbial flocs. An up-flowing stream of liquid is used to suspend or *fluidise* the solids (see Fig. 7.5). Geometrically, the reactor is similar to a bubble column except that the top section

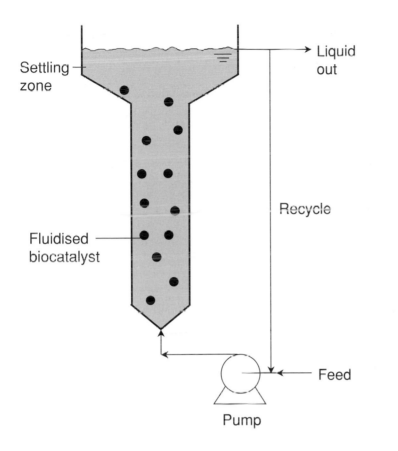

Figure 7.5 A fluidised bed bioreactor.

is expanded to reduce the superficial velocity of the fluidising liquid to a level below that needed to keep the solids in suspension. Consequently, the solids sediment in the expanded zone and drop back into the narrower reactor column below; hence, the solids are retained in the reactor whereas the liquid flows out. A liquid fluidised bed may be sparged with air or some other gas to produce a gas–liquid–solid fluid bed. If the solid particles are too light, they may have to be artificially weighted, for example by embedding stainless steel balls in an otherwise light solid matrix. A high density of solids improves solid–liquid mass transfer by increasing the relative velocity between the phases. Denser solids are also easier to sediment but the density should not be too high relative to that of the liquid, or fluidisation will be difficult.

Liquid fluidised beds tend to be fairly quiescent but introduction of a gas substantially enhances turbulence and agitation. Even with relatively light particles, the superficial liquid velocity needed to suspend the solids may be so high that the liquid leaves the reactor much too quickly, i.e. the solid–liquid contact time is insufficient for the reaction. In this case, the liquid may have to be recycled to ensure a sufficiently long cumulative contact time with the biocatalyst. The minimum fluidisation velocity, i.e. the superficial liquid velocity needed to just suspend the solids from a settled state,

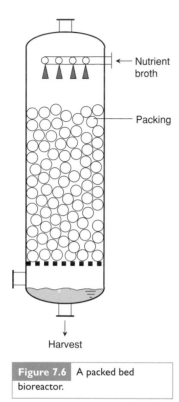

Nutrient broth

Packing

Harvest

Figure 7.6 A packed bed bioreactor.

depends on several factors, including the density difference between the phases, the diameter of the particles and the viscosity of the liquid.

7.2.5 Packed beds

A bed of solid particles, usually with confining walls, constitutes a packed bed (Fig. 7.6). The biocatalyst is supported on, or within, the matrix of solids, which may be porous or a homogeneous non-porous gel. The solids may be particles of compressible polymeric or more rigid material. A fluid containing nutrients flows continuously through the bed to provide the needs of the immobilised biocatalyst. Metabolites and products are released into the fluid and removed in the outflow. The flow may be upward or downward, but downflow under gravity is the norm. If the fluid flows up the bed, the maximum flow velocity is limited because the velocity cannot exceed the minimum fluidisation velocity or the bed will fluidise. The depth of the bed is limited by several factors, including the density and the compressibility of the solids, the need to maintain a certain minimal level of a critical nutrient, such as O_2, through the entire depth, and the flow rate that is needed for a given pressure drop. For a given void volume (i.e. solids-free volume fraction of the bed) the gravity-driven flow rate through the bed declines as the depth of the bed increases. The concentration of nutrients decreases as the fluid moves down the bed and concentrations of metabolites and products increase. Thus, the environment of a packed bed is non-homogeneous but concentration variations along the depth can be decreased by increasing the flow rate. Gradients of pH may occur if the reaction consumes or produces H^+ or OH^-. Because of poor mixing, pH control by addition of acid and alkali is nearly impossible. Beds with greater void volume permit greater flow velocities through them but the concentration of the biocatalyst in a given bed volume declines as the voidage (void volume) is increased. If the packing, i.e. the biocatalyst-supporting solids, is compressible, its weight may compress the bed unless the packing height is kept low. Flow is difficult through a compressed bed because of a reduced voidage. Packed beds are used extensively as immobilised enzyme reactors. Such reactors are particularly attractive for product inhibited reactions: the product concentration varies from a low value at the inlet of the bed to a high value at the exit; thus, only a part of the biocatalyst is exposed to high inhibitory levels of the product.

7.2.6 Photobioreactors

Photobioreactors are used for photosynthetic culture of microalgae and cyanobacteria to produce products such as astaxanthin and β-carotene. Photosynthetic cultures require sunlight or artificial illumination. Artificial illumination is impracticably expensive and only outdoor photobioreactors appear to be promising for large-scale production. Open ponds and raceways are often used to culture microalgae especially in processes for treating wastewater. When a

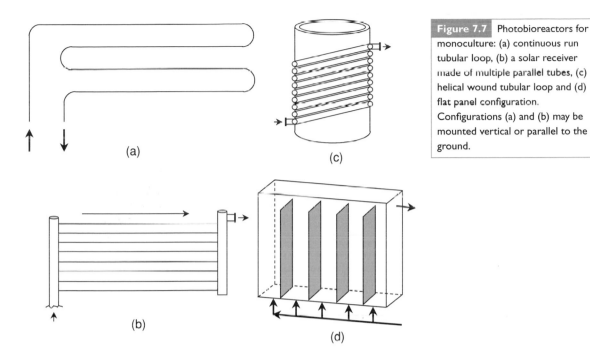

Figure 7.7 Photobioreactors for monoculture: (a) continuous run tubular loop, (b) a solar receiver made of multiple parallel tubes, (c) helical wound tubular loop and (d) flat panel configuration. Configurations (a) and (b) may be mounted vertical or parallel to the ground.

monoseptic culture is required, fully closed photobioreactors must be used. Because it needs light, photosynthesis can occur only at relatively shallow depths. Algal ponds are typically no deeper than 0.15 m. However, too much light causes photoinhibition; a situation in which slightly reducing the light intensity will actually improve the rate of photosynthesis. With increasing cell population, the self-shading effect of cells further limits light penetration. In addition to light, photosynthesising algal cells need a source of carbon, usually carbon dioxide.

Closed photobioreactors for monoculture consist of arrays of transparent tubes that may be made of glass or, more commonly, a clear plastic. The tubes may be laid horizontally, or arranged as long rungs on an upright ladder, as shown in Fig. 7.7. A continuous single run tubular loop configuration is also used, or the tube may be wound helically around a vertical cylindrical support. In addition to the tubes, flat or inclined thin panels may be employed in relatively small-scale operations. An array of tubes or a flat panel constitutes a *solar receiver*. The culture is circulated through the solar receiver by a variety of methods, including centrifugal pumps, positive displacement mono pumps, Archimedean screws and airlift devices. Airlift pumps perform well, have no mechanical parts, are easy to operate aseptically and are suited to shear-sensitive applications.

The flow in a solar receiver tube or panel should be turbulent enough to aid periodic movement of cells from the deeper poorly lit interior to the regions nearer the walls. The velocity everywhere should be sufficient to prevent sedimentation of cells. Typical linear velocities through receiver tubes tend to be 0.3–0.5 m s^{-1}. Because of the need to maintain adequate sunlight penetration, a tubular solar receiver cannot be scaled up by simply increasing the tube diameter. The diameter should not generally exceed 6 cm. Light penetration depends on biomass density, cellular morphology and pigmentation, and absorption characteristics of the cell-free culture medium.

7.3 | Bioreactor design features

Irrespective of the specific bioreactor configuration used, the vessel must be provided with certain common features. Some of the principal features are illustrated in Fig. 7.8. The reactor vessel is provided with a vertical sight glass and side ports for pH, temperature and dissolved O_2 sensors as minimum requirements (see also Chapter 10). Retractable sensors that can be replaced during operation are increasingly used. Connections for acid and alkali (for pH control), antifoam agents and inoculum are located above the liquid level in the reactor vessel. Air, and other gases such as CO_2 or ammonia for pH control, is introduced through a sparger situated near the bottom of the vessel. The agitator shaft is provided with steam sterilisable single or double mechanical seals. Double seals are preferred but they require lubrication with cooled, clean steam condensate. Alternatively, when torque limitations allow, magnetically coupled agitators may be used thereby eliminating the mechanical seals. Most fermentation processes are aerobic and require a continuous supply of sterile air. Consequently, a fermenter is normally provided with air supply and exhaust pipes that are installed with in situ steam sterilisable gas filters. Typically, hydrophobic membrane cartridge filters are used. These filters are rated for removing particles down to 0.45 μm or even 0.1 μm. Thus spores and other micro-organisms are removed from the inlet and exhaust air. Often the gas streams have two filter cartridges in series, with the first serving to protect the final filter. Aeration and agitation will inevitably produce foam which is controlled with a combination of chemical antifoam agents and mechanical foam breakers. Foam breakers are used exclusively when the presence of the chemical antifoam agent in the product is not acceptable or if the antifoam interferes with downstream processing operations such as membrane-based separations or chromatography. The shaft of the high-speed mechanical foam breaker must also be sealed using double mechanical seals.

In most instances, the bioreactor is designed for a maximum allowable working pressure of 377–412 kPa (absolute). Although the sterilisation temperature generally does not exceed 121 °C, the vessel is designed for a higher temperature, typically 150–180 °C. The vessel is designed to withstand full vacuum, or it could collapse while cooling after sterilisation. The reactor can be sterilised in-place using saturated clean steam at a minimum absolute pressure of 212 kPa. Overpressure protection is provided by a rupture disc located on top of the bioreactor. Usually this is a graphite burst disc because it does

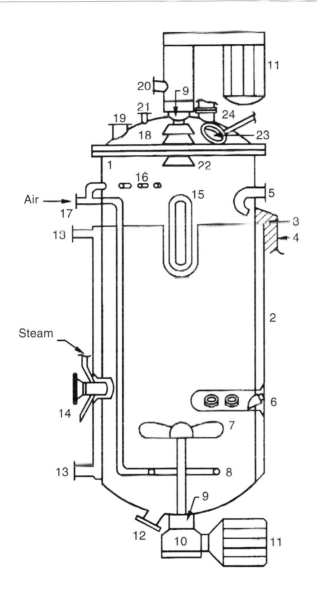

Figure 7.8 A typical stirred tank bioreactor: (1) reactor vessel, (2) jacket; (3) insulation; (4) shroud; (5) inoculum connection; (6) ports for pH, temperature and dissolved oxygen sensors; (7) agitator; (8) gas sparger; (9) mechanical seals; (10) reducing gearbox; (11) motor; (12) harvest nozzle; (13) jacket connections; (14) sample valve with steam connection; (15) sight glass; (16) connections for acid, alkali and antifoam chemicals; (17) air inlet; (18) removable top; (19) medium or feed nozzle; (20) air exhaust nozzle; (21) instrument ports (several); (22) foam breaker; (23) sight glass with light (not shown) and steam connection; (24) rupture disc nozzle.

not crack or develop pinholes without failing completely. Other items located on the head plate of the vessel are nozzles for media or feed addition and for sensors (e.g. the foam electrode), and instruments (e.g. the pressure gauge).

The vessel should have as few internals as practically possible and the design should take into account the needs of clean-in-place and sterilisation-in-place procedures. The vessel should be free of crevices and stagnant areas where pockets of liquids and solids may accumulate. Attention to design of such apparently minor items as the gasket grooves is important. Easy-to-clean channels with rounded edges are preferred, and sometimes essential. As far as possible, welded joints should be used in preference to couplings for all pipe work. Steam connections should allow for complete displacement of all air pockets in the vessel and associated pipe work. Even the exterior of a bio-process plant should be cleanly designed with smooth contours and minimum bare threads.

The reactor vessel is invariably jacketed. In the absence of especial requirements, the jacket is designed to the same specifications as the vessel. The jacket is covered with chloride-free fibreglass insulation that is fully enclosed in a protective shroud as shown in Fig. 7.8. The jacket is provided with overpressure protection through a relief valve located on the jacket or its associated piping. For a great majority of applications, austenitic stainless steels are the preferred material of construction for bioreactors. The bioreactor vessel is usually made in Type 316L stainless steel, while the less expensive Type 304 (or 304L) is used for the jacket, the insulation shroud and other surfaces not coming into direct contact with the fermentation broth. The L grades of stainless steel contain less than 0.03% carbon, which reduces chromium carbide formation during welding and lowers the potential for later intergranular corrosion at the welds. The welds on internal parts should be ground flush with the internal surface and polished.

7.4 | Specific design considerations

Designing a bioreactor is a complex engineering exercise. First, a basic bioreactor configuration needs to be selected (see Section 7.2), based on an understanding of the requirements of the bioprocess of interest. For example, for a highly aerobic microbial growth in submerged culture, the only suitable preliminary bioreactor configurations are the bubble column, airlift devices and stirred tanks. The rheology (i.e. the flow properties, especially the viscosity) of the broth, the shear stress tolerance of the culture, the rate of production of metabolic heat, the oxygen demand and the ability of the cells to withstand brief anaerobic periods, are then used to further narrow down the choice of reactor configuration to, for example, the stirred tank. For the selected configuration, detailed engineering analyses are required to quantify the agitation power and aeration needs to:

(1) satisfy the required oxygen demand (see Chapter 8);
(2) meet the mixing time constraints so that relatively homogeneous nutrient and dissolved oxygen levels are attained in the bioreactor; and
(3) attain a turbulence level that is sufficient to keep the biomass in suspension, remove the heat generated by metabolism and agitation (see Section 7.4.1), but not so intense as to damage the biocatalyst.

Estimation of factors such as the oxygen transfer capability of a bioreactor, the mixing time, the shear stress levels and the heat removal capability, requires different approaches for different types of bioreactor configurations. Here only the removal of heat and estimation

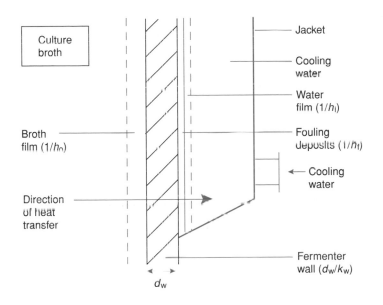

Culture broth

Broth film $(1/h_o)$

Direction of heat transfer

d_w

Jacket

Cooling water

Water film $(1/h_I)$

Fouling deposits $(1/h_f)$

Cooling water

Fermenter wall (d_w/k_w)

Figure 7.9 Heat transfer resistances near a fermenter wall.

of shear stress levels are discussed as important aspects of design. Oxygen transfer is discussed in Chapter 8.

7.4.1 Heat transfer

All fermentations generate heat. Typically, the microbial activity in submerged culture can generate 3–15 kJ m^{-3} s^{-1} of heat. Heat production is especially large when the biomass is growing rapidly in high-density fermentations and when reduced carbon sources such as hydrocarbons and methanol are used as substrate. The metabolic heat generation rate in kJ m^{-3} s^{-1} is numerically about 12% of the O$_2$ consumption rate expressed in mmol O$_2$ m^{-3} s^{-1}. Heat removal in large vessels becomes difficult as the heat generation rate approaches 5 kW m^{-3} (i.e. 5 kJ m^{-3} s^{-1}), corresponding to an O$_2$ consumption rate of about 5 kg m^{-3} h^{-1} (i.e. 43 mmol m^{-3} s^{-1}). In addition to the metabolic heat, mechanical agitation of the broth produces up to 15 kJ m^{-3} s^{-1}. In air-driven fermenters, all energy input due to gassing is eventually dissipated as heat. Consequently, a fermenter must be cooled to prevent the temperature rising and damaging the culture. As the scale of operation increases, heat transfer and not O$_2$ mass transfer becomes the limiting process in bioreactors because the available surface area for cooling decreases as the fermenter volume increases. Temperature is controlled by heating or cooling through external jackets and internal coils. Less frequently, additional double walled baffles, draft tubes or heat exchangers located inside the fermentation vessel are needed to provide sufficient heat transfer surface area.

During cooling, heat flows from the broth side to the cooling water in a jacket or cooling coil (see Fig. 7.9). The rate of heat removal, Q_H, is related to the surface area, A_H, available for heat exchange and the mean temperature difference, ΔT, thus,

$$Q_H = U_H A_H \Delta T \tag{7.1}$$

where U_H is the overall heat transfer coefficient. The coefficient U_H depends on the film heat transfer coefficient of the fluid on either side of the metal wall.

The film heat transfer coefficient is influenced by numerous factors, including:

- the density and the viscosity of the fluid,
- thermal conductivity and heat capacity,
- the velocity of flow or some other measure of turbulence (e.g. power input, gas flow rate, etc.), and
- the geometry of the bioreactor.

The many variables that affect heat transfer can be grouped into a few *dimensionless numbers* to simplify the study and description of those effects greatly. The groups relevant to heat transfer and the corresponding fluid dynamics (e.g. turbulence) are as follows:

$$\text{Nu (Nusselt number)} = \frac{\text{total heat transfer}}{\text{conductive heat transfer}} = \frac{h_o d}{k_T} \tag{7.2}$$

$$\text{Pr (Prandtl number)} = \frac{\text{momentum diffusivity}}{\text{thermal diffusivity}} = \frac{C_p \mu_L}{K_T} \tag{7.3}$$

$$\text{Re (Reynolds number)} = \frac{\text{inertial force}}{\text{viscous force}} = \frac{\rho_L U_L d}{\mu_L} \tag{7.4}$$

$$\text{Gr (Grashof number)} = \frac{\text{gravitation force}}{\text{viscous force}} = \frac{d^3 \rho_L g}{\Delta T \beta \mu_L^2} \tag{7.5}$$

In these equations, d is a characteristic length (e.g. diameter of tube or impeller). These dimensionless groups express the relative significance of the various factors influencing a given situation. The value of the Nusselt number tells us about the relative magnitudes of total heat transfer and that transferred by conduction alone. The Grashof number is important in situations where flow is produced by density differences that may themselves be generated by thermal gradients (hence the $\Delta T \beta$ in the Grashof number). The Reynolds number is employed in describing fluid motion in situations where forced convection is predominant.

Equations for quantifying the heat transfer resistances of the fouling films (dirt deposited on solid walls and particles) and films of heating and cooling fluids are discussed in readily available process engineering handbooks. Suitable correlations for estimating the **heat transfer coefficient**, h_o, for the film of liquid or culture broth in various configurations of bioreactors are summarised in Table 7.1. Note that the correlations given for stirred vessels utilise a Reynolds number that has been defined in terms of the tip speed of the impeller. In some cases, the correlations in Table 7.1 require the thermal conductivity, k_T, and the specific heat capacity, C_p, of the fermentation

Table 7.1 Correlations for the broth-side film heat transfer coefficient in various bioreactor geometries

Bioreactor configuration	Correlation	Ranges
Stirred tanks Coils	$\dfrac{h_o d_T}{k_T}\left(\dfrac{\mu_{Lw}}{\mu_L}\right)^{0.14}=0.87\left(\dfrac{d_i^2 N \rho_L}{\mu_L}\right)^{0.62}\left(\dfrac{C_p \mu_L}{k_T}\right)^{\frac{1}{3}}$	For cooling coils; Newtonian fluids
Jacketed	$\dfrac{h_o d_T}{k_T}\left(\dfrac{\mu_{Lw}}{\mu_L}\right)^{0.14}=0.36\left(\dfrac{d_i^2 N \rho_L}{\mu_L}\right)^{0.67}\left(\dfrac{C_p \mu_L}{k_T}\right)^{\frac{1}{3}}$	For jacketed vessels; Newtonian fluids
Bubble columns	$h_o=9391 U_G^{0.25}\left(\dfrac{\mu_w}{\mu_L}\right)^{0.35}$	Newtonian broths $10^{-3}<\mu_L\ (\mathrm{kg\ m^{-1}\ s^{-1}})<5\times10^{-2};\ U_g\leqslant 0.1\,\mathrm{m\ s^{-1}};\ 0.1\leqslant d_T\,(\mathrm{m})\leqslant 1$
	$\dfrac{h_o}{\rho_L C_p U_G}=0.1\left[\dfrac{U_G^3 \rho_L}{\mu_L g}\left(\dfrac{\mu_L C_p}{k_T}\right)^2\right]^{\frac{1}{4}}$	Newtonian broths
Airlift vessels Draft-tube sparged	$h_o=8710 U_{Gr}^{0.22}\left(\dfrac{A_r}{A_d}\right)^{0.25}\left(\dfrac{C_p \mu_L}{k_T}\right)^{-0.5}$	Newtonian broths $\mu_L=(0.78-5.27)\times10^{-3}\,\mathrm{kg\ m^{-1}\ s^{-1}};$ $0.008\leqslant U_{Gr}\leqslant 0.6\,\mathrm{m\ s^{-1}};\ 0.25\leqslant A_r/A_d\leqslant 1.20.$ The h_o varied from 600 to 2400 $\mathrm{W\ m^{-2}\ ^\circ C^{-1}}$
Annulus sparged	$h_o=13340\left(1+\dfrac{A_d}{A_r}\right)^{0.7} U_G^{0.275}$	Air–water; $0.01\leqslant U_G\leqslant 0.04\,\mathrm{m\ s^{-1}};$ $A_d/A_r=0.242$ and 0.452
Fluidised beds (gas–liquid–solid)	$\dfrac{h_o d_p \varepsilon_L}{k_T(1-\varepsilon_L)}=0.044\left[\dfrac{d_p U_L \rho_L}{\mu_L(1-\varepsilon_L)}\dfrac{C_p \mu_L}{k_L}\right]^{0.78}+2\left(\dfrac{U_G^2}{g d_p}\right)^{0.17}$	All properties are for the liquid phase

broth for estimation of the heat transfer coefficient. For most broths, the values of those parameters are close to those of water. The film heat transfer coefficient generally increases with:

- increasing turbulence,
- increasing flow rate,
- increasing agitation power input;

whilst the coefficient typically declines with:

- increasing viscosity of the culture broth.

The geometry of the bioreactor affects the film heat transfer coefficient mainly by influencing the degree of turbulence or related parameters such as the induced liquid circulation rate in airlift vessels. In bubble columns, the film coefficient is independent of the column diameter so long as the diameter exceeds about 0.1 m. Similarly, in bubble columns, the h_o value is not affected by the height of the gas-free fluid. The value of h_o increases with increasing superficial gas velocity, or power input, but only up to a velocity of about 0.1 m s^{-1}. Furthermore, for identical specific power inputs, bubble columns and stirred vessels provide quite similar values of the heat transfer coefficient.

Literature on heat transfer in airlift reactors is sparse. Equations developed for bubble columns (Table 7.1) may be used to provide an estimate of h_o in airlift vessels when the induced liquid circulation rates are small. Under other conditions, the coefficient in airlift reactors can be more than two-fold greater than in bubble column reactors. When liquid flow velocity does not exceed about 0.015 m s^{-1}, the film heat transfer coefficient is largely independent of liquid velocity. However, for higher liquid velocities h_o increases with liquid velocity as follows:

$$h_o \propto U_L^{1/4} \quad [0.015 \leqslant U_L(\text{m s}^{-1}) \leqslant 0.139] \tag{7.6}$$

A large amount of published data is available on heat transfer in vertical two-phase flows. Some of this information may be applicable to airlift reactors provided that the fluid properties, gas hold-up and relative velocities of the two phases are identical in the airlift and the vertical two-phase flow device. Fungal mycelia-like solids may enhance or reduce heat transfer depending on hydrodynamic conditions in the airlift device. Whereas in bacterial and yeast fermentations the temperature control tolerances are fairly narrow, animal cell cultures demand even more closely controlled temperature regimens. Typically, cells are cultured at 37 ± 0.2 °C. The cells generate little heat and the heat produced by agitation is also small. In addition, the almost water-like consistency of cell culture broths means that heat transfer is relatively easy; however, the temperature differences between the heating/cooling surface and the broth must remain small, or the cells can be damaged.

7.4.2 Shear effects in culture

Shear stress (related to the rate of shear) and other hydrodynamic forces in a bioreactor can damage fragile cells, flocs, biocatalyst particles and multi-cellular organisms such as nematodes. Consequently, establishing the level of the shear rate and other potentially damaging forces in a bioreactor is an important part of bioreactor design. Shear rate is a measure of spatial variation in local velocities in a fluid. Cell damage in a moving fluid is sometimes associated with the magnitude of the prevailing shear rate. But the shear rate in the relatively turbulent environment of most bioreactors is neither easily defined nor easily measured. Moreover, the shear rate varies with location within the vessel. Attempts have been made to characterise an average shear rate or a maximum shear rate in various types of bioreactors. In bubble columns an average shear rate has been defined as a function of the superficial gas velocity as follows:

$$\gamma = kU_G^a \tag{7.7}$$

where the parameter a equals 1.0 in most cases, but the k value has been reported variously as 1000, 2800, 5000 m^{-1}, etc. Equation (7.7) has been applied also to airlift bioreactors using the superficial gas velocity in the riser zone as a correlating parameter; however, that usage is incorrect. A more suitable form of the equation for airlift reactors is

$$\gamma = \frac{kU_{Gr}}{1 + (A_d/A_r)} \tag{7.8}$$

Depending on the value of k, equations such as (7.7) and (7.8) produce wildly different values for the shear rate. In addition, the equations fail to take into account the density and the viscosity of the fluid. Both of these will influence the shear rate.

An average shear rate in stirred fermenters is given by the equation:

$$\gamma = k_i \left(\frac{4n}{3n+1} \right)^{n/n-1} N \tag{7.9}$$

where n, the flow index of a fluid, equals 1.0 for a Newtonian liquid such as water and thick glucose syrup. Typical k_i values are:

- 11–13 for six-bladed disc turbines,
- 10–13 for paddle impellers,
- ~10 for propellers, and
- ~30 for helical ribbon impellers.

The shear rate can be converted to a parameter known as shear stress τ; where

$$\tau = \gamma \mu_L \tag{7.10}$$

Another method of deciding whether the turbulence in a fluid could potentially damage a suspended biocatalyst is based on comparing the dimensions of the cell or the biocatalyst floc with the length scale of the fluid eddies. The mean length, ℓ, of the fluid eddy depends on the energy dissipation rate per unit mass of the fluid in the bioreactor; thus,

$$\ell = \left(\frac{\mu_L}{\rho_L}\right)^{3/4} E^{-1/4} \tag{7.11}$$

In most cases, all the energy input to the fluid is dissipated in fluid eddies and E equals the rate of energy input. Methods for calculating the energy input rate in the principal kinds of bioreactors are noted in Box 7.1. Equation (7.11) applies to isotropically turbulent fluid, i.e. one in which the size of the primary eddies generated by the turbulence producing mechanism is a thousand-fold or more compared to the size of the energy dissipating microeddies. The size of the microeddies is calculated with Eq. (7.11). The length scale of the primary eddies is often approximated to the width of the impeller blade or the diameter of the impeller in a stirred tank. In bubble columns and airlift bioreactors, the length scale of primary eddies is approximated to the diameter of the column (or the riser tube) or the diameter of the bubble issuing from the gas sparger. Generally, if the dimensions of the biocatalyst particle are much smaller than the calculated length, ℓ, of the microeddies, the particle is simply carried around by the fluid eddy; the particle does not experience any disruptive force. On the other hand, a particle that is larger than the length scale of the eddy will experience pressure differentials on its surface and if the particle is not strong enough it could be broken by the resulting forces.

In addition to turbulence within the fluid, other damage causing phenomena in a bioreactor include interparticle collisions; collisions with walls, other stationary surfaces and the impeller; shear forces associated with bubble rupture at the surface of the fluid; phenomena linked with bubble coalescence and break-up; and bubble formation at the gas sparger. Effects of interfacial shear rate around rising bubbles and those due to bubble rupture at the surface can be minimised by adding non-ionic surfactants to the culture medium. These surfactants reduce adherence of animal cells to bubbles; hence, fewer cells experience interfacial shear and rupture events at the surface of the liquid.

In microcarrier culture of animal cells where spherical carriers as small as 200 μm in diameter are suspended in the culture fluid to support adherent cells on the surface of the carrier, interparticle collisions are generally infrequent under the conditions that are typically employed. However, the size of the fluid eddies in microcarrier culture systems may be similar to or smaller than the dimensions of the carriers; hence, the adhering cells may experience turbulence-related damage. Freely suspended animal cells are generally too small to be damaged by fluid turbulence levels that are typically employed

Box 7.1 | Energy input in bioreactors

Depending on the type of the bioreactor, the energy input per unit mass of the fluid is estimated variously as detailed below:

Bubble columns

$$E = gU_G$$

where g is the gravitational acceleration.

Airlift bioreactors

$$E = \frac{gU_{Gr}}{1 + (A_d/A_r)}$$

where A_d and A_b are the cross-sectional areas of the downcomer and the riser, respectively.

Stirred tanks

(i) *Laminar flow*

In stirred vessels the flow is laminar when the impeller Reynolds number Re_i is less than 10. The Re_i can be calculated using the equation

$$Re_i = \frac{\rho_L N d_i^2}{\mu_L}$$

In laminar flow the stirrer power number Po is related to the impeller Reynolds number as follows

$$Po = cRe_i^{-1}$$

where the constant c is ~100 (six-bladed disc turbine) or ~40 (propeller). Because the Power number equals $(P/\rho_L N^3 d_i^5)$, the power input P for the unaerated condition can be calculated. In presence of aeration, the power input is lower. The gassed power input P_G is calculated using the previously determined P value in the equation

$$P_G = 0.72 \left(\frac{P^2 N d_i^3}{Q^{0.56}} \right)^{0.45}$$

where Q is the volumetric aeration rate. Now E is obtained as

$$E = \frac{P_G}{\rho_L V_L}$$

(ii) *Turbulent flow*

The flow in stirred vessels is turbulent when $Re_i > 10^4$. In turbulent flow the power number is a constant that depends on the geometry of the impeller. Some constant Po values are: 0.32 (propeller), 1.70 (two-bladed paddle), 6.30 (six-bladed disc turbine) and 1.0 (five-bladed Prochem® impeller). The unaerated power input P can be calculated using the constant value of the power number. Now the P_G and the E values are calculated as explained for laminar flow.

in cell culture bioreactors. In microcarrier culture, shear stress levels as low as 0.25 N m^{-2} may interfere with the initial attachment of cells on microcarriers.

7.5 | Further reading

Chisti, Y. Animal-cell damage in sparged bioreactors. *Trends in Biotechnology*, **18**: 420–432, 2000.

Chisti, Y. and Moo-Young, M. Fermentation technology, bioprocessing, scale-up and manufacture. In *Biotechnology: The Science and the Business*, second edition, eds. V. Moses, R. E. Cape and D. G. Springham. New York: Harwood Academic, 1999, pp. 177–222.

Doran, P. M. *Bioprocess Engineering Principles*. London: Academic Press, 1995.

Grima, E. M., Fernández, F. G. A., Camacho, F. G. and Chisti, Y. Photobioreactors: light regime, mass transfer, and scale-up. *Journal of Biotechnology*, **70**: 231–247, 1999.

Lydersen, B. K., D'Elia, N. A. and Nelson, K. L. (eds.). *Bioprocess Engineering: Systems, Equipment and Facilities*. New York: John Wiley & Sons, 1994.

Chapter 8

Mass transfer

Henk J. Noorman

DSM Anti-Infectives, The Netherlands

Nomenclature

a	interfacial area per unit liquid volume (m^{-1})
a'	interfacial area per unit total reaction volume (gas plus liquid) (m^{-1})
C	concentration in liquid phase ($mol\,m^{-3}$)
C_i	concentration at liquid side of interface ($mol\,m^{-3}$)
C^*	saturation (= equilibrium) concentration in liquid phase ($= p/H$) ($mol\,m^{-3}$)
C_x	biomass concentration ($kg\,m^{-3}$)
d	liquid film thickness (m)
$\mathbf{D}$	diffusion coefficient or effective diffusivity ($m^2\,s^{-1}$)
D	impeller diameter (m)
H	Henry coefficient ($bar\,m^3\,mol^{-1}$)
H_V	liquid height (m)
J	molar mass flux ($mol\,m^{-2}\,s^{-1}$)
J_g	molar mass flux across gas film ($mol\,m^{-2}\,s^{-1}$)
J_l	molar mass flux across liquid film ($mol\,m^{-2}\,s^{-1}$)
k	mass transfer coefficient ($m\,s^{-1}$)

Basic Biotechnology, third edition, eds. Colin Ratledge and Bjørn Kristiansen.
Published by Cambridge University Press. © Cambridge University Press 2006.

k_g gas film mass transfer coefficient ($m\,s^{-1}$)

k_l liquid film mass transfer coefficient ($m\,s^{-1}$)

$k_l a$ volumetric mass transfer coefficient (s^{-1})

K overall mass transfer coefficient ($m\,s^{-1}$)

K consistency index

n power law index

N impeller rotational speed (s^{-1})

OTR   oxygen transfer rate ($= Ja$ for oxygen) ($mol\,m^{-3}\,s^{-1}$)

p pressure (bar $= N\,m^{-2}$)

p_0 reference pressure ($= 1$ bar) (bar)

p_i pressure at gas side of interface (bar)

p_{in} inlet gas pressure (bar)

p_{out} outlet gas pressure (bar)

P power input (W)

P_s power input by stirrer (W)

q consumption rate ($mol\,m^{-3}\,s^{-1}$)

t time (s)

T_V tank diameter (m)

x distance (m)

v_g superficial gas velocity ($m\,s^{-1}$)

V volume (m^3)

V_g gas volume (m^3)

V_l liquid volume (m^3)

α power law index

$\dot{\gamma}$ average shear rate (s^{-1})

ϵ hold-up or void fraction

μ dynamic viscosity ($kg\,m^{-1}\,s^{-1}$)

μ_0 reference dynamic viscosity ($kg\,m^{-1}\,s^{-1}$)

ρ_l liquid phase density ($kg\,m^{-3}$)

P_o Impeller power number

Re   Reynolds number

8.1 | Mass transfer in bioreactors

8.1.1 Introduction

In a bioreaction process, substrates are consumed and products are formed by action of a micro-organism, or catalytic parts of organisms, for example enzymes. Typical substrates for a living cell are carbon sources such as sugar and oil, nitrogen sources such as ammonia and amino acids, and electron acceptors such as oxygen. Products can be all kinds of organic compounds, from biomass to CO_2. For an optimal rate of reaction, the micro-organism, the academic researcher or the industrial process engineer should see to it that transfer of substrates to the enzyme or cell surface (or the site of reaction inside the cell) and removal of products away from the enzyme or organism is as rapid as possible and, preferably, not rate-limiting. Usually this

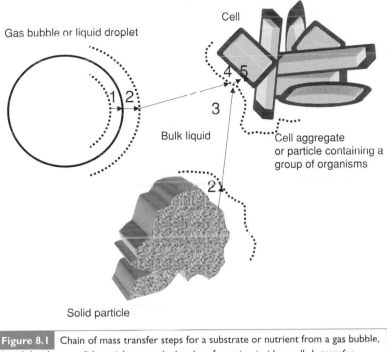

Figure 8.1 Chain of mass transfer steps for a substrate or nutrient from a gas bubble, liquid droplet or solid particle towards the site of reaction inside a cell: 1, transfer (mainly by diffusion) of substrates from gas, liquid or solid phase to the interface with the liquid water phase; 2, transport (usually by a combination of diffusion and convection) across a thin, rather stagnant boundary layer of water phase that surrounds the gas bubble, liquid droplet or solid particle; 3, transport (usually by convection or turbulence) through the bulk liquid phase to a thin boundary layer surrounding a single micro-organism or a particle (clump, pellet, immobilisation carrier) containing a group of organisms; 4, transport (diffusive) across this boundary layer to the cell surface; and 5, transport (passive by diffusion and/or active with a transport enzyme) over the cell envelope to a site inside the cell where the reaction takes place. NB: Products formed take the reverse route.

transfer involves a chain of mass transfer steps as shown in Fig. 8.1. The slowest of these steps will determine the overall mass transfer rate, and its value is to be compared with the slowest kinetic reaction step in order to find out if mass transfer will affect the overall process performance or not. In this chapter, the attention will be focused on reactions involving whole cells. In enzymatic biotransformations, cells are absent and there are less mass transfer steps, but the same concepts can be applied.

8.2 | The mass transfer steps

8.2.1 Effects of transfer limitations

If one mass transfer step is slower than the key kinetic reaction step, it will limit the metabolic activity of the micro-organisms, typically expressed as a reduction in the formation of a desired product from a selected substrate. As a result, two effects may be observed, both with freely suspended cells as well as organisms immobilised inside cell aggregates or solid particles:

(1) *The overall reaction rate is below the theoretical maximum, and the process output is slower than desired.* This is the case in the formation of gluconic acid from glucose by the aerobic bacterium, *Gluconobacter oxydans*. Here, the overall reaction rate is determined by the rate at which oxygen is transferred to the liquid phase. After relieving the limitation, there is no irreversible effect on this particular micro-organism. Another example is a limited supply of sugar to immobilised cells due to slow diffusion inside an immobilisation carrier. The overall rate of production is often reversibly reduced. However, there are also examples of systems where the biosynthetic capacity of a cell is irreversibly damaged after imposing an oxygen transfer limitation (e.g. in penicillin fermentation). Such processes are very sensitive to mass transfer limitations.

(2) *The selectivity of the reaction is altered.* In the formation of baker's yeast from glucose, oxygen serves as an electron acceptor. In the absence of oxygen the electrons will be directed to pyruvate resulting in the formation of ethanol and CO_2 instead of more yeast. *Bacillus subtilis* cultures produce acetoin and 2,3-butanediol when devoid of oxygen. The ratio of the two products is greatly dependent on the dissolved oxygen concentration, and thus on the ratio of oxygen transfer and oxygen consumption rates. Again, the damage can be either reversible or irreversible.

8.2.2 Transfer between phases

The transfer of oxygen from an air bubble to the micro-organism in an aerobic bioprocess is a relatively slow transport step. Oxygen, and other sparingly soluble gases in aqueous solutions (such as hydrocarbons up to four carbon atoms), may become rapidly depleted when it is consumed. If not replaced at the same high rate the situation will be detrimental for the micro-organism. Transfer of material across a liquid–liquid or liquid–solid boundary is similar to gas–liquid mass transfer. An example is the growth on higher hydrocarbons ($>C_6$). The oil phase is present in the form of small droplets and the main resistance to mass transfer lies with the water layer surrounding the oil droplets. Also, the exchange of material between a solid phase (substrate particles, particles that contain micro-organisms) and the liquid phase, obeys similar principles.

8.2.3 Transfer inside a single phase

Inside a gas bubble or oil droplet there is usually enough motion to guarantee a quick transfer of molecules to the interface with the water phase, so the resistance is at the water side of the interface. If the distances in the bulk liquid phase to be bridged are relatively

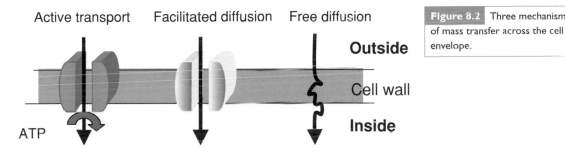

Figure 8.2 Three mechanisms of mass transfer across the cell envelope.

large, a transport resistance can occur in this phase. Such a situation is encountered in large bioreactors where bulk liquid mixing is usually sub-optimal (i.e. the concept of ideal mixing is only applicable in small reactors). In industrial practice, it is important to realise that one has to live with this potential limitation. Therefore its effects on the microbial reaction system should be borne in mind during process development work. Mass transfer limitations inside a solid phase can occur within biocatalyst particles that contain immobilised microorganisms, either as a surface biofilm attached to a carrier, or dispersed throughout the carrier material. Alternatively, the micro-organism itself, particularly if it is filamentous, may be present as a clump or pellet. A substrate entering the particle or pellet may be consumed so fast that nothing enters the inner part of the particle, so that the efficiency of the catalyst is below maximum. Also, the reaction may be slowed down because a toxic or inhibiting product cannot move away quickly enough.

8.2.4 Transfer across the cell envelope

The micro-organism itself can also be considered as a separate (solid or liquid) phase. Transport across the cell envelope (mostly a combination of cell wall and cytoplasmic membrane) can be limited, depending on the size and physical properties (hydrophobicity, electrical charge) of the molecule and whether the organism is equipped with a specific transport mechanism or not. Generally three mechanisms can be distinguished (Fig. 8.2):

- free diffusion: passive transport down a concentration gradient;
- facilitated diffusion: as above but speeded up by a carrier protein;
- active transport: transport by a carrier protein with input of free energy.

The diameter of the microbial cell itself is very small (order of magnitude 1–5 μm) so that diffusion inside the cell is more rapid than transport across the cell envelope. Additionally, in eukaryotic cells there are intracellular organelles (vacuoles, mitochondria), which can present other transport barriers. However, in quantitative terms this type of transport is much more rapid than the consumption rate inside the cell and will normally not limit the overall rate in the chain of transport steps.

8.3 | Mass transfer equations

8.3.1   Fundamental principles

Fick's law (8.1a) states that the mass transfer, J, of a component in single phase will be proportional to the concentration gradient in the direction of the transport. The expression for *steady-state* mass flux is:

$$J = -D \, dC/dx \tag{8.1a}$$

For mass transfer in a solid phase, D is the *effective* diffusivity, a function of the diffusion coefficient, the porosity of the solid and the shape of the channels inside the solid. The relationship between mass flux and concentration difference, ΔC, is:

$$J = D\Delta C/d \tag{8.1b}$$

where D/d is the mass transfer coefficient and the inverse, d/D, can be interpreted as the resistance to transfer. ΔC is the driving force for the transfer. (Strictly speaking this relates to the geometry of a flat sheet boundary layer with thickness d in a stationary fluid but it can be applied to bioreactor systems.) For the *unsteady-state* situation, a mass balance over a layer with diameter dx results in:

$$D\delta^2 C /\delta x^2 = \delta C /\delta t \tag{8.2}$$

These fundamental, theoretical equations can be used to calculate mass transfer by a diffusion process. A pre-requisite is that convective transport is absent and this is rarely the case. More often, a combination of diffusion and convection with phase transfer is encountered but now we have the additional problem that the velocity pattern of the liquid flow is not known. Thus, for gas–liquid and liquid–particle mass transfer in real bioreactors a more empirical approach is required.

For *mass transfer between liquid and gas phases* or *liquid and solid phases* the well-known *two-film theory* (see any standard chemical engineering textbook on mass transfer) can be adopted. Mass flux in both phases must be separately described, whereas the overall transfer is determined by two steps in series across the film, as shown in Fig. 8.3. For gas–liquid transfer the mass flux is described by:

$$\text{Gas film transport:} \; J_g = k_g(p - p_i) \tag{8.3}$$

$$\text{Liquid film transport:} \; J_1 = k_1(C_i - C) \tag{8.4}$$

The concentrations at both sides of the interface, p_i and C_i, are not identical, but related through the Henry coefficient, H:

$$p_i = HC_i \tag{8.5}$$

In practice it is not possible to measure the interfacial values, so it is better to eliminate these from Eqs. (8.3), (8.4) and (8.5) and write the

Boundary layers

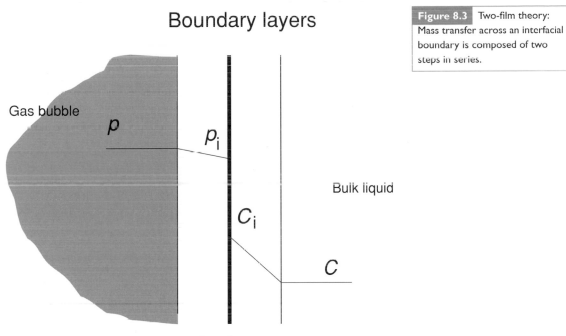

mass flow as a function of the concentrations in both bulk phases:

$$J = K(C^* - C) \tag{8.6}$$

where $C^*(= p/H)$ is the saturation value in the liquid phase. Note that Eq. (8.6) is of the same form as Eq. (8.1b). $(C^* - C)$ is the overall driving force and the overall transfer coefficient, K, results from the sum of the transfer resistances:

$$1/K = 1/(Hk_g) + 1/k_l \tag{8.7}$$

Often this general equation can be simplified as $1/(H\,k_g) \ll 1/k_l$ (i.e. the gas phase film resistance is negligible compared to the resistance in the liquid film). Usually, mass transfer is expressed per unit of volume of the bioreactor, rather than per unit of interfacial area. This is because in many cases, such as when dealing with a sparged and agitated bioreactor, or a packed bed tower reactor, the interfacial area available for mass transfer is not easily determined. The volumetric mass transfer rate then follows from:

$$Ja = k_l a(C^* - C) \tag{8.8}$$

where a is the gas–liquid interfacial area per unit bioreactor liquid volume, or area per unit gas + solid + liquid volume, or area per unit gross vessel volume. When dealing with the transfer of oxygen from gas to liquid, the product $J\,a$ is usually called the oxygen transfer rate (OTR).

For an accurate estimate of $k_l a$, assumptions must be made on the values of C^* (or p) and C. For a laboratory-scale bioreactor (<10 litres operating volume) the bulk liquid phase is assumed to be

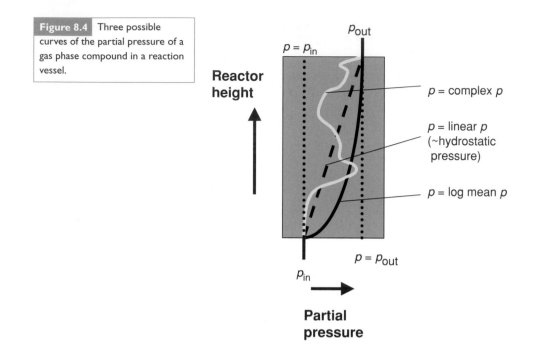

Figure 8.4 Three possible curves of the partial pressure of a gas phase compound in a reaction vessel.

well mixed and hence C is constant throughout the liquid. However, in pilot plants or production-scale vessels (>100 litres) this will not be the case, and local concentration variations need to be taken into account (see also Section 8.5). Therefore, for the gas phase we must assume that one of the following cases will be applicable (Fig. 8.4):

(1) $p = p_{in}$ = constant; there is little or no depletion of the inlet gas, which is often true for small reactors with high gas flow and relatively little transfer;

(2) $p = p_{out}$ = constant; the gas phase is perfectly mixed, which also applies to small systems, but when the transfer rate is high compared to the flow of the gas phase;

(3) p varies inside the reactor; for small reactors p is given by its logarithmic mean value[1], in larger reactors with adequate mixing the hydrostatic pressure determines p, and in large vessels with poor mixing more complex models must be used.

Note that the value of H, and hence C^*, is a function of liquid composition and temperature (gases are generally less soluble at higher temperature). Henry's law also implies that C^* is linearly dependent on p.

There are a number of theories with which the values of k_l and a can be separately estimated. These theories all suffer from questionable assumptions when applied to moving fluids in a real bioreactor, but do give quantitative insight into fundamental aspects of

---

[1] The logarithmic mean concentration: $C_{lm} = (C^* - C)/\ln \frac{C^*}{C}$.

mass transfer. Details on such theories can be found in most standard (bio)chemical engineering textbooks.

8.3.2 Gas–liquid mass transfer in real systems

Much attention has been given to oxygen transfer from the gas phase into the liquid phase in bioreactor processes. Since it is experimentally very difficult to estimate the values of k_l and a separately, $k_l a$ is often treated as a lumped parameter. In bioprocess engineering literature, one can find a large number of expressions for this (volumetric mass transfer) coefficient. Here, a division should be made between the dominant types of reactors used: *bubble columns, airlift reactors* and *stirred tank reactors* (see Chapter 7). In each case the physical properties of the liquid may influence the magnitude of mass transfer. Extreme values are given by:

- A liquid which greatly stimulates bubble coalescence, i.e. a coalescing liquid. The mass transfer will be relatively poor.
- A liquid which suppresses coalescence to a large extent, i.e. a non-coalescing liquid. This gives the highest mass transfer rates.

In a *bubble column* (see Chapter 7, Section 7.2.2) the gas enters through the sparger orifices. If the broth is coalescent and non-viscous (i.e. behaving like distilled or tap water) the bubbles will rapidly take their equilibrium average diameter of $\sim$6 mm. When the air flow rate is high enough the vessel is operated in the heterogeneous flow regime and then hold-up, ε, is a function of the superficial gas velocity ($-$ gas flow per unit cross-sectional area of the reactor), corrected for pressure differences (p_0 is a reference pressure of 1 bar):

$$\varepsilon = 0.6(v_g p_0/p)^{0.7} \tag{8.9}$$

For the mass transfer coefficient, the following correlation has been experimentally verified:

$$k_l a = 0.32(v_g p_0/p)^{0.7} \tag{8.10}$$

In non-coalescing liquids, e.g. ionic solutions and some fermentation broths, the bubbles that originate from the sparger will rise and not mix with other bubbles, provided that the bubble size is smaller than $\sim$6 mm. The interfacial area, and hence $k_l a$, will be higher than when larger bubbles are present. If the bubbles are larger they will break up and take the same equilibrium value as in coalescing liquids. It is noted that in a large bubble column ($>$50 m^3), the bubbles will significantly expand as they rise through the reactor because of the decreasing hydrostatic pressure changes. This will influence mass transfer.

In an *airlift reactor* (Chapter 7, Section 7.2.3), there is a riser section, in which the sparging of bubbles results in an upward liquid flow, a top section, where the bubbles escape from the liquid, and a downcomer section, in which the liquid is recirculated downwards. Although the riser resembles a bubble column, the gas hold-up is lower than predicted by Eq. (8.9) due to the interaction with the liquid flow. Correspondingly, $k_l a$ will be lower, up to one-third of the bubble column value. A precise quantification, however, cannot be easily made.

In a *stirred tank reactor* the flow phenomena are determined by the balance between aeration forces and agitation forces, and large local variations in combination with a number of flow regime transitions make a precise quantification of mass transfer difficult. Sparged gas is usually rapidly collected in the gas cavities formed behind the impeller blades as they rotate. A highly turbulent vortex is established at the trailing end of the cavities from which the gas is dispersed into small bubbles that enter the bulk fluid. These bubbles follow the liquid flow, but will also rise to the surface of the liquid in the tank. They will coalesce in areas that are relatively calm and redisperse in places where the shear stress is high. A part of the bubbles is recirculated into the cavities and the rest escapes at the surface.

There is a correlation available for the average gas hold-up in coalescing liquids:

$$\varepsilon = 0.13(P_s/V_l)^{0.33}(v_g p_0/p)^{0.67} \tag{8.11}$$

For non-coalescing liquids the hold-up value is considerably higher.

Correlations for $k_l a$ are fully empirical. Usually, the extremes of coalescing and non-coalescing liquids are denoted by the following, coarse expressions (accuracy ~30%) valid for P_s/V_l between 0.5 and 10 kW m^{-3}:

$$\text{Coalescing:} \quad k_l a = 0.026(P_s/V_l)^{0.4}(v_g p_0/p)^{0.5} \tag{8.12}$$

$$\text{Non-coalescing:} \quad k_l a = 0.002(P_s/V_l)^{0.7}(v_g p_0/p)^{0.2} \tag{8.13}$$

In a coalescing liquid, $k_l a$ is more sensitive to changes in aeration than changes in agitation, while for a non-coalescing liquid the opposite is true. Note that the correlations are independent of the agitator type. The energy input by agitation is a vital variable in Eqs. (8.11), (8.12) and (8.13). The amount of power drawn by a stirrer of diameter D with a rotational speed N is usually expressed as:

$$P = P_0 \rho_l N^3 D^5 \tag{8.14}$$

The impeller power number, P_0, is a function of the aeration rate, the impeller Reynolds number $(= \rho_l N D^2/\mu)$ and the impeller type (see Fig. 8.5). When a broth is aerated, P_0 generally falls due to the growing size of the cavities behind the impeller blades. For a typical Rushton impeller P_0 falls by a factor of 2, while for a Scaba type (6SRGT) there is hardly any drop.

Example
The oxygen transfer performance of a stirred tank reactor is generally better than that of a bubble column with similar geometry and aeration rate. For a coalescing liquid in a vessel of 100 m^3 reaction volume, with tank diameter 3.5 m, aeration rate 1 vvm (or 1.67 N m^3 s^{-1}),

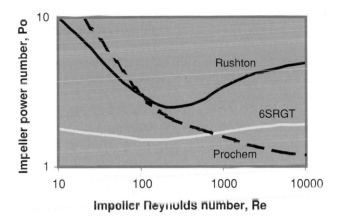

Figure 8.5 Some unaerated impeller power numbers, P_o, as a function of the impeller Reynolds number, Re. In the turbulent flow regime in the absence of aeration the value of P_o for a standard six-bladed Rushton turbine is constant at ~5, for a Scaba 6SRGT impeller it is ~1.7 and for a Prochem agitator it is ~1.0. In the laminar flow regime, there is an inverse proportionality with Re (e.g. for a Rushton impeller $P_o = 64/Re$).

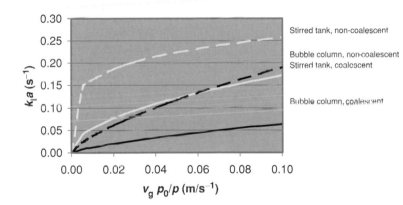

Stirred tank, non-coalescent

Bubble column, non-coalescent
Stirred tank, coalescent

Bubble column, coalescent

Figure 8.6 Illustration of oxygen transfer in different reactors and media as a function of superficial gas velocity using Eqs. (8.10), (8.12) and (8.13). Here it is assumed that k_la in a bubble column with non-coalescent media is three times the value of coalescent media.

head-space pressure 2 bar, impeller diameter 1.75 m, and power input per unit volume $P/V_l = 2$ kW m^{-3}, we get:

Bubble column; Eq. (8.10): $k_la = 0.05$ s^{-1}
Stirred tank; Eq. (8.12): $k_la = 0.14$ s^{-1}

Assuming $(C^* - C) = (0.59$ mol m^{-3} $- 0.10$ mol m$^{-3}) = 0.49$ mol m^{-3}, the bubble column OTR will be 0.024 mol m^{-3} s^{-1}, whereas for the stirred tank it will be 0.070 mol m^{-3} s^{-1}. In spite of this, bubble columns are frequently used in bioprocesses, due to other advantages such as simple construction, even distribution of shear rate, lower energy input, etc. (see also Fig. 8.6).

When high concentrations of filamentous micro-organisms are used, the branched filaments of the mycelium interact with each other and form larger aggregates that decrease the free flow of liquid. This results in high viscosity and pseudoplastic or elastic broth behaviour. Similar observations are made when a micro-organism excretes polymeric substances, such as xanthan. The decrease of mass transfer is partly due to bubble coalescence, which leads to large bubbles in the broth. Also the gas hold-up is reported to be lower due to higher bubble rise velocity. As a consequence the interfacial area will be small. In large bioreactors under extreme conditions, bubbles of 1 m diameter can be observed. Sometimes this effect is partly compensated for by the simultaneous presence of a large number of very small bubbles (diameter <1 mm) which have a long residence time in the broth (15 min or more). There is also an effect of viscosity on k_l. This is due to a decrease of liquid velocity and not a direct consequence of the viscosity itself. Furthermore, in aerated broths the power input may have to be reduced because the size of the cavities behind the impeller blades is larger. This will diminish the shear rates and bubble break-up.

In the literature, these complex, combined effects are described by an extension of Eqs. (8.10), (8.12) and (8.13) with a factor μ^{-n}, where n usually ranges from 0.5 to 0.9. For stirred tanks and non-coalescent media:

$$k_l a = 0.002(P_s/V_l)^{0.7}(v_g p_0/p)^{0.2}(\mu/\mu_0)^{-0.7} \tag{8.15}$$

provided $\mu > \mu_0$, where $\mu_0 = 0.05$ Pa s.

If the broth behaves like a pseudoplastic fluid (viscosity decreases as the shear rate increases) or dilatant fluid (viscosity increases as the shear rates increases), an average viscosity can be taken over the reactor:

$$\mu = K \dot{\gamma}^{n-1} \tag{8.16}$$

The average shear rate can be estimated from:

$$\dot{\gamma} = 10N \tag{8.17}$$

The parameters K and n in the rheology model depend on the biomass concentration, Typically K is proportional to C_x^{α}, with the value of α ranging from 1.5 to 4. For pseudoplastic broths $n < 1$, for dilatant liquids $n > 1$, whereas for Newtonian media $n = 1$.

Example
A pseudoplastic broth in a bioreactor has the following properties: $C_x = 30\,\text{g/l}^{-1}$, $K = 1$, $n = 0.4$. The stirrer speed is 3 revolutions s^{-1}. Using Eqs. (8.16) and (8.17) we find that the apparent viscosity is 0.13 Pa s. According to Eq. (8.15), $k_l a$ is reduced to 51% of the value in a low-viscosity broth. What would happen if the biomass concentration or the impeller speed doubled? (Answer: with double biomass concentration and $\alpha = 2$, $k_l a$ is reduced to 19%; with double impeller speed, $k_l a$ is reduced to 69%.)

8.3.3 Liquid–solid mass transfer

The description of mass transfer through a liquid film to or from a solid surface is much simpler than for gas–liquid mass transfer. In these systems k_l is dependent on the liquid/solid properties, and the value of the interfacial area can be determined experimentally. Usually, liquid–solid transfer applies to situations where mass transfer and reaction are interacting: a substrate is transported through a liquid film to the surface of a particle where micro-organisms are present to consume the substrate. Products formed are transported back through the film and into the bulk liquid. These situations are often treated in terms of apparent kinetics, i.e. the observed rate of reaction is described with standard kinetic expressions, but an *effectiveness factor* (ranging from 0 to 1) is introduced to describe the performance of the reaction compared to the same reaction with no transport limitations.

8.3.4 Mass transfer inside a solid particle

When there are micro-organisms active inside a particle or cellular aggregate, the transport (by diffusion) within the particles may present another resistance. This situation is found in biocatalytic processes when dealing with cells immobilised in alginate or porous solid particles. A proper description of this phenomenon is difficult because the kinetics of the microbial reactions inside the particle may differ greatly from those with freely suspended cells and, hence, will be unknown. This is due to altered physiological conditions for the cells. In addition to an effectiveness factor for external mass transfer, an overall effectiveness factor may be used, also including intraparticle resistance.

8.4 | Determination of the volumetric mass transfer coefficients

If one is interested in approximate $k_l a$ values, or when measurements with real bioreaction systems are impractical or economically not feasible, such as in large bioreactors, model fluids can be used. Information is provided from literature, either more theoretical or more empirical as described above, or a new series of experiments can be designed. The use of model fluids, such as water or salt solutions, if necessary with paper pulp or polymers added to mimic viscous broths, gives extremes of what can be expected in real systems, and qualitative trends as a function of changes. There are a few possible measurement methods:

- *Chemical reaction method.* In order to mimic a microbial reaction, the transferred component can be consumed or produced in a chemical reaction. For oxygen transfer studies, sulphite can be used, as it rapidly oxidises to sulphate in the presence of oxygen and a catalyst. $k_l a$ is found from Eq. (8.8) by measuring the rate of sulphite consumption, $J a(= dC_{sulphite}/dt)$ and $C^*(= p/H$ for oxygen). For most accurate results, conditions should be selected so that C equals zero. Alternatives for sulphite are glucose in combination with the glucose oxidase (oxygen is consumed), or a mixture of

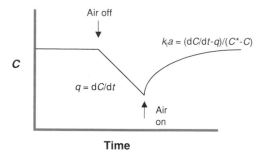

Figure 8.7 Course of the oxygen concentration during a dynamic $k_l a$ experiment. From the linearly falling part, the oxygen consumption rate, q, can be evaluated. From the upward curve then the value of $k_l a$ can be found, for example using a logarithmic plot of $(C^* - C)$ vs. time.

H_2O_2 and catalase (oxygen is produced). Similarly NaOH solutions can be used to study CO_2 transfer (CO_2 rapidly reacts with OH^-).

- *Physical replacement method.* Consider a gas sparged liquid in steady state, so that C^* equals C. The experiment is started when the oxygen level in the gas phase is rapidly changed from one value to another. For example, N_2 gas in a N_2-sparged liquid is replaced by air. Then $J\,a$ in Eq. (8.8) equals dC/dt and, by continuously measuring the oxygen concentration in the liquid, $k_l a$ can be evaluated from this equation. Another possibility is a sudden change in pressure of the component to be transferred. This method is usually very fast, and a rapidly enough responding oxygen electrode is therefore an absolute requirement.

If it is required to have real values for $k_l a$, then theories, model systems or published correlations should not be used. In actively growing cultures, $k_l a$ can be experimentally determined using the following methods:

- *Steady-state bioreaction method.* When using a microbial consuming system in (pseudo) steady state, $k_l a$ can be calculated from Eq. (8.8), when $J\,a$, C^* and C are known, and the difference between C^* and C is large enough. For example, for oxygen, $J\,a$ (OTR) will be equal to the difference in the oxygen mole fractions in the inlet and outlet gas phases multiplied by the inlet and outlet gas flow rates (oxygen transfer rate = oxygen uptake rate, or OTR = OUR). C^* follows from the partial oxygen pressure ($C^* = p/H$), and C can be read from a dissolved oxygen electrode.
- *Dynamic bioreaction method.* When the air flow is temporarily reduced, shut off or replaced by N_2 in a respiring culture, $k_l a$ for oxygen becomes zero and the dissolved oxygen concentration will fall rapidly. The rate of depletion, dC/dt, will become equal to the consumption rate (q). After turning the air flow on again, the concentration will return to its initial value. Again Eq. (8.8) can be used to determine $k_l a$, as $J\,a$ will be equal to $dC/dt + q$ (see also Fig. 8.7). This method is only applicable in small vessels (<100 l), because in larger vessels the gas phase composition will not be uniform after sparging with N_2 (or the gas hold-up must be built up again after shut down of the air flow). In any case, a rapid oxygen electrode is a pre-requisite for accurate results.

8.5 | The effect of scale on mass transfer

8.5.1 Scale-up

In large-scale bioreactors, oxygen transfer is usually better than in a laboratory-scale or pilot plant reactor. This is due to a larger contribution of the gas phase (higher superficial gas velocity), and a larger driving force (high headspace pressure and hydrostatic head).

Example

Consider two geometrically similar, ideally mixed stirred tank reactors, one of 0.1 m^3 reaction volume, and one of 100 m^3. The H_V/T_V ratio is 3.0, and the D/T_V ratio is 0.5. Scale-up is carried out by keeping the power input to the reactors constant at $P/V_1 = 2\,kW\,m^{-3}$, the air flow rate at 1 vvm and a constant average pressure in the broth (determined by the headspace pressure plus the hydrostatic head) of 2.45 bar. Assuming that there is no depletion of the gas phase, the following comparison is made (coalescent broth, $C^* = 0.24$ mol m^{-3} at 1 bar, $C = 0.10$ mol m^{-3}):

$$0.1\ m^3: \ v_s\,p_0/p = 0.007 \text{ m s}^{-1}, \quad k_l a = 0.046 \text{ s}^{-1},$$
$$OTR = 0.022 \text{ mol m}^{-3}\text{ s}^{-1}$$
$$100\ m^3: \ v_s\,p_0/p = 0.071 \text{ m s}^{-1}, \quad k_l a = 0.145 \text{ s}^{-1},$$
$$OTR = 0.071 \text{ mol m}^{-3}\text{ s}^{-1}$$

What would be the OTR difference for a non-coalescing broth? (Answer: OTR $= 0.07$ or 0.12 mol m^{-3} s^{-1}, respectively.)

In a large bioreactor the OTR has maximum limits due to the following restrictive conditions:

- There may be mechanical construction difficulties in very large fermenters ($>300\,m^3$). Furthermore, liquid transport and mixing will become very slow compared to mass transfer and reaction, and thus dominate the overall reaction rate. Cooling limitations may become more significant.
- The average power input should not exceed 5 kW m^{-3}. If it is higher, the micro-organisms may be mechanically damaged and, also, the energy costs and investment costs for the motor will become excessively high.
- The pressure-corrected superficial air velocity should be below 0.10 m s^{-1}. Compressor costs are restricting, and high gas hold-up will increase at the cost of broth space.
- The headspace pressure has a maximum for mechanical reasons. In addition CO_2 partial pressure will also increase, and inhibit growth and production.
- The gas phase cannot be considered ideally mixed. The oxygen partial pressure will fall as the bubbles travel up through the reactor and this reduces the driving force for mass transfer.

Large bioreactor

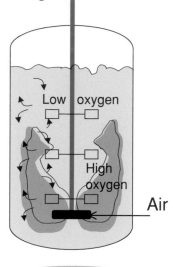

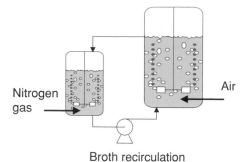

Figure 8.9 An example of a small-scale two-compartment reactor set-up for scaling-down the conditions in the large bioreactor. As an alternative, the N_2-sparged vessel may be in plug flow mode (with some dispersion).

Figure 8.8 Liquid flow and oxygen is transfer in a large bioreactor. Most of the oxygen is transferred in the region near the impeller. In the circulation loop, i.e. the path the broth travels from the impeller, out into the body of the reactor and back to the impeller, more oxygen is consumed than transferred and the oxygen concentration will decrease. In a full-scale stirred tank reactor the liquid circulation loop can be as long as 10 m. With a liquid velocity of 1 m s^{-1} the mean circulation time will be 10 s. As a worst case estimate (no transfer at all outside the impeller region), it will take 10 s before the oxygen will become depleted in the loop. Therefore, the oxygen concentration in the bottom compartment should be so high that local depletion, which can be detrimental for the microbial state and product formation rate, is avoided. Note that Eq. (8.8) predicts that this will reduce the mass transfer rate because the driving force ($C^* - C$) in the bottom part is low as both C^* and C will be high.

In reactors larger than $\sim$10 m^3, the processes of liquid transport and mass transfer become comparably slow. Mass transfer and liquid circulation will interfere, and should be treated together. In a stirred tank reactor with one single impeller, most of the oxygen transfer takes place in the impeller zone. A comparison of oxygen transfer in the bubble column and the stirred tank revealed that outside the impeller zone, the OTR may be only one-third of the value around the impeller. The importance of circulation loops is shown in Fig. 8.8.

8.5.2 Scale-down

As illustrated above, micro-organisms can experience a continuously changing environment when travelling around in a large bioreactor. This may give undesired scale-up effects. To avoid these problems the large scale should be taken as the point of reference, and the possible effects should be studied by simulation of the large-scale variations in a small-scale experimental set-up. Limiting factors on a large scale, such as mass transfer, are thus scaled-down and can be studied and minimised in a practical and economic way. In reality, scale-down cannot be precise, because the large-scale conditions are difficult to determine and are also too complex to be fully understood. Several tools are available to find adequate solutions to down-scaling:

- Two-compartment reactor set-ups can be used, mimicking the two most important reactor zones, and recirculation of broth between the zones, see Fig. 8.9. The size of the two compartments and the circulation rate are critical, as is the flow type in each compartment, i.e. ranging from well mixed to plug flow.
- Development and (large-scale) verification of simple or more sophisticated mathematical flow models for the large vessel can be carried out, and the results used to design the scaled-down experiment.
- Well-characterised microbial test systems can be used, in which the sensitivity to selected variations is known.

In the literature these approaches have been extensively studied for the improvement of oxygen transfer and substrate (feed) mixing in large bioreactors.

8.6 | Further reading

Bailey, J. E. and Ollis, D. F. *Biochemical Engineering Fundamentals*, second edition. New York: McGraw-Hill, 1986. Classic textbook on fundamental aspects of bioprocessing.

Kossen, N. W. F. Scale-up. In *Advances in Bioprocess Engineering*, eds. E. Galindo and O. T. Ramirez. Dordecht: Kluwer Academic, 1994. Illustrations of scale-up in industrial practice, giving a feeling for the fitness of use of the available tools, e.g. scale-down.

Merchuk, J. C., Ben-Zvi, S. and Niranjan, K. Why use bubble column bioreactors? *Trends in Biotechnology* 12: 501–511, 1994. Review on the hydrodynamic, heat transfer and mass transfer characteristics of bubble column bioreactors.

Nielsen, J. and Villadsen, J. *Bioreaction Engineering Principles*. New York: Plenum Press, 1994. A complete and up-to-date textbook. Stoichiometry, kinetics and bioreactor performance aspects (including mass transfer) are separately treated and then integrated. Uses fundamental aspects of microbial physiology with strong emphasis on mathematical tools.

Nienow, A. W. Agitators for mycelial fermentations. *Trends in Biotechnology* 8: 224–233, 1990. Overview on fundamental aspects, use and improvement of different types of agitators, especially for highly viscous mycelial fermentations. Interactions between cell morphology, rheology, mixing, mass and heat transfer processes.

van 't Riet, K. and Tramper, J. *Basic Bioreactor Design*. New York: Marcel Dekker, 1991. Application-oriented book on bioreactor design with lots of useful data, guidelines and rules for practical process engineering.

Chapter 9

Downstream processing

Marcel Ottens

Delft University of Technology, The Netherlands

Johannes A. Wesselingh

University of Groningen, The Netherlands

Luuk A. M. van der Wielen

Delft University of Technology, The Netherlands

Nomenclature

a	acceleration ($m\ s^{-2}$)
A	cross-sectional area (m^2)
B	width (m)
c	concentration solids ($kg\ m^{-3}$)
C	liquid phase concentration ($kg\ m^{-3}$)
C_D	drag coefficient (–)
c_p	specific heat ($J\ kg^{-1}\ K^{-1}$)
D	diffusion coefficient ($m^2\ s^{-1}$)
d_p	particle diameter (m)
d_s	stirrer diameter (m)
g	gravitational acceleration ($9.81\ m\ s^{-2}$)

Basic Biotechnology, third edition, eds. Colin Ratledge and Bjørn Kristiansen.
Published by Cambridge University Press. © Cambridge University Press 2006.

H	height (m)
I	ionic strength ($\mathrm{mol\ m^{-3}}$)
J	flux ($\mathrm{m\ s^{-1}}$)
k	mass transfer coefficient ($\mathrm{m\ s^{-1}}$)
K	constant in Eq. (9.1) (–)
L	feed flow rate ($\mathrm{m^3\ s^{-1}}$)
l	length (m)
L	length (m)
M	mass (kg)
N	rotational speed ($\mathrm{s^{-1}}$)
N	number of passes in Eq. (9.1) (–)
P	power number (–)
P	pressure (Pa)
Q	concentration in auxiliary phase ($\mathrm{kg\ m^{-3}}$)
Q	flow rate ($\mathrm{m^3\ s^{-1}}$)
q	heat flux ($\mathrm{W\ m^{-2}}$)
Q	solid or second liquid phase concentrate ($\mathrm{kg\ m^{-3}}$)
R	radius (m)
r	radius (m)
T	temperature (K)
t	time (s)
U	heat transfer coefficient ($\mathrm{m\ s^{-1}}$)
V	auxiliary or solvent flow rate ($\mathrm{m^3\ s^{-1}}$)
v	velocity ($\mathrm{m\ s^{-1}}$)
V_f	filtrate volume ($\mathrm{m^3}$)
V_p	particle volume ($\mathrm{m^3}$)
x	cartesian coordinate (m)
x	mole fraction (–)
z	length (m)
ΔP	pressure difference (Pa)
ΔT	temperature difference (K)

α	specific filter cake resistance ($\mathrm{m\ kg^{-1}}$)
ε	liquid hold-up (–)
δ	film thickness (m)
ϕ	liquid hold-up (–)
ϕ_v	flow rate ($\mathrm{m^3\ s^{-1}}$)
η	dynamic viscosity (Pa s)
Σ	equivalent settling area ($\mathrm{m^2}$)
ρ	density ($\mathrm{kg\ m^{-3}}$)
ω	angular velocity ($\mathrm{rad\ s^{-1}}$)

Subscripts

s	solid
l	liquid

9.1 | Introduction

After making the product in a fermenter, one might assume that the work is done. But this is not so; we have just begun. The production of biomolecules is governed by the aqueous environment needed for microorganisms. The product can be the micro-organism itself, or a metabolite excreted in the solution or contained in inclusion bodies, but the fermenter may contain up to 95% water and much effort has to be put in concentrating the product. There is a correlation between the concentration of a product in the broth and its price in the marketplace. The more dilute a product, the higher the cost prize. Removal of water is one thing, there are many additional problems in downstream processing (DSP). The product may be intracellular and the cells have to be disrupted to release the product. The fermenter fluid may be complex containing compounds resembling the product, which makes it difficult to purify the product. Even so, a high purity may be needed: in pharmaceutical products up to 99.999% purity is required. These problems govern the approach used to separate the product. Usually the following steps are required:

- *cell disruption* (only when dealing with an intracellular product),
- *clarification* (separation of the cells and cell debris from the liquid),
- *concentration* of the product stream,
- *purification* (often in multiple steps), and
- *product formulation* (giving the product a suitable form).

These steps form the basis of this chapter. Each step requires one or more pieces of equipment. For these we need to know the size, method of operation and use of auxiliaries like solvents, adsorbents and energy. A process may consist of many steps and each step has a yield for the product. Although a yield of 95% might seem high for an individual step, connecting several steps can cause a rapid decay in process yield (0.95^n, n being the number of steps, leading to: 0.95, 0.90, 0.86, . . .). Bioprocesses use large amounts of salts and solvents, and produce huge contaminated wastewater streams. To predict the partitioning and solubility of biomolecules we need thermodynamics. This field is poorly developed for biomolecules (contrary to oil, for example) because biomolecules are complicated, and because there are many compounds in the fermentation fluid. This calls for experimental work on the process: design cannot be based solely on theory. In this chapter many models to describe equipment will be shown besides experimental methods to scale-up a process from laboratory to plant.

9.2 | Cell disruption

Ideally, products are released by cells into the fermentation fluid to allow direct recovery. If the microorganism does not excrete the product, genetic engineering may modify the cells such that the product is excreted. But this is not always possible, and the excreted product may be unstable. So some products have to be released by disruption of cells. Cell walls can be disrupted in several ways. These methods form two main groups: *mechanical* and *non-mechanical*. The non-mechanical methods are used on a small scale. The important ones are:

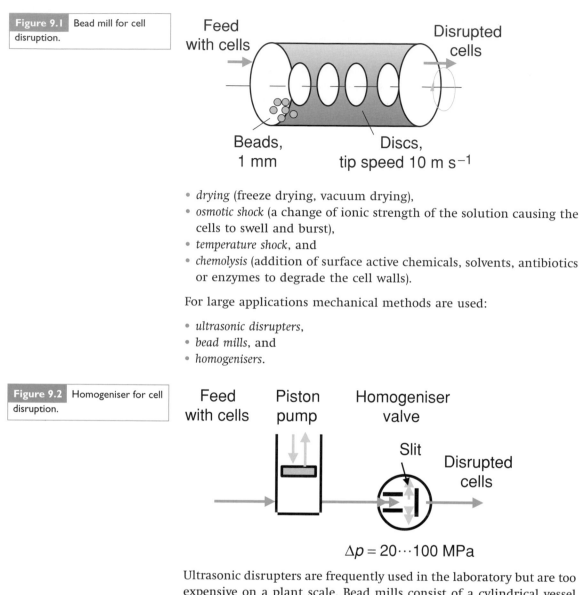

Figure 9.1 Bead mill for cell disruption.

Figure 9.2 Homogeniser for cell disruption.

- *drying* (freeze drying, vacuum drying),
- *osmotic shock* (a change of ionic strength of the solution causing the cells to swell and burst),
- *temperature shock*, and
- *chemolysis* (addition of surface active chemicals, solvents, antibiotics or enzymes to degrade the cell walls).

For large applications mechanical methods are used:

- *ultrasonic disrupters*,
- *bead mills*, and
- *homogenisers*.

Ultrasonic disrupters are frequently used in the laboratory but are too expensive on a plant scale. Bead mills consist of a cylindrical vessel containing rotating discs (with a tip speed of around 10 m s^{-1}) and beads of about 1 mm. The cells in the process fluid are disrupted by shear forces between the beads (see Fig. 9.1). The process is accompanied by heat production and cooling is required. This constrains the size of the equipment. On a production scale the homogeniser is most often used (see Fig. 9.2). This is a valve that can withstand pressures of 40 to 100 MPa. The fluid is forced through the valve slit with a high velocity to disrupt the cell walls. Behind the slit, cavitation causes further disruption. The homogeniser is a simple piece of equipment but has some disadvantages. It is noisy, it can only process large volumes, has a high wear rate, and needs expensive pumps to operate. The effectiveness of the homogeniser depends on the microorganism. Bacterial cells are easily disrupted but yeast cells are not. Homogenising is often done in several passes. The concentration of the released product is given by the following equation:

$$C = C_{max}[1 - \exp(-K N \Delta P^3)] \tag{9.1}$$

where C_{max} is the concentration of the product if all the product is released from the cells; K is a *constant* depending upon the temperature and the type of micro-organism; N is the number of passes through the valve; and ΔP is the pressure drop over the valve. The pressure drop is accompanied by a temperature rise ΔT that can be calculated by applying an energy balance:

$$\Delta T = \frac{\Delta P}{\rho c_p} \tag{9.2}$$

where ρ is the liquid density and c_p the specific heat. The recovery of thermo-unstable proteins may require cooling of the feed and product to avoid denaturation. The temperature rise is independent of the throughput.

9.3 | Clarification

Before concentration and purification of the product, cells or cell debris are removed. This clarification yields a clear liquid containing the dissolved product. Two major techniques are available: *centrifugation* and *filtration*. Large particles can be removed from the liquid by sedimentation but in biotechnology this is only used for large agglomerates.

Box 9.1 | Assignment

A laboratory test reveals that in a certain type of homogeniser 40% of a protein is released after one single passage at a pressure of 40 MPa. Determine the number of passages needed for a conversion of 95% at a pressure drop of 40, 60, 80 and 100 MPa.

9.3.1 Centrifugation

If the gravity is not strong enough to separate the particles in a reasonable time, we can apply a centrifugal field. A laboratory centrifuge is shown in Fig. 9.3. The suspension is put into two identical tubes that are rotated. The acceleration a felt by the particles depends on the distance from the axis of rotation R and the square of the angular velocity ω:

$$a = \omega^2 R \tag{9.3}$$

The angular velocity is given by:

$$\omega = 2\pi N \tag{9.4}$$

with N being the number of rotations per time unit. The acceleration can easily be several thousand times the gravitational acceleration g. *If separation is apparent after 10 minutes of centrifugation at 3000 g, then this separation method can be used on plant scale.* (In larger centrifuges the

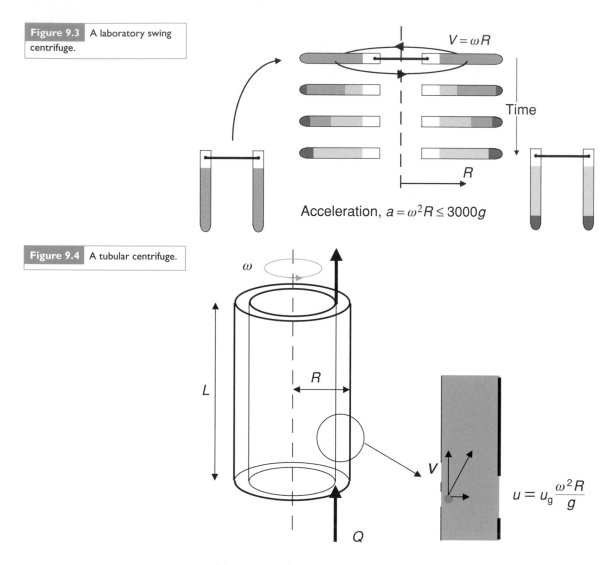

Figure 9.3 A laboratory swing centrifuge.

Figure 9.4 A tubular centrifuge.

residence time is lower but so is the sedimentation distance.) In plant operations, two types of centrifuges are frequently used: the *tubular centrifuge* and the *disc stack centrifuge*. The tubular centrifuge is shown in Fig. 9.4. We will use this centrifuge to demonstrate the *sigma* concept for designing centrifuges. A tubular centrifuge can be seen as a sedimentation vessel turned on its side and with an increased acceleration force. In this case we have to deal with two velocity components: the axial velocity and the radial velocity. The axial velocity is given by:

$$U_{ax} = \frac{\phi_v}{\pi \left(r_o^2 - r_i^2\right)} = \frac{dl}{dt} \tag{9.5}$$

where ϕ_v is the volumetric throughput, r_o the outer tube radius, r_i the inner radius and l the distance in the axial direction. The radial velocity is given by:

$$U_r = U_\infty^c = \frac{dr}{dt} \tag{9.6}$$

where U_∞^c is the terminal settling velocity at the acceleration applied and r the distance in the radial direction. Combining these equations with:

$$\frac{dl}{dr} = \frac{dl}{dt}\frac{dt}{dr} \qquad (9.7)$$

gives:

$$\frac{dl}{dr} = \frac{U_{ax}}{U_r} = \frac{\phi_v}{\pi\left(r_o^2 - r_i^2\right)}\frac{g}{\omega^2 r U_\infty} \qquad (9.8)$$

Integration to obtain the required sedimentation length gives:

$$\int_0^L dl = \frac{\phi_v}{\pi\left(r_o^2 - r_i^2\right)}\frac{g}{\omega^2 U_\infty}\int_{r_i}^{r_o}\frac{1}{r}dr \qquad (9.9)$$

Then substituting Stokes law (giving the terminal settling velocity of a particle in a fluid) gives the maximum throughput:

$$\phi_v = \frac{\pi\left(r_o^2 - r_i^2\right)}{\ln(r_o/r_i)}\frac{\omega^2 L}{g}\left[\frac{\Delta\rho d_p^2 g}{18\eta_l}\right] \qquad (9.10)$$

The centrifuge has the same effect as a gravitational settler with an area Σ:

$$\phi_v = \Sigma U_\infty \qquad (9.11)$$

Using a similar approach, Σ factors for different geometries can be derived.

$$\Sigma = \frac{\pi\omega^2}{g}L_{cyl}\frac{\left(r_o^2 - r_i^2\right)}{\ln(r_o/r_i)}, \qquad \text{tubular} \qquad (9.12a)$$

$$\Sigma = \frac{\pi\omega^2}{g}L_{con}r_i\frac{\left(r_o^2 - r_i^2\right)}{3}, \qquad \text{conical} \qquad (9.12b)$$

$$\Sigma = \frac{\pi\omega^2}{g}\frac{2}{3}\frac{1}{\tan\alpha}\left(r_o^3 - r_i^3\right)z, \qquad \text{disc stack} \qquad (9.12c)$$

Disc stack centrifuges can be compared to a tilted sedimentation vessel with a large area and increased acceleration force, see Fig. 9.5. Disc stack centrifuges contain conical plates (discs) at a short distance from each other (<1 mm). In this way large surfaces can be achieved in small volumes, up to $\Sigma = 0.1\,\text{km}^2$! The feed enters through the axis under the plates, flows to the outside and then back again. The solids leave at the outside, and the clear liquid through a circular slit near the axis. Biomaterials can easily cause fouling and clogging. For aseptic use the material must be well contained and the equipment must be (steam) sterilised. The scale-up of laboratory experiments (I) to plant scale (II) can be done by keeping the ratio of the throughput and the equivalent area constant:

$$\left\{\frac{\phi_v}{\Sigma}\right\}^I = \left\{\frac{\phi_v}{\Sigma}\right\}^{II} \qquad (9.13)$$

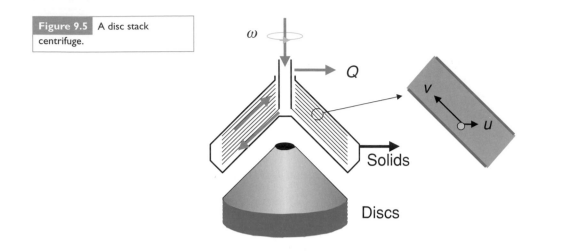

Figure 9.5 A disc stack centrifuge.

Box 9.2 | Assignment

In the initial steps in an insulin production process, solid–liquid separations are necessary. These are cell harvesting, recovery of inclusion bodies and recovery of the precipitated TrpE-Methproinsulin. The company has several disc stack centrifuges equipped with a nozzle discharge of the same type available and we will investigate whether these are suited and how many we require. The (free) water content of the discharged biomass is 60 vol. % to allow it to flow through the nozzle. The disc stack centrifuges have the following dimensions:

> Number of discs $z = 200$; half vertical angle $\alpha = 50°$; external radius $r_u = 0.25$ m; internal radius $r_i = 0.08$ m; distance between discs $\delta = 1$ mm; maximal rotational speed $n = 5000$ rpm.

Characteristics of the feed

> Medium density $\rho_m = 1025$ kg m^{-3}; solids density $\rho_s = 1090$ kg m^{-3}; broth viscosity $\eta_b = 0.035$ Pa s; solids free medium viscosity $\eta_m = 0.001$ Pa s; dissolved product concentration $C_p = 1$ g l^{-1}; cell diameter $d_p = 2 \times 10^{-6}$ m; cell concentration $C = 0.025$ kg kg^{-1}; feed per batch $F = 25$ tons; free water fraction $\varepsilon = 1 - 12\%$.

(1) Calculate the capacity of a centrifuge for the process streams shown above.
(2) How many machines do you require to handle the process with a cycle time of 5 hours?
(3) How much dissolved product do we lose via the biomass stream?

9.3.2 Filtration

Another way to separate particles from suspensions is filtration. The particles are retained by a filter medium, which is a porous fabric or felt. On the surface of the medium the particles form bridges over the pores and create a filter cake: this acts as the medium for the next particles. The liquid is forced through the filter by a pressure

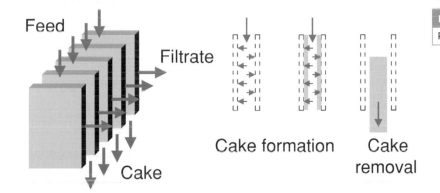

Figure 9.6 Plate filtration principle.

difference. In practice two modes of filtration are used: *batch filtration with plate filters* and *continuous filtration with rotating drum vacuum filters*. The plate filters have a large number of hollow frames (Fig. 9.6). These are covered with the filter medium. The liquid flows from outside to inside: the solids are retained on the filter medium. After a certain time the space between the frames is filled with filter cake and the pressure drop of the equipment increases. The frames are disassembled and the cake removed. This can be done automatically. The rotating vacuum drum filter is a large drum that rotates around a horizontal axis (Fig. 9.7). The filter medium covers the outside of the drum. The drum rotates slowly through a trough containing the feed. The vacuum in the drum sucks in the liquid, leaving the solids as a cake on the outside. Only the lower part of the drum is submerged in the feed, the rest of the surface can be used to wash and dry the filter cake. At the end of the cycle, the cake is scraped off the drum by a knife and collected for further processing.

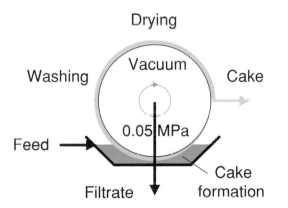

Figure 9.7 Rotating drum filter.

The design of a filter starts in the laboratory with experiments using the same filter medium as in the plant. This can be done with a Büchner funnel. The feed is sucked through the filter at a constant pressure difference, ΔP. At first the filter is clean and the filtration is fast, but as the cake is formed on the filter the rate of filtration decreases. The record of filtrate volume as a function of time is valuable information for scaling up. At the end, the filter cake volume is measured. To describe this experiment we can use Darcy's law for flow through porous media:

$$\Delta P = \eta(R_c + R_m)\phi_v''$$ (9.14)

where R_c is the cake resistance, R_m the medium resistance and ϕ_v'' the liquid flux through the filter in m s^{-1}. The flux is:

$$\phi_v'' = \frac{dV_f}{dt}\frac{1}{A}$$ (9.15)

where V_f is the collected filtrate volume at a specific time and A the surface area of the filter. The cake resistance is the product of the specific cake resistance α and the mass of cake per unit area w:

$$R_c = \alpha w$$ (9.16)

and w can be related to concentration in the feed by:

$$wA = cV_f$$ (9.17)

where c is the concentration of solids in the broth. Substituting Eqs. (9.15), (9.16) and (9.17) in Eq. (9.14) gives:

$$\frac{dV_f}{dt} = \frac{\Delta pA}{\eta\alpha\frac{cV_f}{A} + \eta R_m}$$ (9.18a)

or

$$\frac{dt}{dV_f} = \frac{\eta\alpha cV_f}{\Delta pA^2} + \frac{\eta R_m}{\Delta pA}$$ (9.18b)

Integrating:

$$\int_0^t dt = \frac{\eta\alpha cV_f}{\Delta pA^2}\int_0^{V_f} dV_f + \frac{\eta R_m}{\Delta pA}\int_0^{V_f} dV_f$$ (9.19)

yields

$$t = \frac{\eta\alpha c}{\Delta pA^2}\frac{1}{2}V_f^2 + \frac{\eta R_m}{\Delta pA}V_f$$ (9.20)

By plotting t/V_f versus V_f a straight line is obtained:

$$\frac{t}{V_f} = \frac{\eta\alpha c}{\Delta pA^2}\frac{1}{2}V_f + \frac{\eta R_m}{\Delta pA}$$ (9.21)

From the slope the specific cake resistance is obtained and used for the design of a larger industrial unit. The specific cake resistance can have very large values: 10^{12}–10^{15} m kg^{-1}. If the filter medium resistance is small it can be shown that the filtrate volume versus time has the following behaviour:

$$V_f \sim \sqrt{t}$$ (9.22)

The *specific cake resistance, α,* is a function of the void fraction of the cake and of the diameter of the particles. Small particles give a very high value of α. This is the reason why cell debris alone is difficult to filter. The problem is usually solved by adding filter aids: porous, inert particles with a diameter of 20–50 μm. The added volume of filter aid is larger than that of the particles to be separated. The exact amount can only be determined by experiment. Usually the filter aid is added in two stages: a first small volume as a pre-coat for the filter medium and the bulk volume mixed with the feed. Used filter aid is a waste that may contain a substantial amount of product. The cake resistance α also depends on the diameter of the channels. These can be increased by adding flocculent or changing the pH or ionic strength of the feed.

9.4 | Concentration

After clarification, the feed is still dilute and has to be concentrated before extracting and purifying the product. This usually means removing water. Concentration can also purify the product stream: sometimes this is enough to obtain the desired end-product purity.

Box 9.3 | Assignment

Solid–liquid separation can be done with a rotary vacuum drum filter. To obtain data to design production-scale filter(s), a *Streptomyces* suspension is filtered on a Büchner funnel, which has a circular filter area with a diameter of 20 cm. The pressure difference ΔP across the cake is 0.7 bar (vacuum filtration). Further data: broth density $\rho_b = 1050 \, \mathrm{kg \, m^{-3}}$; broth dynamic viscosity $\eta_l = 0.032 \, \mathrm{Pa \, s}$; biomass concentration $c = 30 \, \mathrm{kg \, m^{-3}}$. A batch experiment yields the following filtrate volumes as a function of time:

t (s): 189, 320, 507, 727, 940, 1204, 1481, 1791, 2116, 2479, 3100

V_f (ml): 100, 150, 200, 250, 300, 350, 400, 450, 500, 550, 600

(a) Plot the experimental values of t/V_f versus V_f.

(b) Determine the average specific resistance of the cake α (in m $\mathrm{kg^{-1}}$) and the medium resistance R_m (in m $\mathrm{kg^{-1}}$). From these data, the rotary vacuum drum filter can be designed. The vacuum here is higher: ΔP is 0.9 bar. Dimensions of the drum filter are: diameter $D = 2 \, \mathrm{m}$, length $L = 4 \, \mathrm{m}$, angle of filtration section $\Delta \gamma = 0.6 \, \pi$ rad.

(c) Calculate the maximum filtration rate that can be obtained theoretically with the rotary vacuum drum filter. The maximum number of revolutions per minute is 5.

(d) The solid–liquid separation steps in the insulin process should handle 50 tons per batch. Can the filter be used for the insulin process?

9.4.1 Evaporation

The oldest and simplest method of concentration is to evaporate water or solvent from the mixture. Biological products tend not to be very stable, so temperature and exposure time should be kept low. The temperature can be kept low by working under reduced pressure. When working at 40 °C, the pressure has to be reduced to 10 kPa.

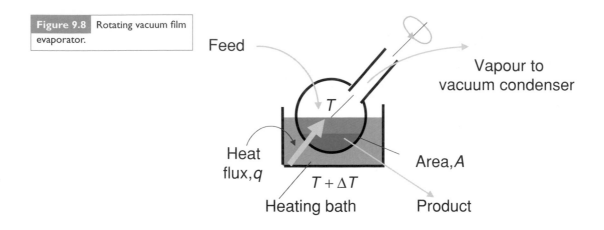

Figure 9.8 Rotating vacuum film evaporator.

The design of an evaporation step requires experimentation in the laboratory. These can be done with a *rotating vacuum film evaporator* consisting of a glass bowl submerged in a heating bath and connected to a vacuum system (Fig. 9.8). The bowl slowly rotates in the heating bath to give equal heating of the volume of the liquid. During an experiment we measure the temperature of the bath and the product, the amount of condensate in time and, if appropriate, the activity of the product as function of time. Valuable information can be gained from this experiment such as the degree of thickening possible, the amount of deactivation of product, the degree of foaming during boiling and a rough idea of the allowable heat flux through the wall.

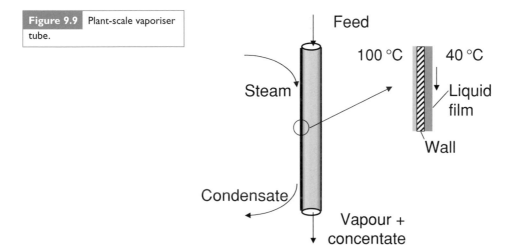

Figure 9.9 Plant-scale vaporiser tube.

In plant equipment the feed is often introduced as a film inside a vertical tube (Fig. 9.9 and Fig. 9.10). A thin film can be heated quickly, reducing the need for long residence times. The heat is supplied by steam condensing at the outside of the tube. The pressure at the outside is higher than at the inside allowing a higher temperature at the outside. Behind the evaporator the concentrated liquid and vapour are separated and the vapour is condensed by heat exchange.

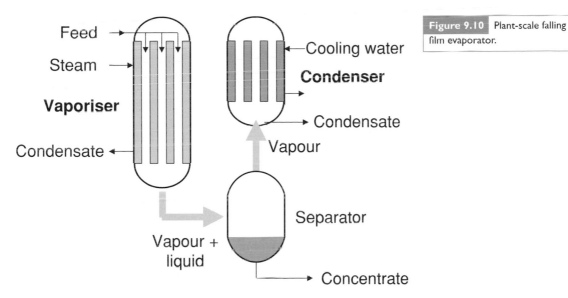

Figure 9.10 Plant-scale falling film evaporator.

During condensing of 1 kg steam 2.2 MJ of energy is released. This is sufficient to evaporate 1 kg of water or several kilogrammes of organic solvent. The generation and use of steam is costly and should be kept at a minimum. This can be achieved by multiple stage evaporators using the vapour obtained to evaporate the liquid feed. The reduction in operating costs (steam) is counteracted by an increase in fixed costs (equipment). There is a limit to the thickening of the process fluid: it will no longer flow if the solids content increases too far. *Tubular falling film evaporators* are well suited to handle viscous products, heat sensitive (enzyme) solutions and foaming products. Several kinds of evaporators are available for plant-scale operation:

- long tube vertical evaporators (natural circulation $1-3\,\text{kW}\,\text{m}^{-2}\,\text{K}^{-1}$; forced circulation $2-13\,\text{kW}\,\text{m}^{-2}\,\text{K}^{-1}$),
- short tube evaporators ($0.5-2.5\,\text{kW}\,\text{m}^{-2}\,\text{K}^{-1}$),
- agitated film evaporators ($2-5\,\text{kW}\,\text{m}^{-2}\,\text{K}^{-1}$),
- centrifugal evaporators ($3-10\,\text{kW}\,\text{m}^{-2}\,\text{K}^{-1}$).

Their selection is based on the following criteria.

- capability of handling a broad range of product viscosity (1–10 000 mPa s),
- capability of handling heat sensitive products,
- limited scale formation,
- limited fouling, and
- foaming.

9.4.2 Precipitation

Precipitation can be used in several parts in the process. Early in the process it can remove water and/or salt and give a stable intermediate. During the recovery process it can be used for concentration, for example, before a chromatography step. In the final stage it can be applied to obtain a solid end-product. During precipitation,

Box 9.4 | Assignment

A yeast extract stream of $0.2\,kg\,s^{-1}$ has to be concentrated by means of evaporation. The solid fraction has to be increased from 0.2 to 0.5% by weight. Measurements have been performed in a bench-scale plant under the following conditions:

Feed: flow rate $F = 0.05\,kg\,s^{-1}$; mass fraction dry material $W_F = 0.2$; temperature $T_F = 40\,°C$.

Concentrate: flow rate $C = 0.02\,kg\,s^{-1}$; mass fraction dry material $W_F = 0.5$; temperature $T_C = 40\,°C$.

Steam: flow rate $S = 0.03\,kg\,s^{-1}$; temperature $T_S = 100\,°C$.

Surface of bench scale evaporator: $A_B = 0.5\,m^2$.

Estimate the steam usage and the surface of the required evaporator in the real plant if we have a feed stream four times higher than in the bench. In the real plant we will use steam at a temperature of $140\,°C$. Assume equal heat transfer coefficients. Use $q = U \cdot \Delta T$.

the solubility of the (un)desired product is lowered until the solution is oversaturated and the product precipitates. The solid precipitate is separated from the solution by a settler, centrifuge or filter. The precipitation can also be performed in a fractionating manner (the precipitates obtained contain different fractions of the different products). The solubility is mostly decreased by adding salts, typically $(NH_4)_2SO_4$, or organic solvents such as acetone or ethanol. Large volumes of these precipitants are needed, causing large waste streams. Salts have several advantages:

• the proteins denature only to a limited extent,
• precipitation can be performed at room temperature,
• a relatively pure precipitate can be obtained in a few steps.

There are three disadvantages:

• large waste streams of salts are produced,
• the salts in the product have to be removed at a later stage (for example by ultrafiltration),
• salts promote corrosion.

The use of solvents as precipitants can cause severe denaturation of the proteins and creates the need to operate at temperatures of 0–5 °C (human plasma: −10 °C). The solvents are, however, easily recovered.

Precipitation is used extensively in the recovery of proteins. The solubilities of proteins are not easily predicted, although the behaviour can be understood qualitatively. A protein consists of both acidic and basic amino acids. In an aqueous environment these groups are ionised and the charge of these groups depends on the pH of the solution (Fig. 9.11). At high pH values the acidic groups are ionised and the charge of the protein is negative. At low pH values the protein is positive. There is one specific value of the pH, the *isoelectric*

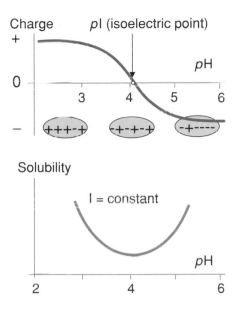

Charge
pI (isoelectric point)

Solubility

I = constant

Figure 9.11 Charge and solubility of proteins.

point pI, where the average charge of the protein is zero. At this pI the proteins do not repel each other and can flocculate and precipitate. Precipitation is mostly performed in stirred vessels. Experiments performed in the laboratory can be used to design large-scale precipitation. For this the geometry of the vessels on the two scales should be the same. A standard stirred baffled vessel with Rushton turbine (see Chapter 7) can be used. Besides the geometry, the power dissipation in the liquid must be kept constant during scaling up. The dissipation is described by the power number P and is determined by the stirring speed N, the liquid density ρ_L and the diameter of the stirrer d_s:

$$P = 5\rho_L N^3 d_s^5 \tag{9.23}$$

The content of the vessel has a mass M of:

$$M = \rho_L \frac{\pi}{4} D^2 H = \rho \frac{\pi}{4} D^3 \tag{9.24}$$

giving

$$\frac{P}{M} = 0.026 N^3 D^2 \tag{9.25}$$

Rapid stirring corresponds to around 1 W kg^{-1} and slow stirring to a factor of, say, one hundred times less. Precipitation is best done in several steps. The precipitant is added near the stirrer and the vessel is stirred rapidly to ensure good mixing. The first particles formed are small and do not suffer from high shear. To let the particles grow, the stirring has to be reduced. At the end, the stirring is stopped to allow the solids to settle. The following things are kept the same in small- and large-scale plants: power input per kg, addition time of the precipitate and the different mixing times.

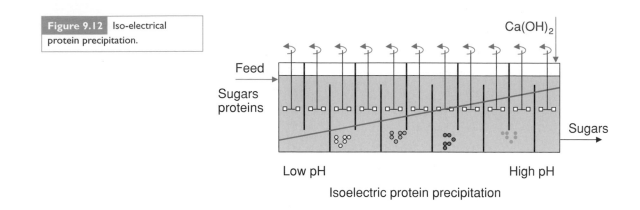

Figure 9.12 Iso-electrical protein precipitation.

Isoelectric protein precipitation

Box 9.5 | Example

An example of isoelectrical precipitation is found in sugar refining. After washing, grinding and filtering of the sugar beets a clarified process stream containing sugars and proteins is obtained. The protein mixture has proteins with varying isoelectrical points. To remove all proteins the process stream needs to experience a pH profile. This is obtained in a baffled/compartmentalised horizontal vessel. The compartments are stirred and allow some back flow. A base is fed at the end of the reactor: it mixes back. This gives a pH profile over the reactor. This profile contains all the pI values of the protein mixture causing the different proteins to precipitate in the different stages (Fig. 9.12).

9.4.3 Ultrafiltration

Concentrating can also be performed using membranes (Fig. 9.13). Two types are frequently used in biotechnology: *microfiltration membranes* (MF) and *ultrafiltration membranes* (UF). MF membranes have pores of 0.2–0.5 μm diameter and thus retain cells. MF resembles ordinary filtration and the theory of Section 9.3 applies. Ultrafiltration membranes have pores of approximately 10 nm diameter and thus retain proteins, but not water and salts. Membranes in the form of porous tubes of 1–5 mm diameter are most common. A thin coating on the surface of the tube is the actual membrane. It can consist of a porous (sponge-like) polymer, porous carbon or porous ceramic. A UF membrane can be used in two ways: to concentrate or to wash out salts from the product (diafiltration). A major difference between ultrafiltration and ordinary (dead-end) filtration is the type of flow along the membrane. In UF the liquid containing the solids flows along the membrane (hence the term cross-flow filtration). A pressure difference of several hundred kPa is applied across the membrane. This is the driving force for transport of water and salt through the membrane. The membrane flux J is small, in the order of 10×10^{-6} m s^{-1}. Increasing the pressure across the membrane initially increases the flux, but only to a limited extent. The water transports protein towards the membrane where it accumulates. At a certain pressure difference the protein precipitates on the membrane.

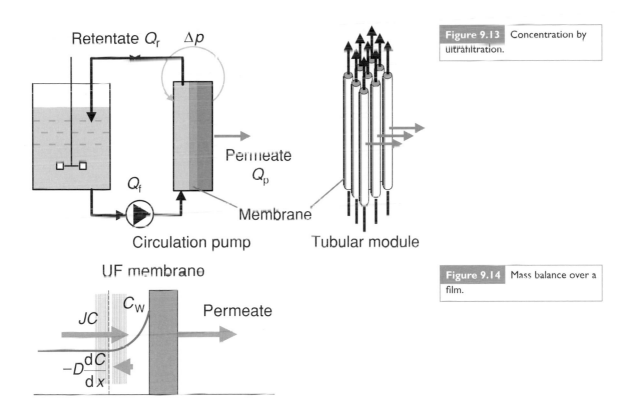

Figure 9.13 Concentration by ultrafiltration.

Figure 9.14 Mass balance over a film.

Increasing the pressure difference further does not increase the flux, but only the gel layer thickness. The relation for the flux can be derived by applying a mass balance over a film near the membrane (Fig. 9.14):

$$J(C - C_p) = -D\frac{dC}{dx} \tag{9.26}$$

Here C is the protein concentration and C_p the protein concentration at the permeate side. Separation of variables and integration and defining the mass transfer coefficient k in terms of the film thickness δ and the diffusion coefficient D:

$$k = \frac{D}{\delta} \tag{9.27}$$

and eliminating the protein concentration in the permeate leads to:

$$J = k \ln\left(\frac{C_w}{C_b}\right) \tag{9.28}$$

From Eq. (9.28) it follows that the flux decreases at increasing bulk concentration. At $C = C_w$ the flux becomes zero. The relation between flux and concentration can easily be measured in a laboratory experiment with a single membrane tube. This requires only a single batch experiment from which the mass transfer coefficient k and the gel concentration C_w can be determined. With these results larger equipment can be designed by using more membrane tubes. In the gel regime, the flux can be increased by increasing the flow in the tube according to Eq. (9.29). Cross-flow velocities, v, of 1–3 m s^{-1} are applied and the resulting mass transfer coefficient can be approximated roughly by:

$$k = 10^{-5} \, v \qquad\qquad (9.29)$$

Box 9.6 | Assignment

An enzyme solution is concentrated by using ultrafiltration. The flux as a function of the concentration is:

C_b (mmol l^{-1}): 1.0, 1.5, 3.0, 5.0, 8.0

J (μm s^{-1}): 14.0, 11.5, 7.7, 4.9, 2.3

Determine the mass transfer coefficient k and the gel concentration C_w.

9.5 | Purification

After releasing the product from the cell and subsequent clarification and concentration of the process stream, a contaminated product stream is available for further processing. In the downstream processing of bioproducts two major groups of purification processes can be distinguished: those for bulk products such as citric acid, enzymes and penicillin and those for small-scale pharmaceutical processes. This section deals with the bulk processes. During bulk purification extreme purity is not required. A few per cent of impurities are often allowed. Two important techniques can be identified: *liquid–liquid extraction* and *crystallisation*. Both make use of an auxiliary phase that selectively extracts a certain component from the mixture.

9.5.1 Extraction

Typical examples of compounds purified by extraction are:

- alcohols and ketones (2-propanol, butanol, acetone),
- carboxylic and amino acids (acetic, gluconic, lactic, citric, some hydrophobic amino acids),
- antibiotics (penicillin, lincomycin, tetracycline, cephalosporin, bacitracin),
- vitamins (A, B, C),
- food components (flavours and aromas, fatty acids from edible oils and fat, caffeine),
- alkaloids and steroids (prednisolone, codeine, morphine, quinine, strychnine, taxol), and
- peptides and proteins (insulin, interferon).

Extraction can be done in the laboratory as shown in Fig. 9.15. Single-stage extraction is often not sufficient and several steps may be needed. For small molecules like citric acid and penicillin, organic solvents such as butanol, butyl acetate or larger amines are used. For

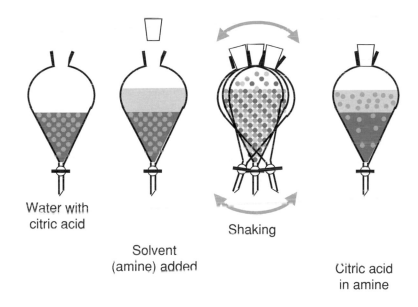

Figure 9.15 Extraction stages in the laboratory.

Water with citric acid

Solvent (amine) added

Shaking

Citric acid in amine

larger and more complex biomolecules, aqueous two-phase extraction can be applied. These systems are composed of an aqueous mixture of a salt (for example $MgSO_4$) and a polymer (polyethylene glycol, PEG) or two polymers (PEG, dextran). In certain concentration ranges these separate into two phases. The dense bottom phase contains most of the salt, whereas the top phase mainly contains the polymer. Both systems are relatively benign to sensitive proteins.

Four factors govern the extraction:

- mass balances (overall, phase, local),
- phase and reaction equilibria (K),
- hydrodynamics, and
- mass transfer and reaction rates (k).

To explain the process we take as an example the extraction of citric acid with an organic solvent. A simple laboratory experiment can show whether extraction can be used. An amount of clarified fermenter liquid, $L(m^3)$, is put into a separation funnel. The concentration of citric acid is c_0 (kg m^{-3}). Then a volume of clean amine solvent V (m^3) is added and the funnel is closed and shaken. Citric acid will be transferred to the organic phase (see Fig. 9.16). After a certain amount of time the system is at equilibrium. After settling, the citric acid contents of both phases are analysed and the ratio gives the partitioning coefficient K. The value of K should be high to make extraction attractive. The partitioning coefficient of the contaminants should be low. The coefficient depends on:

- the nature and concentration of the species,
- the ionic strength I,
- pH,
- temperature, and
- the type of solvent.

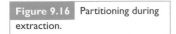
Partitioning during extraction.

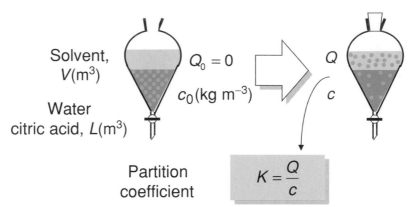

For a first estimate, the value of the partitioning coefficient can be taken as a constant. The ratio of the amounts of citric acid in the two phases is known as the separation (or extraction) factor S:

$$S = \frac{QV}{cL} = K\frac{V}{L} \tag{9.30}$$

If $S_i > 1$, a component moves largely to the auxiliary phase; if $S_i < 1$, the component moves with the feed.

9.5.2 Crystallisation

When a solution is *super-saturated* the solvent contains more product than at equilibrium and as a result the product crystallises. The crystals are separated by filtration or centrifugation. This yields a fairly pure product. A single crystallisation step can often produce the desired purity, but large quantities of the product may be left in the solution. Two ways to obtain super-saturation are cooling (lowering the solubility of the product) and evaporation (increasing the concentration of the product). Crystallisation resembles precipitation but it differs in the way that super-saturation is obtained. Crystallisation makes no use of additives and is the older and more common technique. Inorganic salts such as sodium and ammonium sulphates, and certain organic compounds such as sucrose and glucose, are produced in quantities exceeding 100 millions tons per year. Most bulk pharmaceuticals and organic, fine chemicals are marketed as crystalline products. Crystallisation is important for three reasons:

- the crystals are often very pure – this is important in the finishing step in ultrapurification,
- the production of uniform crystals facilitates subsequent finishing steps like filtration and drying,
- it improves product appearance – which is important for consumer acceptance.

Laboratory scale crystallisation is quite simple to perform, but large-scale crystallisation is more an art than a science. This is because of geometrical constraints of the crystalliser and simultaneous heat and mass transfer in a multi-phase in a multi-component system that

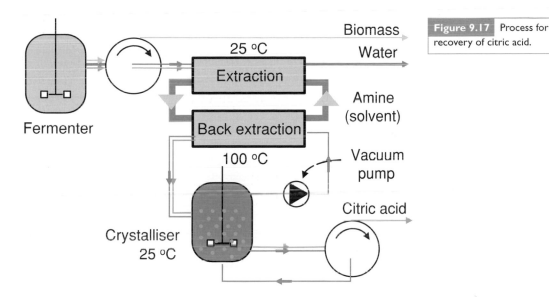

Figure 9.17 Process for recovery of citric acid.

is thermodynamically unstable. Furthermore trace amounts of impurities may have a pronounced effect.

Box 9.7 | Purification example

The production of citric acid will serve as an example to show certain aspects of product purification. Citric acid is used in food: carbonated beverages, dry-packaged drinks, fruit drinks, jams, jellies and canned fruits. It is also used in vegetable oils and for preserving the colour, flavour and vitamin content of fresh and frozen vegetables and fruit. Another application is in cleaning of boilers and heat exchangers. Its chelating ability assists in removal of scale and leads the use of citric acid as a detergent builder, especially in liquid formulations. Citric acid solutions can remove sulphur dioxide from gases and chelate micronutrients in fertiliser.

In the citric acid process, extraction as well as crystallisation is used (Fig. 9.17). Citric acid is an extracellular product of the filamentous fungus *Aspergillus niger*. It is produced with a concentration of $C_o = 50 \ kg \ m^{-3}$. The broth is clarified with a rotating vacuum filter. The process fluid contains a large number of contaminants besides citric acid. So citric acid is extracted with a water-insoluble tertiary amine blend. The amine reacts reversibly with the citric acid:

$$CiH_3 + R_3N \xrightarrow{25 \ °C} R_3NCiH_3 \qquad (1)$$

Most of the contaminants do not react. After settling and separation of the two phases the amine phase is contacted with fresh clean water at a high temperature, where the reaction proceeds in the other direction:

$$CiH_3 + R_3N \xleftarrow[100 \ °C]{} R_3NCiH_3 \qquad (2)$$

The citric acid is back-extracted in the water phase. This phase contains small amounts of contaminants, so the water is evaporated causing super-saturation of citric acid, which crystallises. The crystals are filtered over a vacuum filter. The water vapour from the crystalliser is sent back to the extraction via a vaccum pump and heat exchanger. In this process several cycles are used: the organic solvent cycles from extraction to back-extraction; water from the crystalliser cycles back to the extraction and wash water from the last filter is recycled to the crystalliser. Water from the first filter can be recycled to the fermenter as well, but this is normally not done due to infection hazards in the fermenter. These recycles are needed for economic as well as environmental reasons. The equilibrium of the citric acid is governed by the pH of the aqueous solution. Only the neutral species can be extracted in the organic phase. The complexing reaction is exothermic: it releases heat. At higher temperatures the reaction equilibrium is shifted to the left. This principle is used during extraction and back-extraction. For extraction, several types of equipment can be used. The simplest and most often used is the mixer-settler combination, which can be considered as a single stage.

9.6 | Ultrapurification

Many pharmaceutical products, especially those introduced intravenously into the human body, have to be extremely pure. Purity requirements of 99.999% are not rare. *Sorption processes* that use a solid auxiliary phase are commonly used and the separation of large molecules like proteins will be presented here to illustrate the process of ultrapurification. An example of a separation using a solid sorbent is the following experiment: take a strip of a filter paper and draw a line across the strip with a ballpoint. Put the bottom of the strip in ethanol, see Fig. 9.18. The ethanol will creep up the paper because of capillary forces. When it arrives at the line it will dissolve the ink and transport the components upwards. The colour components in the ink travel at different speeds and separate. The line broadens to a band with different colours. Blue ink is separated into a purple front band and a blue green tail band. This is typical of a chromatography separation. It requires

- a feed (= ballpoint line),
- a porous matrix (= paper),
- an eluent (= ethanol).

In bioprocess technology the matrix consists of *spherical beads* with diameters of 10–100 μm, placed in a column. The beads are made into a gel, appearing as molecular cross-linked fibres with water-filled pores of about 10 nm diameter, which is large enough for proteins to penetrate. Different proteins have a different interaction with the matrix. A protein that interacts strongly will be retarded more than a non-bonding protein. The properties controlling the interactions are:

- pore size,
- polarity or hydrophilic character of the pore surface,
- charge of the surface, and
- shape of the molecules in the surface.

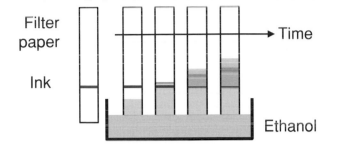

Filter paper

Ink

Time

Ethanol

Figure 9.18 Simple chromatography.

All properties may play a role in a separation, but one property is normally overruling and determines the name of the sorption process. These processes are:

- *gel filtration* (separation on size),
- *adsorption* (hydrophobic interaction, separation on polarity),
- *ion exchange* (separation on charge), and
- *affinity chromatography* (separation on shape: some molecules perfectly fit on the surface).

Interaction of the protein with the matrix also depends on the protein and its concentration; on the concentration of other components in solution; on the characteristics of the solvent; on the pH and I of the solvent and on the temperature T. The partitioning coefficient of a component between the matrix and the solution is an important variable (just like the partitioning coefficient in liquid–liquid extraction). It is given by the relation:

$$K = Q/C \qquad (9.31)$$

where Q is the concentration of the protein in the gel and C the concentration in the solvent. Low K values imply that the protein is repelled by the matrix; high values that it is attracted. At low concentrations, the value of K is independent of the concentration. At higher concentrations the matrix can become saturated. The sorption material has to be:

- insoluble,
- macroporous,
- mechanically stable,
- hydrophilic,
- properly shaped, and
- biochemically stable.

There are several types: organic polymers, inorganic pellets and composite materials (such as reversed-phase sorbents). The inorganic sorbents are applied in colour removal and consist of activated carbon, silica or alumina. The organic polymers are used for amino acid, antibiotic and protein purification and consist of polystyrene, poly(methyl)acrylate or polysaccharides (dextran, agarose, . . .). There are two ways to operate a sorption column: as a *chromatography* column and as an *adsorption/regeneration* system.

Chromatography

In elementary chromatography there is a constant flow of eluent (a suitable fluid) through the column. At a certain moment a pulse of feed is injected at the entrance of the column. This may consist of components A and B, with B travelling faster than A. After some time the *peaks* of both components are collected as separate fractions at the outlet of the column. The separation suffers from *peak broadening* and can be improved by using a longer column or a lower rate of elution. Only a limited amount of feed can be processed in this way. Increasing the throughput can be done by injecting a band of feed into the column. At given eluent velocity more column length will be needed but, on average, better use is made of the column material. Another method is to increase the feed concentration and to enter the area of non-linear chromatography. The bands will form triangular peaks: with a sharp front but a diffuse tail. Again the column length needs to be increased but, on average, the column material is used more efficiently. A gradient in the feed (eluent) composition can also be applied, using variation in pH, I or solvent polarity.

Adsorption/regeneration

The largest throughput per column volume is obtained by using adsorption/regeneration. This is a multiple-step process. This technique can be used when the desired product A binds better to the matrix than the contaminant B. In the adsorption step the feed is pumped through the bed. The fresh beads will mainly adsorb A until the surface is saturated and the small amount of B adsorbed is flushed out during a washing step. The column is regenerated using an eluent with different properties that removes the adsorbed component A from the matrix. Then the cycle starts again. Adsorption fronts are usually sharp and a good separation can be obtained; during regeneration the diffuse tails make separation more difficult.

Gel filtration

In gel filtration molecules are separated based upon their difference in size. The gels have a specific *pore size distribution*. Small molecules can enter the gel pores but larger molecules cannot. So smaller molecules are retarded more. Adsorption at the gel surface is minimised: protein molecules are dissolved in the water in the pores. Gel particles are very open structures and compressible: this limits the allowable column lengths and velocities. Typical values are: particle diameter $d_p = 0.1$–0.2 mm, column length $L = 0.3$–1 m, liquid flux $\phi = 2$–$5 \, 10^{-5}$ m s^{-1}.

Partition equilibrium

The gel in Fig. 9.19 consists of fibres with a thickness F. The space between the fibres has a fraction ε. The centre of a spherical protein cannot approach the fibre closer than the distance of the radius of the protein. Therefore only the light-coloured part of the liquid in

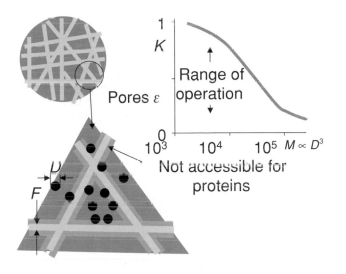

Figure 9.19 Protein partitioning during gel filtration.

the gel can be occupied by proteins. For the larger protein less space is available. For proteins with a diameter D, the available volume is:

$$m = \exp[-(1 - \varepsilon)(1 + D/F)^2]$$ (9.32)

Because adsorption at the pore wall is absent, this equals the partition coefficient. The *partition coefficient* is smaller than one, indicating less protein in the gel than in the surrounding liquid; it is independent of the protein concentration.

Small molecules all have the same retention time, as do very large molecules. The gel is effective only for the separation of molecules with about the same diameter as the fibres. The range covers molar masses, which differ up to a factor of 20. The gel is often named after the maximum molar mass it can effectively retain, for example Sephadex™ G100 can be used up to molar masses of 100 kg mol^{-1}.

Ion exchange

In this sorption process the solid matrix contains charged groups. These can be positive as well as negative. Positively charged exchangers are quaternary ammonium and negative ones are sulfonic acid exchangers. Ions with the same charge as the matrix are repelled. The amounts of free counter ions and charges attached to the matrix are the same. The counter ions can be small ions but also large molecules like proteins. The counter ions can exchange with other counter ions in solution. A positive matrix exchanges negative ions and vice versa. The gels for ion exchange are more open than for gel filtration: the proteins are not separated by size. Proteins can form a monolayer around the fibres in the matrix (see Fig. 9.20) and can occupy up to 10% of the gel volume. The partition coefficient in ion exchange can be much larger than one. Proteins may have a positive

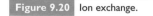

Figure 9.20 Ion exchange.

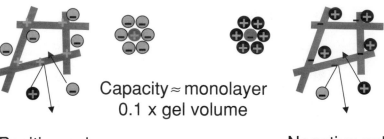

as well as a negative charge depending on the pH of the solution (see Section 9.4). Below the protein pI, the protein has a net positive charge: this changes above the pI. In Fig. 9.21 the maximum capacity of an anion exchanger is shown for a certain protein. Below the iso-electric point the protein is positive and is repelled. Above the pI the protein becomes negative and is attracted. The capacity increases to a maximum value. The maximum capacity is reached at a low ionic strength in the liquid surrounding the particles. At high ionic strength small ions drive out the proteins. The capacity curve of a cation exchanger is the mirror image of an anion exchanger. In this case positively charged proteins (below their pI) bind well.

Figure 9.21 Capacity of an anion exchanger.

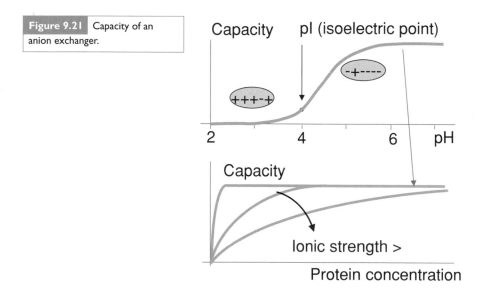

Affinity adsorption/chromatography
Proteins have characteristic shapes, allowing them to fit exactly to counter molecules called *antibodies* or *ligands*. An adsorbent with antibodies on the pore surface can selectively bind one specific molecule. This is called affinity adsorption. The adsorbent has even larger pores

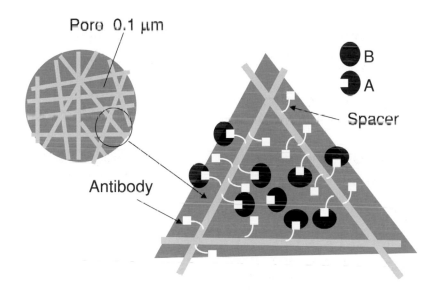

Pore 0.1 μm

Antibody

Spacer

B

A

Figure 9.22 Structure of an affinity adsorbent.

than ion exchange gels because it has to accommodate the antibody besides the proteins. Sufficient space has to be available for this antibody to position itself freely with respect to the protein. So the antibodies are attached to the pore wall by spacers (Fig. 9.22). The gel matrix resembles that used in gel filtration. The spacer should be chosen with care to allow a minimal interaction with feed components. Affinity absorption is an attractive method to isolate a specific component. The column material is used completely, the product obtained is pure and concentrated and the process needs only a small amount of eluent. However, it suffers from the drawbacks that for each component a specific antibody has to be developed, that the adsorbent is expensive and is mostly not very stable. The spacers can detach leading to a loss of efficiency.

Innovations in chromatography

There is an ongoing effort towards better process chromatography. First of all is the development of new stationary phases. These are showing improved mechanical strength, capacity and selectivity (affinity chromatography). Chromatography can use a liquid as the stationary phase, for example in *centrifugal partitioning chromatography*. This technique is widely used in China for extraction of natural products in medicine.

Another development is that of *simulated moving beds*, which are widely applied in food, pharmaceutical and fine chemical industries. These give efficient use of solvents and stationary phase by operating the chromatographic separation continuously (as compared to the batch mode normally applied, see Fig. 9.23). The continuous motion of the solid phase is simulated by switching the feed, extract and raffinate ports in a carrousel of fixed beds. In continuous counter-current contacting, the driving force for mass transfer is

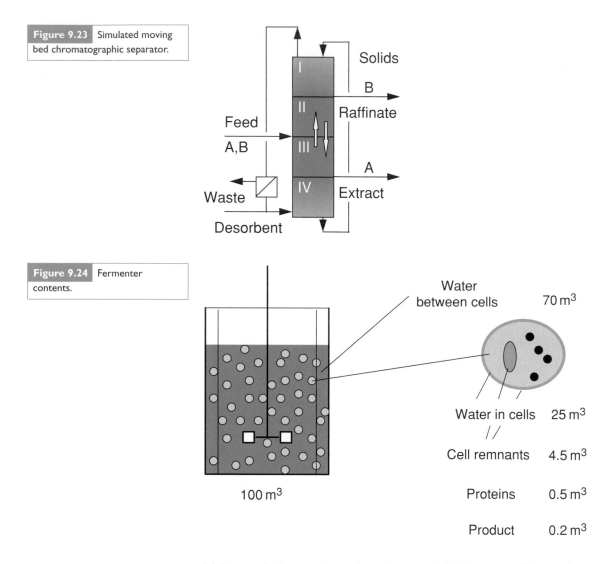

Figure 9.23 Simulated moving bed chromatographic separator.

Figure 9.24 Fermenter contents.

higher and the equipment makes much better use of the column inventory.

9.7 | Sequencing

To develop a good process, we must get *all* pieces of equipment to work together. To illustrate the problem, we consider a process that looks simple in the laboratory, but has to be scaled-up. The example is the downstream processing of an intracellular enzyme. A large fermentation capacity is chosen as it clearly shows the problems in the downstream processing. The fermenter broth (Fig. 9.24) consists for the major part of water. Only a small amount of product is present and a complex mixture of components of secondary metabolites of different sizes and shapes. For simplicity we consider only the following components:

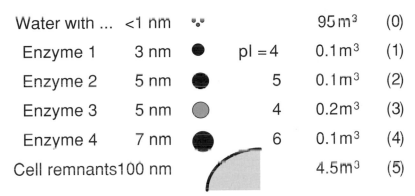

Water with ...	<1 nm			95 m³	(0)
Enzyme 1	3 nm	●	pl = 4	0.1 m³	(1)
Enzyme 2	5 nm	●	5	0.1 m³	(2)
Enzyme 3	5 nm	●	4	0.2 m³	(3)
Enzyme 4	7 nm	●	6	0.1 m³	(4)
Cell remnants	100 nm			4.5 m³	(5)

Figure 9.25 Properties of the six components in the fermenter.

- water with salts and other nutrients,
- four different enzymes,
- cells and cell debris.

The four enzymes have different sizes and iso-electrical points, see Fig. 9.25. Enzyme 3 is the desired product and has to be purified Figure 9.25 suggests a separation on size with gel filtration and afterwards a separation on charge with ion exchange. In the laboratory this can easily be done. An industrial production of 200 tonnes a⁻¹ is chosen which leads to a feed of 100 m³ h⁻¹ of fermentation broth. The process starts with cell disruption with a homogeniser because we are dealing with an intracellular product. A small valve is needed and the costs lie in its energy consumption for cooling and disruption (assumed to be 3 MW). The clarification is done by filtration. Because the debris is so fine it takes a long time to filter. Filtration can be speeded up by adding filter aid. This consists of large particles that make the filter cake more porous thus increasing the flux. A thorough washing step is needed to prevent product loss with the filter cake. A rotating drum vacuum filter can be used with a large filtration area. The main problem is the filter aid: it forms a huge solid waste stream that is difficult to sell, process or dispose. The most important steps in enzyme purification are gel filtration and ion exchange. Gel filtration is based on differences in size. A mid fraction is needed with enzymes 2 and 3. The most difficult separation is the one between enzymes 2 + 3 and 4: this determines the column length and the amount of flush water. In ideal gel filtration there is neither dilution nor concentration. Each fraction leaves the column in a volume equal to the feed volume. That makes for three times the feed. To allow for losses a factor of five times the feed volume is taken. During scale-up of the gel filtration the following factors are kept constant:

- the composition of the feed,
- the gel particles used and their size,
- the liquid velocity.

This leads to broad, flat, pancake-like structures in which liquid maldistribution may become a problem. The process needs a bed surface

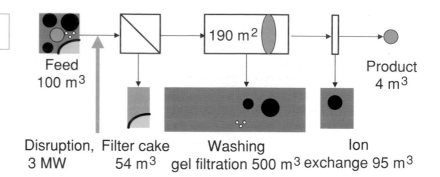

Figure 9.26 Volumes, area and energy needed in the process.

of 190 m²! In the ion exchange step only enzymes 2 and 3 need to be separated. This can be done in an anion exchanger at pH 5. Enzyme 3 binds strongly and enzyme 2 weakly. Regeneration is done with the pH value dropping to 4. An eluent amount of three times the capacity is chosen for enzyme 3, which should suffice. Ion exchange resins have a capacity far greater than gel filtration resins, which is the reason why significantly smaller volumes of ion exchange resin are needed. The enzyme is assumed to concentrate ten times. The results are shown Fig. 9.26. To sum up the process: 0.2 m³ of product in pure form is obtained in a solution of 4 m³. The waste produced is:

• 54 m³ of filter cake,
• 500 m³ of wastewater from the gel filtration, and
• 95 m³ of water from the ion exchange.

The waste has 3000 times the volume of the product (an *E*-factor of 3000)! A huge amount of gel is needed besides the energy input of 3 MW.

The following improvements can be made. The liquid stream to the gel filtration can be reduced by an ultrafiltration step. About nine-tenths of the water can be removed in this way. This reduces the size of the gel filtration column by a factor of 10 together with the wastewater streams. Another obvious improvement is to change the order of the gel filtration and the ion exchange. The ion exchange step may become more complex but only two enzymes need to be removed on the gel column. This reduces the streams even further. When using micro-organisms that are able to produce the enzyme at a higher concentration, a significant reduction in streams can be obtained. The filter cake poses a problem. A possibility might be to adsorb the component of interest directly from the fermentation broth, thereby avoiding the filtration step. The waste broth could be sent for biotreatment. The adsorption cannot be operated in a column due to clogging/blocking problems but could be carried out in a bioreactor operated with a slurry of adsorbent. The adsorption conditions are determined by the fermentation liquid and are probably not ideal for separation of the product. A mixture of components will be adsorbed. However, this method may give a substantial reduction in downstream processing throughputs by early concentration in the process. Some industrial research has been performed along this line but not many processes use this route in practice. The reason lies in poisoning or fouling of the adsorbent by other components in the reactor mixture. The cell debris could be flocculated to increase the particle diameter of the cell debris and make the filtration possible even without filter aid. Of course the filtration problem will disappear for large micro-organisms that can produce an extracellular enzyme. A problem associated with this method is the probable degradation of the enzyme at the gas–liquid interface in the fermenter.

The conclusion from this exercise must be:

- scaling-up of a laboratory recipe may not lead to a good industrial process,
- waste streams have to be considered carefully,
- volume reduction has to be done early in the process, and
- intracellular production and filter aids are to be avoided (if possible).

9.8 | Further reading

Garcia, A., Bonen, M. R., Ramirez-Vick, J., Sadaka, M. and Vuppu, A. *Bioseparation Process Science*. Massachusetts: Blackwell, 1999.

Harrison, R. G. *Protein Purification Process Engineering*. New York: Marcel Dekker, 1994.

Olson, W. P. *Separations Technology: Pharmaceutical and Biotechnical Applications*. Buffalo Grove: Interpharm Press, 1995.

Schügerl, K. *Solvent Extraction in Biotechnology: Recovery of Primary and Secondary Metabolites*. Berlin: Springer-Verlag, 1994.

Seader, J. D. and Henley, E. J. *Separation Process Principles*. New York: John Wiley & Sons, 1998.

Thornton, J. D. *Science and Practice of Liquid–Liquid Extraction*, Vol. 1. Oxford: Clarendon Press, 1992.

ANSWERS TO ASSIGNMENTS

9.1: 6, 2, 1, <1

9.2: 1.59 $m^3 h^{-1}$, 3, 20%

9.3: 8.82×10^{11} m kg^{-1}, 8.78×10^{10} m^{-1}, 22.14 $m^3 h^{-1}$.

9.4: 0.12 $kg s^{-1}$, 1.2 m^2

9.6: 5.59×10^{-6} $m s^{-1}$, 12 mmol l^{-1}

Chapter 10

Measurement, monitoring, modelling and control

Bernhard Sonnleitner

Zürich University of Applied Sciences, Switzerland

10.1 Introduction

It is the cellular activities, such as those of enzymes or nucleic acids, that determine the performance of bioprocesses. Unfortunately, they are difficult or impossible to measure on-line. Consequently, we need to monitor or estimate variables such as the concentrations of biomass, metabolites, substrates, products or regulator molecules. These dependent variables often can represent the process objectives more or less directly. If not, models need to be constructed and exploited to link the variables that can be measured or monitored to the desired process objectives. We also need to know all the relevant operating variables that influence the desired objectives significantly and also how they influence them.

10.2 Terminology

Measuring means to describe a variable qualitatively and/or quantitatively. The variable can be a physical one, which is usually quite simple to measure, a chemical one or a biological one, which can be

Basic Biotechnology, third edition, eds. Colin Ratledge and Bjørn Kristiansen.
Published by Cambridge University Press. © Cambridge University Press 2006.

quite tricky to measure. It involves an analytical method and instrument(s). Measurements of variables of interest are normally indirect measuring methods. To measure glucose concentration, for example, we convert a known aliquot of β-D-glucose in the presence of (dissolved) oxygen using the enzyme glucose oxidase into gluconolactone and hydrogen peroxide, which we eventually oxidise using an amperometric electrode: the final measure is the electric current that we relate to the glucose concentration by using stoichiometric and kinetic models.

Monitoring means to obtain process information without manual or personnel intervention and without disturbing the process. This includes cases where samples must be withdrawn from the process.

Modelling is the crisp or fuzzy description of one or more relations between one or more causes and one or more effects. We need to parameterise the models in order to make them useful: this is done by *calibration* or by *training*, i.e. we pretend to know the cause(s) and effect(s) precisely. In practice, we exploit the models most often in the reverse way: we measure or monitor effects and trace them back to their causes. In this case, models must be validated by means of data sets that are different from and independent of the calibration or instrument training sets. In this context, modelling is simply a tool, not a goal on its own.

Control means take the information obtained from a process, process it with algorithm(s) and use it on the same process to keep one or more measured variables as close to the desired set point(s) as possible. The set points themselves need not necessarily be constant, they may well depend on time and/or other variables.

Many technical terms are inconsistently used in the literature. In this text the relevant terms have the following meaning: *on-line* is used for fully automatic, as opposed to off-line, which implies manual interaction by personnel. *In situ* means strictly built into a reactor or an inlet or outlet line. *By-pass* is used for any action that takes place outside the reactor on a sample aliquot removed from the reactor; this is sometimes also called *at-line*. The treated sample may be returned to the reactor or be discarded. *Off-line* means any action after removing a sample and transport to another place, e.g. an analytical laboratory. *Continuous signal* generation is the opposite of discontinuous or discrete signal availability. A *real-time signal* is generated instantaneously, or at a negligible delay compared to the dynamics of the process, and is well suited for control purposes, whereas a delayed signal, with or without dead time, may be less, or not at all, useful for process control. Many analytical methods do not affect the process or the sample aliquots at all: they are non-invasive; others are destructive and the samples must be disposed of.

Basically, all sensors used in bioprocess engineering must be sterilisable or they must be operated outside a safe sterile barrier and linked to the bioprocess by using an appropriate interface. This is a matter of protection of the process from contaminations or of biosecurity. The sensors must be stable and reliable over days or even

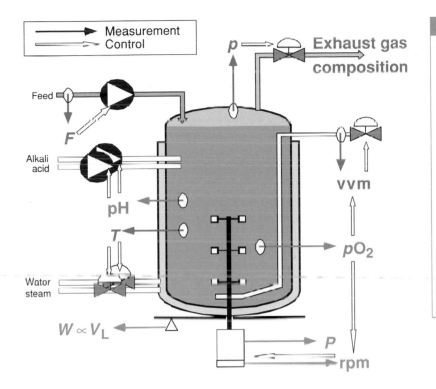

Measurement
Control

p Exhaust gas composition

Feed
F

Alkali
acid

pH

T

Water
steam

$W \propto V_L$

vvm

pO_2

P

rpm

Figure 10.1 Bioprocess variables that are generally regarded as standard: F = (volumetric or gravimetric) feed rate, p = pressure, pH = pH value of liquid, pO_2 = partial pressure of dissolved oxygen, P = electric power drawn by the stirrer motor, rpm = speed of stirrer motor (revolutions per minute), T = temperature of the liquid, vvm = aeration rate (volume of gas per volume of liquid per minute), V_L = volume of liquid, W = weight of reactor. Measurement (or monitoring) is indicated by solid arrows, control actions are identified by arrows pointing towards the respective actuators (valves, pumps, motor).

weeks, and they should have low-maintenance requirements in order to be attractive for industrial use.

10.3 | Measurements generally accepted as standard

There are a few generally accepted standard measurements. Typically, they reflect physical or chemical variables rather than biological ones (Fig. 10.1). Most physical variables can be determined on-line, in situ, continuously and in real time. Biological variables are, with a few exceptions, determined after sampling off-line, discontinuously and often involve manual work and substantial time delay.

10.3.1 Biomass concentration: the key variable?

Biomass concentration is a simple measure of the available quantity of biocatalyst. An ideal measure for the biocatalyst in a bioreaction system of interest would not be just its mass but rather its activity, physiological state, morphology or other typification. As these are difficult to quantify objectively, the biomass concentration is still the key variable, primarily because it provides information on the rates of growth and/or product formation. Almost all mathematical models that are used to describe growth or product formation contain biomass as an important state variable. Many control strategies have the objective of maximising biomass concentration; later we will discuss whether this is always wise.

The *golden standard* for the determination of cell mass concentration is a manual method, namely to harvest a known aliquot of the culture suspension, separate the cells by centrifugation or filtration, wash the cells and dry them to constant weight at a few degrees above the boiling point of the relevant processing fluid in order to overcome capillary condensation of the fluid in the cell paste (i.e. usually at 105 °C at atmospheric pressure for aqueous media; a lower temperature is admissible only when applied under vacuum). After gravimetric determination of the dry mass in the vial or on the filter, the mass concentration in the original sample volume can be calculated if there are neither particulate components in the fresh medium or precipitates formed during cultivation. The result is available with considerable delay. Accelerated drying under infrared heaters or in microwave ovens requires tough standard operating procedures (SOP), but is does reduce the processing time to less than 30 minutes.

There are alternative methods such as relating the biomass level to total and/or viable cell counts. This is quite laborious and error prone. Modern image analysis tools are very helpful (though not inexpensive) for microscopic counting. The cell number result is generally available in shorter time. It must be pointed out that the measured values for cell mass and number concentrations are not equivalent under non-steady-state conditions. So-called standard cells are cells with a constant individual cell mass and composition but these are the exception rather than the rule.

The optical density (OD) of a cell suspension is a widely used substitute for the *golden standard*. It requires sampling, an appropriate dilution of the suspension with a suitable buffer and photometric determination of the turbidity caused by the suspended cells, usually at a wavelength around 600 nm. The OD value reflects a superposition of absorption, reflection and forward scatter of light and, therefore, depends on size, shape, morphology and aggregation of cells as well as on the presence of solutes and particles other than cells in the suspension. Provided a model system, which must be validated for every individual biosystem, exists, this technique yields a very useful and quick estimate of biomass concentration.

10.3.2 Physical and physico-chemical variables

Almost every bioreactor provides information about temperature, pressure, stirrer speed or power consumed, gas flow rate, pH value and partial pressure of dissolved oxygen (pO_2 or DOT for dissolved oxygen tension). Temperature and stirrer speed are invariably closed-loop controlled as a basic requirement. It is, of course, beneficial for the reproducibility and performance of a process to control the other variables listed as well. In many industrial processes, the composition of the exhaust gas is analysed. This is considered as safe (for the process), since the gas analyser is fed with the reactor waste gas, and as beneficial, since the metabolic state of the culture can be estimated from its *respiratory quotient* (RQ, see Section 6.2.2). In addition, an oxygen transfer limitation can be demonstrated by a principally different analytical method than pO_2 measurement with a dissolved oxygen probe. Closed-loop control of variables such as volume (or weight) of the reactor, and flow rates of liquid streams into and out of the reactor, may be decisive for the success of bioprocesses carried out in fed-batch or continuous operation mode.

Temperature and pressure sensors are usually placed in separate stainless steel housings and mounted in a prominent place in the reactor. Most modern pH and pO_2 sensors contain temperature probes in order to compensate for the temperature associated gain drifts of the sensors. Although platinum wire temperature sensitive resistors (Pt-100 or Pt-1000: either 100 or 1000 Ω at 0 °C) are quite stable over time, i.e. they are precise, few laboratories support appropriate references for validating their accuracy.

There are piezo-resistive pressure sensors on the market that have a temperature-dependent gain or off-set shift of less than 2%, many highly temperature-dependent pressure sensors are still in use. We need to know the pressure accurately for safety reasons and to document that no vacuum had occurred during the cooling phase after sterilisation. For bioreactions conducted under pressure, still the exception rather than the rule, accurate signals are mandatory.

The pH value is usually monitored with a single potentiometric glass electrode with a built-in Ag/AgCl reference electrode. Strictly, the signal exploited is the difference in the electrical potentials of the electrodes. Thus, the electrolyte surrounding the reference electrode must be in electrical contact with the measuring solution, i.e. the biosuspension. Between the two there is a diffusion resistance provided by the porous diaphragm in the classical electrodes and a hydrogel in the most modern probes. The diffusion resistance of the hydrogel is large enough to prevent leakage of Ag^+ ions. A problem that sometimes materialises is that the diaphragm clogs due to protein adsorption, precipitations or surface growth; concomitantly, its electrical resistance increases in the order of $G\Omega$ to $T\Omega$ and the signal can drift unpredictably as much as 1 pH unit per day and the response time will deteriorate. In food biotechnology, the risk of glass damage is not acceptable. Many manufacturers are therefore developing proton-sensitive field-effect transistors (pH-FET) as alternatives to glass electrodes. The current problem is the substantial drift of the FETs during sterilisation; this can be as much as 80 mV or roughly 1.5 pH units and is also unpredictable.

Deposits on the detector surface may also be experienced with redox electrodes, which are similarly constructed but have a noble metal (Au or Pt) instead of the proton-sensitive glass at their tip. These electrodes provide some lumped and fuzzy information on the 'general availability of electrons', however, they are very useful for estimation of the quality of strictly anaerobic cultivations.

The pO_2 value is usually monitored with a single amperometric, membrane-covered electrode (so called Clark-type). The signal depends not only on the membrane, but also on the mounting position of the electrode in the reactor because of the possible existence of gradient

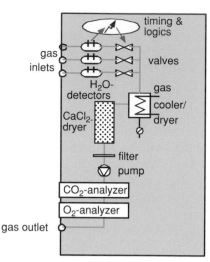

Figure 10.2 Basic concept of an exhaust gas analyser that is robust enough for industrial use. The exhaust gas must be transported towards the analyser gas inlets from where the internal pump takes an appropriate sample stream. More than one inlet is usually present in order to share the investment between more reactors. When suspension or foam is brought to the analyser, it is detected rapidly and individually at every entry. Further intrusion into the instrument is prevented by disabling the respective valves. Depending on the measuring principles of the O_2 and CO_2 analysers, respectively, the gas may have to be dried; this scheme shows a two-step drying sequence. In any case, a reliable gas filter is advisable.

in the reactor. One should take care that no gas bubbles are trapped at the membrane. Growth of biofilms on the membrane is a well-known, but rarely discussed, phenomenon.

Typically, these electrodes are used as a single unit per reactor. Should one deteriorate or malfunction during a process, it cannot be changed unless it is retractably mounted via a secondary housing that can be streamed in situ during the process. Such housing devices are useful in production processes and for large bioreactors.

Exhaust gas analyses is expensive, but worthwhile. Most gas analysers require specific attention when used. Water vapour interferes with CO_2 analyses based on infrared absorption, and ingress of liquid water or foam can be very destructive. Therefore, a simple requirement is that the instrument must be able to cope with foam and dry the gas (see Fig. 10.2). An instrument may serve several gas streams and this substantially reduces the price per channel and reactor. The following variables can then be calculated from the gas analysis values assuming that only O_2 and CO_2 are the reactive gas species (for other reactive gases, analogous procedures are valid): the *oxygen uptake rate* (OUR) and *carbon dioxide evolution rate* (CER) of the reactor are obtained from mass balances. If the working volume (V_L) is known, the *oxygen transfer rate* (OTR) and *carbon dioxide transfer rate* (CTR) can be calculated, and if biomass concentration (x) is known, the *specific rates of oxygen consumption* (q_{O_2}) and CO_2 *production* (q_{CO_2}) can be derived. The calculations are based on *mass balances*. We need two mass balances for each gas, one for the gas phase and one for the liquid phase:

$$\frac{d(V_G y_G)}{dt} - \text{MAFR}^{in} y^{in} - \text{MAFR}^{out} y^{out} \mp \text{transfer}_{G \leftrightarrow L} \quad (10.1)$$

$$\frac{d(V_L c_L)}{dt} = \pm \text{transfer}_{G \leftrightarrow L} \mp q V_L x \, [+\text{transport via liquid phase}] \quad (10.2)$$

where G and L denote the gas or liquid phase, respectively; V is the volume of the respective phase; y is the molar fraction of either O_2 or CO_2 in the gas phase; c is the dissolved gas concentration; MAFR is short for mass-of-air flow rate (assumed to be determined with a mass flow meter); and q is the specific rate of gas consumption (q_{O_2}: negative) or production (q_{CO_2}: positive). Note that the transfer$_{G \leftrightarrow L}$ terms have different signs in the mass balances: in one they are a source, in the other a sink. The transfer via liquid phase may be considered in non-batch cultivations, but even then, may be neglected. Assuming pseudo steady state (i.e. the differentials vanish) and substituting for the transfer$_{G \leftrightarrow L}$ term we get:

$$q V_L x = -\text{MAFR}^{in} y^{in} + \text{MAFR}^{out} y^{out} \quad (10.3)$$

Mass flow meters are not cheap and work more reliably with dry gas, therefore, one usually monitors the MAFR^{in} only but needs MAFR^{out} as well. The equation can still be solved under the assumption that all components of the gas phase are inert apart from O_2 and CO_2: thus the inert gas going in must come out under pseudo-stationary conditions:

$$\text{MAFR}^{in} y_{inert}^{in} = \text{MAFR}^{out} y_{inert}^{out} \quad (10.4)$$

Knowing the y_{inert} values to be equal to $(1 - y_{O_2} - y_{CO_2})$, one can calculate MAFR^{out}.

The respiratory quotient (RQ) is defined as the molar ratio of $|q_{CO_2}/q_{O_2}|$. However, this also holds true for the ratio of production rate to uptake rate over the entire reactor: for calculation of the RQ, one does not need to know the biomass concentration and the working volume. In addition, the mass of air flow rate is not needed and the RQ can be directly calculated from the gas composition data only:

$$RQ = \frac{y_{CO_2}^{out} - y_{CO_2}^{in}}{y_{O_2}^{in} - y_{O_2}^{out}} \quad (10.5)$$

or

$$RQ = \frac{y_{CO_2}^{out} - y_{CO_2}^{in} - y_{O_2}^{in} y_{CO_2}^{out} + y_{O_2}^{out} y_{CO_2}^{in}}{y_{O_2}^{in} - y_{O_2}^{out} - y_{O_2}^{in} y_{CO_2}^{out} + y_{O_2}^{out} y_{CO_2}^{in}} \quad (10.6)$$

The simpler formula (10.5) holds true if the RQ value is close to 1 (or $\text{MAFR}^{in} \approx \text{MAFR}^{out}$); however, if the RQ is significantly different from 1, the inert gas balance must be considered and, then, RQ should be calculated using the extended formula (10.6). Note that, in this context, only the physical solution of gases is considered; it might be necessary to include further chemical reactions in the mass balances, for instance the chemisorption of CO_2 to bicarbonate or even carbonate at higher pH values.

Volumes of gassed and agitated liquids in reactors are difficult to measure accurately by level measurement, especially if there is a foam blanket on top of the liquid. The only reliable solution to this is the determination of the mass of liquid using balances or scales. Knowing the mass makes it also easier to calculate the mass balances. In the case of reactor mass, one has to ensure that all connections to and from the reactor are force-compensated and fixed so that they cannot move during operation.

This also holds true for the determination of flow rates of liquids. A decrease of mass of a supply vessel or an increase of mass of a harvest vessel over time can easily be evaluated into a mass flow rate.

Among the variables most difficult to quantify is foam. The foaming behaviour of a gassed liquid varies with time and has a significant impact on mass transfer due to coalescence of bubbles and on the presence of cells trapped in the foam. Yet, there is no reasonable method available to qualify or quantify these aspects automatically. Foam control is normally carried out by using mechanical foam breakers/separators or the addition of chemical antifoam agents. The addition can be continuous or discrete, actuated in open loop control or triggered by the signal of a foam sensor. These sensors are not very reliable since foam lamellae collapse and stick (stochastically) to the sensors upon foam destruction. There are no a-priori rules for the selection of a most effective antifoam agent: success is a matter of good intuition or trial and error.

10.4 | Non-standard monitoring techniques

Some of the non-standard sensors can be operated *in situ*, most of them are apparatuses rather than sensors and require sampling or sample preparation prior to use (see Fig. 10.3). There are many reasons why these techniques are not yet standard:

- lack of a calibration reference,
- necessity to combine or configure the instruments to a functional entity that is not available on the market,
- complexity of instrument and interface between instrument and process, and
- requirement for specifically parameterised and validated calibration models.

10.4.1 Biomass-related sensors

Sensors designed to determine an *optical density* (OD) also *see* gas bubbles, the intrinsic colour of the medium itself and particulates other than cells, independent of whether they measure the absorbance,

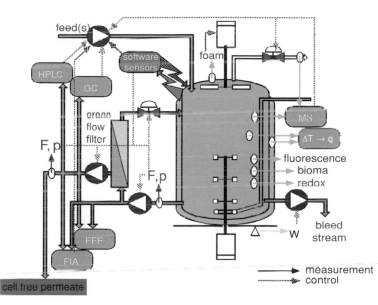

Figure 10.3 Bioprocess variables are generally not monitored, yet they are desirable extensions to the standard: biomass = biomass sensor; fluorescence = fluorescence sensor (F and p are flow rates and pressure, respectively); foam = foam detector and the activation of a mechanical foam compressor; FFF = field flow fractionation; FIA = flow injection analyser; GC = gas chromatograph; HPLC = high-performance liquid chromatograph; MS = mass spectrometer (connected to both liquid and gas phase); redox = redox sensor; software sensors are calculated variables; W = weight; ΔT = temperature difference between biosuspension and jacket water (from which the heat flow, q, can be calculated). Cell-free permeate can be produced by a by-pass stream from the reactor led through a cross-flow filter. Measurement (or monitoring) is indicated by broad arrows, control actions are identified by narrow arrows towards the respective actuators (valves, pumps, motor).

the scatter or the reflection of light. The unwanted effect may exceed the desired signal intensity by much more than an order of magnitude. Usually, the light wavelength chosen is very near infrared as this improves the signal intensity for most microbial cells (spatial dimension approximately four times the wavelength) and reduces the intrinsic light absorption by the medium. Note that if cells exist as larger entities, such as mycelia or pellets, OD readings are of no use. Exclusion of gas bubbles from the optical path is also necessary as is the need to remove attached biofilms or precipitates periodically from the optical window. No biomass sensor can distinguish between live and dead cells or cell debris; they deliver a lumped estimate of biomass but no qualitative information.

Fluorescence is a typical characteristic property of some molecules. Prominent fluorophores in cells are the reduced species of nicotinamide dinucleotides (NADH and NADPH), aromatic amino acids and several vitamins. As long as the (intra-)cellular concentrations of these species are constant, fluorescence intensity should be proportional to the cell density. However, non-linear effects corrupt this concept at higher cell densities. Also, the cellular concentrations of the fluorophores are not constant in praxi, they may change quite significantly and rapidly. This makes it impossible to correlate the fluorescence signal with cell density strictly and accurately. However, the information the fluorescence signal contains is valuable to detect (rapid) physiological changes (rather than biomass concentration).

Electrical impedance spectroscopy is aimed at estimating the sum of liquid volumes enclosed by polarisable membranes (= intact cells) in front of the sensor. The cells behave as microcapacitors in an alternating electrical field. The measurable capacitance change is an estimate of the integral cellular volume. The frequency at which this takes place depends on the individual volume (= size) distribution of the cells in suspension. Again, a tailor-made calibration is necessary. Commercially available instruments work at a single pre-set frequency only. Instruments which can be tuned are being developed and with these chemometric analysis of the spectral data can be applied. This principle circumvents the interferences caused by insoluble or precipitated medium components but is also sensitive towards gas bubbles. However, another interference comes into play: the conductivity of the medium which is variable over time and short-circuits the capacitor.

Another new approach to the optical investigation of biosuspensions is the *in situ* microscope in connection with *image analysis*. Typical applications are cell counting and sizing, and characterisation of shape, texture or mobility of cells. Even different complex filamentous morphologies have been analysed successfully with image analysis techniques.

The message to be learnt from all this is not that these sensors are useless, rather it is that the signals delivered can be translated into useful quantitative information by a tailor-made, i.e. system-specific, off-line calibration while all operating conditions strictly need to be held constant. Absolute values are difficult to obtain, but relative use, for comparison, is valuable. In other words, such signals may be quite useful in (approved industrial) processes that are always operated in the same way.

10.4.2 Methods related to individual components

Relatively new techniques in bioprocess monitoring are *near* and *mid-range infrared spectroscopy*, NIR and MIR. With the spectroscopic methods, analytical information can be obtained non-invasively without direct contact between sample and sensing element (using fibre or conduit optics). Low-maintenance work during operation and simultaneous multi-analyte determination are further advantages. The chemical information in NIR originates from overtone and combination transitions of C–H, O–H and N–H vibrations and is determined in the wave number range from 5000 to 4000 cm^{-1}. Stronger absorbance and more distinct spectral features can be expected from MIR spectroscopy in the wave number range between 800 and 2000 cm^{-1}. However, the strong absorption of water results in very short penetration depth of the radiation (especially around 1600 and 3300 cm^{-1}). Attenuated

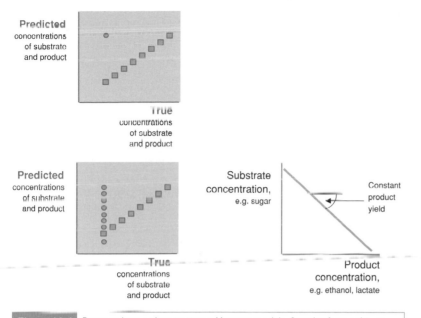

Figure 10.4 Proposed procedure to test calibration models. Samples from cultivations should be spiked with the various substances of interest. Then, one knows the concentration differences of the spiked component exactly (i.e. the true values) and the calibration model must predict this behaviour (squares); at the same time, it must not predict a change in the unspiked components (circle; only one shown in the upper graph). If any other component is predicted to vary (circles in bottom left graph), it is very likely that the model does not predict analytic relations; rather, it has been trained to predict a biological relation, for example, that product concentration increases when substrate concentration decreases (bottom right). In the first case, the model is likely to be useful; in the latter case, the model should be discarded.

total reflection (ATR) elements are therefore preferred. The spectral information is based on vibrations and stretching of various C—O bonds. In all cases, the spectral information from all the medium components overlaps and results in very complex spectra. These spectra must then be analysed by chemometric methods.

Retrospective (off-line) analysis of fermentation data and analysis of synthetic mixtures of analytes of interest is frequently used to establish the tailor-made calibration models. With these models, if validated, the on-line acquired spectra can be interpreted. The calibration model should be based strictly on unique spectral features of a given analyte. This can be tested by spiking real samples (off-line) with various components; a useful model will predict a concentration change of the spiked component only (see Fig. 10.4). Organic acids, sugars, alcohols and biopolymers have been successfully monitored on-line. The same modelling and calibration considerations hold true for the analyses of volatiles done with electronic noses.

Besides the sensors and systems discussed above, there are many established analytical instruments useful for on-line bioprocess monitoring; however, an appropriate interface must be available. The interfaces can work according to one of four different principles:

(1) A sample of the complete biosuspension is taken automatically without affecting the cells, i.e. cells stay alive and active.

(2) A sample of the complete biosuspension is taken automatically with integrated inactivation of cells during sampling.

(3) A sample of the supernatant or permeate is taken after removal of cells.

(4) The analyte of interest is volatile and can be determined from the gas phase sampled after the exhaust gas filter (i.e. beyond the sterile barrier).

In the first two cases, a pump or a valve represents the sterile barrier and must work in a one-way direction only. Furthermore, the valve should have a minimal dead volume and should be designed in such a way that the dead volume can be cleaned and dried *in situ* in order to avoid carry-over from one sample to the next. A few such valves are commercially available. A pump should work continuously with a minimal flow rate to avoid back-growth of contaminants. If no further action is taken and the mean residence time in the sampling line is sufficiently low, cells will remain intact and cellular activities can be determined in the removed samples. Care must be taken to avoid the biosuspension experiencing oxygen limitation in the sample stream.

Case 2 implies an inactivation of cells; this can be achieved by heating or chilling the sample line or by continuously mixing the sample stream with an inactivating solution, e.g. KCN. This inactivates and probably dilutes the sample and makes sense only if substrates or excreted products or metabolites need to be analysed. The sampling line may be periodically rinsed with a cleaning solution, such as alkali or acid, in order to remove biofilms, debris or precipitates.

Case 3 involves the removal of cells from the liquid, most probably by filtration rather than centrifugation. Filters can be mounted *in situ* or in a by-pass. In the first approach, the filter must be mounted in a reactor zone with high turbulence in order to avoid fouling of the filter. The filter can be operated by overpressure in the reactor or by using a suction pump for the permeate. In the latter approach, one needs an extra pump to circulate the biosuspension out of the reactor and across the filter. Cells are enriched in the suspension, when permeate is removed, and circulated back to the reactor; this *analytical cell retention system* leads to an increase of biomass concentration and must be taken into account in appropriate mass balance extensions. The entire set-up should be as close as possible to the reactor, with the stream volume and mean residence time of cells outside the reactor minimised. The liquid velocity should be chosen such that the filtration is operated in tangential flow type (i.e. the sample flow across the membrane is greater than 2 m s^{-1}). The permeate should be pumped actively and continuously in order to avoid back-growth of contaminants, which would change the representative composition of the permeate.

Case 4 is a special case and restricted to volatiles only, e.g. solvents, some esters or acids. Probably, the sample line needs to be heated in order to avoid condensation of water and/or analytes. One can assume saturation of the gas phase provided the aeration rate is reasonably low and, hence, one can calculate the liquid phase concentration from the gas phase concentration provided the partition behaviour between the two phases is known.

Instruments to be connected to bioprocesses via the above-mentioned interfaces can be:

- flow injection analysers (FIA),
- chromatographs (for gases as well as liquids),
- electrophoresis units,
- mass spectrometers,
- electronic noses, and
- field flow fractionation devices.

Unfortunately, most suppliers sell the instruments (including the controlling PC) only, and not in combination with a useful interface or as a dedicated solution of a specific process-analytical problem. Thus specific internal know-how and personnel is required and this is probably the main obstacle to these analytical techniques becoming standard for bioprocessing.

The most general analytical problem solution tool is FIA because it allows the integration of almost any combination of physical and chemical reactions in a flowing system. All others are more specific and, therefore, limited to special, limited groups of analytes. The basic components of FIA equipment are a liquid transport and switching system consisting of tubing, pumps, valves and (a) carrier stream(s) into which a technical system injects a sample automatically. According to the time required for such a sequence, data are produced in a time-discrete manner, not continuously. However, data can be obtained continuously if any injection can be omitted.

The operating principle for FIA is shown in Fig. 10.5. A chemical or biochemical reaction, which is typical for the substance to be measured, takes place while flowing through a tube (i.e. a plug flow type reactor). Physical sample treatment such as dilution, extraction, separation or diffusion can easily be implemented. The most important among those is dilution, where a known volume of sample is injected into a (very small) continuous stirred tank reactor through which a carrier liquid is constantly flowing. The injected aliquot must be perfectly degassed prior to injection and is assumed to be well mixed and diluted by the carrier fluid with time. The residence time distribution of this *dilution reactor* should be determined separately but can be assumed to remain the same under identical operating conditions. The result is, for example, a thousand-fold dilution in less than a minute with an accuracy better than 99% and an even better precision.

Products or residual (co-)substrates are measured by the detection system. The detector is often an optical or electrical device

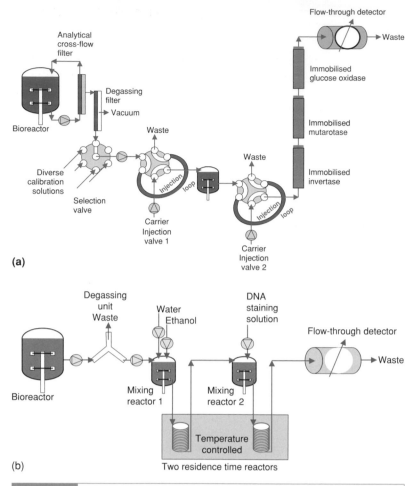

(a)

(b)

Figure 10.5 Two examples for the exploitation of flow injection analysis in bioprocess monitoring. (a) Determination of sucrose. A small sample stream is prepared continuously by cross-flow filtration, subsequently degassed via a solution-diffusion membrane and, in measuring mode, pumped into injection valve 1 in order to load the injection loop (in calibration mode, the selection valve delivers a calibration solution). Periodically, injection valve 1 is switched (for injection clockwise) for a period sufficient to push the sample plug from the loop into the following dilution reactor. After switching back, the carrier stream dilutes the sample in this mixing reactor. The outflow is loaded into the injection loop of valve 2 which is switched (for injection clockwise) an appropriate period after valve 1, namely when the desired sample dilution is reached. After switching back, the carrier stream pushes the diluted sample through three columns packed with immobilised enzymes. In the first, invertase hydrolyses sucrose into α-D-glucose and β-fructose. In the second, mutarotase accelerates the conversion of α-D-glucose to β-D-glucose, which is the only acceptable form for the glucose oxidase in the third column. Together with dissolved O_2, β-D-glucose is converted to gluconolactone and H_2O_2. The latter compound can be determined in the flow through detector, e.g. an amperometric electrode, but other methods are also possible. The co-substrate O_2 must be provided by the carrier stream and must not be limiting. This is why the foregoing dilution step is so advisable: the dynamic range can so be extended over several orders of magnitude. (b) A small sample stream of biosuspension, i.e. containing the cells, is removed from the reactor and subsequently degassed with a simple overflow device. An aliquot is then pumped into a small mixing reactor where the cells are mixed with water (for an appropriate dilution) and ethanol (for fixing the cells) with the ethanol permeabilising the cells. Thereafter, a specific staining solution is added which is allowed to diffuse into the cells for the period determined by the mean residence time in the coil and interact with, in this case, DNA. The following flow-through detector determines the fluorescence intensity, which is a measure for the DNA concentration in the diluted sample stream. If the detector happens to be a flow cytometer, each individual cell is analysed and a population distribution can be evaluated.

(photometer or polarographic electrode), but it can be based on enzymatic or immunological reactions (*biosensors*), redox measurement, or other complex and powerful analytical devices such as *mass spectrometers* or *flow cytometers*. Figure 10.5 illustrates two rather simple examples.

No interference with the sterile barrier is likely since the entire apparatus works outside the sterile space. However, special emphasis must be given to the sampling device interfacing the sterile barrier and to degassing the volume aliquot to be injected. FIA easily meets validation requirements because alternative measuring principles can (theoretically) be run in parallel, which helps to exclude systematic errors that might originate from the complex matrix.

Biosensors are increasingly used as detectors in FIA systems. The biosensor drawbacks of low dynamic range, inability to survive sterilisation, limited lifetime, etc. when used as *in situ* sensors are no longer valid *ex situ* because the FIA interfaces the biosensor, which can be changed anytime, and the FIA can provide samples in optimal dilution. The need for chemicals and reagents can be drastically reduced when employing biosensors.

An outstanding property of FIA is its range of application. It can be viewed as a general solution-handling technique rather than a distinct sensor. This causes high flexibility with respect to analytical methods. However, a high degree of automation is necessary and desirable. FIA is expected to become one of the most powerful tools for quantitative bioprocess monitoring provided that non-linear calibration models can be used and the data evaluation techniques improve, including automatic fault detection of the analytical system. The present tendency is towards using multi-channel FIA systems that work either in parallel or with sequential injection, miniaturisation of FIA devices and automation.

Most of the other analytical instruments listed above can be viewed as special cases of FIA. In *chromatographs* the reactions are omitted and separation of species over an appropriate column occurs. The carrier is either a liquid (HPLC) or a gas (GC). In a *capillary electrophoresis*, separation takes place without a stationary phase. In *field flow fractionation devices*, some species are more retarded on their way along the flow channel than others due to the effect of a perpendicular field, e.g. a gravimetric, magnetic, electric or flow field. The injected sample volumes must be perfectly degassed prior to injection if absolute quantitative information is desired.

On-line *mass spectrometry* and *flow cytometry* are somewhat special. Mass spectrometry works in a high vacuum only. Therefore, a pressure lock must be used together with the sterile sampling interface. This can be a simple capillary with a tiny nozzle for gases or a solution-diffusion membrane for dissolved volatiles. Since the performance of the interfaces changes with time, this must influence the determined signal amplitudes, and it is wise to calculate ratios of the signals of variables to signals caused by inert components, e.g. N_2 or Ar. Then, the signals give also absolute quantitative information, otherwise, relative values only can be derived.

Flow cytometry is an established off-line technique. If combined with FIA as a sampling and sample preparation method, it can also be applied on-line. The strength of this technique is the delivery of segregated information, i.e. quantitative description of a population distribution. The method is based on a high number of measurements of properties of single cells, e.g. 10^4 measurements per second are possible. Individual cells are aligned by means of controlled hydrodynamic flow patterns and pass the measuring cell one by one. One or more light sources, typically laser(s), are focused onto the stream of cells and a detection unit measures the transmitted, scattered and/or fluorescence light. Properties of whole cells such as size and shape can be estimated as well as distinct cellular components. The last requires specific staining procedures which can be achieved in a preceding FIA. Among the items that have been measured are:

- cell vitality,
- intracellular pH,
- DNA,
- RNA content, and
- specific plasmids.

Besides nucleic acids, other intracellular components, e.g. storage materials, enzymes and protein content, can be analysed and the physiological state can be rapidly assessed. With more complex instruments, multi-channel analyses can be performed simultaneously provided the cells are pre-treated appropriately.

10.5 | Control

The main purpose of applying control to biotechnological processes is to keep several state variables at a constant set point or on a predefined trajectory. It is the exception rather than the rule to have a sufficiently accurate process model that permits precise calculation, i.e. prediction, of the individual relevant state variables, such as mass or concentration of substrates, biomass, enzymes or products to meet a desired result, such as maximal productivity or maximal product purity or minimal by-product formation or combinations thereof. A practical solution to this problem is to break the complex system into smaller sub-systems and to try optimising these individually. For instance, forming simple sub-systems concerning operating conditions: growth of a population will be maximum at a given temperature and a given pH (single value or a small range). Therefore, one usually regulates such variables, which are normally easily monitored, by closed-loop control.

However, there are other important process variables that are difficult to monitor or whose impact on the optimality criterion is not well known. In these cases, industrial practices usually apply to open-loop control along pre-defined patterns. For example, glucose concentration could lead to formation of undesired by-product if the former was too high, while it would cause undesired limitation and thus deteriorate the cells' performance if it was too low. The optimal values are usually not exactly known for a given cell type. As these values are not fundamental constants, they must be determined experimentally and individually. However, even the analytical methodology and equipment in research environments do not provide unambiguous and clear data. In production conditions, monitoring is an even greater problem and closed loop control is very unlikely to be applied successfully. Therefore, one tries to make an educated guess as to what the optimal value could be or to determine a desired set point intuitively. In a fed-batch (or a continuous) process, the decisive state variable, in this example the substrate concentration, depends on at least two important effectors: the (volumetric) consumption rate and the flux into and out of the system, as expressed by the mass balance:

$$\frac{d(SV)}{dt} = S_{in}F - r_S V \; (-SF)$$ (10.7)

where S is the substrate concentration, i.e. the state variable that cannot be monitored routinely, V is the volume of the biosuspension (not a constant in a fed-batch process); S_{in} is the substrate concentration in the feed; F is the volumetric feed rate; and r_S is the volumetric substrate consumption rate.

Keeping the concentration at the pre-determined set point means that the differential dS/dt becomes zero and for a fed-batch operation, the mass balance gives the following condition:

$$\frac{d(SV)}{dt} = S\frac{dV}{dt} + V\frac{dS}{dt} = S_{in}F - r_s V$$ (10.8)

where dV/dt is known and equal to F. Rearranging and setting $dS/dt = 0$, and defining $D = F/V$ gives:

$$\frac{dS}{dt} \equiv 0 = S_{in}\frac{F}{V} - r_S - S\frac{F}{V} = D(S_{in} - S) - r_S$$ (10.9)

In other words, the influx must compensate the consumption. According to the simplest kinetic model, the volumetric consumption rate depends on the substrate concentration, the biomass concentration and the maximum specific consumption rate, $q_{S\,max}$, which is assumed to be a (positive) constant parameter, in a first approximation:

$$r_S = q_{S\,max}\frac{S}{S + K_S}x$$ (10.10)

If the specific growth rate, μ, is assumed to be proportional to the specific substrate consumption rate, $\mu = q_S Y_{X/S}$, the necessary trajectory for the feed rate can be derived:

$$F(t) = \frac{q_s}{S_{in} - S}x_0 V_0 e^{(\mu t)}$$ (10.11)

where x_0 is the biomass concentration and V_0 the working volume at the start of the feed and where the numerical value of S is so small in comparison to S_{in} that it can be neglected. These considerations are exploited by reducing the difficult problem of controlling the state variable S to the much simpler problem of controlling the operational variable F. This is frequently done in open-loop control mode, yet closed-loop control of F is straightforward by gravimetric monitoring of the feed reservoir. However, defining an auxiliary variable to control is tricky: one must not forget the numerous assumptions made during the derivation of the feed trajectory, and the variables x_0 and V_0 must be known precisely. This is easy for V_0, but not so for x_0. This risky situation can only be improved if the assumptions are validated experimentally or better models are available and can be applied.

Closed-loop control is usually applied to physical and chemical operating variables such as temperature, pressure, pH, fluxes, volumes and sometimes partial pressures of gases, mainly pO_2. The deviation, ε, between the actual value of the control variable and its set point is used to affect the process by appropriate changes in one or more manipulated variables in such a way that the deviation is minimised. This is done automatically rather than by manual interaction. In some cases, low-level three-point controllers are sufficient; for example, a cooling valve can be switched on if the temperature of the suspension exceeds an upper limit and a heating valve will be activated if the temperature exceeds a lower limit. In other cases, the process may react improperly to such simple step changes of the manipulated variable. Probably, the control variable may start to oscillate around the set point with considerable amplitude. Then, the process dynamics need to be accounted for and the widely applied *proportional integral differential (PID) controller* is based on very simple assumptions about the process dynamics. The PID controller responds to any deviation, ε, of the measured variable from its set point by changing the manipulated variable, y, in the following way:

$$y = y_0 + K_P \left(\varepsilon + \frac{1}{\tau_I} \int \varepsilon \mathrm{d}t + \tau_D \frac{\mathrm{d}\varepsilon}{\mathrm{d}t} \right) \tag{10.12}$$

The four parameters of this controller, the bias y_0, the proportional factor or gain K_P, and the two time constants for the integral and derivative, τ_I and τ_D, must be determined by simple experiments. This is a straightforward procedure as long as the process dynamics remain constant.

In the simplest case, the procedure according to Ziegler and Nicols is useful. In pure proportional mode, the gain is increased systematically until the control variable oscillates stably. The critical gain, $K_{P,crit}$, and the respective time period of oscillations, t_{crit}, are used to determine the parameters as listed in Table 10.1.

In the more common applications, the controller parameters should be continuously updated. In adaptive control, the parameters are changed according to a sensitive indicator of process dynamics. This might be an independently measured variable and, in a first approach, the controller parameters are tuned according to a linear

Table 10.1 Selection of useful PID controller parameters[a] according to Ziegler and Nicols

Desired control mode	K_P	τ_I	τ_D
P	$0.5K_{Pcrit}$	—	
PI	$0.45K_{Pcrit}$	$0.85t_{crit}$	
PID	$0.6K_{Pcrit}$	$0.5t_{crit}$	$0.125t_{crit}$

[a] This procedure is based on practical experience and requires several simple (but permissive!) experiments in which the process is under closed-loop pure proportional control, i.e. with the integral and the differential parts of the controller switched off, such that the controller gain is systematically increased until the process becomes inherently unstable, i.e. the control variable starts to oscillate. The needed parameter values are calculated from the critical gain value and the oscillation period.

relation to the indicator signal. Experience tells us, for example, that the oxygen uptake rate reflects process dynamics quite well. Its value can be simply determined and used to update the parameters of a controller of the specific growth rate continuously by increasing K_P and decreasing τ_I as well as τ_D proportionally. Usually, this leads to significant improvement of controller performance over a longer period or even the entire duration of a bioprocess.

If such a simple black-box approach does not succeed, one needs to employ models. In model predictive control, the model is used to predict the value(s) of the variable(s) to be controlled. Based on this prediction, one can simulate the reaction of the process to an intended change of the manipulated variable. From a variety of changes, the controller picks the best and makes the change accordingly. It is sufficient to make the predictions for a limited time interval ahead, the so-called time horizon, which is updated continuously.

10.6 | Conclusions

Progress in process biotechnology is problem driven. Ever-green problems are to design new bioprocesses in minimal time, to optimise existing processes with maximal efficiency and to operate validated bioprocesses reproducibly with constant high quality. Necessary information is made available by measurement and monitoring, but this is not sufficient. Success requires a sufficiently deep understanding of biological and engineering principles and of all the relevant cause–effect chains. Much of this knowledge can be derived on theoretical grounds, but much is based on practical experience. This expert entity needs to be mapped into clever and safe actions that force the processes to run in the desired way. Modelling and control are most important tools in achieving this goal.

10.7 | Further reading

BellonMaurel, W., Orliac, O. and Christen, P. Sensors and measurements in solid state fermentation: a review. *Process Biochemistry* **38**: 881–896, 2003.

Buziol, S., Bashir, I., Baumeister, A., *et al.* New bioreactor-coupled rapid stopped-flow sampling technique for measurements of metabolite dynamics on a subsecond time scale. *Biotechnology and Bioengineering* **80**: 632–636, 2002.

Feyo de Azevedo, S., Oliveira, R. and Sonnleitner, B. New methodologies for multiphase bioreactors. 3: Data acquisition, modelling and control. In *Multiphase Bioreactor Design*, eds. J. Cabral, M. Mota and H. Tramper. London: Taylor & Francis, pp. 53–84, 2001.

Harms, P., Kostov, Y. and Rao, G. Bioprocess monitoring. *Current Opinion in Biotechnology* **13**: 124–127, 2002.

Komives, C. and Parker, R. S. Bioreactor state estimation and control. *Current Opinion in Biotechnology* **14**: 468–474, 2003.

Lennox, B., Montague, G. A., Hiden, H. G., Kornfeld, G., Goulding, P. R. Process monitoring of an industrial fed-batch fermentation. *Biotechnology and Bioengineering* **74**: 125–135, 2001.

McGovern, A. C., Broadhurst, D., Taylor, J., *et al.* Monitoring of complex industrial bioprocesses for metabolite concentrations using modern spectroscopies and machine learning: Application to gibberellic acid production. *Biotechnology and Bioengineering* **78**: 527–538, 2002.

Schaefer, U., Boos, W., Takors, R., WeusterBotz D. Automated sampling device for monitoring intracellular metabolite dynamics. *Analytical Biochemistry* **270**: 88–96, 1999.

Schügerl, K. Progress in monitoring, modeling and control of bioprocesses during the last 20 years. *Journal of Biotechnology* **85**: 149–173, 2001.

Sonnleitner, B. (ed.) *Bioanalysis and Biosensors for Bioprocess Monitoring. Advances in Biochemical Engineering/Biotechnology*, vol. 66. Berlin: Springer-Verlag, 2000.

Ulber, R., Faurie, R., Sosnitza, P., *et al.* Monitoring and control of industrial downstream processing of sugar beet molasses. *Journal of Chromatography A* **882**: 329–334, 2000.

Chapter 11

Process economics

Bjørn Kristiansen

EU Biotech Consulting, Norway

11.1 | Introduction

This chapter relates to process economics from a processing point of view. It concerns the input *from* the engineering department *to* the whole package necessary for the process engineer to ensure a profitable operation. The starting point for the chapter is as follows: how much will it cost to produce x tonnes per year of a product you have nurtured through to successful pilot scale operation and how much money is it possible to make should the process be scaled-up to industrial operation? This may sound a tall order, but it isn't. You will find that it is remarkably simple to obtain a reasonable estimate of the economic feasibility of your, and any other, process, once you know which tools to use. And what processes are we talking about? Interestingly, the process itself is not that important. To illustrate the economics behind a process, we could have picked any. So if the chapter does not deal with a process you do not recognise immediately, please do not despair. We are dealing with principles, and economic principles are not process specific.

Basic Biotechnology, third edition, eds. Colin Ratledge and Bjørn Kristiansen.
Published by Cambridge University Press. © Cambridge University Press 2006.

Let us take a product we can all relate to. Gemferlin is a health-care product. It is used in the treatment of obesity. What it does and what sort of compound it is, is none of our concern. For us, it is sufficient to know that our laboratory people have demonstrated it can be produced safely and the relevant approval documents are all in order. More important, the marketing people maintain that they can sell x tonnes of the product per year if the price is Y. The fact that Amtrenger plc have produced Gemferlin for a number of years is something else that need not concern us unduly. Their patent has run out and we have developed a process which is a radical improvement to the inefficient Amstrenger process. What we should focus on is determining if we can produce the x tonnes at a production cost that will lead to a sale price of Y or less.

Naturally, we are interested beyond our given task of producing the figures which please our investors. Our investigations reveal that Gemferlin:

- has no known side effects;
- excess intake can be tolerated by the human body;
- can be flavoured;
- has an established market, but still rapidly growing;
- production (our) technology is superior;
- dissolves readily in polar and non-polar liquids.

So our objectives are:

(A) To design a plant for the production of Gemferlin.
(B) To estimate capital and operating costs for the plant.
(C) To work out if the production cost will lead to a competitive sale price.

11.1.1 Where to start?

Given a product and a desired annual production rate there are a multitude of questions that will hit you once you start to work on your objectives, such as:

- What raw materials are required?
- Where can you get them?
- What is the required size of process equipment utilities?
- Do you need a new plant or do you have access to an existing one?
- What will the capital investment be?
- What will the manufacturing cost be?
- What is the optimum batch size?
- Do you need regulatory approval?
- How much product should you produce?
- Are all the stages batch operated or can a number of them be continuous?
- Which process steps or resources constitute bottle-necks?
- What is the environmental impact of the process (i.e. amount and type of waste materials)?
- Can you get the staff?

None of these questions are mutually exclusive, thus you will have no choice but to produce answers to them all. However, the way to tackle them all is to take one question at a time. *The ultimate design criterion is this: how much Gemferlin are we going to produce?* Once this is known, we can start attending all the other, and additional, questions. The production level is given by market consideration, i.e. how much are you planning to sell? For the purposes of this chapter we will assume that the marketing department has come up with a figure of *252 kg of Gemferlin per annum*, based on scientific analysis of the market and intelligence work.

11.2 | Overall production process

Gemferlin is expressed by a modified strain of *Alternaria*, which is cultivated in a suitable medium to produce our product. Thereafter the biomass is removed and discarded. The process liquor containing the extracellular product is subsequently processed to isolate and purify the product. As indicated in Chapter 9, this is basically a matter of removing vast amounts of water to obtain a relatively small molecule at a low concentration. The flow diagram for the whole process is outlined in Fig. 11.1.

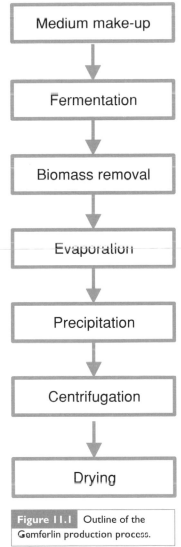

Figure 11.1   Outline of the Gemferlin production process.

Box 11.1

The flow diagram shown in Fig. 11.1 illustrates the processing that must be carried out and not the plant layout. Holding tanks will be required between the different stages to ensure efficient use of the equipment. For example, the production fermenter, which involves the longest stage, must be emptied as fast as possible to minimise turnaround time. Thus, the broth is pumped into a holding tank prior to the biomass removal stage. Also note that the processing units are chosen to illustrate the particular processing operation called for. Thus centrifugation may be replaced by filtration and several intermediate holding tanks and purification steps may be included to give a pure product. However, specialist companies that operate nearer the market end of a process often carry out final product purification.

11.3 | Fermentation steps

11.3.1   Sizing the fermenters

We will take it for granted that the process has been scaled-up successfully (*make sure that this assumption is correct when you come to do this in a real situation as biotechnology is tailor-made for scale-up problems*). The process uses a *synthetic medium*, thus we avoid the use of complex raw materials that may give us problems in the downstream processing and approval procedures. There is no need for especially pure water for the fermentation process: it is sufficient to use tap water. The amount of Gemferlin required is 252 kg per annum. Tests have

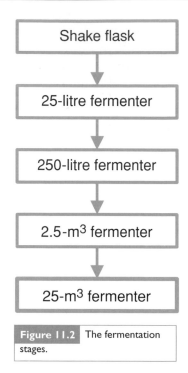

Figure 11.2 The fermentation stages.

shown that the concentration of Gemferlin at the end of a fermentation process is 0.3 kg m^{-3}. There will be product loss in separation and purification stages. If we assume a 10% loss (standard for the processes we are running), we need to produce around 280 kg per annum. Thus our total fermentation capacity will be 1244 m^3 assuming a 75% occupancy (i.e. the operating volume is 75% of the total reactor volume).

We know that reactor cost is proportional to (volume)$^{0.6-0.7}$, thus the larger the volume, the lower the unit production cost will be. However, if we choose a standard reactor volume of 250 m^3 it will run five times a year. Unless you fill it with other processes, the fermenter will be empty for most of the year, and that is expensive. Therefore, we will choose a fermentation volume that means the plant will be running for more than a couple of months. Thus we start by choosing a reactor volume of 25 m^3. It is a good size for cultivating *Alternaria*, both in terms of processing and costs. In addition, the plant will be large enough to take on other projects if we need, or want, to operate as a contract manufacturing organisation (CMO) facility. If we allow some oversizing for the downstream processing stages, we can increase the total capacity of the plant by installing new fermenters only.

Using an *inoculum size of 10%*, the fermentation train will have the steps shown in Fig. 11.2.

Box 11.2

Note that the fermentation stages do not have to use the traditional scale-up factor of 10. An alternative fermenter train could be:

Shake flask → 50-litre fermenter → 1-m^3 fermenter → 25-m^3 fermenter.

This could decrease both your capital costs and your running costs. However, for this scheme to work it is essential that you know the process extremely well, as many fermentation processes are susceptible to a low-inoculum level.

11.3.2 Fermentation time

The following general equation is often used to find the fermentation time (see Chapter 6):

$$\ln x_f/x_o = \mu t$$

where x_f is the final biomass concentration (kg m^{-3}), x_o is the initial biomass concentration (kg m^{-3}), μ is the specific growth rate (h^{-1}), and t is the fermentation time (h).

We know from the experiments in our pilot plant that the final biomass concentration will be 20 kg m^{-3} and as we are using a standard 10% inoculum the initial biomass level is 2 kg m^{-3}. The problem is to find a value for the specific growth rate. Strictly speaking, the above equation is only valid if the cells grow exponentially, something which is not the case for many large-scale fermentation processes

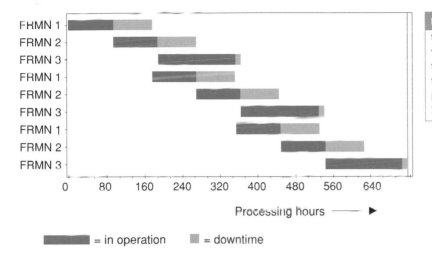

Figure 11.3 Scheduling of the fermenter shown in a Gantt chart, where FRMN 1 is the 250-litre fermenter, FRMN 2 is the 2.5-m^3 fermenter and FRMN 3 is the production fermenter. (The small 25-litre fermenter is not included).

lasting several days and especially not for filamentous fungi such as *Alternaria*. Although the academic exercise of finding the fermentation time is interesting, more often than not we rely on experience to determine the fermentation time. Our tests in the pilot plant have shown that it takes six days for the fermentation process to come to completion and we take that as the fermentation time in the reactor stages where we are producing a product. For the reactor stages where we only want biomass to grow, we may use a smaller number of days.

11.3.3 Scheduling

The product is made in the production vessel only; the smaller vessels are used to produce enough biomass to give a successful inoculum. In our case, the smaller fermenter runs for four days to reach the desired concentration of biomass before the reactor content is transferred to a larger vessel. Thus, the first three stages will each take four days, and the production stage will take six days, with one day turnaround. The scheduling of the fermenters, which ensures the most efficient use of the production vessel, is shown in Fig. 11.3.

Box 11.3

Figure 11.3 shows how to run the smaller fermenters to ensure that a new seed is ready for the production fermenter as soon as this is emptied and made clear from a previous run. It also shows the relatively large downtime for the smaller fermenters. Clearly, there is scope to redesign the plant in order to make more efficient use of the fermenters. This could involve using the smaller fermenter to feed more production vessels or reducing the number of seed stages, as suggested in Section 11.3.1.

11.3.4 Costs for fermentation processing units

Traditionally, costs of fermenters and other processing units were obtained using published indices. A cost index is a way of relating

Table 11.1	Fermenter volumes and purchase cost	
Unit	Volume (m^3)	Cost (1000 × €)
Air compressor		61
Medium make-up tank	10	65
Holding tank for sugar	150	51
Continuous steriliser		205
Seed I	250^a	60
Seed II	2	203
Production	25	687
Total		1332

^{a} Fermenter volume of *Seed I* measured in litres.

present cost to a cost in the past. For example, the chemical engineering plant cost indices for 1986 and 2001 are 318.4 and 394.3, respectively, and if you know that a fermenter costs US$500 000 in 1986, it would have cost 619 200 in 2001. Using cost indices from the literature, you can estimate present-day costs and you can extrapolate to present-day prices. Naturally, costs indices are only average figures, but they have been used successfully for a long time and will continue to do so. However, there are companies that specialise in processing equipment for biotechnological processes and it is much simpler to contact them directly. Once they are willing to suggest a price for the equipment you are after, you can compare their costs with figures available on the Internet and you will have a very good estimate. The fermenters we are going to use are of the stirred tank type. This is a relatively expensive fermenter, both in terms of capital and operating costs, but is probably best suited to the fermentation process we are running. The volumes and costs of different fermenters and associated equipment are given in Table 11.1.

Box 11.4

The prices given in Table 11.1 are ex-factory cost (= price you pay to get your unit out through the factory door) for vessel and agitator. Instrumentation and engineering are additional cost items. Also note that they refer to a basic fermenter with the lowest requirement for containment. If our strain of *Alternaria* had been genetically manipulated we would require a higher level of containment and the increased design specifications will make the processing units more expensive.

11.4 | Downstream processing steps

Holding tank. The fermenter content could go straight to the first stage in the downstream processing. However, we want to empty the production fermenter as quickly as possible to make it ready for the next run, as this fermenter stage is the processing stage that takes the longest time. The downstream processing stages are invariably faster, so we send the content of the fermenter directly to a holding tank. With a fermentation time of six days, it is sufficient for the holding tank to take the content of one production reactor. For faster fermentation processes, the holding tank may take several production reactor volumes.

Removal of biomass. The downstream processing starts by removing the biomass. In our case we have chosen to do this using a rotary vacuum filter (see Chapter 9). This is a well-established and proven technology and probably the method of choice for removing filamentous biomass.

Concentration of the filtrate. To obtain the product, which is a glycoprotein complex, out of the fermentation liquor, we precipitate it with a solvent. To avoid using large volumes of solvent we want to remove as much of the water as possible prior to the precipitation stage. As our product is not heat sensitive, we remove the water by evaporation.

Product precipitation. When the volume of the fermentation liquor has been reduced by 80–90% we add a solvent, which precipitates the product. We could also use salts, notably ammonium salts, for the precipitation

Removing the precipitate. After a short sedimentation time, we concentrate the product in a centrifuge. This results in a product slurry, which must be thoroughly washed.

Washing. The sludge containing the product is washed twice, once with the solvent used in the precipitation and once with water. This is carried out by adding solvent and water to the sludge and centrifuging the resulting solution containing the suspended product.

Drying. After the last wash the product paste is dried. In our case we have chosen a spray drier, but there are a multitude of driers that could be used, depending on the amount of water to be removed and the heat stability of the product.

Packaging. The product emerging from the drier is packed in a suitable container and is ready for shipping.

The downstream processing operation is outlined in Fig. 11.4.

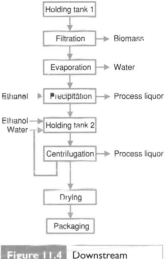

Figure 11.4 Downstream processing of the fermentation broth.

Box 11.5

Recovery of the solvent may be an important part of the process but is not included here. Also note that there will be alternative processing steps that can improve process efficiency and cost. Ultrafiltration is often used to recover proteins and the well-tried technology of rotary vacuum filtration may be replaced by a centrifugation step. In addition, it is also feasible to recover extracellular products, such as Gemferlin without removing the biomass in what is termed *whole broth recovery*. In this case we proceed directly from the holding tank to the extraction process.

11.4.1 Cost of downstream processing units

The cost of units for the downstream processing of the fungal fermentation broth is given in Table 11.2. All the units are conventional

Table 11.2	Purchase costs for downstream processing units
Unit	Ex-factory cost ($1000 \times €$)
Rotary vacuum filter	170
Evaporator	82
Holding tank 25 m^3	36
Holding tank 10 m^3	22
Centrifuges (2)	156
Dryer	64
Total	530

Table 11.3	Plant investment cost	
ITEM	Multiplication factor	Cost ($1000 \times €$)
Equipment purchase cost (EPC)		1862
Installation	$0.3 \times$ EPC	535
Piping	$0.5 \times$ EPC	892
Instrumentation	$0.3 \times$ EPC	535
Building work	$0.3 \times$ EPC	535
Yard improvement	$0.1 \times$ EPC	178
Land purchase	Assumed price	25
Fees, licences	$0.04 \times$ EPC	71
Planning	$0.25 \times$ EPC	446
Site management	$0.05 \times$ EPC	89
Start-up	$0.07 \times$ EPC	125
Contingencies	$0.4 \times$ EPC	714
Working capital	$0.3 \times$ EPC	535
Total fixed capital		6464

and must not be seen as optimal processing units for the downstream processing operations.

11.5 Capital costs

The plant layout is shown in Fig. 11.5.

Note that Fig. 11.5 is a layout of the processing operations. The washing and centrifugation steps can all be carried out in the same units by using similar volumes of solvent and wash water. However, when using centrifuges it is quite common to have a stand-by unit, so our plant will have two centrifuges. To estimate the total plant investment, it is common to relate this to the purchase costs for the main process units, which were shown in Sections 11.3.5 and 11.4.1. The calculations to obtain the capital investment required is shown in Table 11.3 below.

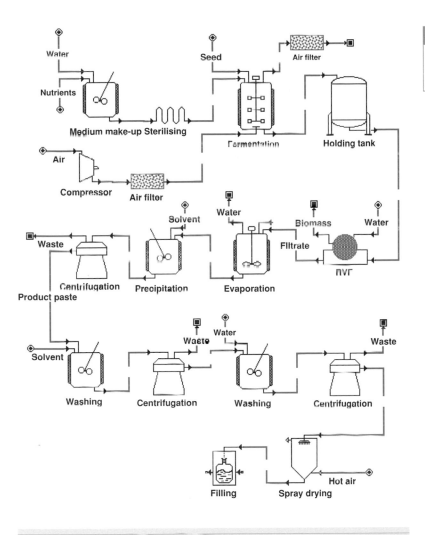

Figure 11.5 Processing steps for the fermentation plant (produced using Superpro Designer, Intelligen, Inc., USA, with permission).

Box 11.6

The cost estimates in Table 11.3 are very dependent on the value of the multiplication factors. Although presented in the table as a fixed value, the multiplication factors are within specific ranges. As with cost indices, these are based on actual figures and averaged out. The value to choose will be influenced by type and size of plant, and its location. For example, should the level of containment be very high, the multiplier for instrumentation could be as great as 0.8. Thus, when searching the literature for values for the multiplication factors it is important to bear in mind the aspects that influence the magnitude of the factors.

11.6 | Operating costs

The next step is to find out how much it will cost to run the plant. This includes the cost of all chemicals, use of steam, water and electricity, staff costs, insurance, maintenance, interest on the loan you took out to pay for the equipment, etc. It is possible to work out all the items individually and add up the total, but it is a mammoth task and is much simplified using process simulators. These are PC-based programs that will provide cost estimates. There are also ones that will help you design and run the plant (see Further reading section). In our case, we simply feed in the details of the plant we have designed to obtain reasonable estimates of materials consumption, staffing and associated costs. However, it is important to bear in mind that even the best process simulators are very dependent on the input you can provide.

11.6.1 Consumption of chemicals

It is often claimed that raw material costs, including substrate costs, contribute more to plant operating costs for biotechnological processes than for conventional chemical processes. However, it is more differentiated than that as the value of the product will play a part. For high-value therapeutic products, the raw materials will normally not be a significant part of the processing costs, whereas for low-value products, such as bulk enzymes or organic acids, plant economics are very dependent on keeping the costs of the raw materials down. Germferlin is a relatively high-value product and keeping substrate cost down is not essential, but is helpful to improve the profitability of the process. As for most fermentation processes, the carbon source will be the major cost substrate. At this stage we are using sucrose, but cheaper materials such as molasses and corn syrups are alternatives that must be considered. In addition to the demand for low-cost substrates, it must also be remembered that the substrate should not interfere with any of the post-fermentation stages. In our case, we have left this stage behind us, for tests in the pilot plant have come up with a medium composition that is cheap, has high bio-availability and supply is constant throughout the year. The only chemical required in addition to the substrates is the solvent used in precipitating the product. We use ethanol. The overall consumption of chemicals is given in Table 11.4. Note that the prices quoted in the table are bulk prices; they are far removed from the exorbitant prices paid for laboratory-grade materials.

Box 11.7

One good reason for going into detail with the medium cost is that for large-scale operation it is important to optimise the medium. While poor utilisation of ingredients may be tolerated in laboratory-scale operation, it is not so for large-scale processes. This is particularly true for the most expensive medium ingredient, which in our case is the sucrose. The table also shows that solvent recovery (see Section 11.4) should be considered as a part of a cost efficiency exercise.

We will now look at all the other items that contribute to the overall running costs.

Table 11.4 Medium composition and annual costs

Ingredient	Concentration (kg m^{-3})	Price kg^{-1} (€)	Annual cost (€)
Sucrose	50	0.8	35 640
$(NH)_2SO_4$	5	1.8	8 091
KH_2PO_4	2	4.11	7 324
$MgSO_4$	1	0.36	321
$FeSO_4$	5×10^{-3}	0.35	2
$ZnSO_4$	2×10^{-3}	1.23	1
$CuSO_4$	1×10^{-3}	1.44	1
Thiamine	10×10^{-3}	34.34	306
Ethanol		0.2	91 106
Total			142 790

11.6.2 Labour costs

Fermentation plants are run on a three 8-hour shifts and seven days per week basis. The labour costs are very scale dependent, but the extent of instrumentation and automation is so high in modern plants that the overall labour requirement is relatively low. To obtain labour costs it is essential that the location of the plant is known, as salaries are much influenced by geography. For our cost exercise, we have assumed a mid-European location and a social cost factor of 0.3 (national insurance, holiday pay, etc.), i.e. cost = salary × 1.3. Each shift will have a supervisor who costs 1.4 × shift worker.

11.6.3 Utilities

Electricity

Fermentation plant operations such as aeration, agitation, heating, cooling and pumping are all consumers of electricity: lots of it too! As a rule of thumb, a stirred tank fermenter requires an electrical input of 1 HP 100^{-1} gallons for the agitation with another 5 kW m^{-3} liquid for the aeration. With the production fermenters running for 168 hours per batch, the electricity bill will be high. The other main contributor to the large electricity bill is the evaporator; the remaining units are either low-energy demanding or run for too short a time to contribute much to the total.

Water

Water is traditionally considered a major cost factor because most types of plant and fermentation processes consume a lot of water. Therefore it would be beneficial to have your own well on site and have tuned the fermentation process to accept tap water (remember we have opted for a mid-European location) so that the water does not require specific purification processing.

Steam

High-pressure steam is used in the steriliser and the evaporator. For the continuous steriliser, we require about 2 kg of steam per

Table 11.5	Operating costs	
ITEM	Details	Cost (1000 × €)
Chemicals		143
Plant operators	Three shifts of three people	502
Electricity	€ 0.08 kW^{-1} h^{-1}	92
Chilled water	€ 35.00 per 10^6 kcal	21
Cooling water	€ 5.00 per 10^6 kcal	2
Steam	€ 10.00 per 10^6 kcal	8
Maintenance	10% of plant cost	646
Insurance	0.25% of plant cost	16
Water	For processing	20
Depreciation	Assume a flat rate of 10%	646
Local taxes	1% of plant cost	65
Administration	15% of operator cost	75
Cost of sales	2% of operating costs	47
Laboratory	15% of staff costs	75
Total		2358

sterilisation cycle. In general, steam is an essential utility as we need to operate aseptically, but is not a significant cost factor.

All the items to include in our calculations to obtain an estimate for the running costs are given in Table 11.5.

It can be seen from Table 11.5 that the capital dependent items, depreciation and maintenance, are the most expensive contributing factors, followed by labour costs and chemicals. As you now know what it will cost to reach the annual production target of 252 kg of Gemferlin, you have to convince your finance people that they can make a good business out of your process.

11.7 | The economic case for investment

To converse with our finance colleagues, we must have some economic parameters with which they can get an initial estimate of the profitability of our process. These are payback time, gross margin and return on investment, and are defined below:

$$\text{Payback time (years)} = \frac{\text{Total investment}}{\text{Net profit}}$$

$$\text{Gross margin (\%)} = \frac{\text{Gross profit}}{\text{Revenue}}$$

$$\text{Return on investment (ROI)} = \frac{\text{Net profit}}{\text{Total investment}}$$

To obtain the information on which to base the economics of your project we will use the internal rate of return method (IRR) for

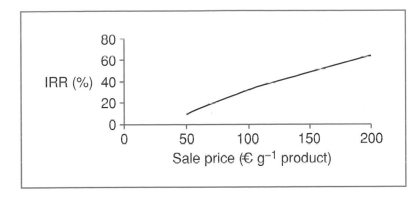

Figure 11.6 The influence of sale price on the internal rate of return.

the financial analysis, but we could equally well have used either of the other two. The IRR is the return a company would earn if they expanded or invested in themselves, rather than investing that money externally. It is the return of investment that results in a present value of the plant equal to the cost of the investment; the present value of all cash flow is zero at the discounted cash flow rate of return. Figure 11.6 shows the relationship between the sale price of our product and the resulting IRR.

From Figure 11.6 we will find that for the production process presented above, a sale price of €100 per gram of your product will give you a return of 32%. If we increase the sale price, the process will look more attractive on paper, but it may be very difficult to find customers who will accept the higher prices. In any case, for the type of process we have designed here, an IRR of 32% would be a very acceptable rate and chances are that you will be given the funding to start building your plant. However, before you start building, you will be asked if you can make the plant even more profitable. To find an answer to this you must carry out a cost sensitivity analysis.

Cost sensitivity
Is it possible to improve the process or can the magnitude of the individual cost factor be reduced? According to Table 11.5, the major cost contributing factors are:

- depreciation,
- maintenance,
- labour costs, and
- chemicals.

On paper, using an old plant that has been written off should reduce the depreciation factor, but your finance people will not always allow you to do that as there are other finance issues that may come into play. It is also very likely that the maintenance cost will be high in an old plant and any benefit will be lost.

Labour costs may be reduced if you consider another location, but you must bear in mind that you require highly skilled operators and moving to another location may not be feasible. Alternatively, you can hire production facilities from outside your company. Out-sourcing by way of contract manufacturing is becoming more accepted for production of high- to medium-value products. What is very likely is that you can reduce chemical costs. Solvent recovery as a means of reducing solvent costs has already been mentioned, as has the use of molasses and/or corn as a carbon source.

Price mark-up

Whilst you work out possible ways of improving your process there is something else you should be aware of. You are a producer and not a distributor of your product. Before it reaches the consumer your product has to be blended with a suitable inert ingredient and placed in an attractive packaging. As yours is a health-care industry product you can multiply your sale price by a factor of four to five to get the price the user has to pay. Will your average customer be willing to pay between €400 and €500 for your product? If not you will have a hard time trying to find a distributor who will take your product at €100 per g^{-1}. So you must settle for an IRR below 32%, in which case you have to work harder trying to convince your finance people to invest in your process.

11.8 | Conclusion

To estimate the process economics or the economic potential of any biotechnological process is relatively straightforward. There are many tools, such as process simulators, books and WWW publications that provide all the help you will need. The more specific details related to your process you can provide, the more relevant the estimate will be. What is also extremely important is that you must communicate with those concerned with other aspects such as process verification and approval, sales and marketing. Unless they have cleared your way, any figure you may come up with will have no relevance to the actual situation you dream of, namely seeing your product hit the market.

11.9 | Further reading

Peters, M. S. and Timmerhaus, K. D. *Plant Design and Economics for Chemical Engineers*, fourth edition. New York: McGraw-Hill, 1980. It may be beginning to show its age, but it is still a very valuable and informative textbook.

Reismann, H. B. *Economic Analysis of Fermentation Processes*. Boca Raton FL: CRC Press, 1988. Basic textbook with lots of practical information. The presentation is very dated but it is still a good read if you need help.

Kalk, J. P. and Langlykke, A. F. Cost estimates for biotechnology projects. In *Manual of Industrial Microbiology and Biotechnology*, eds. A. L. Demain and N. A. Soloman. Washington, DC: American Society for Microbiology, pp. 363–385, 1986. Another text that is still used extensively in spite of the years gone by since its publication

Petrides, D. Bioprocess design and economics. In *Bioseparation Science and Engineering*, eds. R. G. Harrison, P. W. Todd, S. R. Rudge and D. Petrides. Oxford: Oxford University Press, 2003. Good on production details, but you might be better off buying the intelligent simulation package if you can afford it.

PROCESS SIMULATION SOFTWARE

BioPro and SuperPro Designer. From Intelligen, Inc., USA, handles material and energy balances, equipment sizing and costing, economic evaluation, environmental impact assessment, process scheduling, and de-bottle-necking of batch and continuous processes.

Biotechnology Design Simulator (BDS). Developed by Life Sciences International (Philadelphia, PA) focuses on scheduling of batch operations and resource utilisation as a function of time.

Batches. From Batch Process Technologies (West Lafayette, IN) is a batch process simulator that has found applications in pharmaceutical, biochemical and food processing industries. It is especially useful for fitting a new process into an existing facility and analysing resource demand as a function of time.

Biokinetics. From Alfa Laval, modular designs that mainly focus on mammalian cell cultures. The modules are predominantly bioreactor modules, cell harvesting modules, purification modules and biodeactivation modules.

Part II

Practical applications

Chapter 12

High-throughput screening and process optimisation

Steven D. Doig
University College London, UK

Frank Baganz
University College London, UK

Gary J. Lye
University College London, UK

12.1 Introduction

The biological production of active compounds, ranging from small molecules, such as organic acids, vitamins or antibiotics, through to macromolecules, such as therapeutic proteins or plasmid gene therapy vectors, is of great commercial and social value. The cornerstone of any such bioprocess is the cell cultivation step where a highly selected, and usually engineered, cell-line is grown under carefully controlled conditions. The term *cell-line* is used here to represent both microbial and mammalian cells. The aim of the cultivation step is to yield the product in as an efficient and cost-effective manner as possible. However, the design and implementation of a cell cultivation process is often a complex, lengthy and costly task. The development of a cell cultivation process typically involves four stages, as shown in Fig. 12.1. *Stage 1* involves the initial identification of a native, or wild-type, cell-line that produces the compound of interest, though

Basic Biotechnology, third edition, eds. Colin Ratledge and Bjørn Kristiansen.
Published by Cambridge University Press. © Cambridge University Press 2006.

Figure 12.1 Schematic representation of a typical cell screening and cultivation development process. The dotted arrows represent possible iterative cycles arising from the process interactions between stages. Highlighted in the shaded boxes are the key inputs and factors to be considered at each stage.

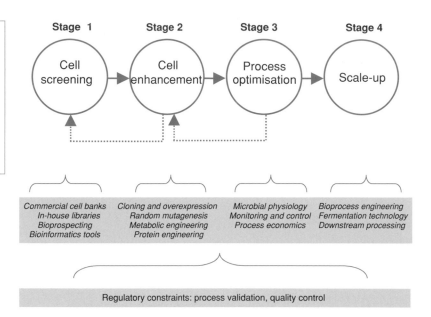

usually slowly and at low levels. This is followed by *Stage 2* in which the productivity of the chosen cell-line [g product (g cells)$^{-1}$ h^{-1}] is enhanced using a variety of microbiological and molecular biology techniques. *Stage 3* involves optimisation of the growth media composition and culture conditions; while in *Stage 4*, scale-up of the process from laboratory, through pilot plant to manufacturing scale occurs.

12.1.1 High-throughput experimentation

Traditionally cell culture development has been carried out following a sequential series of experiments, using conventional apparatus with a high labour requirement. Conventional experimentation usually involves carrying out one or only a few experiments at a time. Such experiments are usually monitored in detail and once the data collected are analysed, the knowledge gained leads to the next series of experiments. Although this approach at first appears entirely rational, it is clearly inadequate in circumstances where very large numbers of experiments are required. It is also apparent that these established methods are no longer adequate commercially since speed-to-market is critical in order to maximise the return on research investment for each new drug (see Chapters 11 and 13). As a consequence, the biotechnology industry has embraced a new approach termed *high-throughput experimentation*, or HTE, which implies parallel experimentation where automation and operation at smaller scales are combined in order to provide better quality information both quicker and more cheaply.

High-throughput approaches, regardless of the experimental goal, enable many variables, such as type of cell-line, carbon and nitrogen sources, nutrient concentrations, pH and temperature, to be examined simultaneously. This necessarily requires *parallelism*, i.e. that many experiments are carried out side-by-side rather than sequentially. Due to the experimental intensity, HTE is often performed using

Table 12.1 Some generic examples of the utility of HTE at each stage of the cell culture development process

Experimental objective	Comments	Examples
Identification of a wild-type cell-line displaying a novel enzyme activity	• In-house cell banks might range from tens to many thousands of cell-lines • Cell banks can be routinely tested for biocatalytic activity against novel intermediates in a synthetic pathway	• Lipases for production of chiral alcohols and acids • Oxidative and reductive whole cell biocatalysts • Enzymes capable of asymmetric C—C bond formation
Screening a cell library for enhanced metabolite production	• Traditional techniques, such as random mutation, produce many cell-lines with potential enhancements • Combinatorial biocatalysis/ metabolic engineering	• Higher antibiotic titres from fungal cell cultures • Improved yields of primary metabolites such as acids and alcohols
Enzyme evolution for improved specificity	• Using a variety of genetic techniques, enzyme activities can be modified and tested very quickly • Directed evolution generates thousands of cell-lines each expressing enzyme variants	• Enzymes with increased activity, altered specificity or broader pH and temperature optima
Optimisation of media composition and process conditions	• Media composition affects cell cultivation performance and process economics • Experimental designs can be used to optimise conditions with typically 10 to 100 experiments still being required	• Quantification of the best C and N sources and concentrations and their interaction • Testing and comparing complex growth media, e.g. corn steep liquor, protein hydrolysates, etc.
Determination of growth kinetics, yields and oxygen requirements	• Kinetic and yield parameters are crucial for scale-up • Well-defined conditions (oxygen and pH) required for control of optimal process	• Measurement of process kinetic parameters • Establishment of dissolved oxygen and pH set-points

laboratory robotic platforms that enable experiments to be automated so that the supervision of vast numbers of simultaneous experiments becomes manageable. Moreover, because of the large number of experiments it is possible to perform, the volume of each is ideally reduced in order to minimise development costs. Table 12.1 highlights some of the typical applications of high-throughput experimentation.

12.2 | Generic considerations for cell cultivation

There are several factors fundamental to successful cell-line cultivation that need to be considered regardless of the scale of operation or experimental throughput. Aseptic operation is considered essential for most applications. Also generally taken for granted is the need to control physical and engineering parameters regardless of whether the development process is carried out in a high-throughput or conventional way. Similarly, the type of output information, such as data on cell growth rates and product yields, on which process decisions are made, is the same regardless of the level of throughput.

12.2.1 Aseptic operation

Aseptic operation of a bioprocess implies that the cell-line of choice is cultured free from contamination by unwanted and opportunistic organisms. This is especially important when using engineered cell lines since they usually grow more slowly than wild-type strains. Such contamination results in, at best, a reduced yield of the desired product and at worst means that an experiment must be abandoned. For cell cultivations producing therapeutic products the growth of a monoculture is an absolute requirement.

12.2.2 Control of the physical and engineering environment

Efficient cell cultivation processes require the control of key physical parameters and bioreactor designs that can supply oxygen at adequate rates. Unfortunately the saturation concentration of oxygen in aqueous media is very low (typically 5 to 7 mg l^{-1}) and, therefore, an efficient and continual supply of oxygen, usually in the form of air, is paramount. Oxygen supply is key to the successful design and operation of a bioreactor, particularly at large scale. Under conditions of oxygen limitation many potentially detrimental phenomena can occur. It is therefore desirable that during the cell-line screening (Stage 1) and cell enhancement (Stage 2) stages of the development process an understanding of the dissolved oxygen level during cultivation is known. During the process optimisation (Stage 3) it is vital that it is measured and controlled as a basis for subsequent scale-up (Stage 4).

Other key physical parameters affecting cellular performance are pH and temperature. Optimal pH and temperature exist for each cell culture and thus these parameters must be measured and controlled in order to make a proper assessment of growth and product formation kinetics. Since most biological processes are neither very exothermic nor endothermic, control of temperature during cell screening and optimisation is not usually a problem, except at large scale (see Chapter 7). On the other hand, pH control can be challenging, particularly at small scales, and is very important during all stages of cell screening and cell cultivation optimisation.

12.2.3 Determination of cell growth and product formation parameters

Several parameters that quantitatively evaluate the performance of a cell-line have been defined earlier (see Chapters 3 and 6). Cell growth

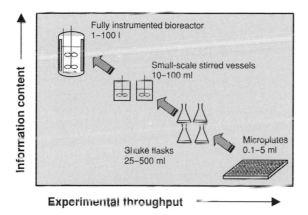

Figure 12.2 The relationship between experimental throughput, scale of operation and output information of various cell cultivation vessels (figure adapted from commercial literature by DasGip, www.dasgip.de).

kinetics, the yield of biomass on carbon, oxygen and nitrogen and specific product formation can be described using quantitative parameters and are the key output data from any cell-line screening and cultivation optimisation programmes. Normally they must be determined for many different cell-lines grown on many different media under various different environmental conditions. To illustrate the importance of a quantitative comparison it might be considered that selection of a cell-line with the highest yield of product per mass of cells is ideal. However, such a cell-line may be very slow growing, or grow inefficiently on the carbon or nitrogen source, and therefore it may not be the ideal choice. For example, a wild-type cell-line expressing a catabolic enzyme of interest for use in a bioconversion process may provide a high yield of product on biomass, but only grow slowly. However, a recombinant E. coli cell-line engineered to heterologously express the same enzyme may be much easier and quicker to grow, but give a lower specific yield. The choice of which of the two scenarios is better is very much down to the economic issues of the specific product and process, but the example shows that quantification of these biological parameters is essential in any high-throughput development process.

12.3 | High-throughput cell cultivation equipment

A variety of semi-specialised bioreactor designs are available for high-throughput cell cultivation. These can be categorised according to their scale of operation: (a) conventional bioreactors, (b) shake flasks and (c) microtiter plates. Figure 12.2 illustrates the scale and level of experimental throughput that is achievable for each design against the amount, accuracy and utility of the information that can be gathered on cell growth and product formation. As discussed below, and summarised in Table 12.2, there is a strong relationship between the level of experimental throughput and the amount of information that can be obtained.

Table 12.2 Overview and comparison of conventional and high-throughput equipment currently used for cell cultivation process development

Cell cultivation equipment	Typical experimental throughput	Level of monitoring and control	Cost of operation
Conventional stirred tank bioreactor: 1–100 l	Low: 1–5 per technician	High: pH, oxygen, T, biomass and product	High: capital, raw materials, labour
Miniaturised stirred bioreactor: 10–100 ml	Low/medium: 20 per technician	High: pH, oxygen, T, biomass and product	Medium: capital, labour
Shaken flask: 25–500 ml	Medium: 50 max. per technician	Low: T, biomass, product	Low
Microtiter plate: 0.1–5 ml per well	Very high: thousands per technician	Low: T, biomass, product	Medium: capital, increased use of disposables

12.3.1 Bioreactors

For operating with culture volumes above 1 litre, bioreactors, and in particular the *stirred tank bioreactor*, is the cultivation vessel of choice since it is relatively easy to instrument. It provides a well-defined environment for cell growth and it has long been accepted by the industry. More importantly, a lot of information about this type of reactor has been gained over years of use. The engineering environment is well defined and the output information from such equipment is directly applicable to scale-up as laboratory-scale stirred tanks are geometrically similar to pilot- and manufacturing-scale vessels. Moreover, since large sample volumes can be taken, the use of the most accurate analytical equipment is possible and the level of process knowledge obtained is unrivalled.

The main drawbacks with laboratory-scale stirred tank bioreactors are the low level of experimental throughput and the high level of raw materials requirement due to the volume of operation. Setting up a fully instrumented stirred tank bioreactor, including cleaning, preparation of media, sterilisation, calibration of probes and inoculation is also a time-consuming job requiring a highly skilled technician. Therefore, the number of experiments that can be performed simultaneously is typically limited to 1–5 per person. Media costs during the development process can be significant, especially for mammalian cell processes, and therefore the larger scale of these vessels can limit the number of experiments that can be performed.

To circumvent these limitations the use of *miniaturised stirred tanks* (typically 10 to 100 ml) is becoming increasingly popular. Miniaturised stirred tanks are quite literally scaled-down versions of conventional stirred tanks. They are normally geometrically similar to conventional vessels and offer the advantages of the well-defined environment and aseptic operation. However, since they are of smaller scale they offer the advantage of raw material savings and thus reduce process

Table 12.3 Advantages and disadvantages of shaken cultivation vessels compared to standard stirred bioreactors

Advantages	Disadvantages
Easy to operate	Lower oxygen mass transfer efficiency
Lower material requirement and capital investment	Less accessible to monitoring and control
Higher throughput	Scale-up criteria not well established
Lower labour requirement	Lower information content per experiment

development costs. Moreover, they are more amenable to parallelism as many more vessels, typically up to sixteen, can be operated at one time per technician. These vessels also offer relatively high oxygen mass transfer rates ($k_l a$ of up to 500 h^{-1}) due to the continued use of a rotating impeller for mixing.

Unfortunately, the conventional pH and oxygen electrodes commonly used with larger-scale stirred tank bioreactors, cannot be employed in miniaturised vessels. Therefore, specialist and often more expensive *alternative probes* are necessary. For example, oxygen- and/or pH-sensitive dyes, can be immobilised on the ends of fibre optic cables to make very small (1–2 mm diameter) probes. These dyes and their application to monitoring of small-scale cell cultivations are discussed further below.

12.3.2 Shake flasks

The ubiquitous conical *Erlenmeyer* flask has been used for cell-line cultivation for many years and is probably still the most commonly used cultivation vessel at the early stages of process development. Typically shake flasks are operated with between 25 and 500 ml working volume. Shaking confers both advantages and disadvantages when compared to conventional stirred tank vessels as summarised in Table 12.3. Mixing and oxygen mass transfer are both promoted by shaking. The rate of both processes is determined by the geometry of the flask, the fill volume and the intensity of shaking (frequency and amplitude of shaking). Typically a shaking frequency of 100–400 rpm is used and a shaking amplitude of between 1 and 5 cm is common. *Shaker-incubators* are widely available commercially and shake the vessel in either an orbital or reciprocal (linear) pattern. Orbital shaking is generally favoured as it reduces the amount of splashing and wall growth. Shaker-incubators are also available with humidity control, thus limiting water evaporation from the flasks.

Shake flasks are typically operated with a fill volume of 10–25%. In this way a surface area to volume ratio of between 100–500 m^2 m^{-3} is generated. This is important since oxygen mass transfer occurs solely via surface aeration in this type of vessel, resulting in cell cultivations in these devices being more susceptible to oxygen limitation than those in stirred tanks. In the commonly used orbital shaking motion, the liquid medium will move around the vessel as a wave and hence liquid phase mixing is not as efficient as in stirred vessels. A common approach to minimise this problem and to increase the oxygen mass transfer rate is to use flasks with *inserted baffles*. These baffles are usually made out of glass folded in from the wall of the flask. Their design is rarely well defined and significant variation in mixing, oxygen mass transfer and thus cell growth is apparent. Furthermore, splashing of the medium can occur and this can lead to exacerbated *wall growth*, an undesirable phenomenon, and wetting of the seal at the neck of the vessel. Such wetting usually blocks the passage of oxygen through the seal and therefore the use of baffled shake flasks comes with some risks.

In terms of their operation, shaken vessels are generally simpler to set up and operate than stirred tank bioreactors. However, due to their smaller size and mode of agitation they are more difficult to instrument. Therefore the level of information generated by these systems is not as high as with conventional stirred tanks. Although miniaturised dissolved oxygen and pH probes can be fitted in shake flasks, their use is troublesome due to the complexity of the mechanical attachment. Nevertheless, some commercial systems are available and pH control via automated additions of acid and/or base is becoming possible. However, this level of sophistication is not common and control of dissolved oxygen is still not possible.

A further problem is *sampling*. Due to the small volume, only small samples can be taken and therefore extensive analysis of cell growth and product formation is not feasible. Moreover, sampling of shaken flask cell cultivations requires that the sterile barrier is removed and this can result in problems of contamination. Alternatively, sacrificial flasks can be used for sampling, but this can cause problems with variability between different flasks.

12.3.3 Microtitre plates

Given the need for higher-throughput experimentation, microtitre plates are now being used routinely for cell-line cultivation. These vessels are also mixed by shaking and therefore in some ways are similar to shaken flasks. However, as shown in Fig. 12.3, their geometry is very different and they are produced with a standard footprint of 82 × 125 mm per plate. Plates are available with between 6 and 1536 wells per plate and individual cells can have either a circular, square or rectangular cross-section and can be of variable depth between 0.8 and 6 cm. Fill volumes vary from as low as 10 μl, for a single well in a 1536-well plate, up to 20 ml in a deep 6-well plate. Microtitre plates are fabricated in a range of materials including polystyrene, polypropylene and glass.

Seals are available for microtitre plates to help maintain aseptic operation and limit the rate of *evaporation*. The latter can be quite significant at elevated temperatures and over long cultivation periods

(a)

(b)

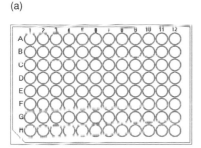

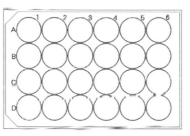

Figure 12.3 Typical microtitre plate geometries. (a) Plan view of a standard 96-well microtitre plate. Cross-sections show relative heights of standard shallow well and deep well formats. (b) Plan and cross-section of a 24-well microtitre plate. Dimensions of plates and well volumes are given in Section 12.3.3.

if not controlled. Commercially available seals are usually thin films of plastic and use either adhesive or thermal contacting in order to provide a barrier impervious to liquid at the surface of each well. However, these seals can limit the rate of oxygen mass transfer and therefore for rapidly growing cultures the wells are often left unsealed. Under such circumstances the cultivation is carried out in a microbiological safety cabinet both to limit the contamination risk as well as to reduce the exposure to the technician.

The mechanism of liquid phase mixing and oxygen mass transfer in microtitre plate cell cultivation is the same as for shake flasks. However, because of the smaller scale the intensity of shaking needs to be somewhat different: smaller amplitude (1–3 mm) and higher frequency is normal (500–1500 rpm). Oxygen mass transfer rates of between 100 and 200 h^{-1} are reported in a standard round 96-well microtitre plate operated with a working volume of around 200 μl. In order to increase oxygen transfer rates, the use of square wells has proven valuable since the corners of the well are thought to act like baffles and oxygen transfer values can be twice those observed in round wells, making oxygen transfer rates higher than those that can be achieved in shake flasks.

The primary advantage of the microtitre plate as a cell cultivation vessel is the potential for HTE and automation. The microtitre plate is available in a standard format and as such it is highly amenable to automation. Using a number of 96-well microtitre plates, it is quite realistic to carry out 500–1000 *simultaneous cell cultivations* with minimal manual intervention (discussed further in Section 12.3.4). The major drawback, however, is the difficulty of instrumentation compared to larger-scale systems (see Table 12.2). Therefore, per experiment, the quality and quantity of data are not as great as achieved in larger-scale cultivations. As the use of conventional dissolved oxygen and pH probes is not possible, alternative probes have been developed based on fluorescent dyes. An oxygen-sensitive fluorescent ruthenium dye can be used as a means of quantifying the dissolved oxygen concentration. This dye can either be coated onto the end of a fibre optic cable, or can be immobilised in an adhesive silicone patch fitted within each well of the plate. When excited by a light-emitting diode at a specific wavelength, the dye gives off a characteristic fluorescence that can be quantitatively related to the oxygen concentration. The dye does not consume oxygen and is highly responsive to changes in dissolved oxygen levels. The narrow diameter of the fibre optic probes (1–2 mm) means that they can be inserted into a variety of small-scale cultivation vessels. Similar developments are also available for pH measurement. In this way it is possible to measure on-line, the pH during the growth of a cell-line in a microtitre plate. Moreover, pH control via the automated addition of acid or base by a robotic arm is possible although with limitations on the number and frequency of additions that can be made.

For the parallel analysis of all the wells on a microtitre plate, *automated plate readers* can be used. These are spectrophotometric devices that are specifically designed to read the optical density, fluorescence or luminescence in individual wells of a microtitre plate. Typically these devices are programmed to read and record over a range of wavelengths (180–900 nm) in each well on a microtitre plate in a period of 15–30 seconds. These devices can be used to make measurements of cell growth via measurement of the optical density at 600–660 nm and therefore provide a relatively simple and efficient method for monitoring biomass growth. Dissolved oxygen and pH can also be measured using the fluorescent probes described above. However, for the majority of plate readers currently available, shaking must be stopped before the reading is carried out and this can have undesirable affects on the growing cell culture.

12.3.4 Automation and parallel operation

Automation implies the use of *robotics* and computer software to assist in the execution of the cell cultivation experiment by collecting and analysing a wide variety of data automatically. The use of automation with miniaturised small-scale stirred vessels allows the control and data logging of several experiments in parallel (up to 16 bioreactors at once) in a similar manner from a single computer. Microtiter plates are routinely handled in robotic systems due to their standard footprint and simple design. For example, automated microtitre plate experiments are the norm in high-throughput screening of drug candidates, where up to 250 000 different compounds can be evaluated per day. Liquid handling robots controlled by computers can easily deal with microtitre plates. In this case the laboratory robots can carry out far more than just data collection and

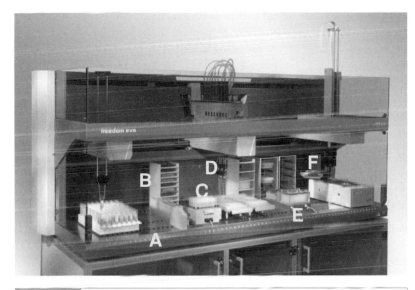

Figure 12.4 Photograph of a commercial robotic platform for performing high-throughput cell screening and optimisation experiments in microtitre plates. The items on the robotic deck (A) are mapped in the controlling software. The cultivation itself is performed on a heated plate shaker (C) and growth media, or culture broth, are dispensed using the liquid handling pipettes (D) into secondary microtitre plates housed in the *hotel* (B). Some preliminary cell harvesting stages can also be performed in microtitre plates and centrifuges and filtration devices (E) can be incorporated onto the platform. The microtitre plate grabber (F) is used to move plates around the deck and between the various unit operations and analytical devices. In this way it is possible to perform the entire cultivation process without human intervention whilst data collection is fully automated (image courtesy of Tecan UK Ltd).

analysis. In fact most of the steps in the cell cultivation process itself can be automated, including inoculation, preparation and dispensing of the growth medium to each well, shaking, measurement of biomass and dissolved oxygen concentration, and control of medium pH. It is also possible to integrate an automated primary cell recovery step, such as filtration or centrifugation, once growth has ceased. Such automation is not possible using conventional vessels and equipment. Neither stirred tanks nor shake flasks can be handled robotically due to their complex geometries and the lack of commercial platforms.

A robotic platform for use in microtitre plate-based cell screening and process optimisation should include the following key components: a deck providing space for location of equipment items at specific coordinates, an *XYZ* robotic arm incorporating pipette tips (typically 4–96 pipettes per arm) for accurate liquid handling, a second robotic arm for grabbing and moving plates around the deck, several pieces of robot friendly equipment (shakers, plate readers) and a computer to control and monitor the whole process. Figure 12.4 shows a photograph of a typical robotic platform.

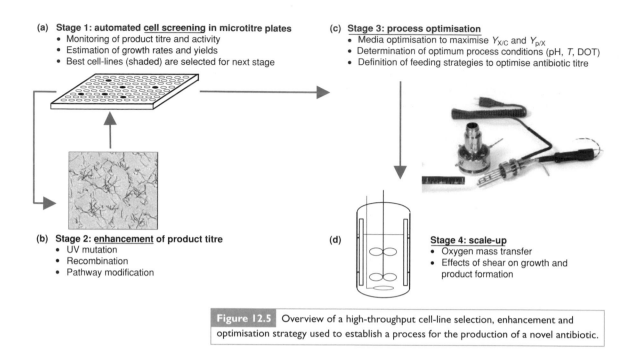

(a) Stage 1: automated <u>cell screening</u> in microtitre plates
- Monitoring of product titre and activity
- Estimation of growth rates and yields
- Best cell-lines (shaded) are selected for next stage

(b) Stage 2: <u>enhancement</u> of product titre
- UV mutation
- Recombination
- Pathway modification

(c) Stage 3: process optimisation
- Media optimisation to maximise $Y_{X/C}$ and $Y_{p/X}$
- Determination of optimum process conditions (pH, T, DOT)
- Definition of feeding strategies to optimise antibiotic titre

(d) Stage 4: scale-up
- Oxygen mass transfer
- Effects of shear on growth and product formation

Figure 12.5 Overview of a high-throughput cell-line selection, enhancement and optimisation strategy used to establish a process for the production of a novel antibiotic.

12.4 | The high-throughput development process

A typical high-throughput development process is discussed below within the context of the four stages shown in Figure 12.1: cell screening, cell enhancement, process optimisation and scale-up. To illustrate the development process an example of a novel antibiotic produced by a filamentous microorganism isolated from the natural environment will be used. Figure 12.5 gives an overview of the development process. Antibiotic synthesis is a function of several factors: genetic (expression levels of key enzymes), physiological (e.g. carbon fluxes) and environmental conditions (e.g. oxygen concentration). Each of these factors must be considered during the cell cultivation development process.

12.4.1 Cell-line screening

The aim of cell-line screening is to identify the best available native cell-line for the production of a given bioactive compound or enzyme. Cell-lines available for inclusion in these initial screens either come from *in-house cell libraries* or from commercial *culture collections*. In addition, specific databases, such as those detailing microbial metabolic pathways can be used to identify cell-lines that are capable of specific biochemical conversions or the synthesis of particular compounds. Alternatively entirely new cell-lines can often be identified by sampling and enrichment from the natural environment, a procedure often termed *bioprospecting*. Regardless of the origin, the number of cell-lines that might be included in an initial screen could range from tens to several thousands. These large numbers are one of the key challenges in this first stage of the development process. Equally important is the selection and employment of a suitable analytical tool. Although precise quantification of product formation is not essential at this stage, any analytical technique must be rapid and give a clear positive or negative response for each cell-line being evaluated.

In order to handle such large numbers in a high-throughput manner the fully automated microtitre plate approach is most usually employed for cell-line cultivation and evaluation. The lower level of output information (less quantitative and obtained in a less well-defined engineering environment) is not as critical at this stage of the development process.

Box 12.1 | Production of a novel antibiotic: Stage 1

A group of antibiotics with important antimicrobial activity are the polyketides, the best-known example is erythromycin. Most commercially available polyketide antibiotics are produced by *Streptomyces* sp. and related filamentous microbial cell-lines that occur naturally in the soil. During the first stage of the development process, a collection of wild-type cell-lines that may produce a polyketide antibiotic with the desired antimicrobial activity, is obtained. Each of these cell-lines is then cultured in a chemically defined media either on agar plates, or in liquid culture in microwells as shown in Fig. 12.5(a). Determination of the cell-lines producing the most potent antibiotic might be carried out using an agar diffusion test such as the Kirby–Bauer test where inhibition of the growth of a susceptible microorganism is measured.

12.4.2 Cell-line enhancement

Following the initial screening stage, a number of the most promising cell-lines are chosen to go forward to the next stage of the development process, cell-line enhancement. At this point a variety of molecular biology techniques (as described in Chapters 4 and 5) can be used specifically to enhance the performance of the native cell-lines, as shown in Fig. 12.5 (Stage 2). Several techniques can be applied including: *cloning and recombination*, *site directed mutagenesis*, *directed evolution* and *metabolic pathway engineering*. Alternatively, if little is known about the genetics of the most promising cell-lines, *random mutagenesis* may be employed by exposure to UV irradiation or chemical agents. The choice of the most appropriate technique is very much case specific. For example, a catabolic enzyme of potential use as an industrial biocatalyst can first be isolated from a wild-type cell-line identified in the screening stage, cloned and expressed in a more amenable host such as *E. coli*. The specific activity of the enzyme can then be enhanced by directed evolution. The number of cloned cell-lines that might be generated in such a process will normally be in the order of tens of thousands. Again, due to the large numbers of new cell-lines to be evaluated, microtitre plates are most often used.

Box 12.2 | Production of a novel antibiotic: Stage 2

The most promising cell-lines identified from the initial screen are next subjected to a range of techniques whereby the antibiotic titre is increased, as shown in Fig. 12.5 (Stage 2). This enhancement stage is almost always necessary since wild-type cell-lines usually grow slowly and have a low yield of antibiotic on biomass. Simple techniques such as UV mutagenesis are often used to improve antibiotic titres from *Streptomyces* and related species. However, more sophisticated approaches involving the identification and enhancement of key enzymes and fluxes involved in the biosynthetic pathway are also possible. Directed evolution has been used to improve specificities and metabolic engineering has also been used to model and optimise carbon fluxes from feed sources through to product. Furthermore, these techniques can be used to alter enzyme specificity and thus change the structure of the polyketide molecules synthesised in order to provide novel antibiotics that overcome the resistance mechanisms of the target bacteria.

Whatever techniques are employed, the number of modified cell-lines is again vast and therefore cultivation and testing of each is best carried out in microtitre plates handled using robotic platforms. Individual colonies growing on agar plates are robotically transferred to individual wells of a microtitre plate containing a liquid growth media and then incubated at 25–30 °C for five to seven days. A colony-picking robot uses a digital camera to create an image of the cell-line library on the agar plate and then a robotic arm *punches* out an individual colony and transfers it to the cultivation-ready microtitre plate. All stages of the cultivation are automated. Selection of the enhanced cell-line yielding the highest product concentration is carried out using either an integrated chromatographic assay or possibly an *in-situ* analysis technique such as near-infrared spectroscopy that can be used non-invasively. The best cell-lines are kept for further cycles of enhancement.

12.4.3 Process optimisation

Once a limited number of the most promising cell-lines have been identified, normally 5–10, the next stage is to optimise growth and product formation for each. The specific objectives of this stage of the development process include: (a) optimisation of the growth medium composition; (b) determination of growth and product formation kinetic parameters; and (c) establishment of a defined protocol for larger-scale operation, such as the optimum culture pH, temperature, dissolved oxygen level and specific nutrient feeding strategies. Precise quantification is essential so that sufficient information is available for rational scale-up. In conventional approaches these experiments would certainly be carried out in fully instrumented and well-defined bioreactors at scales between 1 and 20 litres. In the high-throughput approach, miniaturised stirred bioreactors operated in parallel are increasingly favoured.

For growth studies, the large number of carbon and nitrogen sources that can potentially be tested and the wide range of concentrations over which each might be considered, mean that the number of

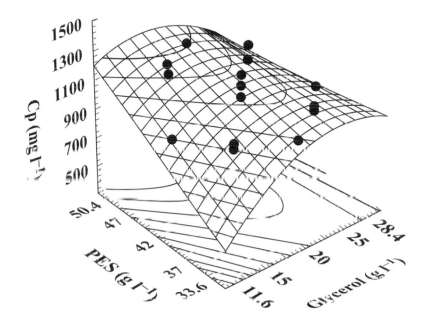

Figure 12.6 Use of experimental design in the optimisation of carbon and nitrogen source concentrations for antibiotic production by *Streptomyces clavuligerus*. Graph shows increase in antibiotic concentration (Cp) at various glycerol (carbon source) and soybean extract (PES, complex nitrogen source) concentrations. The curvature of the graph shows the strong interaction between carbon and nitrogen levels in the broth with regard to optimal antibiotic production (reproduced with permission from Gouveia, E. S., Baptista-Neto, A., Badino, Jr, A. C. and Hokka, C. O., 2001. Optimisation of medium composition for clavulanic acid production by *Streptomyces clavuligerus*. *Biotechnology Letters* **23**: 157–161.)

experiments is again potentially very large. Experimental design tools have been developed, for example, software packages based on statistical approaches that aim to minimise the number of experiments to be performed by allowing a number of factors to be varied simultaneously. Statistical treatment of the data within the software can help identify specific interactions between the factors being investigated that would normally be missed in traditional experiments where only one factor is varied at a time. An example of the interaction between carbon and nitrogen source concentrations for antibiotic production by *Streptomyces clavuligerus* is shown in Fig. 12.6.

12.4.4 Scale-up

Scale-up is an engineering methodology that involves transferring a cell cultivation process to successively larger scales of operation. It normally involves increasing the scale of the cultivation from laboratory or pilot plant (1–1000 litres) up to manufacturing scale, which can be up to several 100 m^3. This is not a procedure that can be tackled in a high-throughput manner, due to the large media and labour

> ### Box 12.3 | Production of a novel antibiotic: Stage 3
>
> Having identified and engineered a cell-line making a potentially interesting new antibiotic, 100-ml scale miniaturised stirred tanks are used to define and optimise the best conditions for growth as shown in Figure 12.5 (Stage 3). For the production of novel polyketide antibiotics, values for the specific growth rate and yield factors for the biomass and substrate must be determined using a range of growth media and individual operating conditions. Moreover, time profiles of growth and product formation are obtained and this is important because the two processes rarely occur simultaneously. The objectives are to select the best combination of carbon and nitrogen sources and the ideal feeding strategies. Complex carbon and nitrogen sources such as corn steep liquor and soya flour, respectively, are typically chosen as they are cheap and although growth rates are low, product yields are high. Protocols of carbon and nitrogen feeding during the antibiotic production phase are also determined at this stage of the development process.

costs associated with each experiment; however, it is an essential part of the development process.

12.5 | Summary

The time taken to develop and evaluate the economic viability of a cell cultivation process is essential to commercial success. During the period intervening the initial discovery of a novel bioactive compound (Stage 1) and the point at which the product is released onto the market (post Stage 4), a project is using valuable company resources, in terms of labour and materials, but is not yielding any revenue. It is therefore ideal that this period is as short as possible.

Clearly, to define a manufacturing process a large number of experiments are required in order to screen a wild-type library, select and optimise a single cell-line and design a robust large-scale cell cultivation process. Any approach that can shorten the time taken to perform these experiments reduces the commercial risk and enhances potential revenue. By using emerging high-throughput technologies during Stages 1, 2 and 3 of the cultivation development process the time taken to acquire sufficient process information can be considerably shortened and therefore the chances of commercial success greatly enhanced.

12.6 | Further reading

Buchs, J. Introduction to advantages and problems of shaken cultures. *Biochemical Engineering Journal* 7: 91–98, 2001.
Chartrain, M., Salmon, P. M., Robinson, D. K. and Buckland, B. C. Metabolic engineering and directed evolution for the production of pharmaceuticals. *Current Opinion in Biotechnology* 11: 209–214, 2000.

Devlin, J. P. *High Throughput Screening: the Discovery of Bioactive Substances*. New York: Marcel Dekker, 1997.

Hilton, M. D. Small-scale liquid cell cultivations. In *Manual of Industrial Microbiology and Biotechnology*, second edition, eds. A. L. Demain and J. E. Davies. Washington, DC: ASM Press, 1999.

Kumar, S., Wittmann, C. and Heinzle, E. Minibioreactors. *Biotechnology Letters* **26**: 1–10, 2004.

Lye, G. J., Ayazi-Shamlou, P., Baganz, F., Dalby, P. A. and Woodley, J. M. Accelerated design of bioconversion processes using automated microscale processing techniques. *Trends in Biotechnology* **21**: 29–37, 2003.

Chapter 13

The business of biotechnology

Jason Rushton
Merlin Biosciences Ltd, UK

Chris Evans
Merlin Biosciences Ltd, UK

13.1 | Introduction

Biotechnology is the exploitation of biological processes for industrial or other purposes. In this chapter we will discuss the biotechnology industry's development from its initial manifestation – the *biotech start-up company* through its maturation and development to yield integrated companies contributing products on a global scale – and what factors contribute to the success and failure of the entrepreneurial application of the science described elsewhere in this volume. This industry appeared in the 1970s, initially in the USA (an opportunity created by intellectual resource and inherent entrepreneurial spirit allied to a powerful capitalist environment) and soon afterwards in Europe and Asia as well. Our aim in this chapter is to give you a feel for what you need to have, and what you need to do, if you are to start up and successfully run a biotechnology company.

Basic Biotechnology, third edition, eds. Colin Ratledge and Bjørn Kristiansen.
Published by Cambridge University Press. © Cambridge University Press 2006.

13.2 | What is biotechnology used for?

As an introduction, we will review what companies are using biotechnology for, to see why some areas have been successful and others have failed.

13.2.1 The applications: medicine

The significant proportion of biotechnology investment has been directed to health-care, and specifically in the discovery of new drugs. Patents provide legal protection and mean that an effective new drug can be sold at high price for as long as the patent on it prevents someone else from making and selling it at a lower price. Once a drug comes *off patent* it can be manufactured as a *generic*, and sales and profit margins for the originator rapidly plummet. Patents do not last forever: usually it is 20 years, although in the USA the time is only 17 years. Therefore, if a drug takes 15 years to develop, a patent will only protect its manufacturer from competition for a further 5 years. This means that the original inventor of the drug must have invented a new one every five years (ideally more often), if they are to sell high-value, high-profit drugs. Thus discovery or invention of new drugs is critical to the commercial strategy of many big pharmaceutical companies. In fact, the drug *super-companies* formed by the mergers that created such companies as GlaxoSmithKlein and Astra Zeneca must launch several new drugs each year just to keep their competitive position and their shareholders happy.

The majority of this book is about the technologies of biotechnology, not about their application to drug discovery, so we will summarise here how the latter is done. The most commonly used approach is outlined in Fig. 13.1. A wide range of discovery techniques can identify a molecular target, including the disciplines of genomics, proteomics, X-ray crystallography and computational design. This *target* is a molecular entity whose activity is considered important in a disease. The discovery process is then run to generate or find a small molecule compound that will interfere with the effects of that target. The approach to this process is usually a combination of *bottom–up* investigation (where the target is dissected and profiled in detail followed by a chemistry design process) and a *top–down* approach (where the target details are initially less important and the activity is focused on screening large numbers of chemical molecules with the hope of finding a winner). The result of this process is a candidate drug, which, after much analysis and modification, is developed into the active ingredient of a medicine.

This process has a high failure rate: only around one in 13 drugs discovered and placed in pre-clinical trials will ever reach the launch stage. To add to the challenge the development cost has risen significantly in the last decade, driven by more rigorous regulatory requirements, complex disease states and higher attrition rates. A study by the Tufts Center for the Study of Drug Development put the

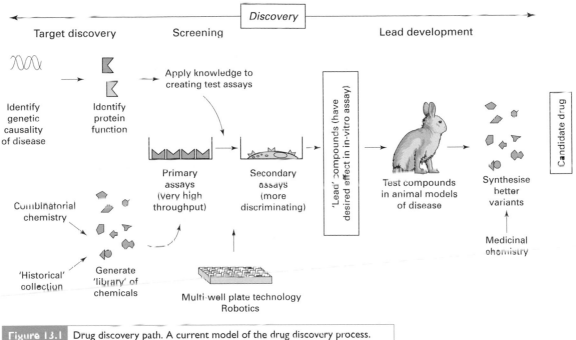

Figure 13.1 Drug discovery path. A current model of the drug discovery process. Process flows from left to right. The process starts with genomics-driven discovery of a *target* gene, and hence protein, and with the generation of a diverse set of chemicals from combinatorial libraries or from collections of chemicals accumulated during a company's history. The chemicals are assayed for their ability to block (or sometimes enhance) the target protein's action initially in a high-throughput, usually biochemical, assay, and then in more complex *secondary* assays, usually cellular function assays. The result is a screen *lead*. These are tested in whole animal disease models, and tested for pharmacological properties, and if necessary modified by directed medicinal chemistry to produce a candidate drug.

average drug development cost in 1987 at US$231m, the same study conducted in 2001 put this cost at US$802 million; even accounting for inflation this is a huge increase. Typical costs for drug discovery programmes are given in Table 13.1.

The risk return profile means that the pharmaceutical industry spends huge sums of money on research and development, which yield things that do not work. Unsurprisingly they are willing to pay significant sums to biotechnology companies that can provide science or technology that:

- enhances the understanding of disease (and hence lowers the inherent risk in the approach);
- increases the efficiency of the process in the discovery, development or clinical stages; and
- gives a competitive advantage in the above.

This is a continuum of activity from basic biomedical research to commercial drug development, and the drug discovery biotechnology industry occupies the middle of this space. Thus some companies

Table 13.1 Comparative numbers of biotechnology companies: numbers of biotechnology companies in different countries and their employment and R&D expenditure compared to the countries' populations

Country	Population (millions): mid 1990s average	Number of biotechnology companies (1998)	Total biotech employees (1998)	Total biotech R&D spend (million €)
USA	260.5	1274	140 000	8268
UK	57.9	245		
Germany	80.9	165		
France	57.6	141	39 000	1910
Sweden	8.7	85		
Rest of EU and Scandinavia	175.3	400		

Source: Ernst and Young's European Life Sciences 99, 6th Annual Report. London: Ernst and Young International, 1999.

are essentially applied extensions of academic groups, others are fully integrated and indistinguishable from small drug companies. In between are companies providing specific technological skills or services, such as genomics, combinatorial chemistry and molecular design technology. In addition, in the striving for higher success and reduced cost, some companies are seeking to alter radically the order in which these steps are undertaken, for example performing some aspects of the conventional development (Fig. 13.2) as part of discovery (Fig. 13.1).

Medical diagnostics are devices used to identify diseases and various patient conditions. These have a quite different dynamic in terms of their development and market. It is hard for an academic researcher to discover and develop a new drug; however, the process engaged to discover and develop a new diagnostic *marker* for the difference between sick and healthy people is more straightforward and in many cases less capital intensive. The main limitation on the commercialisation of diagnostics is making them reliable and simple enough to be used on a large scale and, ideally, to be performed by automated machinery, thus removing the need for skilled assay technicians. In addition, as the results from using diagnostics may be used in making important decisions they must still be approved by regulatory authorities and be of reproducible high quality. As a result, the diagnostics industry is dominated by a small number of companies with powerful marketing and distribution abilities, usually allied to their *platform* instrumentation, large automated instruments that can perform a wide range of tests, or to their particular brand identity. Small companies can only gain a foothold in this market by finding specialist niches.

Genomics-driven drug discovery may change this, with drugs being increasingly targeted according to diagnostic tests that have been developed for those drugs and sold together (an idea called the RxDx tandem). The diagnostic-drug combination of the future may take into account the particular patients genome, examine the genes

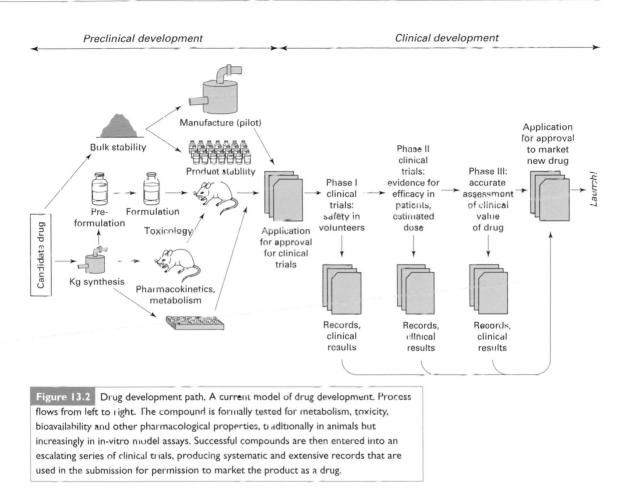

Figure 13.2 Drug development path. A current model of drug development. Process flows from left to right. The compound is formally tested for metabolism, toxicity, bioavailability and other pharmacological properties, traditionally in animals but increasingly in in-vitro model assays. Successful compounds are then entered into an escalating series of clinical trials, producing systematic and extensive records that are used in the submission for permission to market the product as a drug.

for a particular response profile and lead to adaptation of treatment accordingly. In the prevention of disease, diagnostics may indicate an enhanced risk of, for example, heart disease allowing lifestyle changes and drug treatments years before any symptoms could have been detected. The power of diagnostics also exposes ethical issues: if you were diagnosed as having an increased risk of heart disease or Alzheimer's disease years before any symptoms, should you be offered health and life insurance?

13.2.2 The applications: food and agriculture

Food and agriculture are more important economically than health-care, even in Western countries, and are clearly of much greater concern to the rest of the world. However, these areas have not attracted so many biotechnology companies. At root, this is because a new food cannot be sold at US$1000 a meal in the same way that a new drug can be sold at US$1000 a bottle. Food is price sensitive: the higher the price, the less you sell. Above a certain price, you sell none (price limited). So it is hard to justify expending very substantial amounts of money on developing new food materials because that money cannot be reclaimed in a premium price on the food. The main exception is in plant breeding, where the cost of generating a new strain of plant can be off-set both by sales of a very large amount of seed-stock and in the premium price the farmer can charge for the resulting produce, or in the savings he can make in growing the crop (using less fertiliser, less pesticides or herbicides). In principle, the cost of developing a transgenic crop plant that is resistant to pests (an exercise costing tens to hundreds of millions of dollars) can be recovered by charging extra for the seed: farmers would pay more for the seed because they would have to spend less on pesticides.

A similar economic argument makes animal reproduction technologies valuable, either in the generation of *transgenic* animals or, more recently, cloning them. The scientific and commercial value of such *cloning* explains some of the excitement over the 1997 announcement of the birth of *Dolly* the cloned sheep. Dolly was not a product in her own right but more a proof of concept demonstration of a technology that may yield products. Dolly died in February 2003 at the age of six from a common disease – sheep pulmonary adenomatosis (SPA), a lung tumour brought on by a virus but, although this was an early demise in sheep terms (they may live until 12 years or so), there was no evidence that her cloned status played a significant part in her early death.

Product-orientated biotechnology in agriculture has been most successful when it focuses on added value in the final product (rather than increased bulk). Typical of food and agricultural biotechnology programmes are the use of genetically engineered enzymes in food processing (added value can be the development of more attractive food flavours, for example), transgenic fruit and vegetables to prolong shelf-life (the FlavrSavr tomato was the first such product), and bacterial silage additives and nodule stimulants for legumes to increase productivity.

The creation of these so-called *Frankenstein foods* has generated much political and ethical debate and views on their utility and safety can vary widely between countries, governments and between people as a whole. Opinions on this subject run strong and even result in illegal activities where experimental or commercial crops are damaged in protest. It is still fair to say that whilst there are those that protest, many people across the world consider genetically engineered tomatoes delicious and the risk to health as nil!

Even so, the raw material cost in many consumer products is a small fraction of costs of packaging, transport, storage and selling: for example, in the *over-the-counter* pregnancy tests, the majority of the manufacturing cost lies not in the antibody reagents, but in the plastic casing. And this is itself a small fraction of the cost of storage and transport of the packaged tests. So the biotechnological product must add exceptional value to be worth developing.

Two other areas of biotechnology have had successful application in plant sciences. Both are applications of the *new* biotechnology to very extensive, established *old* industries. The first area is in the use of enzymes and, to a lesser extent, micro-organisms in food preparation.

The other is in horticulture, where micropropagation technologies have now become so widely accepted for developing new decorative plant types that they are mainstream horticultural practice. Gardeners will tolerate levels of pesticide use and *crop failure* greatly in excess of those allowed a farmer: their *crop* only has to look pretty. For crop plants these techniques have proven only occasionally successful in large-scale production, although they are part of the panoply of technologies used in plant breeding.

13.2.3 The applications: other industries

Many other industries could, in principle, benefit from biotechnology and may have already incorporated such technologies in their operations. The fabric and textiles industries are using biotechnology quite substantially, for example textiles and leather are treated with enzymes to improve their finish. Biological washing powders in the home employ enzymes (proteases and sometimes also lipases) that can then be used in low-temperature washes to achieve better results than with just ordinary detergents. The paper pulp industry is taking up biotechnology rapidly as a cleaner (and hence cheaper) alternative to chemical and mechanical processes. The plastics industry uses the polymers made by micro-organisms, although in practice materials such as the polyhydroxyalkanoates (such as polyhydroxybutyrate mixtures – *Biopol*) – see Chapter 16 – have gained only marginal industrial use.

Other biomaterials such as xanthan gums (see Chapter 16) are used in some specialised industrial applications, but this is rare, and opportunistic, and usually does not exploit our systematic knowledge of biological systems, but only our accidental knowledge of their properties and products. This is because the chemical industry bases most of its technology on using petroleum oils and gases, or products derived from these sources, and is consequently very cheap; the industry for converting these materials into a huge variety of products is flexible, efficient and sophisticated.

13.3 Biotechnology companies, their care and nurturing

The *biotechnology company* is a company that is set up specifically to turn the science of biotechnology into a commercial product and sell the result. It is the science base of the company that is defining. In the next section we will discuss what it takes to move a biotechnology company from that initial scientific idea to a flourishing commercial enterprise.

13.3.1 General rules

Successful biotechnology companies must combine scientific creativity and market need alongside the formal processes of the industrialisation of a technology.

Scientific creativity

The science in a new biotechnology company generally falls into *discovery* – you have discovered something wonderful – or *platform technology* – you can do something wonderful. In either case, first-rate science is needed to found a first-rate company. Good science is not necessarily *leading-edge* science. Research has *fashions* and, to an extent, the biotechnology industry follows the fashion because these areas of research or technologies are where senior researchers have chosen to work and where funding can be obtained. Emerging science and new methodologies, although exciting, are not necessarily the only means of progressing a research pathway, the old methodologies must also be employed, and tried and tested routes of discovery can still yield results.

Nor, unfortunately, does high-quality research necessarily mean science that is captivating for the bench scientist to perform. It must conform to what most people would recognise as scientific *good practice*. This is taking care that your experiments test your hypothesis rigorously and using all the data and knowledge available to put the results in context. The acid test for quality is often by peer review prior to publication in a journal as a paper.

Market need

Science on its own is not enough. We must sell it to someone – a *market*. But what is a *market need*? A general statement that, for example, *people want a cure for AIDS* is not useful. Which people? Who will pay for it? How? How much? Will your product cure all cases of AIDS or only some? Just as scientific creativity cannot occur in a vacuum, so market research must find out something specific. Biotechnology research and development is expensive, so it is important that a market for the intended product is big enough to give a return on all the investment needed.

Industrialisation

If success in biotechnology is defined as achieving a commercial return then a company must have a product that someone wants to purchase. As with the majority of goods that we buy day-to-day there must be an implied quality to the product. For example you assume that if you buy a new car, it will do the job correctly and you trust that the manufacturer, in the development of the vehicle, tested and modified the car to allow it to perform its job safely and well. Drug development is the stage between discovery and commercialisation that covers this testing and optimisation, combined with the manufacture of the product to high quality. This area is highly regulated by several authorities such as the Food and Drug Agency (FDA), European Medical Evaluation Agency (EMEA) and for devices achieving the Certificate of Excellence (CE) mark of quality. Even at the laboratory bench, scientists are expected to work to good laboratory practice (GLP) standards, which means that work is highly controlled and the recording of results is meticulously performed and laboratory books inspected, sometimes weekly.

Drug products must be shown to be non-toxic, effective and safe for use in people. The drug development stage is one which can consume significant time and money and also one that companies can find the most challenging to complete.

13.3.2 The basic components

The market is the commercial environment in which the company operates: it is not a component of the company. Science is a central, critical component, but it is not the only one. For the biotechnologist, it is important to remember that the scientist does not have to provide all of the other features that makes a successful biotechnology company. If the team initiating a biotechnology programme cannot see or provide the route through to the commercialisation of their technology, then they should team up with someone else who can. Whilst this may be achieved via partnering with another company it is also a role that seed venture companies can provide, as can *business angels* – individuals who can bring their own wealth and business experience to a company as joint investors and directors.

13.3.3 People

A new company's need for excellent, motivated people who have commitment as well as skill and knowledge is paramount. Who is going to be the entrepreneur who makes this company happen? It may be the founding scientists, but they are not going to do it in their spare time remaining from an academic job. It is not going to be the scientific advisory board, who are there to advise and support the scientists. It is not going to be the Board of Directors. It needs someone to jump with both feet into the science and business and make sure that things happen.

In Europe the cultural fear of failure has limited academics' inclination to make the leap, although the emergence of commercialisation teams within many British universities has provided a route and support structure to enable this to happen. To a limited extent, the USA supports entrepreneurship even at the cost of failure – it is seen as meritorious to have *had a go* and failed, because it proves motivation and drive, and the scientist who has tried and failed is unlikely to fail again in the same way, thus increasing the chances of success. In Europe, cultural conservatism means that failure is considered more significant than effort. People are therefore not willing to try for a major success if there is a significant risk of failure. This cultural barrier is disappearing slowly; the high media profile of successful scientific entrepreneurs is encouraging this cultural change and an increasing number of scientists are *having a go*. But, in our personal experience, many researchers who want to see their science commercialised also are unwilling to jump whole-heartedly into that enterprise themselves.

Although the central, driving entrepreneur is often a founding scientist with a *good idea*, it need not be. Packard Inc. were turned into a leader in the field of scientific analytical instrumentation by two business-school graduates who, at the start, knew almost no science at all. Against the background of failures and successes in Europe and the USA in the last ten years, experience shows that both business and scientific skills are essential for the success of a company, and that it is a rare scientist indeed who can combine both roles. As the biotechnology sector matures there are now a number of individuals with a *been there, done that* background – individuals who have learned from their mistakes, made significant successes and are hungry for more. The so-called serial entrepreneurs are the rare breed of science and commercial skill coupled with an insatiable desire to chase down even more achievement.

13.3.4 Attitudes and culture

This *jump-in-feet-first* approach from academia requires a major culture change. Academic science focuses on the subject, commercial science on the object. Academics typically address a topic or discipline, and follow it wherever it goes. The output of this intellectual endeavour is expressed in publications and it is the process and progress of research and knowledge that is important. Commercial science addresses a specific objective with a market and consumer in mind; it then uses any tools or disciplines that are appropriate in order to generate that product.

These apparently small differences in emphasis have major cultural effects. For example, there is little reward for an academic to be part of a multi-disciplinary team but it is essential for most commercial programmes. It is impossible for an academic scientist to be *redundant* as, by definition, what they do is what they are meant to be doing. (They may be incompetent or unfundable, but that is different.) Industrial scientists can most definitely be redundant in the sense that their science, no matter how excellent, is no longer needed to achieve the company's aims. This is made more acute by the need for a company to focus on a small number of products or projects, while it is worth an academic group having at least as many projects as it has Ph.D. students.

This is not the same as the choice between *blue sky* and *applied* research. Many companies carry out highly speculative research; indeed, much academic work in biomedicine is, in essence, applied.

Some academics believe that these differences make science, in a commercial context, less attractive to the career scientist. This view is flawed because the industrial/commercial environment can be an extraordinary place to do science for several reasons:

• the environment is intellectually stimulating and many of the world's top brains work in industry;
• the commercial pressures and multi-faceted challenges mean the environment is rapid and exciting;

- state-of-the-art equipment and materials can be in plentiful supply;
- there is a real opportunity for career development into any or all of the areas of science, technology or business the company is involved with;
- there is the chance of making substantial financial gains whilst still pursuing the interesting science

13.3.5 Strategy

Having found the people, and the great science, you must decide what you are going to do. This is your strategy: what you mean to do in the mid and longer term, beyond the exigencies of day-to-day research. The strategy of a company is, of course, specific to that company, but we can frame the things that the strategy should address as questions. Some key strategic questions for a small company start-up are:

- What is your company's specific aim?
- What is your first product going to be? This is absolutely essential. Out of the cornucopia that your science could create, you must choose one thing to start with and focus most of your energies on. This *focus* is critical for new science-driven companies with limited resources. This means hard choices and may mean dumping some *pet projects*.
- How do you deal with success? Success in a research programme usually means having to start a development programme that may lead to clinical trials. Do you have the skills or funds to do this? If not, how are you going to get them?
- What will you do next? After your initial research programme has concluded (with success or failure), do you have to make all the scientists redundant or do you have another programme for them to move on to? Remember that commercial science is focused on a particular product, not on a discipline or process. Whatever those scientists have to do, it must fit in with the overall aims of the company and the company's competitive advantage (see below). Define what the scientific advantage of the company is and where the advantage may be deployed and hence what the scientists are going to be doing.

13.3.6 Product versus service versus technology

A key aspect of your strategy is how your company is going to form and develop itself in order to make money. In the 1980s it was every biotechnology company's dream to become a FIPCO, a *fully integrated pharmaceutical company*, like Pfizer or Roche, performing numerous roles from basic discovery to shipping products to doctors. To achieve this aim for a small biotechnology company is in fact very unrealistic as it takes years and costs billions to build such infrastructure and the pitfalls along the way are numerous. Over time biotechnology companies have evolved their strategies to become partners to the larger pharmaceutical companies both in terms of providing a source of new products and as providers of allied technology and services.

The types of companies and their offerings are varied but can include the following.

- *Product company.* Your aim is to discover or invent products, take them as far through development as your funding allows, and then sell or license them to someone with experience in the later stages of development, clinical trials, manufacturing and distribution. Examples include all the larger *first wave* biotechnology companies such as Amgen, Celltech and Chiroscience.
- *Tools company.* You develop tools or technologies that help other people develop products. Examples of such *toolsets* include bioinformatics software, compound screening technology and combinatorial chemistry libraries. These are often also called *technology platform* companies.
- *Fee for service company.* You have a technology and/or a skilled technical personnel resource that are essentially available for hire on a contract research basis. This may include chemical synthesis, drug screening, biological testing and many aspects of pre-clinical and clinical development work.
- *Hybrid Company.* You have range of the above approaches giving a blend of near-term cash generating activities and coupled with more long-term research and development projects. Examples include companies that sell diagnostic devices and services while they pursue therapeutic drug research.

You should also be aware that your strategy will probably change. The most successful companies have evolved their strategy and the shape of their business significantly over time to make the best of success, reduce the impact of failure and to accommodate the ever-changing external environment. It is useful to have a good idea as to the approaches different companies can take and use this to establish the route by which you feel your business can achieve success.

13.3.7 Success

A strategy must be able to define *success* in a useful, meaningful way. Ask yourself what is your ultimate goal and work out if this is SMART, i.e. specific, measurable, achievable, realistic and time orientated. What are the significant steps along the way, and how will you show that you have passed them?

Success is typically defined as commercial in a capitalist economy. By different criteria, the biotechnology industry as a whole either has been very successful or a dismal failure. Only a small fraction of biotechnology companies have become profitable on the basis of sales of their products – seemingly the remainder would then be regarded as commercial failures; however, over 90% are still in existence as active, science-based companies and over 60% would have given their initial investors an internal rate of return (IRR, a measure of the financial success of the investment – see below) of over 10% – an overall investment success. For your start-up company, you may more easily define success and progress towards it in terms of achieving

milestones, e.g. by signing a major collaboration with a pharmaceutical company, by entering your first product into clinical trials or achieving the proof of concept with your development.

13.3.8 Competitive advantage

This is a trendy phrase from the management manuals of the 1980s that means that you can do something better than your competitors or is something that you can do and no-one else (or, more realistically, very few other people) can do. For the budding biotechnology entrepreneur ask 'What is it that, rather than merely being good at, you excel at and how can you exploit this to your commercial advantage?' *Excellence* is the watchword here and it may be classed in five areas.

You hold the patent on doing it. This is a powerful argument. Scientists should always patent an idea, process or invention that they think might be of some use to themselves or someone else. The patent prohibits anyone else from *practising* your patented invention without your agreement. It does not physically prevent anyone from copying your invention, but it makes it illegal to do so, and you can sue them if you have the time and money. Patents are crucial in the commercial world of biotechnology, venture capitalists are very nervous about investing in a company with weak or no patents and once your invention becomes publicly known there are a whole host of people who will set about copying it and trying to steal your idea and the potential financial rewards. An example is the patent on polymerase chain reaction (PCR) owned by Hoffman–La Roche to whom anyone in the world using PCR for commercial purposes must pay a licence fee or Roche will sue them.

You have the tools necessary to do it. This is as good as holding the patent in the short term, as it means that, while in theory someone else could copy your process or invention, in practice they cannot. Examples would be owning key cell-lines, gene clones or production equipment. This, however, is only a competitive advantage until your competitors can either duplicate your tools, or find a way around the need to use them; in time and with enough money and effort this is often possible.

You have the skills necessary to do it. This is a powerful competitive weapon until someone else learns how to do it. The skills base of this sort is sometimes called the company's *intellectual capital*. Early practitioners in the science of in-vitro fertilisation were in that position until the rest of the competition learnt the art and caught up.

You have a lot of resources or money to do it. This is a weaker form of competitive advantage in biotechnology because the industry is often a knowledge-based one and not a resources-based one; however, the advantages of scale can still apply. Many companies have lots of resources, especially major pharmaceutical or agricultural companies, and if your sole competitive advantage is that you have bought 20 DNA automatic synthesisers and lots of computers and technicians to run them then you will shortly be out-competed by another company which can afford 30 DNA synthesisers. Of course, if you don't know how to employ these resources effectively then the advantages of scale are eliminated.

You are the first to do it. This is the least attractive of all, but it is often where biotechnology companies start. They see an opportunity and set up a company to exploit it. Their advantage is that they can move faster than anyone else, but this only lasts while you keep moving and being the first is always difficult.

Other forms of competitive advantages include having efficient factories to compete on price and ease of supply or the development of a recognised *brand name*, however, these only come into full force when products are launched and the manufacturing and marketing teams take over.

The only way to show you have a competitive advantage and benchmark yourself against the competition is to demonstrate that what you want to do can actually work. In therapeutics discovery, this means proving that your material has some effect in people (remember that most drug discovery programmes fail). As it takes tens of millions of pounds to develop a product to the point of proving therapeutic efficacy, companies often have to accept a less-rigorous proof, such as a sound scientific reason, for supposing that it will work, evidence that it works in vitro, evidence that it works in animals, evidence that it is not actually harmful in humans (Phase I data). Each step along the path in Figs. 13.1 and 13.2 adds to the evidence and support for your competitive advantage.

13.3.9   Competitive intelligence

Part of proving that you have a competitive advantage is knowing how good you currently are compared to how good you have to be. This is competitive intelligence. Is there a medical need that you are going to satisfy and is someone else already filling that need? Is that need still going to be there in ten years' time? Who else is working to meet that need and are they ahead of you? This is a combination of finding out what the competition is doing, and what the market is. A surprising number of business proposals we have seen contain no evidence that their authors realise that the outside world exists, even less that it might contain competitors.

13.3.10   The business plan

Much of the above goes beyond *strategy* and into tactics. Tactical planning should be carried out by a team of people bringing scientific, product development, business and financial skills together, because all of these things are essential. The end-product of this planning process is a detailed roadmap of what your business is going to do – a business plan. But the business plan is a product of planning, not an end in itself. No matter how colourful or typographically creative it is, it is worthless if the planning behind it is not rigorous and the plan itself is not followed.

During the construction of a biotechnology company business plan, scientists must be aware that not only will bankers, accountants and the like be telling them what experiments they can and cannot do in the company, but that these people actually have a valid and useful viewpoint that can sharpen and focus a company's plan substantially. Typically, the stages that this process goes through are summarised below: we have considered several of them already.

- *Identify* the science that will go into the company, according to the criteria summarised above.
- *Define* what you are going to do with that science. This is the first part of the *business plan*, a document that should literally describe what the business plan does. It should include consideration of:
  - What can the science really do?
  - Who is going to do it, and where?
  - Who is going to manage them (i.e. make sure that everything happens)?
  - Are there bits the company cannot do, or it is not sensible to do, and if so who is going to do them, and how will you pay them?
  - Who will own the new intellectual property?
  - Who will manage the development programmes?
  - What are the key milestones?
- *Identify* the company's competitive advantage.
  - How will the company be funded, and specifically, how much money do you need to get started?
  - Where will you be when that runs out, and then who will give you some more?
  - Who do you sell your product to and, by implication, what is your product?
  - What happens if (when) it doesn't work?

The last point can be hard for some scientists to accept, but it is a statistical fact that most science on its way to commercialisation fails and you have to ask what happens to your company then. If it is a *one product company*, when the product fails, the company fails, and everyone is out of a job. So it is wise to look round for other technologies you can bring into the company. It is possible that, after a year, half of the brilliant science that led to forming the company has been abandoned! This should be viewed as evidence of growth and evolution, not failure, providing it has been replaced by something better.

The whole process boils down to identifying the shortest route between where you are and where you want to go (but not taking scientifically unjustified short-cuts), with suitable options for when all does not go to plan. This is why the strategy is important – you cannot define the shortest path to where you want to be until you know where that is. It also shows that in a company you cannot separate science from business issues.

The result of this process is a detailed plan of what the business will be doing, why it will survive and, preferably, flourish if given a

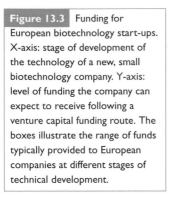

Figure 13.3 Funding for European biotechnology start-ups. X-axis: stage of development of the technology of a new, small biotechnology company. Y-axis: level of funding the company can expect to receive following a venture capital funding route. The boxes illustrate the range of funds typically provided to European companies at different stages of technical development.

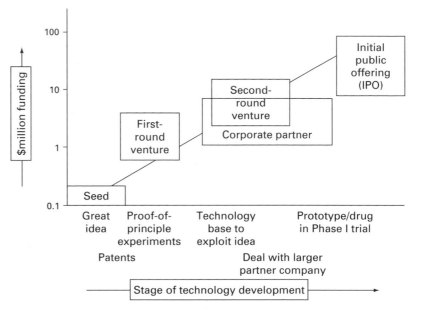

certain amount of money. In addition to being a working document for the planning and guidance of the company, the business plan also forms the basis of an investment proposal. In order to raise money to make all the plans happen, you take the plan to a funder and say 'I propose you invest in this company because it will do this with the money and we can make more money as a result'.

It is impossible for the business plan to be 100% accurate and, in fact, many elements will almost certainly be wrong. Unforeseen events, from scientific breakthroughs or failures to stock market crashes, will risk the derailment of your carefully laid plans. Unexpected challenges on the way should be expected, even embraced; but if you cannot plan a path for success, it's better that you don't try in the first place.

13.4 | Investment in biotechnology

Having defined what your company is to do, you need money to allow you to start. Very few biotechnology ideas can be realised in a way that requires no investment. Sometimes the investment is *only* a few tens of thousands of pounds to make the first material you can sell. More usually it will take tens or hundreds of millions. Very few individuals can afford such sums, so you must convince other people to invest money into you and your idea. These other people are the investors. There are several different types of investor and depending on the stage your company is at, they will fund you in stages. Figure 13.3 illustrates the stages on a typical company funding path. Understanding this path and the motivations of the people that you will meet along its way is important if you are to source investment for your biotechnology company.

Ideally an investor should not only be a source of funding. Certain investors will help you establish and run the business by contributing their time and experience in your support not only as board members but in day-to-day operational matters as well. This is a valuable resource particularly at the early stages when small teams have gaps in certain skills and are undoubtedly stretched as they try to manage several tasks at once. Such *hands on* investors can provide help with issues such as employment contracts, location/facilities, securing the intellectual property with university technology transfer officers, patent lawyers, hiring additional skilled staff from their networks and business development activities.

13.4.1   Seed investment

The first steps to developing an idea into a company (which includes all the processes we alluded to above) is to seek seed funding. Seed funding provides enough money to set the company up, acquire key patents, negotiate the graceful exit of the founding scientists from their current jobs and create a corporate entity. It also pays for planning and writing the business plan, a time-consuming and skill-intensive business involving hiring lawyers, patent agents and accountants. Such seed funding is provided by private investors (see below) or specialist, professional seed funding companies, which are still rare in Europe, although more common in the USA. There is a shortage of seed funding to take potential companies from *I have this great idea* to *this is a company you can believe in*. In part this is because the risks at this stage are huge and the rewards very uncertain. The so-called funding gap is one in which a company can raise enough capital to become established, yet has not achieved the size or demonstrated enough potential to attract the interest of larger venture capital institutions.

13.4.2   Private funding for biotechnology

Once you have a company established it will need substantial amounts of money to continue to pursue its product development goals. Start-up companies are usually funded privately through investment by private transactions between the company and individuals or groups of individuals. Typically, such investments are through the issue of new shares, so new investors become shareholders and all the previous shareholders are *diluted* (i.e. have their share in the company reduced). From a founder point of view owning fewer shares may seem a bad idea; however, it is better to hold fewer shares in a more valuable and viable business than a large slice of a company that is worth very little and about to go bust.

Once the company exists, it can work to attract more substantial funding to carry out its plans as articulated in its business plan. This *first round finance* (seed funding does not count as real investor money) comes from one of two sources.

Private investors

These are people with sufficient wealth to be able to put substantial amounts (usually at least US$250 000) into the company, take some active part in helping the company in financial or commercial terms and, most importantly, take the risk that they may lose their investment.

Venture capitalists (VCs)

These are people or companies who specialise in investing in risky propositions. They set up a fund into which people put their money and then the venture capital *fund managers* invest that capital in high-risk ventures. This is exactly analogous to the investment trusts and funds that are common savings routes for the general public, but with far higher risks and, the investors hope, far higher returns.

Both types of investor will want to evaluate your business against certain criteria, which include the people involved, their *due diligence* study on the science, the return on investment, exit route and whether anyone else is willing to fund the idea. This due diligence process can take some time (often months) and can be demanding on company and investor alike.

People

Most VC groups will invest in people as much as in science. In addition to the technical aspects, VCs look for teams that have the right skill sets (business and science), work well together and have demonstrable evidence that they can deliver on the investment promise. *Good* things in the characteristics of the scientific founders of a company are a demonstrated willingness to learn new expertise, collaborate with people from different disciplines, think laterally when challenged and remain focused on the business objectives of the company. A degree of commercial acumen and a desire to make a lot of money is also useful.

Often a VC will also look for additional externally sourced *management* to support the business, specifically a Chief Executive Officer (CEO). This person will have experience in running a science-based, commercial operation, will be accepted by the scientists as their company leader and is a credible person to put in front of bankers, accountants and other city professionals, vital as the company matures and seeks further funding.

Due diligence

After assuring themselves that the people are at least potentially suitable, the VC will carry out an external test of the science, by calling up experts, having any patents checked out by lawyers, asking around at meetings and conferences, and checking the perceived strength of the company's science, technology and people. This is known as *due diligence* (after a legal phrase meaning in essence *I have done whatever I can*). Due diligence can vary from a few chats in a bar to gain an informal impression to a full-scale consultancy project costing hundreds of thousands of pounds.

The due diligence process gives the VC an estimate for how reliable the current science is and what the market might be and the risks to be addressed along the way. Usually this due diligence view will differ materially from the scientists' view. It is also worthwhile for an entrepreneur to do *due diligence* on the VC to see what they have done for people in the past, in terms of help with management, guidance in business and scientific strategy, building the company up so it can cope with its own success and contacts in the world of finance. Ultimately, due diligence is about decision making and risk: an investor usually performs enough due diligence to get to the point where he can decide whether a particular investment opportunity (despite its inherent risks) is a worthwhile one to take or that all things considered the best thing would be not to invest.

Exit route

No-one putting money into a start-up biotechnology company expects to be paid back from the company's profits, at least for a minimum of five years, so there must be some other *exit route* by which they get their money back. This can be

- privately selling your share in the company to someone else;
- getting bought by another company (merger or acquisition being different versions of a similar process);
- floating on the stock exchange and so in effect selling your shares to the general public.

All of the above are possible for a company if they are successful with their research and products, so the question here is: 'when will it happen?' For investors the *when* is critical for calculation of the return on investment (ROI): a 100% gain in value in 1 year is 100% per annum ROI, a 200% gain in 4 years is a 50% ROI, even though the absolute amount of the latter is higher.

Funding stages

VCs invest when a company has already gained some seed funds, has developed its business plan and hired its core team. This is known as *first-round* or *first-stage* finance, and is typically between £0.5 million and £3 million. This is the riskiest end of venture capital. This money will typically take a company engaged in drug discovery and development through 1.5–3 years' work, and take the science from some basic research to a proof of principle. Then the company will need to raise more money, arranged in a second-round finance with companies that specialise in that stage of investment. Second-stage finance houses tend to lean more heavily on formal due diligence studies, look for an experienced management team in place, and look to the detailed timing of when they can float the company and so get their money back. Second-round funding usually raises between £8 million and £15 million. If all goes well, the company will then be floated

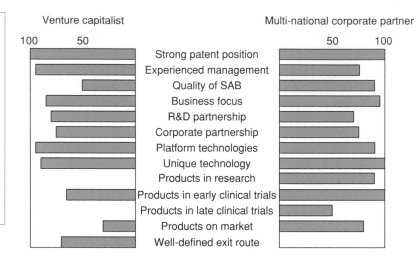

Figure 13.4 What they look for in biotechnology companies. Summary of Ernst and Young survey of the fraction of venture capital investors (left) and multi-national partner company licensing negotiators (right) who have stated that specific aspects of a biotechnology company are essential to consideration of funding or collaborating with them respectively. Length of bar is proportional to percentage who considered this aspect important.

on a stock exchange in another two or three years. This should raise £10–30 million. However it may need a *top-up* funding to get it there: this is termed Mezzanine financing.

13.4.3 Corporate partners

The other main source of funds for your new company is other companies, and usually much larger ones. These may be clients (i.e. who buy your products) but, in the early days, most biotechnology companies have no products, so larger companies may become partners with you in order to help you develop products in so-called co-development deals. They benefit because you have something that can help them innovate and they get access to new technologies and products early on. You benefit because they provide skills or infrastructure you do not have. Often corporate partners will also fund, organise and perform later-stage clinical trials (which can be hugely expensive and complicated) as well. In essence a corporate partner is a combination of collaborator and client. You get funds and resources, they get new programmes or products. There are a huge variety of corporate partnership arrangements, from simple purchase of goods to outright purchase of the company. However, the things that corporate partners will look for in your company are surprisingly similar to those a VC will look for, as illustrated in Fig. 13.4. Bear in mind that few companies have all of these: however, if your start-up has none of them, you will have some problems getting it funded.

13.4.4 Grants

Occasionally agencies that provide grants to academics to perform research will also provide grants to biotechnology companies. However, much more common is other types of government-grant support aimed at such small-to-medium-sized enterprises (SMEs). The biotechnology industry is knowledge-based, clean, rapidly growing, and based in the West's long investment in its scientific and technological infrastructure. Also, much of it is addressing health-care, probably the only sector of the economy to grow every decade in the twentieth century. So biotechnology is seen as good, both socially and economically, and is encouraged with various degrees of vigour by governments.

This has led to a profusion of types of government support for new biotechnology from which start-up companies can benefit. These include:

- *Technology transfer schemes.* These are schemes to help transfer science or technology from (usually) a university setting into a commercial one. Following US models, European technology transfer offices are now becoming better equipped and better skilled to find the most appropriate route for commercialisation.
- *Small company support schemes,* such as for example the SMART and SPUR schemes in the UK. These are generic schemes to help small companies get off the ground using direct government financial assistance. Similar schemes occur in many other countries including the USA and are available through specific government funding agencies. The conditions for obtaining one of these awards vary with the country concerned but in most cases no pay-back of the funding is required. (This will come later via indirect increased taxes to be paid by the company if it prospers and grows!)
- *Regional development support.* This is government support to try to encourage industry to settle in one region rather than another. Only occasionally are these places where the best science and scientists are already based.
- *National and international coordination efforts.* These are attempts to get the technology policy or regional support geographically integrated. There are some commercially based schemes, such as EUREKA, to encourage pan-European commercial developments.
- *Major infrastructure programmes* with biotechnology relevance. In both Europe and the USA the government supports major programmes of work which have biotechnology spin-offs, such as genome projects. These are usually *pre-competitive.*

Many government grants can provide very substantial sums for companies especially if they are in areas being targeted for economic development. In Europe, such areas would include places like Liverpool in the UK, or Sicily in Italy. However, it is generally true that if the company is dependent on grants to survive, then it was a bad economic idea from the start.

13.4.5 The stock market and biotechnology
More-established companies can raise money from the general public by selling shares on a stock market where suitably regulated brokers trade shares on behalf of their clients. Public funding in this way has very different constraints from private funding. It is very closely regulated to stop companies or brokers defrauding the public.

Shareholders have statutory rights that mean that they are the ultimate arbiters of the company's future, and many company brochures will talk about *increasing shareholder value* as recognition

Table 13.2 Typical[a] costs and success rates for drug discovery

Stage	Cost (US$, millions)	Time (years)	Success rate (%)
Target discovery	3.5	3	65
Screening	5	1	
Medicinal chemistry	7	1	60
Pre-clinical development	6	1	50
Phase I clinical trial	10	}	}
Phase II clinical trial	10	} 5	} 25
Phase III clinical trial	140	}	}
Total	180	10	4

[a] Column 1: stage in drug discovery and development process (see Figs. 13.1 and 13.2); Column 2: cost in US dollars; Column 3: time taken for this phase; Column 4: typical success rate for that stage of the process for a project.
Source: Figures compiled by Merlin from several pharmaceutical company sources, 1997–1999.

that these people actually own the company. In principle, shareholders can fire the board of directors (see below), or demand the company accounts for its actions; although in practice only major investment funds, which hold large blocks of shares, are in a position to exert any control over how the company is run.

In order to get a biotechnology company *listed* (i.e. have their name put on the list of shares available for trade), the company has to demonstrate that it is suitably stable. In the UK this means having a trading record for several years, or having at least two products in clinical trials, or a number of other criteria. It also means having a prospectus that has been verified by lawyers to say that every statement in it is demonstrably true, even down to the definition of chemical or medical terms. Part of this process requires an external group of experts to write a report on the company, which in essence says that they, experts in the field, agree that what the company says makes sense – this is known (unsurprisingly) as *the experts report*. Accounts have to be presented and audited, company directors have to sign legal forms that they are suitable people, and have to be checked out for past fraud offences and so on. This is all to protect the public from the worst excesses of entrepreneurship.

When and where you float your company is an arcane art. There are many different stock markets that can list a company (Table 13.2); listing in one market does not imply listing in any of the others as they all have slightly different rules and constituencies. Although their enthusiasm for biotechnology investments waxes and wanes, there can be substantial differences.

13.4.6 Valuing biotechnology companies

Public and private financing is by selling shares in your company. In essence, you sell a part of the company to someone in exchange for funds. But what are your shares worth? If someone is willing to give you £4 million, does this buy 5% of your company, or 95%? It depends on whether your company is worth £80 million or £4.2 million. Valuing your company appropriately is therefore important.

The details of how a value is placed on a company is beyond the scope of this article. In summary:

- There is no rational way of valuing a start-up company. You have some ideas, some patents, some people and no premises, products, established programmes or track record. The overwhelming objective factor is the chance that your crucial first product will fail, scientifically or commercially, and this probability is a matter of opinion. Values are dominated by *feel* and your credibility.
- When the company has been in business for 3–4 years, has 40 employees and two products in late development, we can *guesstimate* its value by working out what the company will be worth when it reaches its final goal and the chances it will make it there. Your goal may be to be bought out for US$550 million or to generate a stream of new drugs that you will sell to a big pharmaceutical company. This gives you a final figure and a guess for how long it will take to get there. You then multiply this by the probability of achieving it, divide this by the expected return that you could have earned investing the same money in a *safe* investment over the same time, and that is the value of the company.
- If you are a public company, your value is the number of outstanding shares multiplied by whatever people will pay for them. This can lead to your company suddenly losing value because the share price drops and is the reason that reporters say that falls in the stock market have *wiped billions off the value of industry*.

13.5 | Who needs management?

Management is a word that has come up several times above. Why are investors so keen on management?

The scale of operations of a company is larger than in a research group. A drug discovery and development company can expect to grow to 30–50 people in 18 months, possibly to over 100 people in three years, all working on essentially the same product or related groups of products. This cannot happen by chance – it must be organised. It must also be focused on a very specific goal. Company funding is based on success, not on activity. If a line of research is not working someone has to make the hard decisions about what to do about it including, in extremis, firing the scientists involved.

This needs professional management – people who know how to organise and run a scientific programme with such defined goals. Sometimes the scientists can grow into this role. Sometimes they can accept it from an outsider recruited to the company specifically to manage it. But filling that role is an absolute condition of setting up a company, and companies without effective management almost always fail. Sometimes they take a long time and a lot of money before they fail, which is why investors look for good management as part of the company team: without it, there is a very high probability that their money will be wasted.

This imposition of management is sometimes resented by scientists used to academic freedom because they feel that they are *giving up control* of their science. This is a fallacy for three reasons.

- They are not giving up control of anything – before the company was founded there was nothing there to control. No-one was developing the product, hiring the scientists, performing the work.
- It is not *their* science. A successful company must be assembled from many scientific and technical strands, for reasons outlined above. They are a contributor, not a sole author.
- No one person is in control of a small company if it is to perform with the energy, flexibility and enthusiasm that will carry it to success. It must be a team, not a dictatorship.

13.5.1   Where is management?

Finding appropriate management is difficult. You need quite different sorts of people at different stages of a company. The senior management, and particularly the Chief Executive Officer (CEO), of a new start-up with ten employees must be able and willing to do everything, to do without formal reporting structures, and to know everything that goes on in the company. The manager of a public company of 400 employees must delegate nearly all of that and instead control a reporting and responsibility system that has several layers between him and the bench scientist. A company's management becomes more obvious, more structured and includes more people as the company grows.

As a company grows, the people who ran the company very well at one stage have to give way to ones who are competent to run it in the next. One of the skills of the entrepreneur who starts a small company is to know when their skills should be replaced by someone suited to run a more mature organisation.

Finding people who can perform these tasks, and particularly the many-sided and changing task of running a new start-up company, is hard. As in science, the only evidence that you can do it is a *track record* of having done it before. The CEO is particularly critical as he or she has overall responsibility for making the company work. CEOs for new biotechnology companies come from a variety of backgrounds, where their experience in management, in directing science and in relating to the needs and concerns of the board of a company fit them for the role. Academic research does not usually fit a scientist for such a role. Neither does being a management consultant (criticising how someone is performing is not the same as performing well yourself), nor does *experience* of business gained solely through an MBA (Masters of Business Administration) course.

Critical tests for a CEO of a new biotechnology start-up could be caricatured as:

- *The nature test*. Can they read *Nature* and understand what they are reading? This is critical, as the fundamental of the start-up is good science. (They probably will not have time to read *Nature*, but that is another problem.)
- *The light-bulb test*. Can they (and are they willing to) change the light-bulb if it blows, i.e. do anything practical needed to keep the company running. There may be no-one else around to fix it.
- *The cat-herder test*. Can they convince a group of disparate scientists that what the CEO wants them to do is more worthwhile in scientific terms than what the scientists thought they wanted to do? (He or she can threaten to fire them, but that will not capture the creativity and dedication of which the best scientists are capable.)
- *The deal test*. Can the CEO go out and make deals that will bring the company money in return for a small amount of its technology or products? Such deals are critical for funding, but also to show that someone else has faith in you.
- *The suit test*. Can the CEO put on a metaphorical (or literal) dark suit and convince investors that he or she is really on their side and that their investment is safe in his or her hands?

These general criteria apply to all the senior people in a small company. The *head of molecular biology* in a start-up may find themselves watching the pilot plant or presenting to an investment banker who does not know what DNA stands for; there are few well-defined job descriptions in such an environment. This is half the fun of it.

As well as people who run the company as a whole, your start-up will need more specialist management functions such as financial and personnel management. Initially these will be provided by someone outside the company, such as the venture capital company backing the company, or by the CEO in his *spare time*. As the company develops, a more specialised type of manager with less concern for science and more concern for management as a process and skill in its own right is needed. Scientists should note that these people are needed: they are not hired purely to make your life at the bench harder. Without them you might wake up one day and find that the company has run out of money.

This brings us into the realm of general management theory and practice, which this chapter will not discuss further. There are many books and courses on this available, some of them relevant to the unique environment of a small, science-based company.

13.5.2 Directors and others

In law, every company must have a Board of Directors. These people do exactly what their name implies: they direct the company so that its value to its shareholders is maximised. There are stringent laws about what company directors can and cannot do in general terms, and some financial scandals in major companies have involved directors abusing their position for their own gain.

The directors should add substantial value to the company, in terms of contacts, experience, advice and business acumen. Their role should emphatically not be just to rubber stamp what the CEO wants to do and for that reason it is considered bad practice for the Chairman of the Board to be the CEO. A venture capitalist looking to fund a company or a scientist looking to join it at a senior level will look at the Board to see whether they are there as window dressing or whether they will really help the company flourish.

Parallel to the Board, and often answering to it, most biotechnology companies have a Scientific Advisory Board (SAB). It should advise the CEO and directors on any technical aspect that the company needs guidance over and, specifically, provide perspective, contacts and advice on all areas of science that might be relevant to the company. For example, an agricultural genetics company might have an agrochemicals expert and a farmer among theirs.

13.6 | Patents and biotechnology

Patents are critical to a small company based on knowledge. If you make an invention and it is not patented, anyone with suitable resources is free to come along and copy it. For a small company, many of your competitors will have far greater resources than you do and so can simply take your ideas and use them themselves. For this reason, investors and professional management are very eager to protect your intellectual property (IP) with suitable legal walls and, ideally, with patents.

The process of patenting in the UK is beyond this article. In summary, the scientist, advised by someone who knows the language and law of patenting, has to submit (*file*) a description of the invention to the patent office. The office's own examiners then check that the patent fulfils the three critical criteria:

• *Novelty*. No-one has done it before, or even talked about it in a realistic way.
• *Utility*. It must be useful for something. This means that the gene you discovered is not patentable in its own right but must be related to a product.
• *Enablement*. You must describe how someone else could do it (whatever it is).

If it passes, then the patent is granted. The process takes a long time, and costs a lot of money. In a novel field like biotechnology there is also a lot of debate (much of it carried out in the law courts) about just what *an invention* is.

The critical part of the patent is the exact wording of the claims. The claims are a set of statements, usually at the end of the patent, which define exactly what it is you are patenting. If your claims are very *broad* (i.e. general), you can succeed in getting a patent on a number of potential applications of your idea, not only one. The wording here is critical. Thus *a nucleic acid* is broader than *DNA* or *a gene*; *a molecule* is broader than *an alcohol*, which is broader than *2-methylbutan-1-ol* and so on. Of course, if your claim is too broad then the patent office will not allow it because it will not be novel: use of 2-methylbutan-1-ol as a cure for cancer may be novel but use of *a molecule* certainly is not.

Your role in patenting is therefore to make sure that you have described your invention in terms of a final product – in the case of a gene sequence, maybe a diagnostic test for a genetic defect or a drug that blocks the action of that gene's protein product – and in terms that meet the criteria above. A good patent agent can be very helpful in this process and their help should be encouraged.

13.7 | Conclusion: jumping the fence

This chapter has not been about *entrepreneurship*. An entrepreneur is someone who can see a way to make all the things we describe above actually happen, and does it. The former needs knowledge, breadth of experience and contacts, but the latter is the most important, and really can be summed up in three words: *Just Do It*. Three words do not a chapter make, so we have focused on what an entrepreneur or business person should do to create a successful biotechnology business rather than the personal characteristics that make a scientist into an entrepreneur. But without the will to make it happen, none of this is relevant. This is why we have returned many times to the nature of the people involved rather than a formal process that will lead them gently and inevitably to success.

This is an extremely favourable time in history for new, fast-moving companies in high technology. Investors, regulators and governments all want to see your small company succeed. It is also a time of unprecedented technological change in the life sciences, and so the environment has never been better to build a life-science-based company. For all its commercial failings and public misconception, the biotechnology industry will continue to be as dynamic and exciting a business sector as any in the next decade. It is a superb environment for a scientist to enter, for good science, the potential of substantial reward and just plain fun.

13.8 | Further reading

Southon, M. and West, C. *The Beermat Entrepreneur: Turn your Good Idea into a Great Business.* Harlow: Pearson Education, 2002.

Robbins, C. *From Alchemy to IPO: The Business of Biotechnology.* New York: Perseus Publishing, 2001.

Ernst & Young. *Beyond Borders: A Global Perspective*, *2004 Biotechnology Report*. New York: Ernst & Young, 2004.

USEFUL WEBSITES

Association of the British Pharmaceutical Industry (ABPI), http://www.abpi.org.uk

Bioindustry Association, http://www.bioindustry.org/index.shtml

British Venture Capital Association, http://www.bvca.co.uk

The Pharmaceutical Research and Manufacturers of America (PhRMA), http://www.phrma.org

Chapter 14

Amino acids

L. Eggeling
Research Centre Jülich, Germany

W. Pfefferle
Degussa AG, Germany

H. Sahm
Research Centre Jülich, Germany

14.1 | Introduction

The story of amino acid production started in Japan in 1908 when the chemist, Dr K. Ikeda, was working on the flavouring components of kelp. The specific taste of the kelp preparations, kombu and katsuobushi, is traditionally very popular with the Japanese (Fig. 14.1). After acid hydrolysis and fractionation of kelp, Dr Ikeda discovered that one specific fraction he had isolated consisted of glutamic acid which, after neutralization with caustic soda, developed an entirely new delicious taste. This was the birth of the use of

Basic Biotechnology, third edition, eds. Colin Ratledge and Bjørn Kristiansen.
Published by Cambridge University Press. © Cambridge University Press 2006.

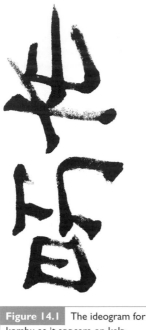

monosodium glutamate as a flavour-enhancing compound. The production of monosodium glutamate (MSG) was soon commercialised by the Ajinomoto Co. Ltd based on its isolation from vegetable proteins such as soy or wheat protein. However, with this process the waste fraction was high, and also the chemical synthesis of D,L-glutamate was of little use since the sodium salt of the D-isomer is tasteless.

The breakthrough in the production of MSG was the isolation of a specific bacterium by Dr S. Udaka and Dr S. Kinoshita at Kyowa Hakko Kogyo in 1957. They screened for amino-acid-excreting microorganisms and discovered that their isolate, No. 534, on a mineral salt medium excreted L-glutamate. It soon became apparent that the isolated organism needed biotin and that L-glutamate excretion was triggered by an insufficient biotin supply. A number of bacteria with similar properties were also isolated, which are today all known by the species name *Corynebacterium glutamicum* (Fig. 14.2). *Corynebacterium glutamicum* is a Gram-positive bacterium which can be isolated from soil. Together with genera like *Streptomyces*, *Propionibacterium* or *Arthrobacter*, it belongs to the actinomycetes sub-division of Gram-positive bacteria. The successful commercialisation of MSG production with this bacterium provided a big boost for amino acid production with *C. glutamicum* and later with other bacteria like *E. coli* as well. Nucleotide production also developed rapidly in the 1970s with *C. ammoniagenes*, which is closely related to *C. glutamicum*. The production mutants and the processes developed also resulted in a demand for sophisticated fermentation devices. Consequently, the development of amino acid technology was an incentive for the fermentation industry in general.

14.2 | Commercial uses of amino acids

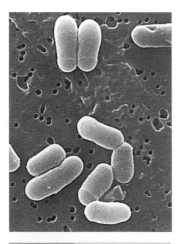

Figure 14.2 Electron micrograph of *Corynebacterium glutamicum* showing the typical V-shape of two cells as a consequence of cell division.

Amino acids are used for a variety of purposes. The food industry requires L-glutamate as a flavour enhancer, or glycine as a sweetener in juices, for instance (Table 14.1). The pharmaceutical industry requires the amino acids themselves in infusions – in particular the essential amino acids – or in special dietary foods. And last, but not least, a large market for amino acids is their use as feed additives. The reason is that typical animal feed, like soybean meal for pigs, is poor in some essential amino acids, like methionine and lysine. This is illustrated in Fig. 14.3 where the nutritive value of soybean meal is depicted by a barrel but the use of the total barrel is limited by the shortest stave, that is by the stave representing methionine. Amino acids are added therefore to increase the effectiveness of the feed. The addition of as little as 10 kg methionine per tonne of feed increases the protein quality of the feed just as effectively as adding 160 kg soybean meal or 56 kg fish meal. The first limiting amino acid in feed based on plant crops and oil seeds is usually L-methionine, followed by L-lysine, and then by L-threonine. Another important aspect of feed supplementation is that with a balanced amino acid content the manure from the animals contains less nitrogen (because more

Table 14.1 Amounts of amino acids being currently produced

Production scale (tonnes y^{-1})	Amino acid	Preferred production method	Main use
1200000	L-Glutamic acid	Fermentation	Flavour enhancer
600000	L-Lysine	Fermentation	Feed additive
550000	D,L-Methionine	Chemical synthesis	Feed additive
40000	L-Threonine	Fermentation	Feed additive
16000	Glycine	Chemical synthesis	Food additive, sweetener
14000	L-Aspartate	Enzymatic catalysis	Aspartame, polymer
13000	L-Phenylalanine	Fermentation	Aspartame
4500	L-Cysteine	Reduction of cystine, fermentation	Food additive, pharmaceutical
3500	L-Cystine	Extraction, fermentation	Cysteine, pharmaceutical
2000	L-Arginine	Fermentation, extraction	Pharmaceutical
1500	L-Alanine	Fermentation, extraction	Sweetener, building block
1200	L-Tryptophan	Fermentation	Feed, pharmaceutical
1200	L-Leucine	Fermentation, extraction	Pharmaceutical
1000	L-Valine	Fermentation, extraction	Pesticides, pharmaceutical
500	L-Isoleucine	Fermentation, extraction	Pharmaceutical

of the nitrogen in the improved feed has been used by the animal) thus reducing environmental pollution.

Over the past three decades, the demand for amino acids has increased dramatically. The market is growing steadily by about 5–10% per year. Thus, within ten years the total market has approximately doubled (Fig. 14.4). Some amino acids, such as L-lysine, which is required as a feed additive, display a particularly great increase. The world market for this amino acid has increased more than 20-fold in the past two decades. Other amino acids have appeared on the market such as L-threonine, L-aspartate and L-phenylalanine, the last two being required for the synthesis of the sweetener Aspartame. Estimates for current worldwide demand for the most relevant amino acids are given in Table 14.1. L-Glutamate continues to occupy the top position followed by L-lysine together with D,L-methionine, while the other amino acids trail behind at a considerable distance.

There is a close interaction between the prices of the amino acids and the dynamics of the market. More efficient fermentation technology can provide cheaper products and hence boost demand. This in turn will lead to production on a larger scale with a further reduction of costs. However, since the supply of some amino acids, e.g. L-lysine, as a feed additive is directly competitive with soybean meal (the natural L-lysine source) there are considerable fluctuations in the amino acid demand depending on the crop yields. The amino acids produced in the largest quantities are also the cheapest (Fig. 14.5). The low prices in turn dictate the location of the production plants. The main factors governing the location of production plants are the price of the carbon source and the local market. Large L-glutamate production plants are spread all over the world, with a significant presence

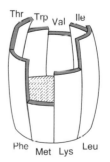

Figure 14.3 The barrel represents the nutritive value of soybean meal, which is first limited by its methionine content.

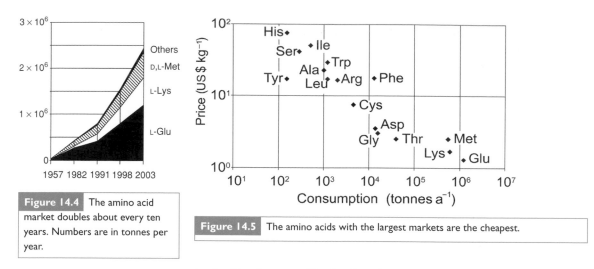

Figure 14.4 The amino acid market doubles about every ten years. Numbers are in tonnes per year.

Figure 14.5 The amino acids with the largest markets are the cheapest.

in the Far East, e.g. Thailand and Indonesia. For L-lysine the situation is different. Since one-third of the world market is in North America and there is convenient access to maize as a feedstock material for the fermentation process, about one-third of the L-lysine production capacity is located there. In almost all cases, the companies producing L-lysine are associated with the maize milling industry, either as producers, in joint ventures or as suppliers of cheap sugar. This illustrates the fact that the commercial production of amino acids is a vigorously growing and changing field with many global interactions.

14.3 | Production methods and tools

Some amino acids are chemically synthesised, such as glycine which has no stereochemical center, or D,L-methionine. This latter sulphur-containing amino acid can be added to feed as a racemic mixture, since animals contain a D-amino acid oxidase, which together with a transaminase activity converts D-methionine to the nutritively effective L-form. The classical procedure of amino acid isolation from acid hydrolysates of proteins is still in use for selected amino acids with a low market volume (Table 14.1). Other methods use precursor conversion with bacteria, or enzymatic synthesis. However, for L-amino acids required in large volume, fermentative production by engineered bacteria is the method of choice.

Classical strain development
Bacteria do not normally excrete amino acids in significant amounts because regulatory mechanisms control amino acid synthesis in an economical way so that the needs of the cell (for protein synthesis) are exactly matched by the synthetic processes. There are no surplus amino acids and only a small pool of them exists within the cell to meet its immediate needs. Therefore, mutants have to be generated that oversynthesise the respective amino acid. A great number of amino-acid-producing bacteria have been derived by mutagenesis and

Table 14.2 A genealogy of strains obtained by classical mutagenesis and screening, showing improved yield and some of the phenotypic characters of the mutants

Strain	Character	Yield of L-lysine (%)
AJ 1511	Wild type	0
AJ 3445	AEC^r	16
AJ 3424	AFC^r Ala$^-$	33
AJ 3796	AEC^r Ala$^-$ CCL^r	39
AJ 3990	AEC^r Ala$^-$ CCl^{r}ML^r	43
AJ 1204	AEC^r, Ala$^-$ CCL^{r}ML^r FP^s	50

AEC^r, resistant to S-(β-aminoethyl)-L-cysteine; Ala$^-$, L-alanine-requiring; CCL^r resistant to α-chlorocaprolactam; ML^r, resistant to γ-methyl-L-lysine; FP^s, sensitive to β-fluoropyruvate.

screening programmes. This has involved the consecutive application of:

- undirected mutagenesis,
- selection for a specific phenotype, and
- selection of the mutant with the best amino acid accumulation.

Taking the best resulting strain, the entire procedure was repeated in several additional rounds to increase the productivity each time and, eventually, resulted in an industrial producer (Table 14.2). Due to this iterative optimisation over decades, excellent high-performance strains are now available. However, due to the repeated mutagenesis steps, such producer strains might carry, in addition to the necessary mutations, also disadvantageous mutations influencing growth and reducing the speed of sugar conversion to amino acid. Speed is of course essential to reduce individual fermentation times and thus to increase the number of total fermentations per unit time to achieve most profitable use of the fermentation equipment.

Genomic techniques
To get rid of disadvantageous mutations, it is now common practice first to compare the genome sequence of the producer with that of the wild type and then to introduce those mutations by genetic engineering that are really necessary. This *re-building* ensures high productivity of the final mutant, together with high speed of sugar conversion, to give the simplest and most effective strain possible (see Fig. 14.6). Other genomic tools are *transcriptomics* using DNA microarray technology to characterize producers of different efficiency rapidly, or to qualify variations in fermentation processes, thus resulting in still further improvements and consolidations of the entire production processes.

Intracellular flux analysis
An entirely different approach in strain development is the reliable quantification of the carbon fluxes in the living cell. A great deal

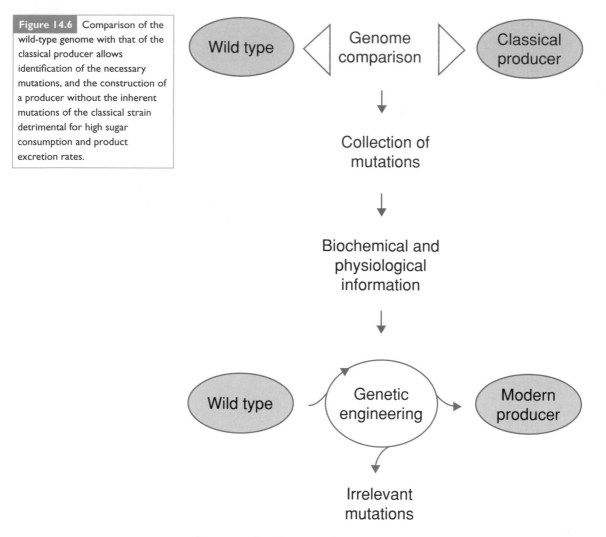

Figure 14.6 Comparison of the wild-type genome with that of the classical producer allows identification of the necessary mutations, and the construction of a producer without the inherent mutations of the classical strain detrimental for high sugar consumption and product excretion rates.

of progress has been made recently in developing to a high level of sophistication the old isotope labelling technique. In particular, with ^{13}C-NMR spectroscopy the intracellular fluxes can now be quantified with very high resolution. For instance, in *C. glutamicum* it has even been possible to quantify the back fluxes as present in the anaplerotic reactions. The method is described in detail in Chapter 2 of this book. Such flux quantifications are of major assistance in selecting the reactions in the central metabolism to be modified by genetic engineering.

14.4 ∣ L-Glutamate

14.4.1 Biochemistry

As already mentioned, L-glutamate was the first amino acid to be produced. Production invariably uses *C. glutamicum*. For its fuelling pathways, this bacterium uses the glycolysis, the pentose phosphate pathway, and the citric acid cycle to generate precursor metabolites and reduced pyridine nucleotides (Fig. 14.7).

This bacterium displays a special feature in the anaplerotic reactions, however. Since L-glutamate is directly derived from α-ketoglutarate, a high capability for replenishing the citric acid cycle is, of course, a pre-requisite for high-glutamate production. It was originally assumed that only the phospho*enol*pyruvate carboxylase (PEPC) was present as a carboxylating enzyme serving this purpose. However, molecular research, in close conjunction with ^{13}C-labelling studies, showed that an additional carboxylating reaction must be present. The pursuit of this enzyme activity resulted in the detection of pyruvate carboxylase activity, PyrC, and the identification of its gene. Therefore, *C. glutamicum* has the pyruvate dehydrogenase (PyrDH) shuffling acetylCoA into the citric acid cycle, and two enzymes supplying oxaloacetate: pyruvate carboxylase (PyrC) together with a phospho*enol*pyruvate carboxylase (PEPC; Fig. 14.7). Both carboxylases can basically replace each other to ensure conversion of carbon-three units to oxaloacetate. This is different from *E. coli*, which has exclusively the phospho*enol*pyruvate carboxylase serving this purpose, or *Bacillus subtilis*, where only the pyruvate carboxylase is present. Since it is in possession of both enzymes, *C. glutamicum* has an enormous flexibility for replenishing citric acid cycle intermediates upon their withdrawal.

The reductive amination of α-ketoglutarate to yield L-glutamate is catalysed by the glutamate dehydrogenase. The enzyme is a multimer, each sub-unit having a molecular weight of 49 100. It has a very high specific activity of 1.8 mmol min^{-1} (mg protein)$^{-1}$, and L-glutamate is present in the cell in a rather high concentration of about 150 mM. In the case of other amino acids, in contrast, the intracellular concentrations are usually below 10 mM. The high concentration serves to ensure the supply of L-glutamate directly required for cell synthesis and also for the supply of amino groups via transaminase reactions for a variety of cellular reactions. As much as 70% of the amino groups in cell material stems from L-glutamate.

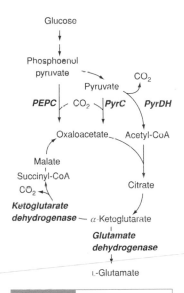

Figure 14.7 Sketch of main reactions of *C. glutamicum* connected with the citric acid cycle and of relevance for L-glutamate production. PyrDH, pyruvate dehydrogenase; PyrC, pyruvate carboxylase; PEPC, phospho*enol*pyruvate carboxylase.

14.4.2 Production strains

For the biotechnological production of L-glutamate, the intracellularly synthesised amino acid must be released from the cell. This requires specific treatments to result in export of the amino acid by a presumed carrier. A specific carrier must be present since otherwise, in addition to the charged L-glutamate, other metabolites and ions would also leak from the cell and the cell would not be viable. However, L-glutamate formation is still not fully understood. The reason for this is that a wide range of treatments lead to the secretion of glutamate. These include: (i) growth under biotin limitation, (ii) addition of penicillin, (iii) addition of lysozyme, (iv) addition of surfactants, (v) use of oleic acid auxotrophs, and (vi) use of glycerol auxotrophs. All these treatments apparently have the cell wall or the lipid membrane as the target in some way or another. Furthermore, the phospholipid

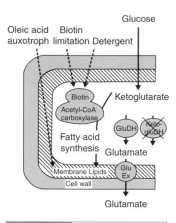

Figure 14.8 Model of the action of a selection of techniques (dashed arrows) to induce L-glutamate excretion and which are linked to the cell envelope. Also shown is the flux from glucose to extracellular L-glutamate involving an export carrier.

composition is significantly changed in the case of biotin limitation. Accordingly, a relation thus exists between:

• a disorder of the cell wall,
• the lipid composition of the membrane, and
• the putative carrier localised in the membrane.

A plausible model is shown in Fig. 14.8 that makes a causal relation between the classic biotin effect and glutamate export. Biotin is a coenzyme of acetyl-CoA carboxylase and thus directly involved in fatty acid synthesis. Under biotin limitation the phospholipid content of the membrane is drastically decreased from 32 to 17 nmol mg^{-1} (DW)$^{-1}$, and the content of the unsaturated oleic acid increased relative to the saturated palmitic acid by 45%. This altered lipid composition results in a favourable lipid environment of the carrier and thus in high export of L-glutamate. The membrane composition is similarly affected by oleic acid or glycerol auxotrophic mutants. Surfactant addition also acts on the acetyl-CoA carboxylase activity, since its addition results in dissociation of the multi-enzyme complex. The altered fatty acid composition of the membrane then provokes the carrier to become active and L-glutamate is excreted.

Apart from the export process and high glutamate dehydrogenase activity, a third component in L-glutamate production is α-ketoglutarate dehydrogenase (Fig. 14.7). Those unnatural conditions resulting in L-glutamate efflux also reduce the activity of this enzyme. Exposing the cell to either penicillin, surfactants or biotin-limitation reduces the α-ketoglutarate dehydrogenase activity up to a residual activity of only 10%, whereas the activity of the glutamate dehydrogenase is hardly affected. The competing α-ketoglutarate dehydrogenase activity is therefore lowered, thus preventing an excess conversion of α-ketoglutarate to succinyl-CoA and, therefore, favouring its conversion to L-glutamate.

14.4.3 Production process

The most relevant factors influencing L-glutamate formation are the ammonium concentration, the dissolved O_2 concentration and the pH. Although, in total, a large amount of ammonium is necessary for sugar conversion to L-glutamate, a high concentration is inhibitory to growth as well to the production of L-glutamate. Therefore, ammonium is added in a low concentration at the beginning of the fermentation and is then added continuously during the course of the fermentation. The oxygen concentration is controlled, since under conditions of insufficient oxygen, the production of L-glutamate is poor and lactic acid as well as succinic acid accumulates, whereas with an excess oxygen supply the amount of a-ketoglutarate as a by-product accumulates. A flow diagram of the process is shown in Fig. 14.9.

For the actual fermentation, the production strains are grown in fermenters as large as 500 m^3 (Fig. 14.10). After pre-cultivation, the onset of L-glutamate excretion is controlled by the addition of

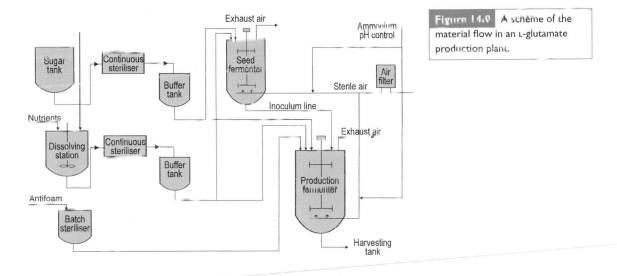

Figure 14.9 A scheme of the material flow in an L-glutamate production plant.

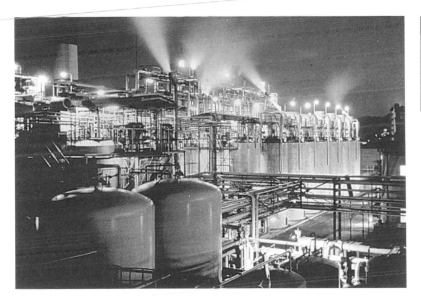

Figure 14.10 Amino acid production plant of Kyowa Hakko in Japan showing on the right seven large fermenters each 240 m³ in size, suitable for L-glutamate production.

surfactants such as polyoxyethylene sorbitan monopalmitate (Tween 40). Yields of between 60 and 70% L-glutamate, based on the glucose used, have been reported. At the end of the fermentation the broth contains L-glutamate in the form of its ammonium salt. In a typical downstream process, the cells are separated and the broth is passed through a basic anion exchange resin. L-Glutamate anions will be bound to the resin and ammonia will be released. This ammonia can be recovered via distillation and reused in the fermentation. Elution is performed with NaOH to form monosodium glutamate (MSG) directly in the solution and to regenerate the basic anion exchanger. From the eluates, MSG may be crystallised directly followed by further conditioning steps like decolorisation and sieving to yield a food-grade quality.

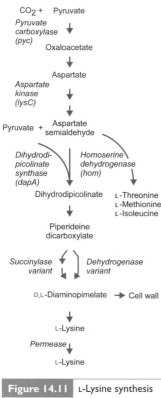

Figure 14.11 L-Lysine synthesis in *C. glutamicum* with the carboxylation reaction supplying oxaloacetate. Also shown is the central role of aspartate semialdehyde distribution and the link to cell-wall synthesis.

14.5 L-Lysine

14.5.1 Biochemistry

The second amino acid made exclusively with *C. glutamicum* is L-lysine. The carbons of L-lysine are derived in the central metabolism from pyruvate and oxaloacetate (Fig. 14.11). In contrast to the special situation with L-glutamate, where practically only a single reaction represents the synthesis pathway, L-lysine is synthesised via a long pathway. Moreover, the first two steps of L-lysine synthesis are shared with that of the other members of the aspartate family of amino acids: L-threonine, L-methionine and L-isoleucine.

The kinase-initiating lysine synthesis is feedback-inhibited by lysine plus threonine

The first reaction initiating L-lysine synthesis is catalysed by aspartate kinase. As is typical of an enzyme at the start of a lengthy synthesis pathway, the activity of aspartate kinase is tightly controlled. The enzyme is inactive when L-lysine plus L-threonine together are present in excess, thus providing a feedback signal (see Chapter 2) concerning the availability of these two major metabolites of the aspartate family of amino acids. The kinase has an interesting structure (Fig. 14.12). It consists of two α-sub-units of 421 amino acid residues each, and two β-sub-units of 171 amino acid residues. An exciting discovery was that the amino acid sequence of the β-sub-unit is identical to that in the carboxyterminal part of the α-sub-unit. The molecular basis is that the gene for the smaller β-sub-unit, *lysCβ*, is an in-frame constituent part of the larger α-sub-unit. Thus two promoters are present at this locus: one driving *lysCα* expression together with that of the downstream gene, *asd*, and one driving *lysCβ* and *asd* expression. The regulatory features of the kinase reside in the β-sub-unit. Thus specifically altering the β-sub-unit structure, or those of both sub-units together in their carboxy-terminal part, results in a kinase which is always active and no longer inhibitable. With such an insensitive kinase, *C. glutamicum* already excretes some L-lysine, showing the rather simple type of flux control in this organism.

The synthase limits flux

A further important step of flux control within lysine biosynthesis is at the level of aspartate semialdehyde distribution. The dihydrodipicolinate synthase activity competes with the homoserine dehydrogenase for the aspartate semialdehyde (Fig. 14.11). Graded overexpression of the synthase gene, *dapA*, together with enzyme activity measurements have shown that with an increasing activity of synthase a graded flux increase towards L-lysine is the result. Therefore, the synthase acts as a barrier to control the flux of aspartate semialdehyde towards L-lysine. This barrier can also be overcome when an increased aspartate semialdehyde concentration is available, as can easily be obtained by reducing the flux towards the homoserine-derived amino acids. This can be achieved with mutated homoserine dehydrogenase enzymes which have very weak catalytic activity.

Lysine synthesis is split which ensures proper cell-wall formation

A remarkable feature of *C. glutamicum* is its possession of a split pathway for L-lysine synthesis. At the level of piperideine-2,6-dicarboxylate, flux is possible either via the succinylase variant of D,L-diaminopimelate synthesis or the dehydrogenase variant (Fig. 14.11). In contrast, *E. coli*, for example, has only the succinylase variant and *Bacillus macerans* only the dehydrogenase variant. The flux distribution via both pathways has been quantified in a study using NMR spectroscopy and $[1-^{13}C]$-glucose as the substrate. Surprisingly, the flux distribution is variable (Fig. 14.13). Whereas at the start of the cultivation about three-quarters of the L-lysine is made via the dehydrogenase variant, at the end of the process the newly synthesised L-lysine is almost exclusively made via the succinylase route. There is a mechanistic reason for this. As kinetic characterisations have shown, the dehydrogenase has a weak affinity towards its substrate, ammonium, with a K_m of 28 mM. Thus at low ammonium concentrations, as are present at the end of the fermentation, the dehydrogenase cannot contribute to L-lysine formation. Instead, flux via the succinylase variant is favoured, where after succinylation of piperideine-2,6-dicarboxylate, a transaminase incorporates the second amino group into the final L-lysine molecule.

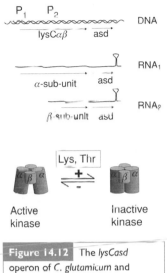

Figure 14.12 The *lysCasd* operon of *C. glutamicum* and allosteric control of the kinase. The second promoter within *lysC* results in formation of the β-sub-unit constituting the regulatory sub-unit of the kinase protein of $\alpha_2 \beta_2$-structure.

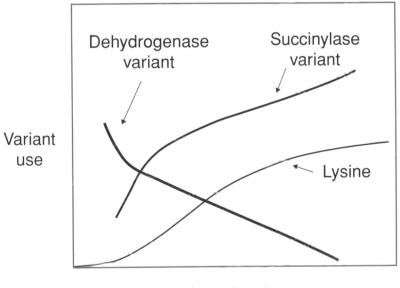

Dehydrogenase variant

Succinylase variant

Variant use

Lysine

Fermentation time

Figure 14.13 At the beginning of the L-lysine fermentation use of the dehydrogenase variant prevails over that of the succinylase variant, whereas at the end the succinylase variant is used almost exclusively. Variant use is from 0 to 100%.

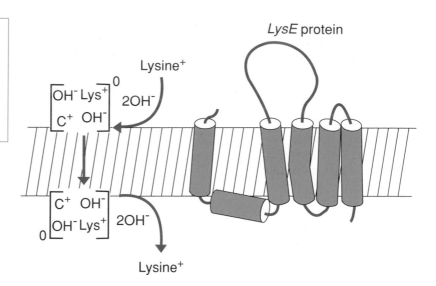

Figure 14.14 Topology of the L-lysine exporter showing its five membrane spanning helices and the additional hydrophobic segment. The formally distinct steps of the translocation process driven by the membrane potential are included.

If either the succinylase or the dehydrogenase variant is inactivated, L-lysine accumulation is reduced to 40%. Thus both variants together ensure in fermentations a high flux towards L-lysine. The natural function of this split pathway is always to provide a proper supply of the penultimate intermediate of L-lysine synthesis. This is D,L-diaminopimelate, which is a crucial linking unit within the peptidoglycan of the cell wall. The split pathway in *C. glutamicum* is an example of an important principle in microbial physiology: pathway variants are generally not redundant but evolved to provide key metabolites under different environmental conditions.

Export of L-lysine

The molecular basis for bacterial amino acid export was completely unknown until 1996 since a specific export process appeared nonsensical. The breakthrough was achieved by the cloning of the lysine export carrier from *C. glutamicum*, which at one blow enabled amazing discoveries concerning the nature and relevance of such a new type of exporter. The L-lysine carrier, *LysE*, is a comparatively small membrane protein of 25.4 Da. It has the transmembrane spanning helices typical of carriers and is probably active as a dimer (Fig. 14.14). Several distinct steps are involved in the translocation mechanism. These are: (i) the loading of the negatively charged carrier with its substrate L-lysine together with two hydroxyl ions, (ii) substrate translocation via the membrane, (iii) the release of L-lysine and the accompanying ions at the outside of the membrane, and, finally, (iv) the reorientation of the carrier. The driving force for the entire translocation process is the membrane potential.

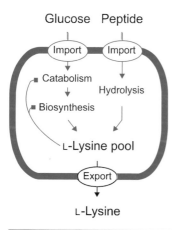

Figure 14.15 Amino acid exporters serve as a valve to release an excess of amino acid present, as can be the case in producers or in the natural situation during growth on peptides.

Access to the lysine-exporter gene, *lysE*, has also made it possible to solve the puzzle as to why *C. glutamicum* has such an exporter at all. In a *lysE* deletion mutant supplied with glucose and 1 mM of the dipeptide, lysyl-alanine, an extraordinarily high intracellular L-lysine concentration of more than 1 M accumulates, abolishing growth of the mutant (Fig. 14.15). Thus, the exporter serves as a valve to excrete any excess intracellular L-lysine that may arise in the natural environment in the presence of peptides. As in the case of other bacteria, too, C. glutamicum has active peptide-uptake systems as well as hydrolysing enzymes giving access to the amino acids as valuable building blocks. However, C. glutamicum has no L-lysine-degrading activities and therefore must prevent any piling up of L-lysine. As genome projects have now shown, there are indeed numerous similar carriers present in various Gram-negative and Gram-positive bacteria. Therefore, this type of intracellular amino acid control by an exporter is expected to be present in other bacteria, too.

14.5.2 Production strains

L-Lysine producer strains have been derived over the decades by mutagenesis to give strains excreting more than 170 g l^{-1} L-lysine. It is clear that these strains may carry an extensive list of phenotypic characters to achieve this massive flux directioning (Table 14.2). Typically, the strains are resistant to some analogue of lysine or diaminopimelate. A typical feature of L-lysine producers is their resistance to the lysine analogue S-(2-aminoethyl)-L-cysteine (Fig. 14.16). In these mutants, the aspartate kinase (see Fig. 14.12) is mutated so that it is no longer inhibited by L-lysine. Dozens of other chemicals structurally related to L-lysine, such as γ-methyl-L-lysine or α-chlorocaprolactam, have been used in screenings to obtain improved producers. At this stage of strain development it was often not known how phenotypic characters correlate with overproduction and which was the molecular basis for that. However, with the advent of whole-genome sequencing classical producers can be sequenced now, and the mutations recognised can be used to assay for their importance and relevance to derive a good producer (see Fig. 14.6). Using this genomic-based approach, just three point mutations were introduced into the genome of the wild type to derive an excellent L-lysine producer. By introducing alleles of the genes coding for aspartate kinase (lysC-Thr311Ile), pyruvate carboxylase (pyc-Pro458Ser) and homoserine dehydrogenase (hom-Val59Ala) production of 80 g l^{-1} L-lysine with a productivity of 3.0 g l^{-1} h^{-1} was achieved.

14.5.3 Production process

The most common carbon sources for L-lysine fermentation and also other amino acids are molasses (cane or sugar beet molasses), high test molasses (inverted cane molasses), or sucrose and starch hydrolysates. In contrast to E. coli, the wild type of C. glutamicum can utilise both glucose and sucrose. In the past, molasses was mostly used for production since it is a relatively cheap carbon source. However, the utilisation of molasses has severe disadvantages:

* waste is exported from the sugar company to the fermentation plant and causes additional costs there;
* the seasonal availability of molasses causes ageing effects in its quality during storage.

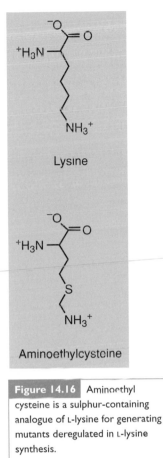

Lysine

Aminoethylcysteine

Figure 14.16 Aminoethyl cysteine is a sulphur-containing analogue of L-lysine for generating mutants deregulated in L-lysine synthesis.

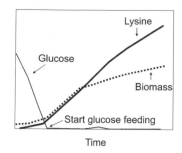

Figure 14.17 Time course of L-lysine accumulation in a production process. There are three phases of growth and L-lysine accumulation.

Therefore, there is a clear tendency away from molasses towards refined carbon sources such as hydrolysed starches. Profitable nitrogen sources are ammonium sulphate and ammonia (gaseous or ammonia water). The growth factors required are provided from plant protein hydrolysates, cornsteep liquor or by the addition of the defined compounds. A typical lysine fermentation is shown in Fig. 14.17. After consumption of the initial sugar, the substrates are added continuously and L-lysine accumulates up to 170 g l^{-1}. Ammonium sulphate provides the counter-ion to neutralise the accumulating basic amino acid. Therefore, L-lysine is present in the fermentation broth as its sulphate. As a convention in the literature, lysine is usually given as lysine·HCl. Due to the high sugar cost, the conversion yield is a very important criterion for the entire production process. Technical processes have been published with a yield of 45–50 g lysine 100 g^{-1} carbon source.

For the recovery of L-lysine, several basically different processes have been developed. Three processes are currently in use to supply L-lysine in a form suitable for feed purposes:

- A crystalline preparation containing 98.5% L-lysine·HCl. It can be made by ion exchange chromatography, evaporation and crystallisation. Also direct spray-drying of the ion exchange eluate is possible.
- An alkaline solution of concentrated L-lysine containing 50.7% L-lysine. It is obtained by biomass separation, evaporation and filtration.
- A granulated lysine sulphate preparation consisting of 50% L-lysine. It consists of the entire fermentation broth conditioned by spray-drying and granulation.

These processes differ significantly in investment costs, losses during downstreaming, amount of waste volume and user friendliness. All this, together with the fermentation itself, decides the success of the various competitors producing L-lysine.

14.6 | L-Threonine

14.6.1 Biochemistry

The commercial production of L-threonine is done with *E. coli* mutants. The synthesis of L-threonine proceeds via a short pathway comprising only five steps (Fig. 14.18). As already mentioned, the first steps are shared with that of L-lysine and L-methionine synthesis. Furthermore, L-threonine is also an intermediate in the L-isoleucine synthesis. This naturally requires special metabolic regulation. In *C. glutamicum* this was solved in such a way that the sole aspartate kinase present was only inhibited by the joint presence of L-lysine and L-threonine. In the case of *E. coli*, however, three isoenzymes are present each of which is separately inhibited by a different end-product: one by L-threonine, one by L-lysine and one by L-methionine. There are furthermore two homoserine dehydrogenase activities: one is inhibited by L-threonine and one by L-methionine. Additionally, the corresponding genes are grouped into transcriptional units, thereby ensuring a balanced synthesis of the appropriate amino acid at the level of gene expression. The relevant operon for L-threonine synthesis in *E. coli* is *thrABC*. It encodes three polypeptides, with *thrA* encoding an apparently fused polypeptide of aspartate kinase plus homoserine dehydrogenase. A strong expression control of this operon is provided by a transcription attenuation mechanism. The corresponding leader peptide at the beginning of the transcription unit is Thr-Thr-Ile-Thr-Thr-Thr-Ile-Thr-Ile-Thr-Thr, serving to sense the availability of L-threonine and L-isoleucine. When the corresponding tRNAs are uncharged, the leader peptide formation does not occur, and transcription of the operon is increased at least ten-fold.

14.6.2 Producer strains

Based on this pathway structure and regulation there is a clear focus on two major targets for the design of a producer strain: the prevention of L-isoleucine formation and stable high-level expression of *thrABC*. Therefore, in one of the first steps of strain development, chromosomal mutations were introduced to produce an isoleucine leaky strain (Fig. 14.19). The isoleucine mutation located in the threonine deaminase is a very specific and important one. L-Isoleucine is required only at low L-threonine concentrations but, at high concentrations of L-threonine, growth is independent of added L-isoleucine. This is the case with a threonine deaminase mutated to have a low affinity. This mutation has several advantageous consequences. In the first place, it prevents an excess formation of the undesired by-product L-isoleucine. Additionally, it prevents the L-isoleucine-dependent premature termination of the *thrABC* transcription due to limiting tRNA^{Ile}.

A third consequence of the isoleucine mutation is more subtle. It relates to the stability of the plasmid-containing producer strain in the various pre-cultivation steps. Starting from a single clone, a pre-culture is inoculated for each production and is then enlarged in several stages. This means that the clone is fermented for about 25 generations so that there is a great danger of the plasmid that contains the *thrABC* operon being lost. This would, of course, be a complete disaster if it happened in the final production stage. In the presence of the isoleucine leaky mutation, however, cells that have lost the plasmid now are clearly disadvantaged since they are not synthesising a high concentration of L-threonine. Their further proliferation is halted, thereby stabilising a culture where almost all the cells that are growing contain the plasmid. Further engineering during strain evolution involved the introduction of resistance to L-threonine and L-homoserine, which turned out to result in increased expression of a carrier protein exporting L-threonine from the cell into the medium. Subsequently, *tdh*, which encodes the threonine dehydrogenase, was inactivated thus preventing threonine degradation. To obtain very high activities of the *thrABC*-encoding enzymes, the operon was cloned

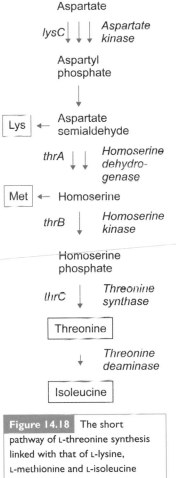

Figure 14.18 The short pathway of L-threonine synthesis linked with that of L-lysine, L-methionine and L-isoleucine synthesis. *Escherichia coli* has isoenzymes, as indicated by the parallel arrows, each of them separately regulated by either inhibition or gene expression involving the individual amino acids of this pathway.

Wild type
↓
Introducing the Ile⁻ mutation.
↓
Selecting for Thr^r, Hom^r
↓
Inactivation of threonine
dehydrogenase *(tdh)*
↓
Overexpression of
thrABC with pBR322
↓
Overexpression with pRS10
↓
Engineering
sugar uptake

Figure 14.19 Relevant steps in the development of an *E. coli* strain suitable for L-threonine production involving undirected mutagenesis, gene inactivation and use of different plasmids.

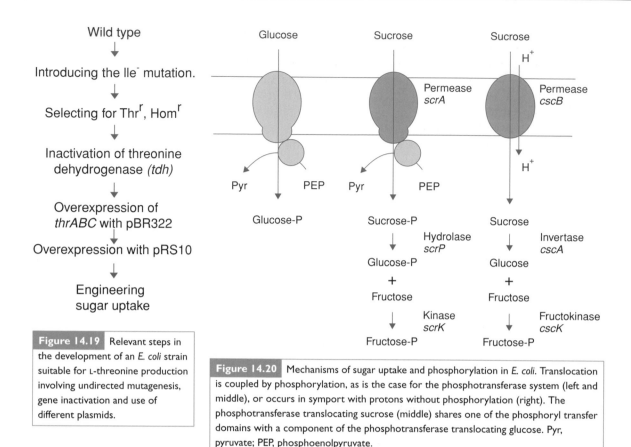

Figure 14.20 Mechanisms of sugar uptake and phosphorylation in *E. coli*. Translocation is coupled by phosphorylation, as is the case for the phosphotransferase system (left and middle), or occurs in symport with protons without phosphorylation (right). The phosphotransferase translocating sucrose (middle) shares one of the phosphoryl transfer domains with a component of the phosphotransferase translocating glucose. Pyr, pyruvate; PEP, phosphoenolpyruvate.

from a strain whose aspartate kinase and homoserine dehydrogenase activities are resistant to L-threonine inhibition. In addition the transcription attenuator was deleted. In fermentations the operon engineered in this way was successfully used with pBR322 as a vector, but a further improvement was obtained by replacing this plasmid by a pRS1010 derivative, resulting in an even more stable high-level expression.

Substrate uptake

Since the cost of the sugar has a decisive influence on the price of the amino acid produced, it is essential to be able to switch between glucose and sucrose as substrates. However, K-12 *E. coli* strains cannot use sucrose, as was also the case with the originally developed L-threonine producer. Fortunately, two different sucrose-utilising systems of other strains are available to engineer sugar utilization (Fig. 14.20). One of them is represented by the *scr* regulon of *E. coli* strain H155, where the actual translocator consists of the phospho*enol*pyruvate : sugar phosphotransferase system (PTS). Introduction of the *scr* genes into a K-12 strain results in the uptake and phosphorylation of sucrose. Due to subsequent hydrolase and fructokinase activities, the sugar is then channelled into the central metabolism. An alternative sucrose utilisation system is provided by the *csc* regulon of some *E. coli* strains. In this case, sucrose is translocated by the *cscB* encoded translocator in symport with protons. Using transposition, the sucrose-utilisation capability of the *csc* regulon was introduced into a glucose-utilising strain. Although originally without uptake of sucrose, this strain now imported sucrose at a rate of 9 pmol min^{-1} (mg DW)$^{-1}$. With the plasmid-encoded regulon the rate obtained was 43 pmol min^{-1} (mg DW)$^{-1}$, which was almost identical to that of the strain from which the *csc* regulon had been isolated.

14.6.3 Production process

The fermentation of the engineered L-threonine producer is in a simple mineral salts medium with either glucose or sucrose as the substrate with addition of a small amount of a complex medium component like yeast extract. After inoculation and consumption of the initially provided sugar, continuous feeding of sugar begins. Additionally, ammonia has to be fed in the form of gas or as NH$_4$OH which is regulated via pH control. Thus the feeding strategy in the case of L-threonine fermentation is quite easy as compared to L-lysine fermentation where the accumulation of the basic product requires the feeding of sulphate as the counter-ion. After 77 h of fermentation L-threonine is present at about 100 g l^{-1} with a conversion yield of up to 60%. The fermentation is characterised by low by-product formation, which is an advantage for downstream processing. Cystallization of L-threonine is easy due to its low solubility and the low salt concentration present. A process is described where the cells are initially coagulated by a heat- or pH-treatment step, followed by filtration. Subsequently, the broth is concentrated and crystallisation initiated by cooling. The separation and drying of the crystals leads to an isolation yield of 80–90% with the L-threonine having a purity of more than 90%. A recrystallization step may be required for high-purity L-threonine.

14.7 | L-Phenylalanine

14.7.1 Biochemistry

L-Phenylalanine can be produced with *E. coli* or *C. glutamicum*. The L-phenylalanine synthesis is shared in part with that of L-tyrosine and L-tryptophan. The three aromatic amino acids have in common the condensation of erythrose 4-phosphate and phospho*enol*pyruvate to 3-deoxy-D-arabino-heptulosonate 7-phosphate (DAHP) with further conversion in six steps up to chorismate. L-Phenylalanine is then finally made in three further steps (Fig. 14.21). There are three DAHP synthase enzymes in *E. coli* encoded by *aroF*, *aroG* and *aroH*. These enzymes play a key role in flux control. Their regulation of catalytic activity, in each case by one of the three aromatic amino acids, recalls the specific regulation of aspartate kinase in the synthesis of threonine. About 80% of the total DAHP-synthase activity is contributed

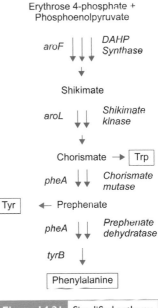

Figure 14.21 Simplified pathway of L-phenylalanine synthesis involving ten individual enzyme-catalysed reaction steps. In addition, isoenzymes operate in *E. coli* as indicated by the parallel arrows. Selected key enzymes and key genes are given.

by the *aroG*-encoded enzyme. Interestingly, there are two bifunctional polypeptides, each encoding chorismate mutase-prephenate dehydratase. That encoded by *pheA* is inhibited by L-phenylalanine, and that encoded by *tyrA* by L-tyrosine. The *pheA* gene expression is dependent on the level of tRNA^{Phe}.

14.7.2 Production strains

Producer strains have a feedback-resistant DAHP activity encoded either by *aroF* or *aroG* and a feedback-resistant chorismate mutase-prephenate dehydratase encoded by *pheA*. As a rule, the producers are L-tyrosine auxotrophic mutants. There are very good reasons for this, one of which is that enzymes of the common pathway from DAHP to prephenate are no longer regulated by L-tyrosine and enzyme activities are no longer feedback-inhibited. Another reason is that in this way tyrosine accumulation is prevented, which would otherwise undoubtedly result as a by-product since there are only two additional steps from prephenate to L-tyrosine. An essential aspect is that due to the auxotrophy: a beneficial growth limitation is possible by appropriate tyrosine feeding (see below). In some *E. coli* strains, the temperature-sensitive cI$_{857}$ repressor of bacteriophage λ has been used together with the λP$_L$ promoter to enable inducible expression of the key genes *pheA* and *aroF*. This enables extremely high enzyme activities to be adjusted solely in the actual production runs thus eliminating the inherent problems of strain stability due to the resulting high metabolite concentrations. It enables the pre-cultivation steps up to the seed fermenter to be performed with low expression of the key genes but in the actual large production fermenter the genes are now induced to a high level of expression.

14.7.3 Production process

As with the other amino acids, effective L-phenylalanine production is the joint result of genetically engineering cellular metabolism and tight control of the production process in the fermenter. Control of metabolic regulation is necessary for two reasons. First, the carbon flux has to be optimally distributed between the four major products of glucose conversion, which are L-phenylalanine, biomass, acetic acid and CO$_2$. The second reason is that the cellular physiology is not constant during the course of fermentation, which correspondingly requires an adaptation of fermentation control during the process. Figure 14.22 shows the typical time curve of L-phenylalanine production. The major problem is that *E. coli* tends to produce acetic acid which has a strong negative effect on process efficiency. To prevent this, researchers have developed an ingenious sugar-feeding strategy, which first collects on-line data and fluxes such as O$_2$ concentration, sugar consumption and biomass concentrations. These are then counterbalanced during the process to control the optimum sugar concentration. The feeding of sugar starts when the cells enter Stage 2 of the fermentation where the glucose initially provided has almost been consumed. The trick is to prevent too high a glucose concentration occurring since this would result in acetic

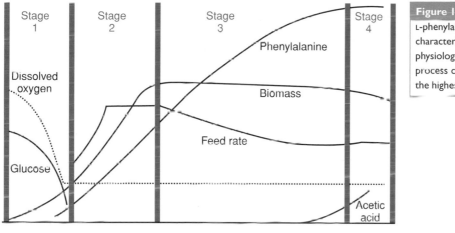

Figure 14.22 The four stages of L-phenylalanine production characterised by different physiology requiring different process control regimes to give the highest yields in shortest times

acid formation and, at the same time, to prevent too low a glucose concentration since this would result in an excess of CO_2 evolution. Thus the feeding rate is a compromise where the process is run at the highest possible feeding rate which still provides a sufficiently strong limitation to prevent acetic acid excretion. When the L-tyrosine initially present has been consumed, the cells proceed to Stage 3. As already mentioned, almost all L-phenylalanine producers are tyrosine auxotrophs. The L-tyrosine concentration selected at the start of the culture therefore fixes the minimum amount of biomass necessary to metabolise the pre-determined amount of glucose efficiently. In Stage 3, the metabolic capacity of the cells decreases which brings about a consequent decrease of the glucose feeding rate. At the end of Stage 3, acetic acid excretion begins and the cells enter Stage 4 where no further L-phenylalanine accumulation occurs and the process is eventually terminated. This example of amino acid production shows that by the sophisticated application of feeding strategies with adaptive control a very high L-phenylalanine concentration can be achieved with a high yield within 2.5 days. Values of 50.8 g l^{-1} L-phenylalanine with a yield of 27.5% have been reported.

14.8 | L-Tryptophan

14.8.1 Biochemistry

L-Tryptophan is a high-price amino acid which still has a rather low market volume. It is one of the candidate amino acids to be used for further improvement of animal feed. Effective production processes are available with mutants of *E. coli*, *C. glutamicum* and *Bacillus subtilis*. However, still in use is the effective enzymatic synthesis of L-tryptophan from cheap precursors yielding a product of highest purity. This type of production is based on the activity of the biosynthetic tryptophan synthase (Fig. 14.23). This enzyme catalyses the last step in the tryptophan synthesis, which in fact consists of

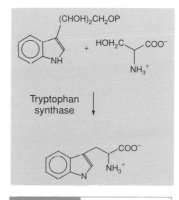

Figure 14.23 Tryptophan synthase naturally uses indole 3-glycerol phosphate plus L-serine, but in the production process indole plus L-serine are used as substrates.

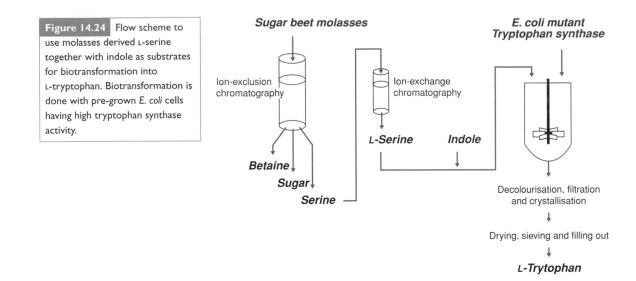

Figure 14.24 Flow scheme to use molasses derived L-serine together with indole as substrates for biotransformation into L-tryptophan. Biotransformation is done with pre-grown *E. coli* cells having high tryptophan synthase activity.

two partial reactions:

Indole-3-glycerol phosphate

$\rightarrow$ indole + glyceraldehyde 3-phosphate (α-sub-unit)

Indole + L-serine $\rightarrow$ L-tryptophan + H_2O (β_2-sub-unit)

These separate reactions are catalysed by separate sub-units of the enzyme: α and β. The enzyme of *E. coli* is an $\alpha_2\beta_2$-tetramer, which can be dissociated into functional α-sub-units and a β_2-sub-unit. The α-sub-unit catalyses the cleavage of indole-3-glycerol phosphate, whereas the β_2-sub-unit catalyses the condensation of L-serine with indole to form L-tryptophan. It is this latter reaction which is advantageously used in the industrial production.

14.8.2 Production from precursors

The production is based on *E. coli* cells which have a high tryptophan synthase activity. The α and β-sub-units encoding genes *trpA* and *trpB*, respectively, are located on the *trpEDCBA* operon which is regulated by repression and attenuation. In the *E. coli* mutant used, the repressor of that operon has been deleted as it is part of the attenuator region together with the first structural genes of the operon. As a consequence, about 10% of the total protein is tryptophan synthase with an excess of β-sub-units present. Although indole is not the true substrate, with a sufficiently high concentration the synthase as well as the β-sub-units present will react with it. Indole is available from the petrochemical industry as a comparably cheap educt, whereas the second educt, L-serine, is recovered from molasses during sugar refinement using ion-exclusion chromatography, and further purification steps (Fig. 14.24). The resulting L-serine is fed to the previously cultivated *E. coli* cells, and indole is added continuously at a concentration adjusted to 10 mM, which is controlled on-line. This type of process ensures an almost quantitative conversion of indole

Table 14.3 Comparison of the productivity of immobilized *E. coli* cells for the production of L-aspartate

Immobilisation method	Aspartase activity (Ug⁻¹ cells)	Half-life (days)	Relative productivity (%)[b]
Polyacrylamide	18 850	120	100
Carrageenan	56 340	70	174
Carrageenan (GA)[a]	37 460	240	397
Carrageenan (GA + HA)[a]	49 400	680	1498

[a] GA, glutaraldehyde; HA, hexamethylene diamine.
[b] Considers the initial activity, decay constant and operation period

to yield L-tryptophan with a space–time yield of about 75 g l⁻¹ day⁻¹. Further processing of the L-tryptophan solution can be taken from Fig. 14.24 leading to a pyrogen-free pharmaceutical product of the highest quality.

14.9 | L-Aspartate

14.9.1 Biochemistry

L-Aspartic acid is widely used as a food additive and in pharmaceuticals. Demand increased rapidly with the introduction of aspartame as an artificial sweetener. This is a dipeptide consisting of L-aspartate and L-phenylalanine which is about 200-fold sweeter than sugar and was successfully introduced into the market as a low-calorie sweetener. Although L-aspartate was originally produced fermentatively, it is currently produced exclusively using aspartase due to the high productivities and the cost effectiveness of the process. In fact, the use of aspartase to make L-aspartate represents one of the highest productivities known for an enzyme used in biotechnology (see also Chapter 24). The method developed allows re-use of the enzyme to the extent that over 220 000 kg of product can be produced per kilogram of enzyme.

Aspartase catalyses the interconversion between L-aspartate and fumarate plus ammonia (Fig. 14.25). The reaction favours the amination reaction. The enzyme of *E. coli* is a tetramer with a molecular weight of 196 000, which has an absolute requirement for divalent metal ions. A severe disadvantage at the beginning of the studies by the Tanabe Seiyaku Co. Ltd, which now successfully uses aspartase, was the instability of the enzyme. After incubation of the enzyme in solution for just half an hour at 50 °C, activity is no longer detectable. Nevertheless, a residual activity of 10% is present when the enzyme is immobilised in polyacrylamide. Such a physical confinement of cells in space turned out to be the method of choice. Table 14.3 shows that with the natural polymer κ-carrageenan, resulting from a screening of different polymers and use of appropriate cross-linking, exceptional improvements were obtained in the relative productivity as well as

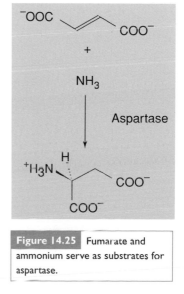

Figure 14.25 Fumarate and ammonium serve as substrates for aspartase.

in the stability of the catalyst. The final material has a half-life of almost two years. This represents an almost unimaginable progress in comparison to the initial situation where the enzyme in free solution only had a half-life measured in minutes. An initial disadvantage of the original cells used was their fumarase activity, which results in the partial conversion of fumarate to L-malic acid. To solve this problem a heat treatment step of the cells is used which eliminates the fumarase activity almost completely. Using such conditioned cells and starting from 1 M ammonium fumarate, the final product solution contains 987 mM L-aspartate, 10.7 mM non-reacted fumarate and only trace quantities (1.9 mM) L-malic acid.

For the production process the immobilised cells are packed into a column designed as a multi-stage system. The stages introduced, each consisting of a set of parallel horizontal tubes, serve two purposes. On the one hand, they allow effective cooling to prevent decay of the catalytic activity since the aspartase reaction is exergonic. About 6 kcal heat mol^{-1} substrate evolves in the actual large-scale production process which is very close to that calculated from the standard free energy change of the aspartase reaction of 4 kcal mol^{-1}. On the other hand, the flow properties of the column are increased. Any compacting of the bed over time is prevented, and the preferred plug-flow characteristics are obtained. With such a column, flow rates of two column volumes per hour are possible. The continuous process enables full automation and control to achieve an optimum throughput with the highest product quality. Yet another advantage of such a controlled continuous process is its reduced waste production. A typical volumetric activity is about 200 mmol h^{-1} (g cells)$^{-1}$. Assuming a 1000-litre column, the yield of L-aspartate is 3.4 tonnes per day, which is 100 tonnes per month. The final product is eventually purified by crystallisation.

14.10 | Outlook

Although amino acids are now among the classical products in biotechnology, their demand is increasing enormously. Constant development of the processes is required, new processes have to be established and understanding of the exceptional capabilities of producer strains deepened. Surprising new information, of general interest for cellular physiology, has been gathered such as the existence of specific export carriers or cyclic fluxes within the anaplerotic reactions. Moreover, much information has been obtained from strain development in conjunction with fermentation technology, with the new science of metabolic engineering at the interface between them. In fact, amino acid production is an outstanding example of the integration of many different techniques. In this way, the early Japanese activities on the taste of kelp laid the foundation for the continuing very successful and flourishing production of amino acids.

Acknowledgements

We would like to thank the following for providing material for this article: R. Faurie, Amino CmbH; K. Ikeda, Ajinomoto Ltd; N. Kato, Kyoto University; Y. Kawahara, Ajinomoto Ltd; W. Leuchtenberger and G. Thierbach, Degussa AG; T. Shibasaki, Kyowa Hakko Kogyo; T. Tosa, Tanabe Seiyaku.

14.11 | Further reading

Bongaerts, J., Krämer, M., Müller, U., Raeven, L. and Wubbolts, M. Metabolic engineering for microbial production of aromatic amino acids and derived compounds. *Metabolic Engineering* **3**: 289–300, 2001.

Chibata, I., Tosa, T. and Shibatani, T. The industrial production of optically active compounds by immobilized biocatalysts. In *Chirality in Industry*, eds. A. N. Collins, G. N. Sheldrake and J. Crosby. London: John Wiley & Sons, 1992.

Debabov, V. G. The threonine story. *Advances Biochemical Engineering* **79**: 114–136, 2003.

de Graaf, A. A. Metabolic flux analysis of *Corynebacterium glutamicum*. In *Bioreactor Engineering, Modeling and Control* eds. K. Schügerl and K. H. Bellgardt. Berlin: Springer-Verlag, 2000, pp. 506–555.

Eggeling, L. and Bott, M. *Handbook of Corynebacterium glutamicum*. Boca Raton, FL: CRC Press, 2005.

Hodgson, J. Bulk amino acid fermentation: technology and commodity trading. *Bio/Technology* **12**: 152–155, 1994.

Eggeling, L. and Sahm, H. New ubiquitous translocators: amino acid export by *Corynebacterium glutamicum* and *Escherichia coli*. *Archives of Microbiology* **180**: 155–160, 2003.

Ikeda, M. Amino acid production processes. *Advances Biochemical Engineering* **79**: 1–35, 2003.

Konstantinov, K. B., Nishino, N., Seki, T. and Yoshida, T. Physiologically motivated strategies for control of the fed-batch cultivation of recombinant *Escherichia coli* for phenylalanine production. *Journal of Fermentation and Bioengineering* **71**: 350–355, 1990.

Ohnishi, J., Mitsuhashi, S., Hayashi, M., *et al.* A novel methodology employing *Corynebacterium glutamicum* genome information to generate a new L-lysine-producing mutant. *Applied Microbiology and Biotechnology* **58**: 217–223, 2002.

Chapter 15

Organic acids

Christian P. Kubicek

Institut fur Verfahrenstechnik, Umwelttechnik und Techn, Austria

Levente Karaffa

University of Debrecen, Hungary

15.1 | Introduction

Various organic acids are accumulated by several eukaryotic and prokaryotic micro-organisms. In anaerobic bacteria, their formation is usually a means by which these organisms regenerate NADH, and their accumulation therefore strictly parallels growth (e.g. lactic acid, propionic acid, etc; see Chapter 2). In aerobic bacteria and fungi, in contrast, the accumulation of organic acids is the result of incomplete substrate oxidation and is usually initiated by an imbalance in some essential nutrients, e.g. mineral ions. Despite the completely different physiological prerequisites for the formation of these products, no distinction will be made between these two types of products in this chapter. The organic acids described below are those that are manufactured in large volumes (see Table 15.1), and marketed as relatively pure chemicals or their salts.

Basic Biotechnology, third edition, eds. Colin Ratledge and Bjørn Kristiansen.
Published by Cambridge University Press. © Cambridge University Press 2006.

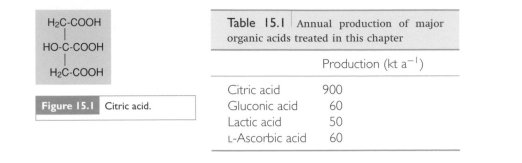

Figure 15.1 Citric acid.

Table 15.1 Annual production of major organic acids treated in this chapter

	Production (kt a^{-1})
Citric acid	900
Gluconic acid	60
Lactic acid	50
L-Ascorbic acid	60

15.2 | Citric acid

Citric acid (2-hydroxy-propane-1,2,3-tricarboxylic acid; Fig. 15.1) was first discovered as a constituent of lemons, but is today known as an intermediate of the ubiquitous tricarboxylic acid cycle (see p. 31) and therefore occurs in almost every living organism. Originally produced from lemons by an Italian cartel, the discovery of its accumulation by *Aspergillus niger* (then named *Citromyces*) in the early 1920s led to a rapid development of a fermentation process that, 15 years later, accounted for more than 95% of the world's production of citric acid.

15.2.1 Microbial strains and biochemical pathways of citric acid accumulation

Most of today's citric acid is produced by *A. niger*. Industrial strains of this fungus are among the most secretly kept organisms in biotechnology and this also precludes the knowledge of the strategy used for their isolation during strain selection and improvement. Several mutant isolation procedures, on the other hand, have been reported by academic laboratories, which include tolerance against high sugar concentrations, 2-desoxyglucose, respiratory chain inhibitors, fluoroacetate, low pH and others, but the significance of these strategies to the industrial know-how has not been revealed. Other obvious strategies have been focused towards decrease or elimination of by-product formation, such as oxalic acid and gluconic acid (see below). More recently, sequencing of the *A. niger* genome has been completed (see http://www.gene-alliance.com/start1.htm). Over 13 000 genes encoded in approximately 34.5 million base pairs have been identified using an eight-fold coverage of the complete sequence. This information now allows the design of DNA arrays (see Chapter 5), which could then be used to identify genes whose up-and-down regulation correlates with strain improvement, fermentation success and the influence of detrimental parameters.

In addition to *Aspergillus*, several yeasts have been described that form large amounts of citric acid from n-alkanes and also – albeit in lower yields – from glucose. These include *Candida catenula* (former *C. brumptii*), *C. guilliermondii*, *Yarrowia lipolytica* and *C. tropicalis*. A disadvantage in the use of these yeasts is their simultaneous production of isocitric acid, which can be up to 50% of the citric

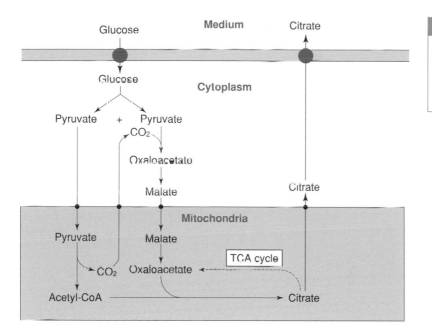

Figure 15.2 Simplified metabolic scheme of citric acid biosynthesis. Side reactions and intermediates not relevant to citric acid biosynthesis have been omitted. TCA cycle, tricarboxylic acid cycle.

acid produced, particularly when n-alkanes have been used as feedstock substrate. (Although isocitric acid is just as useful as citric acid for most purposes, it cannot be sold as 'citric acid' because, clearly, it is not the same.) Mutant selection has therefore frequently sought to select for mutants with very low (approximately 1% of the wild type) aconitase activity (see Figs. 2.9 and 15.2), using resistance to monofluoroacetate as a selection criterion.

The biochemical pathways of citric acid formation involve glycolytic catabolism of glucose to two moles of pyruvate and their subsequent conversion to the precursors of citrate, oxaloacetate and pyruvate (Fig. 15.2). A key in this process is the use of one mole of pyruvate and the CO_2 released during the formation of acetyl-CoA to form oxaloacetate (the Cleland–Johnson reaction). The importance of this step becomes obvious by a simple calculation: if the oxaloacetate required for biosynthesis of citrate had to be formed by one turn of the tricarboxylic acid cycle, two moles of CO_2 would thereby be lost and, consequently, only two-thirds of the carbon of glucose accumulate as citric acid, i.e. 0.7 kg kg^{-1} sugar. Practical yields, however, are much higher, yet are perfectly consistent with the synthesis of oxaloacetate by an anaplerotic CO_2 fixation (i.e. a reaction, normally destined to balance the carbon needed for biosynthetic purposes; see p 34) by pyruvate carboxylase. In addition, the pyruvate carboxylase reaction has a further important implication in citric acid biosynthesis: unlike in several other eukaryotes, pyruvate carboxylase of A. niger is localised in the cytosol, and the oxaloacetate formed is therefore converted further to malate by cytosolic malate dehydrogenase (Fig. 15.2), thereby also regenerating 50% of the glycolytically produced NADH. This provision of cytosolic malate as an 'end-product' of glycolysis is of utmost importance to citric acid

Table 15.2	Optimal conditions for citric acid production
Sugar concentration, g l^{-1}	120–250
Trace metal ion limitation	
Mn, M	$<10^{-8}$
Zn, M	$<10^{-6}$–10^{-7}
Fe, M	$<10^{-4}$
Dissolved oxygen tension, mbar	>140
pH	1.6–2.2
Phosphate concentration, g l^{-1}	0.2–1.0
Ammonium salts, g l^{-1}	>2.0
Time, h	160–240

overflow because it is the co-substrate of the mitochondrial tricarboxylic acid carrier in eukaryotes.

While the biochemical pathway for citric acid biosynthesis, as shown in Fig. 15.2, is experimentally well supported, the reason for accumulation of citric acid in molar yields of up to 90% of the consumed glucose is still not fully understood. In the past, it was thought that inactivation of an enzyme degrading citrate (e.g. aconitase or isocitrate dehydrogenase) would be the key to the accumulation of citric acid, but since then solid evidence for the presence of an intact citric acid cycle during citric acid fermentation has been presented and hence these explanations have been abandoned. More likely, fine regulation of one or more of the enzymes degrading citrate by metabolites may be relevant for citric acid accumulation. However, equally likely, citrate accumulation may be the result of enhanced (deregulated) biosynthesis rather than inhibited degradation. A more detailed description of the various mechanisms proposed and the evidence presented in favour of them can be taken from some of the reviews and papers given in Section 15.6.

15.2.2 Regulation of citric acid accumulation by nutrient parameters

While citric acid can accumulate in extremely high amounts, this accumulation is only observed under a set of rather strictly controlled nutrient conditions (i.e. excessive concentrations of carbon source, H$^+$ and dissolved O$_2$, sub-optimal concentrations of certain trace metals and phosphate). In fact, during growth of *A. niger* in standard media for the cultivation of fungi, little if any citric acid is accumulated. The conditions required for optimum yields vary with the type of fermentation (see below), and are most critical in the submerged fermentation process. Optimal conditions are given in Table 15.2, and are explained below.

Sugar type and concentration

The type and concentration of the carbon source is the most crucial parameter for successful citric acid production as it applies both to the submerged as well as to the surface production process. Only

Table 15.3 Raw materials which have been reported as carbon sources for citric acid production

Blackstrap molasses	Cotton waste
Cane molasses	Whey permeate
Bagasse	Brewery waste
Starch	Sweet potato pulp
Date syrup	Pineapple waste water
Apple pomace	Banana extract
Carob sugar	

sugars that are rapidly catabolised by the fungus – such as sucrose, maltose or glucose – allow high yields as well as high rates of acid accumulation. In the currently used industrial processes, beet and cane molasses predominate as carbon source raw materials. However, both beet and cane molasses are very variable in quality both from season to season and from refinery to refinery. Several components present in molasses have been identified to affect citric acid production but, as the whole composition is so complex, as yet no general strategy for quality assessment can be claimed. Their selection for use in the fermenation process, therefore, still depends on how they perform in small-scale fermenters (~5 to 10 m³). (Often a 'good' batch of molasses will be blended with a 'poor' batch in order to use up the latter material.) A variety of alternative raw materials have been proven applicable on a laboratory scale as well (Table 15.3). Among them, the use of glucose syrup was previously more or less restricted to the USA because of fiscal and other restrictions in Europe. This attitude has been changing, however, in view of the increased availability (and pressure for use) of various waste materials containing glucose polymers.

The concentration of the carbon source used for citric acid production is very high (100 to over 200 g l⁻¹), which seems logical when a bulk product is produced economically. However, the carbon source concentration has also been shown to have an influence on the regulation of citrate overproduction, as the yields from glucose (g g⁻¹) significantly decrease when the carbon concentration decreases below 100 g l⁻¹ (Fig. 15.3). Only very little citric acid is produced at sugar concentrations below 50 g l⁻¹.

With respect to the biochemical basis for the relationship between citric acid accumulation and sugar concentration, a high sugar concentration induces an additional glucose transport system. The increased uptake of glucose under conditions of high sugar supply will then counteract the inhibition of hexokinase by trehalose 6-phosphate. Support of this theory is obtained from the fact that *A. niger* strains in which the gene encoding trehalose 6-phosphate synthase has been knocked out, now accumulate citric acid at an increased rate even at lower sugar concentrations. Furthermore, the intracellular concentration of fructose 2,6-bisphosphate ($F2,6P_2$) is elevated using high sugar concentrations. $F2,6P_2$ is the strongest

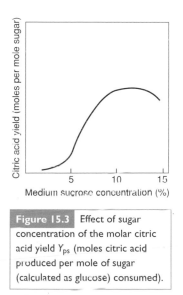

Figure 15.3 Effect of sugar concentration of the molar citric acid yield Y_{ps} (moles citric acid produced per mole of sugar (calculated as glucose) consumed).

stimulator of phosphofructokinase, which may increase the overall glycolytic flux.

Trace metal ions

The effect of trace metal nutrition has been known for a long time and has been the key to the establishment of successful fermentation processes, although the effect is much more pronounced in the submerged fermentation process as opposed to the surface process (see Section 15.2.3). While all usual trace metal ions (Fe, Zn, Cu, Mn, Co) are essential for *A. niger* growth, some of them – particularly Mn^{2+}, Fe^{3+} and Zn^{2+} – have to be present in the medium at growth-limiting concentrations to give high citric acid yields. The effect of manganese ions is particularly striking, as even concentrations as high as $2 \, \mu g \, l^{-1}$ will decrease citric acid accumulation by about 20%. The concentration of metal ions below which citric acid is accumulated in high amounts is not absolute, however, but depends on their relative proportion to other nutrients, particularly phosphate.

Since the concentrations of those metal ions that affect citric acid production are adventitiously introduced into the medium by the high concentrations of the carbon source, all carbon sources to be used in citric acid fermentation have to be purified so they are free of metal ions. This can be done in various ways, e.g. by precipitation or cation exchange treatment. The latter is usually performed only with glucose syrups. Purification of industrial carbon sources such as sugar beet or sugar cane molasses is even more essential, and is mostly carried out by complexation with ferrocyanide and subsequent precipitation, which also seems to have a beneficial effect on the citric-acid-forming metabolism of *A. niger*. Alternatively, the effect of trace metals can be antagonised either by the addition of copper, which blocks manganese transport into the mycelia, or by the addition of lower alcohols or of lipids, which may facilitate citric acid export from the cells.

Several different hypotheses have been offered to explain the biochemical basis of this requirement for trace metal ion limitation but no single convincing explanation can yet be offered. The influence of Mn^{2+} has been most thoroughly studied. The effect seems to be a multiple one, as it has been reported that a limiting concentration of Mn^{2+} increases the flux of carbon through glycolysis, alters the composition of the *A. niger* plasma membrane, impairs DNA synthesis and protein turnover, including that of a component of the standard respiratory chain, and hence leads to impaired respiration. Increased protein degradation also elevates intracellular NH_4^+ concentration which, in turn, stimulates phosphofructokinase activity. This effect, together with the increased $F2,6P_2$ concentration (see above), will counteract the inhibitory effect of citrate on phosphofructokinase. A further striking effect of manganese deficiency on several fungi, including *Aspergillus* spp., is its effect on the morphology of the fungus: manganese-deficient grown mycelia are strongly vacuolated, highly branched, contain strongly enthickened cell walls

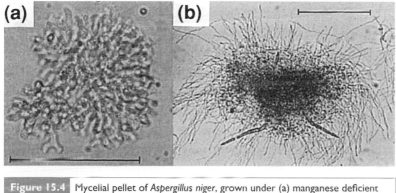

Figure 15.4 Mycelial pellet of *Aspergillus niger*, grown under (a) manganese deficient conditions and (b) manganese sufficient (0.1 mM) conditions. Marker bars indicate 50 (a) and 250 (b) μm. (Reproduced with permission from Roehr, M., Kubicek, C. P. and Kominek, J., 1996, Further organic acids. In *Biotechnology*, 2nd edition, Vol. 6: *Products of Primary Metabolism*, ed. M. Roehr. Weinheim: Verlag Chemie, pp. 364–379.)

and exhibit a bulbous appearance (Fig. 15.4). The attached reading list (Section 15.6) provides more detailed information on the existing literature in this area.

The influence of other metal ions on the accumulation of citric acids by *Aspergillus* spp. is even less clear: some workers have claimed a particularly strong influence of Fe^{3+}, which is, however, not supported by others.

pH

Citric acid accumulation has been reported to accumulate in significant amounts only when the pH is below 2.5. Because of the pK values for citric acid (3.1, 4.7 and 6.4), a pH of 1.8 is automatically reached when certain amounts of it accumulate in the medium in the absence of any other buffering agent and hence there is no problem in reaching this point. However, some carbon sources used (e.g. sugar beet molasses) contain a significant amount of several amino acids (particularly glutamate) which strongly buffer the medium between pH 4 and 5. The reason for the requirement of a low pH is that it prevents production of other acids like gluconic acid and oxalic acid. Glucose oxidase is induced by high concentrations of glucose and strong aeration in the presence of low concentrations of other nutrients, i.e. conditions which are otherwise typical for citric acid fermentation and will thus inevitably be formed during the starting phase of citric acid fermentation and convert a significant amount of glucose into gluconic acid. However, due to the extracellular location of the enzyme, it is directly susceptible to the external pH and will be inactivated once the pH decreases below 3.5. Also, some strains of *A. niger* accumulate oxalic acid at pH 6, which must be avoided because of its toxicity. Its formation has been attributed to the hydrolysis of oxaloacetate, but a possible involvement of the glyoxylic acid cycle under certain conditions has still not been completely ruled out. An *A. niger* mutant strain lacking both glucose oxidase and oxaloacetate hydrolase accumulated citric acid at pH 5 and, under these conditions, production is completely insensitive to manganese ions. However, in a medium at low pH, the mutant did not produce any citric acid when Mn^{2+} was added, indicating that the requirement for Mn^{2+} deficiency is related to specific conditions.

Another explanation suggested that the effect of pH may be related to the energetics of citrate biosynthesis by *A. niger*, as the exclusive operation of citric acid accumulation (as occurs during the idiophase of fermentation) yields 1 ATP and 3 NADH, whose turnover is limited by the absence of biosynthetic processes of equivalent capacity. Hence, while part of the NADH pool can be re-oxidised by the alternative, salicylhydroxamic acid (SHAM)–sensitive respiratory pathway described below, at a low external pH ATP will be consumed by the plasma-membrane-bound ATPase for maintainance of the pH gradient between the cytosol and the extracellular medium (see also p. 41).

Dissolved O_2 tension

Accumulation of high amounts of citric acid is dependent on strong aeration. A dissolved O_2 tension higher than that required for vegetative growth of *A. niger* is essential, and even sparging with pure O_2 is in use. Most recently, the use of oxygen vectors, such as 5% n-dodecane, for the improvement of citric acid production was reported. Sudden interruptions in the air supply on the other hand (as may occur with power failures) cause an irreversible impairment of citric acid production without any harmful effect on mycelial growth. The biochemical basis of the high dissolved O_2 tension appears to be the induction of an alternative respiratory pathway which is required for re-oxidation of the glycolytically produced NADH. This pathway allows the sites of energy conservation to be by-passed and thus decreases the energy yield of cells. Instead of the establishment of the chemical bonds for ATP, changes in the free enthalpy during alternative electron transport result in the release of heat. As a consequence, citric acid production requires extensive cooling, which accounts for a fair share of the production costs. The physiological function of this uncoupled respiration is thought to be the removal of the reducing equivalents in excess without concomitant ATP production.

Nitrogen

Nitrogen sources used in media for citric acid production have included ammonia salts, nitrates and the potential ammonia source, urea. No one material has been shown to be definitely superior to another, as long as it was guaranteed that the compounds did not increase the pH. It should be noted that the effect of nitrogen sources is mainly observed in chemically defined media, as no further nitrogen is necessary when beet molasses are used as carbon source. On the other hand, several authors have described that the exogenous addition of ammonium ions during citric acid fermentation even stimulates citrate production.

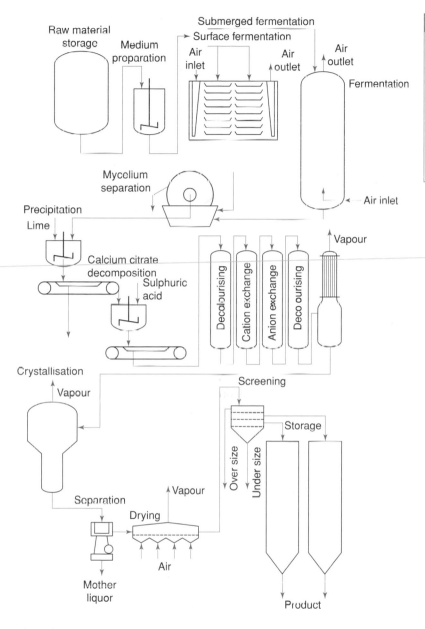

Figure 15.5 Flow-sheet of citric acid manufacture by surface or submerged process (Reproduced with permission from Roehr, M., Kubicek, C. P. and Kominek, J., 1992, Industrial acids and other small molecules. In *Aspergillus Biology and Industrial Applications*, eds. J. W. Bennett and M. A. Klich. Reading, MA: Butterworth-Heinemann, pp. 91–131.)

Phosphate

The concentration of the phosphate source is usually kept low in the media. Moreover, an appropriate balance of nitrogen, phosphate and trace metals appears to be important for the accumulation of citric acid in batch cultures.

15.2.3 Production processes for citric acid

Basically, there are two different types of fermentations carried out for the production of citric acid, e.g. the surface process and the submerged process (see Fig. 15.5). In addition, some citric acid is also produced, particularly in some East Asian countries, by solid-state

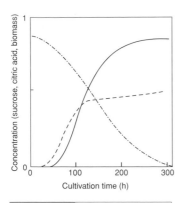

Figure 15.6 Time course of a typical industrial citric acid fermentation showing citric acid monohydrate (___), biomass (---), and sugar (-·-). Typically, in 250–280 hours, 8–12 g l^{-1} biomass dry wt and 110–115 g l^{-1} of citric acid are obtained from 140 g l^{-1} sucrose.

fermentation called the 'koji' process. The Japanese wheat bran process accounts for about 20% of the annual citric acid production in Japan. Similar processes, frequently on a relatively small scale, are also carried out in China and South East Asia. The process uses solids from potato starch processing or wheat bran, adjusted to a pH of 4–5 and with a water content of 70–80%. Addition of several materials such as α-amylase or the filter cake of a glutamic acid fermentation have proven beneficial. After 5–8 days, the koji is harvested and placed in percolators, and the citric acid is extracted with water. Further purification occurs by the same procedures as for the surface or submerged fermentation (see below).

Surface fermentation is the older and more labour-intensive version of citric acid fermentation, yet it is still in use, even by some major producers of citric acid. The main reasons for this are the lower power requirements and the higher reproducibility of the process due to its lower susceptibility to interference by trace metal ions and variations in the dissolved O_2 tension. The fermentation is usually carried out in aluminium trays, filled with nutrient medium to a depth of between 50 and 200 cm. Each tray holds about 100 litres of medium. Spores are distributed over the surface of the trays, and sterile air (serving both as an O_2 supply as well as a cooling aid) is passed over them. The mycelium develops as a coherent felt, becoming progressively more convoluted. A final yield of 0.7–0.9 g g^{-1} supplied sugar is obtained within a period of 7 to 15 days.

The submerged fermentation process is desirable because of its higher efficacy due to higher susceptibility to automatisation. Yet the severe influence of trace metal ions and other impurities present in the carbohydrate raw materials and the disturbance of the process by variations in O_2 supply make it more difficult to manage, particularly since the quality of the carbohydrate source is variable. There are two types of fermenters in use: stirred tanks and aerated tower fermenters. Both types are constructed of high-grade stainless steel and contain facilities for cooling. Sparging with O_2 occurs from the base.

One of the most prominent features of submerged fermentation is the mycelial development, which shows a characteristic pattern: the germinating spores form stubby, forked and bulbous hyphae, which aggregate to small (0.2–0.5 mm) pellets, which have a firm, smooth surface and sediment quickly when harvested (see Fig. 15.4). This striking morphology has been shown to be critical for attaining high yields by submerged fermentation and is dependent on an appropriate nutrient composition. It is therefore a convenient indicator for the progress of fermentation, e.g. by automated image analysis. A final yield of 0.8–0.9 kg kg^{-1} is obtained after 7 to 10 days (Fig. 15.6).

Citric acid production by yeast is exclusively done by submerged cultivation, and is carried out with either n-alkanes or glucose syrup as carbon sources. Various fractions of straight-chain paraffins (about C_9 to C_{20}) are preferred substrates. The pH should be kept above 5 and the P/C-ratio of the medium should be between 0.0001 and 0.002.

However, the world oil crisis in 1973/1974 almost entirely ended the exploitation of this process, because then sugars became the cheaper carbon source.

Recovery of citric acid from the surface process usually starts with filtration of the culture broth and thorough washing of the mycelial cake, which may trap up to 15% of the citric acid produced. Filtration of the mycelium from the submerged process often requires the use of filter aids due to the by-production of a slimy heteropolysaccharide, formed as a protective layer against shear stress caused by the impeller. In several cases, lime at pH 3 is added to the broth to precipitate any oxalic acid. Recovery of citric acid from the broth is then generally accomplished by three basic procedures: (1) precipitation, (2) extraction and (3) ion exchange adsorption. Several workers have also proposed solvent extraction, which makes use of various aliphatic alcohols, ketones, amines or phosphines. Obviously, the extractants require approval by the respective food and drug authorities. Crystallisation of citric acid is finally performed in vacuum crystallisers. Citric acid monohydrate, the main commercial product in Europe, is formed at temperatures below 36 °C, and citric acid anhydride is formed at higher temperatures.

15.2.4 Applications of citric acid

Due to its pleasant taste, low toxicity and excellent palatability, citric acid is widely used in industry for the preparation of food and sugar confectionery (21% of total production) and beverages (45%). Other major applications are in the pharmaceutical and detergent/cleaning industry (8 and 19%, respectively). It is also able to complex heavy metal ions, such as iron and copper, and therefore is applied in the stabilisation of oils and fats or ascorbic acid against metal ion-catalysed oxidation. It is useful as a buffer over a broad range of pH values. In addition, citric acid esters of a wide range of alcohols are known and can be employed as non-toxic plasticisers. Finally, some of its salts have commercial importance, e.g. trisodium citrate may be used as a blood preservative, which prevents blood clotting by complexing calcium, or as a stabiliser of emulsions in the manufacture of cheese.

Today, citric acid is produced in bulk amounts with an estimated worldwide production of 900 000 tonnes per year, most of which is produced by fermentation with A. niger. The bulk of production occurs in Western Europe (41%) and North America (28%).

15.3 | Gluconic acid

D-Glucono-δ-lactone, the simplest of the direct dehydrogenation products of D-glucose, and its free form – gluconic acid – are produced by a large variety of bacteria and fungi. The equilibrium of the lactone and the free acid in solution is dependent on pH and temperature.

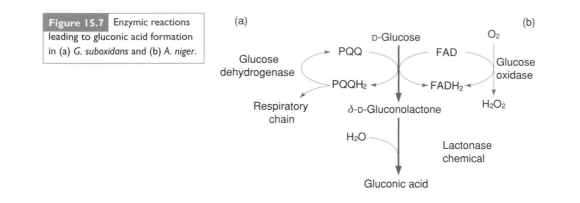

Figure 15.7 Enzymic reactions leading to gluconic acid formation in (a) *G. suboxidans* and (b) *A. niger*.

15.3.1 Biology, biochemistry and biotechnology of gluconic acid accumulation

Microbial accumulation of gluconic acid was first observed in cultures of acetic acid bacteria, and a bacterial parasite of olive trees, *Pseudomonas savastanoi*. With regard to fungi, gluconic acid formation by *A. niger* was observed in 1922. Subsequently, gluconic acid has been shown to be produced by several prokaryotic as well as eukaryotic micro-organisms, such as members of the bacterial genera *Pseudomonas, Vibrio, Acetobacter* and *Gluconobacter*, as well as species of the fungal genera *Aspergillus, Penicillium* and *Gliocladium*.

Bacterial gluconic acid formation mainly occurs by a membrane-bound D-glucose dehydrogenase, which uses PQQ (pyrroloquinoline quinone) as a coenzyme (Fig. 15.7a), and converts extracellular glucose into extracellular gluconic acid. Another enzyme, an intracellular NADP-dependent glucose dehydrogenase, does not seem to be involved in gluconic acid accumulation. Gluconic acid is not usually an end-product, but will normally be transported into the cell and be further catabolised via the reactions of the pentose phosphate pathway. However, the pentose phosphate pathway is repressed by extracellular glucose concentrations >15 mM and a pH below 3.5 (the latter also prevents the formation of 2-oxogluconate), and gluconic acid is therefore accumulated when these conditions are applied.

Gluconic acid formation in fungi is a two-step process involving oxidation of β-D-glucose to D-glucono-δ-lactone by glucose oxidase and the subsequent hydrolysis of the lactone to gluconic acid, which can be either spontaneous or catalysed by lactonase. Glucose oxidase is extracellular, i.e. partially cell-wall bound in *Penicillium* spp., but is secreted into the medium by *Aspergillus* spp. Glucose oxidase is a tetrameric, glycosylated flavoprotein, which uses O_2 in its reaction (Fig. 15.7b). The enzyme is most actively induced by high glucose concentrations, high aeration and at a pH above 4. In *A. niger*, glucose oxidase, lactonase and two of the catalases are induced by H_2O_2 in a coordinated way, probably mediated by the product of the regulatory gene, *goxB*. The requirement for a relatively neutral pH is caused by the fact that glucose oxidase is inactivated at pH values below 3 (see Section 15.2.1) and hence not induced since no H_2O_2 is formed. Physiologically, glucose oxidase formation may be involved in the antagonistic reaction of A. niger against other micro-organisms, resulting in glucose withdrawal and formation of hydrogen peroxide. To protect itself against the arising hydrogen peroxide, A. niger also secretes multiple forms of catalase.

15.3.2 Fermentation processes for production of gluconic acid

Several processes for the production of gluconic acid have been developed, almost all of which use either A. niger or Gluconobacter oxidans as producer organisms.

Gluconic acid production with A. niger was developed in the 1930s and is traditionally achieved by the calcium gluconate process. This name stems from the use of calcium carbonate for neutralisation of the fermentation broth; unless carried out, the decrease in pH would inactivate glucose oxidase and hence stop gluconic acid accumulation. The production medium contains up to 120–150 g glucose l^{-1} (most frequently derived from corn); further increases in the glucose concentration are hampered by the limited solubility of calcium gluconate, which would precipitate on the mycelia and inhibit both O_2 and substrate uptake by the fungus. Other components of the nutrient medium – particularly salts to supply phosphorus and nitrogen – are added in limiting amounts in order to restrict growth of the fungus. Contrary to citric acid production, glucose oxidase formation and thus a high-yield gluconic acid fermentation requires the presence of a relatively high concentration of manganese ions. Application of increased O_2 pressure has been shown to be advantageous, which is easily understandable by considering the stoichiometry of the reaction (see Fig. 15.7b). Fermentations with almost quantitative yields (corresponding to >90% on a molar basis) are usually completed in less than 24 h.

The sodium gluconate process has been used as a superior alternative to the calcium gluconate process as it enables the fermentation of even higher glucose concentrations (up to 350 g l^{-1}). In this process, the pH is maintained close to pH 6.5 by the addition of NaOH. In other respects, the process is similar to the calcium gluconate process. This process has been employed for the development of continuous fermentations in Japan, which claimed the conversion of 35% (w/v) glucose solutions with 95% yield. In addition, a continuous production employing the osmotolerant yeast *Aureobasidium pullulans* was also described, with the advantage of having extremely high (>350 g l^{-1}) glucose concentrations in the medium.

Several different bacterial gluconic acid fermentation processes have been described but only a few of them are actually performed on an industrial scale. As already mentioned, a high glucose concentration (>15%, w/v) and a pH below 3.5 are necessary for high yields. Several workers have also shown the possibility of using immobilised cells for gluconic acid production.

Methods for product recovery are similar for both fungal and bacterial fermentations but depend on the type of carbon source used and the method of broth neutralisation. Calcium gluconate is precipitated from hyper-saturated solutions in the cold and is subsequently released by adding stoichiometric amounts of sulphuric acid. By repetition of this step, the clear liquid is concentrated to a 50% (w/v) solution of gluconic acid. Sodium gluconate is precipitated by concentration to a 45% (w/v) solution and raising the pH to 7.5. Today, sodium gluconate is the main manufactured form of gluconic acid and, hence, free gluconic acid and δ-gluconolactone are prepared from it by ion exchange. As gluconic acid and its lactone are in a pH- and temperature-dependent equilibrium, either or both can be prepared by appropriate adjustment of these two conditions.

15.3.3 Commercial applications of gluconic acid

Gluconic acid is characterised by an extremely low toxicity, low corrosivity and the ability to form water-soluble complexes with a variety of di- and trivalent metal ions. Gluconic acid is thus exceptionally well suited for use in removing calcareous and rust deposits from metals or other surfaces, including milk or beer scale on galvanised iron or stainless steel. Because of its physiological properties it is used as an additive in the food, beverage and pharmaceutical industries, where it is the preferred carrier used in calcium and iron therapy. In several food-directed applications, gluconic acid 1,5-lactone is advantageous over gluconic acid or gluconate because it enables acidic conditions to be reached gradually over a longer period, e.g. in the preparation of pickled goods, curing fresh sausages or leavening during baking. Mixtures of gelatin and sodium gluconate are used as sizing agents in the paper industry. Textile manufacturers employ gluconate for de-sizing polyester or polyamide fabrics. Concrete manufacturers use 0.02–0.2% sodium gluconate to produce concrete highly resistant to frost and cracking. In pharmacy it is used as a counterion in iron and calcium salts for therapy of deficiencies for these metals. According to recent estimates, its annual worldwide production is >60 000 tonnes.

15.4 | Lactic acid

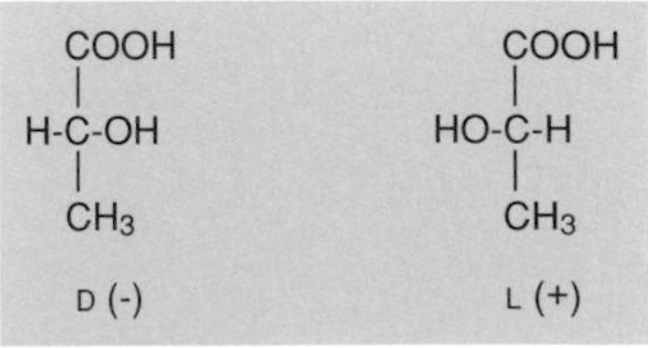

Figure 15.8 D (−) and L (+) lactic acids.

Lactic acid (Fig. 15.8) was first isolated from sour milk in 1798 by Scheele, and subsequently shown to occur in two isomeric forms, i.e. L (+) and D (−) isomers, and as a racemic mixture of these. The capital letters prefixed to the names indicate configuration in relation to isomers of glyceraldehyde, and the (+) and (−) symbols indicate the direction of rotation of a plane of polarised light. The mixture of isomers – the racemate – is called D,L-lactic acid. [The strict, and more recent, chemical nomenclature of these two stereoisomers is

S- and R-lactic acid for the L and D forms, respectively. However, most biologists (and biotechnologists) continue to use the older system.

15.4.1 Production organisms and biochemical pathways

Lactic acid was the first organic acid to be manufactured industrially by fermentation (1881, Littletown, Massachusetts, USA). Lactic acid bacteria are acid-tolerant, facultative anaerobic micro-organisms. Traditionally, they are functionally classified into hetero- and homofermentative bacteria, each of which in turn can be divided according to their coccoid or rod-shaped form.

Homofermentative lactic acid bacteria produce almost exclusively lactic acid as the end-product of glucose catabolism, while heterofermentative bacteria, in addition to lactic acid, also form considerable amounts of acetic acid, formic acid and ethanol. Most heterofermentative strains lack aldolase activity, resulting in an increased flux via the hexose monophosphate pathway during glucose catabolism (see Chapter 2). In contrast, glucose catabolism in homofermentative strains occurs by an intact glycolytic hexose bisphosphate pathway and subsequent regeneration of the gained NADH by reduction of pyruvate. However, under growth conditions in which the glycolytic flux is low, the homolactic behaviour is lost and increased amounts of other metabolites (see above) are produced. Theoretically, 2 mol. lactic acid can be formed from 1 mol. hexose, resulting in a theoretical yield of 1 kg lactic acid kg^{-1} hexose. For practical reasons, however, highest yields are in the range of 90–92%.

Application of molecular genetic techniques to determine the relatedness of food-associated lactic acid bacteria has resulted in significant changes in their taxonomic classification. The lactic acid bacteria associated with foods now include species of the genera *Carnobacterium*, *Enterococcus*, *Lactobacillus*, *Lactococcus*, *Leuconostoc*, *Oenococcus*, *Pediococcus*, *Streptococcus*, *Tetragenococcus*, *Vagococcus* and *Weisella*. The genus *Lactobacillus* remains heterogeneous with over 60 species, of which one-third are heterofermentative. Heterofermentative lactic acid bacteria are involved in most of the typical fermentations leading to food or feed preservation and transformation, whereas the homofermentative bacteria are used for bulk lactic acid production. Generally, strains operating at a higher temperature (45–62 °C) are preferred to the latter, as this reduces the power requirements needed for medium sterilisation. *Lactobacillus* spp. (e.g. *L. delbrueckii*) are used with glucose as the carbon source, whereas *L. delbrueckii* spp. *bulgaricus* and *L. helveticus* are used with lactose-containing media (whey). *Lactobacillus delbrueckii* spp. *lactis* can ferment maltose, whereas *L. amylophilus* can even ferment starch.

Most lactic-acid-producing micro-organisms produce only one isomer of lactic acid; however, some bacteria, which unfortunately can occur as infections during lactic acid fermentations, are known to contain racemates and are thus able to convert one isomeric form into the other.

In addition to lactic acid bacteria, other micro-organisms can produce lactic acid, e.g. *Rhizopus nigricans* and *Bacillus coagulans*. These organisms are not used for commercial purposes, however.

15.4.2 Lactic acid production

Although the molecular genetics of lactic acid bacteria are well advanced, strain selection is still carried out in traditional ways. Besides high yields of lactic acid, industrial strains are selected particularly for acid tolerance and phage insensitivity.

Raw materials used should meet certain criteria of purity as this strongly aids the final purification procedure of lactic acid, but this depends on the quality of the brand to be manufactured. As lactic acid has a very low selling price, appropriate selection of the carbon source is an important point. Materials frequently used include glucose syrups (e.g. derived from starch hydrolysis), maltose-containing materials, sucrose (e.g. from molasses) or lactose (whey).

Lactic acid is classically produced as its calcium salt. Most fermentation protocols in use today are only slight modifications of those developed in the early 1950s. They are carried out in reactor volumes up to 100 m^3, using the carbon source between 120 and 180 g l^{-1}, and appropriate concentrations of nitrogen- and phosphate-containing salts and micronutrients. As lactic acid bacteria display complex nutrient requirements for B-vitamins and some amino acids, appropriate supplements (crude vegetable materials, such as malt sprouts) have to be added. Fermentations are run at 45 °C with gentle stirring (lactic acid bacteria are anaerobic organisms and the introduction of O_2 therefore has to be avoided). The pH is maintained between 5.5 and 6.0 by the addition of sterile calcium carbonate. As an alternative to neutralisation with calcium carbonate, ammonia can be used, which also aids in the recovery of lactic acid by esterification (see below), but this results in a more expensive process. Due to the corrosive properties of lactic acid, wood or concrete were used as materials for the construction of the fermenters in the past. Today, however, stainless steel is used in the majority of cases, particularly at larger production volumes. Conversion yields of 85–95% of the theoretical maximum are usually obtained after 4–6 days.

Process variants using continuous cultivation or immobilised cells have been described in the research literature, but as yet industrial applications have not been realised.

Several techniques to purify lactic acid have been developed which are necessary to satisfy the different purity requirements. It is very important that the residual sugar concentration has dropped to below 0.1% (w/v) when higher purity lactic acid is to be obtained. A standard procedure for recovery from rather pure nutrient media is given in Fig. 15.9. Broths from the fermentation of lower quality raw materials require even more extensive purification steps, including pre-purification by filtering the hot calcium lactate solution, and its repeated recrystallisation. Alternatives used are solvent extraction (e.g. using isopropyl ether, 2-butanol or trialkyl tertiary amines in

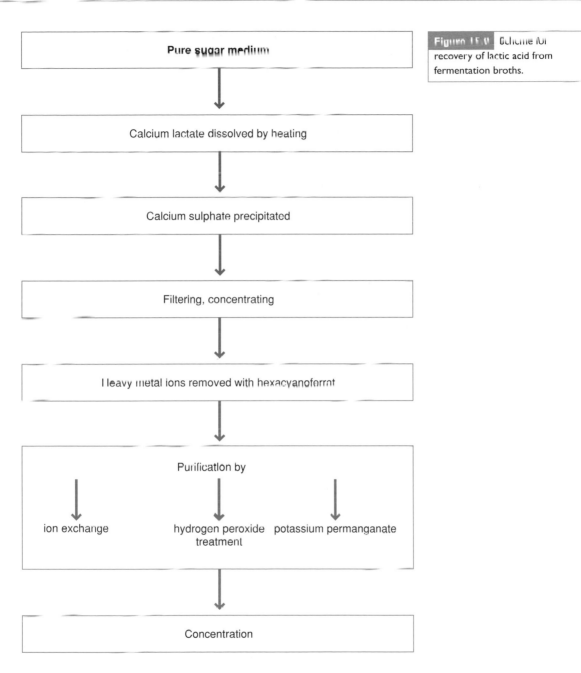

Pure sugar medium

↓

Calcium lactate dissolved by heating

↓

Calcium sulphate precipitated

↓

Filtering, concentrating

↓

Heavy metal ions removed with hexacyanoferrat

↓

Purification by

ion exchange   hydrogen peroxide   potassium permanganate
               treatment

↓

Concentration

Figure 15.9 Scheme for recovery of lactic acid from fermentation broths.

organic solvents), or esterification with methanol and subsequent distillation.

15.4.3 Applications

Lactic acid is a highly hygroscopic, syrupy liquid and is technically available in various grades, i.e. technical grade, food grade, pharmacopoeia grade and plastic grade. The properties of these grades and their respective applications are given in Table 15.4. Recent estimates of the current market volume of lactic acid are around $50\,000\ \text{t}\,\text{a}^{-1}$,

Table 15.4 Commercial grades of lactic acid and their uses

Quality	Property	Application
Technical grade	Light brown colour Iron free 20–80% lactic acid	Deliming hides, textile industry, ester manufacture
Food grade	Colourless, odourless >80% lactic acid	Food additive, acidulant, production of sour flour and dough
Pharmacopoeia grade	Colourless, odourless >90% lactic acid <0.1% ash	Intestine treatment, hygienic preparations, metal ion lactates
Plastic grade	Colourless <0.01% ash	Lacquers, varnishes, biodegradable polymers

70% of which is from fermentation, and the remainder from chemical manufacture.

15.5 | Other acids

In addition to citric acid, gluconic acid and lactic acid, a number of other acids are commercially produced by fermentation in minor amounts.

15.5.1 Itaconic acid

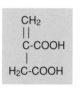

Figure 15.10 Itaconic acid.

Itaconic acid (methylene succinic acid, Fig. 15.10) was originally known as a product of pyrolytic distillation of citric acid. In the 1940s, it was found that this acid could be produced by fermentation using *Aspergillus terreus*. Chemically, itaconic acid is a structurally substituted methacrylic acid. Because of its slight toxicity, it is mainly used in the manufacture of styrene butadiene co-polymers but it has to compete with similar petrochemistry derived products that are cheaper, but not as effective, in producing the right polymers.

Commercially, itaconic acid is produced by a submerged fermentation process employing strains of *A. terreus* or *A. itaconicus*. The biochemistry of its formation occurs by reactions similar to that involved in the accumulation of citric acid, e.g. carbon catabolism via the glycolytic pathway and anaplerotic formation of oxaloacetate by CO_2 fixation (Fig. 15.11). In addition – and in contrast to *A. niger* – *A. terreus* contains an additional enzyme, aconitate decarboxylase, which forms itaconate from *cis*-aconitate. As this reaction is localised in the cytosol, and because citrate synthase and aconitase are localised in the mitochondria, it has been implied that *A. terreus* transports *cis*-aconitate, rather than citrate, in exchange with malate out of the mitochondria (Fig. 15.11). Analogous to the presumed citrate exporter in *A. niger*, *A. terreus* probably has a transport protein capable of excreting itaconic acid. During fermentation, itaconic acid formation is also accompanied by varying amounts of succinic, citramalic and itatartaric acid. Data currently available suggest that these are not

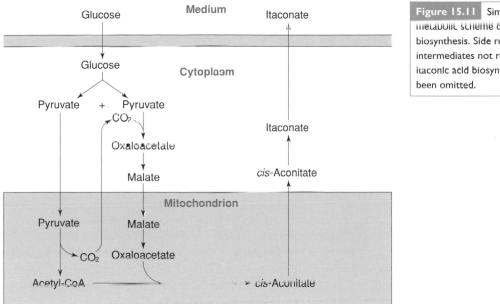

Figure 15.11 Simplified metabolic scheme of itaconic acid biosynthesis. Side reactions and intermediates not relevant to itaconic acid biosynthesis have been omitted.

degradation products of itaconic acid but rather are formed by other pathways.

The fermentation production of itaconic acid is largely similar to that of citric acid, i.e. it requires an excess of an easily metabolisable carbon source (glucose syrup, crude starch hydrolysates, molasses), high dissolved O_2 tensions, and a limitation in metal ions by the aid of complexation and/or precipitation with ferric hexacyanoferrate (Prussian blue) or addition of copper (see Section 15.2.2). Growth is usually restricted by phosphate limitation. However, no data are available on the Mn^{2+} effect. The effect of pH is also different: several workers reported that the pH has to be maintained between 2.8 and 3.1, and lower pH values favour the formation of the by-product itatartaric acid. Yields of 85% (w/w) of the theoretical maximum have been reported to be obtained within 5 days of cultivation at rather high temperatures (39–42 °C). Promising attempts for the production of itaconic acid by immobilised biomass was also reported.

Recovery is usually performed by evaporation, active carbon treatment followed by crystallisation/recrystallisation. Itaconic acid is sold in two grades: refined, which is a pale tan to white crystalline solid, and industrial grade, which is darker in colour. The main potential for the utilisation of itaconic acid is the manufacture of styrene butadiene co-polymers, and for lattices and paint emulsions, to improve adhesion of the polymer. Due to its acid groups, the resulting heteropolymers have hydrophilic properties. Itaconic acid is also added in small (<2%) amounts to vinylidene chloride coatings where it leads to improved adhesion to paper, cellophane and poly(ethylene terephthalate) films in packaging and photography.

The total market size is approximately $15\,000\ \mathrm{t\,a^{-1}}$. While the demand for substitution of acrylic or methacrylic acid in polymers is

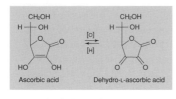

Figure 15.12 L-Ascorbic acid in equilibrium with dehydro-L-ascorbic acid. [O] means oxidation, [H] reduction.

high and the potential market for itaconic acid is growing, expansion of the market is only possible by reduction of production costs, which currently yields a price of approximately US$ 4 kg^{-1}.

15.5.2 L-Ascorbic acid (vitamin C)

Ascorbic acid is the official IUPAC designation for vitamin C. It was discovered as an extract from peppers in 1928 by Szent-Györgyi. Its most significant characteristic is the reversible oxidation to dehydro-L-ascorbic acid (Fig. 15.12), with which it forms a redox system. A number of enzymes are stimulated by ascorbic acid, notably iron-containing dioxygenases and copper-containing monooxygenases. One of the best known symptoms of ascorbic acid deficiency – scurvy – can be explained by the malfunctioning of these oxidases required for collagen biosynthesis. However, ascorbic acid also protects the body against formation of carcinogenic nitrosamines and oxygen radicals, and has essential functions in iron uptake. These properties, together with its nutritional qualities and low toxicity, are the main reasons for the numerous applications of vitamin C in the food and pharmaceutical industries.

Commercially, ascorbic acid is mainly produced by a combination of five synthetic organic chemical and one biotransformation steps, known collectively as Reichstein synthesis. Its basic principle is reduction of C-1 of D-glucose, and oxidation at C-5 and C-6, while simultaneously preserving the chirality at C-2 and C-3. The classical scheme is shown in Fig. 15.13. The microbially catalysed step is the oxidation of D-sorbitol to L-sorbose, which is carried out by *Acetobacter xylinum*. Large-scale fermentations occur at 30–35 °C and pH 4–6. All six steps of Reichstein's synthesis generally have a yield of >90%, and thus the final yield of ascorbic acid is about 60%. Estimates of current industrial production are at 80 000 t a^{-1} with a global market of over US$ 600 million with an annual growth rate of 3–4%. The bulk of this amount is produced as free ascorbic acid.

There have been several attempts to produce ascorbic acid directly by fermentation but none of these has so far advanced to a commercial process. Microalgae of the genus *Chlorella* can directly form L-ascorbic acid from D-glucose, although at very low yield. Their ascorbic-acid-enriched biomass is currently used as an aquaculture fish feed or additive.

As a consequence, despite being energy consuming, requiring high temperatures and pressures for several steps and involving considerable quantities of organic and inorganic solvents with huge waste disposal costs, no alternative to the Reichstein synthesis has been established yet. However, there have been several trials to reduce the number of organic chemical synthetic steps by microbially producing more appropriate starting substances. The most successful ones are shown in Fig. 15.13: one possibility is the fermentative production of 2-keto-L-gulonic acid from L-sorbose with *Bacillus megaterium* or *Pseudogluconobacter saccharoketogenes*. Yields are in the range of 75–90% and

Table 15.5 Other organic acids, for which microbial production is possible

Acid	Producer	Potential application
Tartaric acid	*Gluconobacter oxydans*	Beverages, drug uses
Fumaric acid	*Rhizopus nigricans*	Polyester manufacture
	R. arrhizus	L-Aspartate manufacture
Malic acid	*Aspergillus wentii*	Beverages, flavour
trans-2,3-Epoxysuccinic acid	*Paecilomyces* spp.	β-Lactam precursor
	A. fumigatus	
	A. clavatus	
Succinic acid	*A. niger*	
Kojic acid	*A. oryzae*	Cosmetics, insecticides
Gallic acid	*A. wentii*	Blue pigments

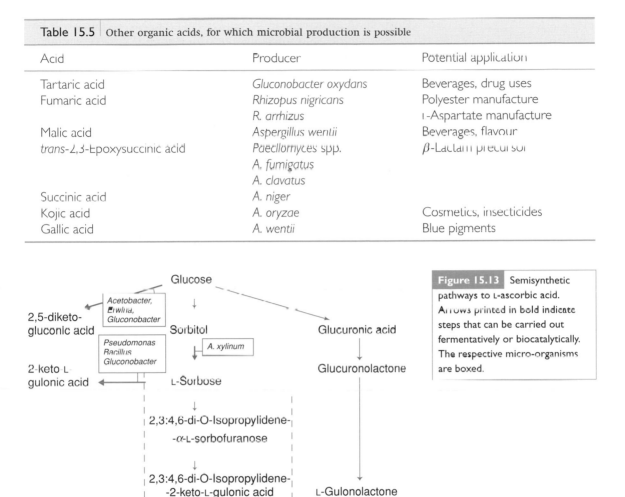

Figure 15.13 Semisynthetic pathways to L-ascorbic acid. Arrows printed in bold indicate steps that can be carried out fermentatively or biocatalytically. The respective micro-organisms are boxed.

will therefore, once scaled up, enable a cheaper production route to L-ascorbic acid.

A promising continuous biocatalytic system for the synthesis of Reichstein intermediates is based on glucose first being converted to gluconate via an NADP-dependent glucose dehydrogenase from *Thermoplasma acidophilum*. Further conversion to 2,5-diketo-D-gluconate is achieved using cell preparations containing membrane-bound gluconate/2-keto-D-gluconate dehydrogenase and the cytochrome C cofactor. Finally, 2,5-diketo-D-gluconate is converted to 2-keto-L-gulonate by a NADPH dependent 2,5 diketo D gluconate reductase with resultant regeneration of $NADP^+$ by gluconate dehydrogenase.

Another very short, mostly biocatalytic pathway to ascorbic acid would be possible via L-gulonolactone, which can be directly converted to ascorbic acid by L-gulonolactone dehydrogenase. While L-gulonolactone is readily obtained by chemical hydrogenation of D-glucuronolactone, the latter can be obtained from glucose or starch only in low yields.

15.5.3   Other acids

A small number of other tricarboxylic acid cycle-related acids can be produced in commercially attractive amounts; none of which, however, has so far received industrial practice. They are shown in Table 15.5. Some of these, such as fumaric acid, have in the past been produced by fermentation on an industrial scale, but are currently unable to compete with the chemical productions.

15.6 | Further reading

Cocain-Bousquet, M., Even, S., Lindley, N. D. and Loubiere, P. Anaerobic sugar catabolism in *Lactococcus lactis*: genetic regulation and enzyme control over pathway flux. *Applied Microbiology and Biotechnology* **60**: 24–32, 2002.

Hancock, R. D. and Viola, R. Biotechnological approaches for L-ascorbic acid production. *Trends in Biotechnology* **20**: 299–305, 2002.

Karaffa, L. and Kubicek, C. P. *Aspergillus niger* citric acid accumulation: do we understand this well-working black box? *Applied Microbiology and Biotechnology* **61**: 189–196, 2003.

Kascak, K., Kominek, J. and Roehr, M. Lactic acid. In *Biotechnology*, 2nd edition, Vol. 6, *Products of Primary Metabolism*, ed. M. Roehr. Weinheim: Verlag Chemie, pp. 294–306, 1996.

Roehr, M., Kubicek, C. P. and Kominek, J. Citric acid. In *Biotechnology*, 2nd edition, Vol. 6, *Products of Primary Metabolism*, ed. M. Roehr. Weinheim: Verlag Chemie, pp. 308–345, 1996.

Roehr, M., Kubicek, C. P. and Kominek, J. Further organic acids. In *Biotechnology*, second edition, Vol. 6, *Products of Primary Metabolism*, ed. M. Roehr. Weinheim: Verlag Chemie, pp. 364–379, 1996.

Roehr, M., Kubicek, C. P. and Kominek, J. Gluconic acid. In *Biotechnology*, second edition, Vol. 6, *Products of Primary Metabolism*, ed. M. Roehr. Weinheim: Verlag Chemie, pp. 347–362, 1996.

Roehr, M., Kubicek, C. P. and Kominek, J. Industrial acids and other small molecules. In *Aspergillus: Biology and Industrial Applications*, eds. J. W. Bennett and M. A. Klich. Reading, MA: Butterworth-Heinemann, pp. 91–131, 1992.

Stiles, M. E. and Holzapfel, W. H. Lactic acid bacteria in food and their current taxonomy. *International Journal of Food Microbiology* **36**: 1–29, 1997.

Willke, T. and Vorlop, K. D. Biotechnological production of itaconic acid. *Applied Microbiology and Biotechnology* **56**: 289–295, 2001.

Chapter 16

Microbial polysaccharides and single cell oils

James P. Wynn
Martek Biosciences Corp., USA

Alistair J. Anderson
University of Hill, UK

16.1 Introduction

When micro-organisms are provided with a surplus of glucose, or another source of carbon and energy, they may produce one or more intracellular storage compounds that will then be usable by the microorganism should it subsequently face deprivation of a carbon source, i.e. starvation. Some yeasts, fungi and a few microalgae accumulate large amounts of oil, or lipids. Bacteria more commonly accumulate a polymer known as polyhydroxyalkanoate (PHA). Both types of storage compound can be seen (under the microscope) as forming distinct inclusions within the cells. Concentrations of them can reach 70%, or even more, of the cell dry weight in certain species. Glycogen (a polymer of glucose that is sometimes referred to as bacterial starch) and trehalose (a disaccharide) are other well known examples of microbial storage compounds. Some microorganisms may, instead of producing PHA or lipids, synthesise large amounts of polysaccharides – the amounts are often so large that they are excreted from the cells and, in contrast to the other storage compounds, are thus extracellular.

The synthesis of all these products is promoted when growth is restricted by the availability of an essential nutrient other than

Basic Biotechnology, third edition, eds. Colin Ratledge and Bjørn Kristiansen.
Published by Cambridge University Press. © Cambridge University Press 2006.

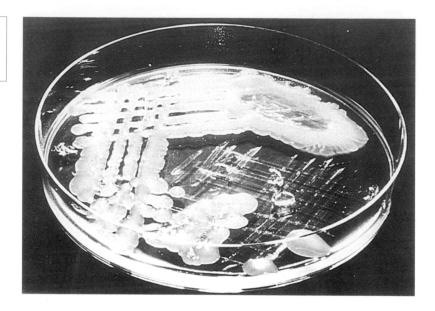

Figure 16.1 An alginate-producing strain of *Pseudomonas mendocina* growing on agar.

carbon. Usually nitrogen is chosen as the limiting nutrient. Thus when the cells run out of nitrogen they still continue to assimilate the carbon source but, because cell growth can no longer occur as nitrogen is essential for protein and nucleic acid synthesis, this incoming carbon is channelled into a storage compound. The choice of which storage compound is produced is, of course, entirely dependent upon the genetic make-up of the organism.

In this chapter, we have focused our attention on those microbial storage products of commercial (biotechnological) value. This means that, unlike our chapter in the previous second edition of this book, we no longer cover the production of polyhydroxyalkanoates, as commercial interest in these materials has considerably diminished. Polysaccharides and oils, though, continue to be biotechnologically important materials.

16.2 | Microbial polysaccharides

16.2.1 Introduction

Many micro-organisms produce substantial amounts of polysaccharide when surplus carbon source is available. Some of these polysaccharides accumulate within the cell and act as storage compounds, glycogen being a well-known example. Other polysaccharides, known as *exopolysaccharides* (EPS), are excreted by the cell and are generally the microbial polysaccharides of commercial interest. They may remain associated with the cell, as a capsule or slime, or simply dissolved in the medium. This depends on various factors, including the chemical structure of the polysaccharide and how vigorously the culture is agitated. On solid media, large slimy colonies may be produced (Fig. 16.1).

While some microbial exopolysaccharides, or *gums* as they are generally known in industry, are well established as commercial products, they must compete with plant polysaccharides, some of which are manufactured on a vast scale and at a low price. Production of microbial exopolysaccharides by fermentation can continue throughout the year, unlike production of plant polysaccharides, and fermentation, if carefully controlled, can yield a very consistent and reliable product. However, fermentation is a relatively costly process, which is not ideally suited to the manufacture of cheap products, even at high volume.

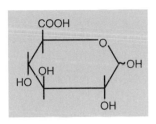

Figure 16.2 Structure of glucuronic acid, which is commonly found in microbial exopolysaccharides.

16.2.2 General properties

Microbial polysaccharides are, like plant and seaweed polysaccharides, of value because they can be used to modify the rheology (i.e. flow characteristics) of solutions. They increase viscosity and are commonly used as thickening, gelling and suspending agents.

Some polysaccharides, such as dextran and scleroglucan, are *neutral* and lack ionisable groups. Others, such as xanthan and gellan, are *acidic*. Acidic polysaccharides, which are of greater industrial importance, are polyelectrolytes, and possess carboxyl groups from uronic acids, such as glucuronic acid (Fig. 16.2) and/or pyruvate residues.

The conformation (shape) of polysaccharide molecules in solution is affected by the ionic strength (salt concentration), pH and the concentration of the polysaccharide. The acidic polysaccharides are generally more affected by the presence of cations in solution. Divalent cations can cross-link polysaccharide chains to produce a strong gel.

16.2.3 Xanthan

Xanthan is produced by the Gram-negative bacterium, *Xanthomonas campestris*. It is the best-studied and most widely used exopolysaccharide. Xanthan is a large polymer, having an M_r in excess of 10^6 daltons. It is a branched polymer with a β-(1→4)-linked glucan (i.e. polymer of glucose) backbone with a trisaccharide side chain on alternate glucose residues (Fig. 16.3). The pyruvate and acetate content depend on the bacterial strain, culture conditions and processing of the polymer. These substituents do not have a great influence on the properties of the polymer.

Xanthan is a polyelectrolyte due to the glucuronic acid residues in the side chains. Despite being an acidic polysaccharide, the viscosity of xanthan is relatively independent of the salt concentration.

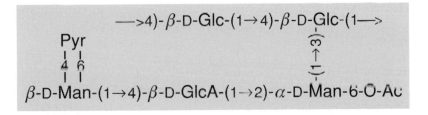

Figure 16.3 The structure of xanthan. The extent of acetylation of the mannose unit adjacent to the backbone is commonly 30%, but can be significantly lower or higher.

—>6)-α-D-Glc-(1—>

—>2)-α-D-Glc-(1—>

—>3)-α-D-Glc-(1—>

—>4)-α-D-Glc-(1—>

Figure 16.4 Structure of dextran. The predominant linkage is α-(1→6).

Xanthan is the most important commercial microbial polysaccharide, and current production is around 20 000 t a^{-1}. Kelco, now part of Monsanto, is the principal manufacturer. Xanthan was first used in 1967 and approved for food use in the USA in 1969. It is widely used for stabilisation, suspension, gelling and viscosity control in the food industry. These properties are also exploited for water-based paints and a wide variety of other domestic and industrial applications. Crude xanthan is employed as a suspending and lubricating agent in drilling muds used by the oil industry.

16.2.4   Dextran

Dextran (Fig. 16.4) is an α-glucan containing various linkages, depending on the producing organism. It is produced by a wide variety of Gram-positive and Gram-negative bacteria, including *Leuconostoc mesenteroides* and *Streptococcus* species.

Unlike most exopolysaccharides, which are synthesised within the cell, dextran is produced from sucrose by an extracellular enzyme, dextransucrase, which acts on sucrose polymerising the glucose units and liberating free fructose into the medium.

The properties of dextrans are manipulated by hydrolysis of the solvent-precipitated polymer using *exo-* or *endo-*dextranases or mild acid treatment, to generate a product with the desired molecular weight range. Dextran was the first commercial microbial polysaccharide and has been manufactured by Pharmacia for almost 50 years. It was first used as a blood plasma extender. Dextrans now have many clinical applications, including the prevention of thrombosis and use in wound dressings to absorb fluid. Sephadex remains a well-known gel filtration medium and dextrans now have many other laboratory applications. Dextrans are also used in foodstuffs.

16.2.5   Gellan

Gellan (Fig. 16.5) is a linear heteropolysaccharide whose repeating unit contains two glucose, one glucuronic acid and one rhamnose residue. Gellan is an acidic gel-forming polysaccharide produced by *Pseudomonas elodea*. It was developed by Kelco Inc., USA, as *Gelrite* by deacetylation of native gellan gum (by heating at pH 10), which is partially *O*-acetylated on one of the two glucose residues. The deacetylated product forms firm, brittle gels, which have the potential to replace agar and carrageenan. Gellan offers various advantages over agar for microbiological applications: it is resistant to enzymatic degradation and has a high gel strength at low concentration. Gel formation is influenced by temperature and the presence of cations

—>3)-β-D-*Glc-(1→4)-β-D-GlcA-(1→4)-β-D-Glc-(1→4)-α-L-Rha-(1—>

Figure 16.5 Structure of gellan.*This glucose carries *O*-acetyl and glyceryl residues in the native polymer.

...u) β-D-Glc-(1→3)-β-D-Glc-(1→3)-β-D-Glc-(1→
$$\uparrow$$
$$(1→6)$$
$$|$$
β-D-Glc

Figure 16.6 Structure of scleroglucan.

——>3)-β-D-Glc-(1——>

Figure 16.7 Structure of curdlan.

and the polymer undergoes a coil to double helix transition upon gel formation.

Gellan is approved for use in food and is widely used, at low concentrations, as a thickener.

16.2.6 Scleroglucan

Scleroglucan (Fig. 16.6) is a neutral polysaccharide with a 1→3-β-glucan backbone and branches consisting of a single glucose residue attached in an apparently regular sequence to every third glucose unit in the polymer chain.

Scleroglucan is a fungal exopolysaccharide, and is produced by various *Sclerotium* species. *Sclerotium rolfsii* and *Sclerotium glucanicum* are the most important species for commercial production of scleroglucan.

Scleroglucan is a soluble polysaccharide and is pseudoplastic over a broad pH and temperature range, and is unaffected by various salts. It is used to stabilise drilling muds, latex paints, printing inks and seed coatings.

16.2.7 Curdlan

Curdlan (Fig. 16.7) is a 1→3-β-glucan produced as an exopolysaccharide by *Alcaligenes faecalis* var. *myxogenes*. Similar polysaccharides are produced by *Agrobacterium radiobacter* and *A. rhizogenes*, and *Rhizobium trifolii*.

Unlike scleroglucan, curdlan is insoluble in water and forms a strong gel on heating above 55 °C and this gel formation is irreversible. Curdlan can be used as a gelling agent in cooked foods and as a support for immobilised enzymes. The properties of curdlan resemble those of the 1→3-β-glucan, laminarin, which is found in many brown algae.

16.2.8 Pullulan

Pullulan (Fig. 16.8) is an α-glucan with a trisaccharide repeating unit. It is produced commercially using the fungus *Aureobasideum*

——>6)-α-D-Glc-(1→4)-α-D-Glc-(1→4)-α-D-Glc-(1——>

Figure 16.8 Structure of pullulan.

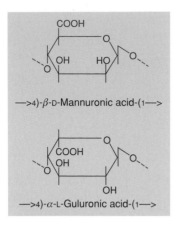

—>4)-β-D-Mannuronic acid-(1—>

—>4)-α-L-Guluronic acid-(1—>

Figure 16.9 Alginate is composed of mannuronic acid and guluronic acid. The proportions and sequence of these monomers depend on the source of the polymer.

pullulans. The fermentation is relatively slow (5 days) compared with the production of bacterial exopolysaccharides but 70% of the substrate (glucose) is converted to polysaccharide.

Pullulan forms strong, resilient films and fibres, and can be moulded. The films have a lower permeability to O_2 than cellophane or polypropylene and, being a natural product, the pullulan is biodegradable. Similar polymers are produced by some bacteria.

16.2.9   Alginate

Alginate is a linear polymer composed of mannuronic and guluronic acids (Fig. 16.9). It is produced by the Gram-negative bacteria *Azotobacter vinelandii* and *Pseudomonas* species. The bacterial exopolysaccharide is similar to algal (seaweed) alginate, except that some of the mannuronic acid residues are *O*-acetylated.

The relative abundance of mannuronic and guluronic acids and the degree of acetylation depends on the organism and growth conditions. Polymers containing a high mannuronic acid content are elastic gels, whereas those with a high guluronic acid content adopt a different conformation and are strong, brittle gels. Alginates are not random co-polymers of mannuronic and guluronic acids, and regions containing a single monomer (i.e. -M-M-M-M-M-M- and -G-G-G-G-G-G-) may be present in the chain. These are known as block structures and also affect the shape and properties of the polymer.

Seaweed alginates are widely used in the food industry as thickening and gelling agents. Alginate beads provide a simple and effective method of immobilising cells and enzymes. The cell suspension or enzyme solution is mixed with a calcium salt and allowed to drip into a solution of alginate. The polysaccharide chains are cross-linked by interaction of the divalent cation with the carboxyl groups, forming a gel. Alginate is a useful matrix for immobilising cells, but may not retain enzymes efficiently.

Bacterial alginates are not used commercially because the producing strains are relatively unstable and they also excrete a degradative enzyme which decreases the molecular weight of the product. They have, however, considerable potential for commercial use because polymers with a wide range of properties can be produced by appropriate selection of the producing strain and fermentation conditions.

16.2.10   Biosynthesis of polysaccharides

The biosynthesis of xanthan is shown in Fig. 16.10. Each monomer is assembled on a lipid carrier (Fig. 16.11), anchored in the cytoplasmic membrane, prior to transfer to the growing polymer chain. The lipid carrier is similar, or the same as, the C_{55} isoprenyl phosphate used in the biosynthesis of peptidoglycan and lipopolysaccharides in bacterial cell walls.

In xanthan biosynthesis, sugar nucleotides, for example uridine diphosphate glucose (UDP-glucose), act as activated precursors, providing the energy for the formation of glycosidic bonds between adjacent monosaccharides.

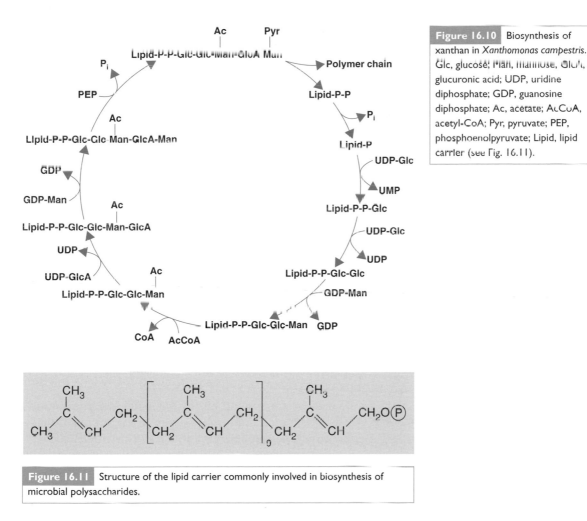

Figure 16.10 Biosynthesis of xanthan in *Xanthomonas campestris*. Glc, glucose; Man, mannose, GlcA, glucuronic acid; UDP, uridine diphosphate; GDP, guanosine diphosphate; Ac, acetate; AcCoA, acetyl-CoA; Pyr, pyruvate; PEP, phosphoenolpyruvate; Lipid, lipid carrier (see Fig. 16.11).

Figure 16.11 Structure of the lipid carrier commonly involved in biosynthesis of microbial polysaccharides.

The biosynthesis of most exopolysaccharides is essentially similar to that of xanthan and differences are beyond the scope of this chapter. Dextran synthesis is, however, quite different and is synthesised outside the cell. A single extracellular enzyme, dextransucrase, cleaves the disaccharide sucrose to glucose and fructose, and polymerises the glucose units to form dextran.

16.2.11 Production of polysaccharides

Microbial polysaccharides are produced in batch culture in aerated stirred tank reactors. Polysaccharide synthesis generally commences during growth and continues after cessation of growth. Excretion of polysaccharide increases the viscosity of the culture. This limits the attainable polysaccharide concentration because it becomes increasingly difficult to achieve adequate mixing and O_2 transfer in the viscous cultures. Furthermore, the power required to stir viscous cultures is high and consequently the cost of heat removal to maintain the required temperature is increased.

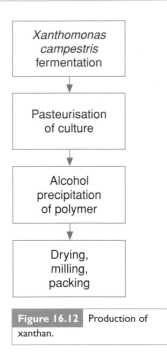

Figure 16.12 Production of xanthan.

Production of microbial polysaccharides is generally favoured by a high carbon/nitrogen ratio in the medium. The nitrogen source is the growth-limiting nutrient and its concentration is set to produce the required biomass concentration. Additional carbon source may be added after cessation of growth. Since cations can affect the rheological properties of polysaccharide solutions, care must be taken in optimising the concentrations of salts provided as nutrients in the medium.

Continuous culture is not used for production of microbial polysaccharides. At higher growth rates, which are desirable for high productivity, an increasing proportion of the carbon source is used to produce biomass rather than polysaccharide. Furthermore, some polysaccharide-producing micro-organisms are not stable in continuous culture and can be outgrown by variants that produce little polysaccharide. Strain stability is less of a problem in batch cultures that are of shorter duration.

The stages of xanthan production are summarised in Fig. 16.12.

16.3 | Single cell oils (SCOs)

16.3.1 Introduction

Lipids are defined by their solubility in non-polar organic solvents (hexane, diethyl ether, etc.) and insolubility in water. With this being a definition of physiochemical properties, rather than their biochemical origins, the term *lipids* encompasses a range of biochemically unrelated compounds (including sterols, carotenoids, fatty acyl lipids as well as polyhydroxyalkanoates). In order to restrict the length and breadth of the present section, the lipids being described here are restricted to fatty acyl lipids and, more specifically, triacylglycerol lipids (TAG) – see Fig. 16.13 – which are produced by microorganisms *via* fermentation processes and now used for human consumption. These then are the **single cell oils**.

Synthesis of fatty acids, the basic building blocks of acyl lipids, is a process undertaken by essentially all living cells, the only exception being certain obligate parasites that obtain lipids from their host. The biochemistry underlying lipid synthesis is well documented in biochemistry text-books (see Section 16.4) and will not be covered here in any detail though a brief outline of the process in lipid-accumulating microorganisms is shown in Fig. 16.14. It is sufficient to point out the basic tenet of lipid accumulation is that significant TAG accumulation does not occur in actively growing cells. It occurs after cells have depleted some critical nutrient from the culture medium, usually nitrogen (N), while carbon (C) remains available (see Fig. 16.15). Therefore all SCO fermentations must include a period of active growth in nutrient replete conditions (to generate biomass) followed by a period of restricted growth in the presence of a C source, where one (at least) nutrient (usually N) is depleted during which TAG is produced.

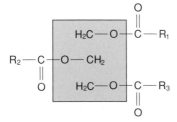

Figure 16.13 Structure of a triacylglyceride molecule: the glyceryl backbone is inside the shaded box. Attached to this backbone are three fatty acyl residues containing aliphatic chains R_1, R_2 and R_3, respectively, which may all be identical or all different.

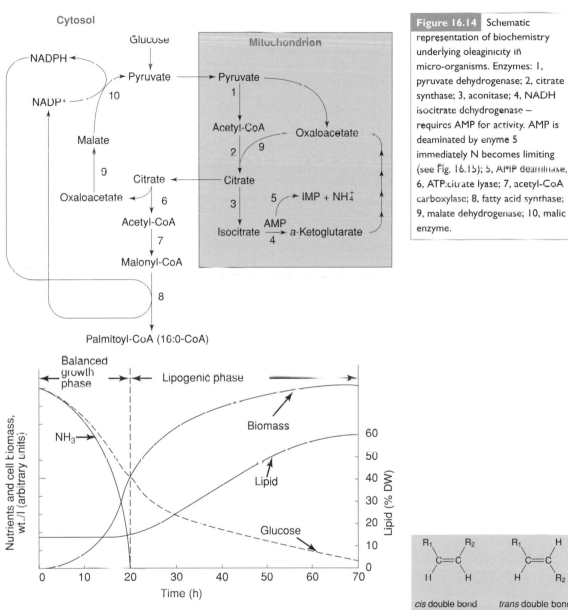

Figure 16.14 Schematic representation of biochemistry underlying oleaginicity in micro-organisms. Enzymes: 1, pyruvate dehydrogenase; 2, citrate synthase; 3, aconitase; 4, NADH isocitrate dehydrogenase – requires AMP for activity. AMP is deaminated by enyme 5 immediately N becomes limiting (see Fig. 16.15); 5, AMP deaminase, 6, ATP:citrate lyase; 7, acetyl-CoA carboxylase; 8, fatty acid synthase; 9, malate dehydrogenase; 10, malic enzyme.

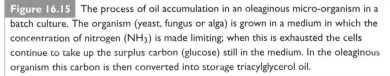

Figure 16.15 The process of oil accumulation in an oleaginous micro-organism in a batch culture. The organism (yeast, fungus or alga) is grown in a medium in which the concentration of nitrogen (NH_3) is made limiting; when this is exhausted the cells continue to take up the surplus carbon (glucose) still in the medium. In the oleaginous organism this carbon is then converted into storage triacylglycerol oil.

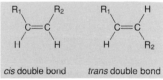

cis double bond   trans double bond

Figure 16.16 Structure of cis and trans double bonds. Double bonds 'lock' the fatty acid structure and lead to the existence of cis and trans isomers. Fatty acids in biological systems are almost exclusively the cis isomer. R_1 and R_2 represent acyl chains, in a fatty acid molecule one will possess the terminal methyl (CH_3) group while the other will possess the carboxylic acid (COOH) group.

Bacteria produce fatty acids that have a variety of structures including branched chains, cyclopropane rings and *trans* double bonds. However, all fatty acids synthesised by eukaryotic microorganisms, plants and higher animals, and this then includes all fatty acids of dietetic and nutritional importance, are straight chain fatty acids that contain only *cis* double bonds (see Fig. 16.16) that are usually

Table 16.1 Fatty acid structure and nomenclature

Trivial name	Molecular structure	Systematic name	Numeric designation
Palmitic acid	$CH_3(CH_2)_{14}COOH$	Hexadecanoic acid	16:0
γ-Linolenic acid	$CH_3(CH_2)_4(CH=CH.CH_2)_3(CH_2)_3COOH$	All *cis*-6, 9, 12-octatrienoic acid	18:3(n-6)
Arachidonic acid	$CH_3(CH_2)_4(CH=CH.CH_2)_4(CH_2)_2COOH$	All *cis*-5, 8, 11, 14-eicosatetraenoic acid	20:4(n-6)
DHA	$CH_3CH_2(CH=CH.CH_2)_6CH_2COOH$	All *cis*-4, 7, 10, 13, 16, 19-docosahexaenoic acid	22:6(n-3)

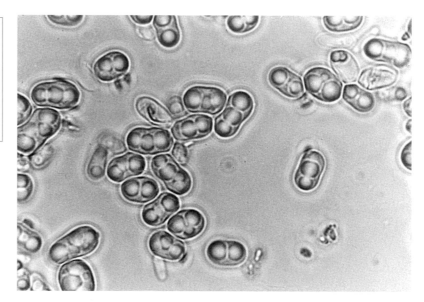

Figure 16.17 A photomicrograph of a typical oleaginous micro-organism. This is a photograph of *Cryptococcus curvatus*, formerly known as *Apiotrichum curvatum*. Cells are packed with oil droplets up to 70% of the total mass.

spaced at intervals of three carbon atoms with each double bond being separated by a methyl carbon, (referred to as *methylene interrupted*), i.e. —CH=CH—CH₂—CH=CH— (for examples see Table 16.1).

Although essentially all organisms synthesise fatty acids, the accumulation of significant amounts of TAG is not universal. Prokaryotes generally do not produce TAG as a storage material – they tend to produce the polyhydroxyalkanoates or polysaccharides as described earlier – the vast majority of the acyl lipid they contain is in the form of phospholipid (PL). TAG production among eukaryotes is variable by species. Those that do accumulate significant TAG (above an arbitrarily set 20% w/w of their dry weight) are described as the **oleaginous microorganisms** while those not accumulating significant TAG are described as non-oleaginous. Clearly, it is the oleaginous species that are the subject of this section. The biochemical basis for microbial oleaginicity has been well defined (see Fig. 16.14 and also Section 16.4). A photomicrograph of a typical oleaginous yeast is shown in Fig. 16.17.

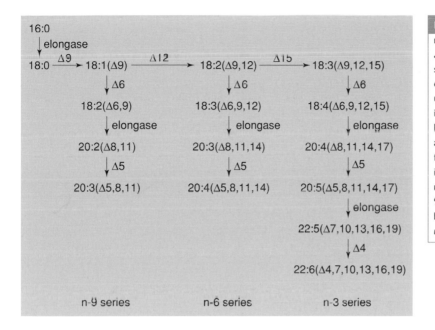

Figure 16.18 Overall scheme of modifications made to fatty acids after de novo synthesis. *Elongases* serve to increase the fatty acid chain length by addition of a C_2 unit (acetyl-CoA). *Desaturases*, indicated by Δ, introduce a double bond between two adjacent C atoms. Only the position of the first C atom is given and this is indicated by the number: thus $\Delta 9$ means that the bond from C atom 9 to C atom 10 is now a double bond. The fatty acid has become *unsaturated*.

This then outlines the boundaries of the present section in that the oils discussed are triacylglycerols containing straight chain fatty acids with double bonds in the *cis* configuration and which are separated from one another by a methylene carbon atom.

16.3.2 Nomenclature of fatty acids

The naming of fatty acids can appear confusing as in most cases any one of three names can be used, depending on the personal preference of the writer. These names can be thought of as (i) a systematic name, (ii) a trivial name or (iii) a numerical designation. The different names of selected fatty acids are shown in Table 16.1. The systematic names, though precise, tend to be long and confusing to those not familiar with lipid chemistry, as a result these names are seldom used. In contrast the trivial names give no direct information about the structure of the fatty acid yet are still widely used both in scientific and non-scientific circles. The numerical designation has the dual benefits of being concise while explicitly denoting the chemical structure of the fatty acid. In the numerical designation (see Table 16.1), the number before the colon indicates the number of carbon atoms making up the acyl chain, while the number after the colon gives the number of double bonds that the fatty acid contains. The n-3, n-6 or n-9 designation informs the reader to which series the fatty acid belongs (see Fig. 16.18) and indicates the position of the last double bond (counting from the methyl end of the fatty acid). As all double bonds are *methylene interrupted* (see above), once the position of the final double bond is assigned then the position of all other double bonds can be inferred.

Table 16.2 Fatty acyl composition of an oil and a fat

Fatty acid	Lard	Canola oil
Appearance at room temperature	Solid (fat)	Liquid (oil)
Saturated fatty acids (% total fatty acids)		
16:0	25	3
18:0	13	1
Monounsaturated fatty acids (% total fatty acids)		
16:1	3	–
18:1	43	64
22:1	–	1
Polyunsaturated fatty acids (% total fatty acids)		
18:2	11	22
18:3n-3	<0.5	8
Summary		
Total % saturated fatty acids	38	4
Total % polyunsaturated fatty acids	11	30
Total % short chain fatty acids (<18 carbons)	27	3

16.3.3 Functional roles of cell lipid

The majority of cell *acyl* lipid exists in one of two forms, either triacylglycerol (TAG), Fig. 16.13, which is a cell storage compound as it is energy rich (more so than both protein and carbohydrate), or phospholipid (PL), Fig. 16.19, which is a key structural component of all biological membranes (making up the *lipid bilayer*). TAG is essentially physiologically inert playing a storage role (as against future starvation) or a protective function against cold (blubber in sea mammals) or as padding around vital organs. In contrast, the PL in cell membranes plays a key role in maintaining and regulating the activity of the cell. Rather than being simply barriers between different cellular compartments, biological membranes are the site of numerous fundamental biochemical reactions – many enzymes are either membrane bound or membrane associated (e.g. electron transport chains) and depend on a suitable membranous environment for activity. Membrane fluidity is a key factor in determining membrane-associated enzyme activity. The key factor in regulating the fluidity of the membrane environment is the fatty acyl composition of the PL in the lipid bilayer. The longer and/or fewer double bonds (desaturations) contained in an acyl chain, the higher the melting point of that fatty acid and the higher the melting point of any lipid (be it TAG or PL) containing that fatty acid. This phenomenon can be seen in the difference between fats (e.g. animal lard) and plant oils (e.g. Canola oil, also known as rapeseed oil) – see Table 16.2. Fats (solid at room temperature) contain higher levels of long chain saturated fatty acids (no double bonds) attached to the glycerol backbone (see Fig. 16.13). In contrast, oils

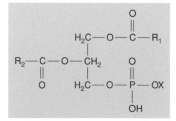

Figure 16.19 Structure of a phospholipid molecule: X can be H, ethanolamine, serine, inositol, choline, glycerol, etc. When the attached group is H the molecule is phosphatidic acid, the others are named phosphatidyl X (i.e. phosphatidylethanolamine, etc.).

(liquid at room temperature) contain a greater predominance of double bonds (unsaturated fatty acids) and, when the chain length of a fatty acid reaches 18 or 20 carbons, there are usually several double bonds (i.e. they are known as the **polyunsaturated fatty acids –** PUFA) in the molecule to maintain them in a liquid or fluid form.

As this phenomenon extends to PL and therefore to membranes, the fatty acid composition of a membrane PL has a major influence on membrane fluidity. Indeed, it is a recognised fact that many microbial cells respond to a decrease in growth temperature by increasing the level of unsaturated fatty acids in their cell membranes. In so doing these microbes counteract the decrease in membrane fluidity that would occur at decreased temperature by producing membranes that are more fluid.

As well as their structural and storage roles, certain fatty acids are precursors for a range of cell signalling molecules. Arachidonic acid (20:4n-6, ARA) and eicosapentaenoic acid (20:5n-3, EPA) are precursors of a variety of potent cell signalling compounds (the eicosanoids, prostaglandins and leukotrienes) in higher animals including ourselves. These signalling molecules are involved in the regulation of many cellular processes including inflammatory responses, blood coagulation and reproductive function. ARA and EPA are corresponding members of the n-6 and n-3 series of fatty acids (Fig. 16.18) and the signal molecules derived from them are synthesised by the same enzymes in spite of this difference in structure. Therefore ARA and EPA *compete* for the enzyme active sites. As the signal molecules synthesised from ARA and EPA often regulate the same cellular processes, but in an antagonistic fashion, the cellular ARA/EPA ratio can have a profound impact on certain homeostatic responses.

Of particular relevance to the current chapter is the role played by ARA and another very long chain PUFA, docosahexaenoic acid (22:6n-3, DHA), in the development of neural and eye tissue. Although these two fatty acids are relatively minor fatty acids, in nature they are the most common PUFA in phospholipids of neural tissue, including the brain, and also of the eye. Both of these fatty acids are present in human breast milk and their addition to infant formula (normally devoid of DHA and ARA) has been shown to be beneficial to both visual and intellectual development. These two fatty acids are now included in infant formula in more than 60 countries worldwide.

16.3.4 Advantages and disadvantages of SCOs

That micro-organisms produce a wide range of fatty acids has been known since the beginning of the twentieth century and attempts to produce oil in significant quantities from microbial sources dates back to the Second World War in Germany. However, it was not until 1985 that the first commercial process for SCO production commenced (Oil of Javanicus, produced using the fungus *Mucor circinelloides*) and it was not until the beginning of the twenty-first century that SCO became a commercial success.

The key reason for the initial failure of microbial sources of oils to compete with oils from traditional sources (plant and animal/fish) was their cost and difficulty of production. In order to produce SCO, it is necessary to cultivate large amounts of microbial biomass as the oil is invariably stored within the cells. Although fat levels of >70% dry wt. have been reported, it is more typical for the most oleaginous micro-organisms to accumulate approx. 50% of their dry weight as lipid. Furthermore, fermentations generally cannot generate >200 g dry mass per litre of culture. As a result for every tonne (1000 kg) of oil to be produced >10 000 litres of culture must be grown. Initially, the technology to carry out this type and scale of microbial culture was unavailable and was only developed in the 1940–1960s as part of the drive to produce single cell protein (a microbial substitute for meat) using various bacteria and yeasts growing on hydrocarbons or methanol. It is of note that the name single cell oil was coined to draw the comparison with single cell protein and to use less emotive words than *microorganism* or *microbe*, which tended to arouse distaste in the minds of the public if they were to buy the microbial protein or oil.

Even with the advent of technology for the cultivation of high-density microbial cultures on a large scale, the commercialisation of SCO was not easy. The fermentation technology was expensive both to install and operate. As a consequence SCOs were (and still are) expensive to produce and must attract a premium price to be commercially viable.

Attempts to utilise phototrophic micro-organisms (various micro-algae) to decrease the cost of SCOs, on the basis that the carbon (CO_2) and energy source (sunlight) are free, have proved unfounded. Low culture cell densities, as a result of *self-shading* (only the cells at the surface of the culture getting full sunlight), gas exchange (to remove the O_2 evolved during photosynthesis) and the need to harvest vast volumes of culture broth (due to low cell densities) have resulted in the costs of photosynthetic production exceeding that of heterotrophic fermentation (feeding glucose or another suitable carbon source) in conventional fermenters.

In order to capture a market, SCOs have to have a definitive and recognised advantage over other oils (plant or animal/fish) that can be produced at a fraction of the cost. For the first SCO, *Oil of Javanicus*, this advantage was that it was very rich in γ-linolenic acid (18:3n-6, GLA). GLA is the active ingredient in evening primrose oil, which has been highly valued (and therefore priced) as a *folk remedy* for a range of maladies (including pre-menstrual syndrome and eczema). While evening primrose oil contains only 8% GLA, the SCO contained 18–20% GLA (Table 16.3). Although this advantage was sufficient to warrant commercial development of this SCO the longevity of the process was severely compromised by the subsequent commercialisation of borage oil, an alternative plant source richer in GLA than the SCO. Even though borage was not an ideal agronomic crop, borage oil was able to out-compete *Oil of Javanicus* to such a degree that production was halted in 1990 after just six years.

Table 16.3 The fatty acid composition of selected plants, fish and single cell oils

Source	Saccharomyces cerevisiae	Mucor circinelloides	Mortierella alpina	Crypthecodinium cohnii	Schizochytrium sp.	Borage oil	Evening primrose oil	Soybean oil	Cod liver oil
Type of organism	Yeast	Fungus	Fungus	Microalga	Microalga	Plant	Plant	Plant	Animal/fish
				Fatty acid profile (relative % of total fatty acids)					
16:0	15	22	14	20	29	10	6	12	13
16:1	42	1		1	12				6
18:0	5	6	5	1	1	4	2	3	2
18:1	35	40	4	14	2	16	8	23	27
18:2	–	11	4	–	3	40	75	56	10
18:3n-3	–	–	–	–	–	Tr.	Tr.	6	3
18:3n-6	–	18	3	–	–	22	8	–	–
20:4n-6	–	–	55	–	–	–	–	–	1
20:5n-3	–	–	–	–	–	–	–	–	10
22:5n-6	–	–	–	–	12	–	–	–	
22:6n-3		–	–	30	26	–			5

Table 16.4 Advantages and disadvantages of single cell oils

Advantages	Disadvantages
Simple fatty acid profile	High cost
Not effected by geographical or environmental factors	Limited production capacity
Quality and supply can be guaranteed	Potential adverse public perception
Very rich in fatty acid of interest	

This example demonstrates an important feature of SCOs, they can never financially compete directly with similar oils from plant or animal sources. Other recent attempts to make a microbial competitor to cocoa butter and/or cocoa butter equivalent, though displaying some impressive science, have again served to highlight this point. Through the use of inhibitors, substrate feeding and strain selection, yeasts were persuaded to synthesise and accumulate an oil with a reasonable approximation to the composition of cocoa butter. However, even when a process was developed that could use waste products from the dairy industry (at zero cost) this product was still not economically viable.

Despite the high cost of the fermentation technology required to produce SCOs, these oils can and have become a commercial reality and, indeed, can have certain advantages over oils from traditional sources as a result of their fermented origin (Table 16.4).

The microbial world contains huge diversity and this diversity is reflected in the range of fatty acids found in microbial cell lipids. While plant oils do not contain polyunsaturated fatty acids with carbon chains >18, microbial lipids containing high levels of DHA

(22:6n-3) are known (Table 16.3). Certain animal/fish oils also contain very long chain PUFA but, in these cases, the fatty acids are at low levels (generally <10% of total fatty acids) and constitute a component within a complicated lipid profile. It should be noted that the very long chain PUFA composition of animal/fish oils is a reflection of their dietary intake rather than synthesis by the organism. Animal oils are, therefore, not only complex but also variable, due both to geographical and climatic factors. Microbial oils reflect solely the organism's biochemical capacity for fatty acid biosynthesis. This results in oil which has a simple fatty acid profile, is potentially very rich in the fatty acid desired and which is very reproducible (Table 16.3).

The biotechnological origins of SCO, the biomass being grown in enclosed tanks under controlled conditions and as a culture containing only a single organism (i.e. an anexic culture), also means that the quality of the product can be closely controlled and precludes the possibility of contamination with either environmental pollutants, pesticide and herbicide residues and even toxins from microbial contamination, issues that have caused concern in some quarters over the quality of oils from traditional (plant and some animal) sources.

As fermentation runs last only a matter of days, not only the quality but also the quantity of product can be guaranteed. Climatic conditions, be it drought or flood, and other factors such as overexploitation of resources (e.g. overfishing) do not threaten the productivity of a fermenter. Therefore SCO production is reproducible, its quality can be safe-guarded to a very high level, and its supply can be rapidly increased (or decreased) to match the prevailing market requirements.

16.3.5   Current SCO production

As stated above, SCO can only compete with traditional oils if a distinct benefit for the microbial oil can be demonstrated and that benefit can support a premium price. Currently microbial oils that are *very* rich in two fatty acids meet these requirements and these are in current (2005) production. These fatty acids are arachidonic acid (ARA, 20:4n-6) and docosahexaenoic acid (DHA, 22:6n-3). These fatty acids are important due to their role in infant nutrition, and a SCO blend containing ARA and DHA is thus being added to infant formula worldwide. In the USA, since its introduction in February 2002, infant formula containing the DHA/ARA blend has achieved greater than 70% market penetration.

Neither DHA or ARA are available in a suitable oil from any traditional source – plant or animal. Plants do not synthesise very long chain (VLC) PUFAs (chain length >18) and, while animal sources are known that contain both of these fatty acids, they contain these VLC PUFA at modest levels and are not suitable for inclusion in baby formula. Fish oils, in particular, are well known for their content of n-3 fatty acids, including DHA; however, these fish oils also always contain eicosapentaenoic acid (EPA, 20:5n-3). Eicosapentaenoic acid

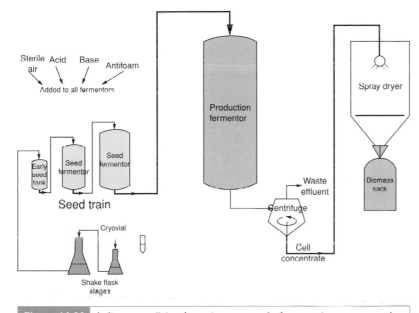

Figure 16.20 A diagram outlining the various stages of a fermentation process used to produce a single cell oil. The organism of choice is grown through a series of fermenters using inoculum volumes of about 10% at each stage. Only in the final stage will the composition of the medium be made with a low concentration of NH_3 and a high concentration of glucose (see Fig. 16.15) as, up to this stage, the organism is grown in the seed fermenters to give the maximum cell density, not lipid levels. The cells after being harvested from the production fermenter are harvested, dried and, finally, extracted with hexane to remove the oil.

should not be included in infant formula as it has been found to impair neonate growth. Thus there is a need for a DHA-rich oil that does not contain EPA.

Microorganisms that accumulate impressive amounts of cell lipid (in the form of triacylglycerol, the preferred lipid form for food use and the form of lipid naturally contained in human breast milk) very rich in either ARA or DHA are known and at least three of these microorganisms have been developed to commercial reality. All SCO production processes follow essentially the same steps (Fig. 16.20) involving a seed train of cultures of increasing volumes to inoculate a final large-scale fermentation vessel. Once the microbial culture has obtained a suitable cell density and lipid content, the tank is drained (for cleaning, sterilisation and re-batching). The culture broth is then harvested to remove the microbial biomass, which is dried and extracted with hexane in a process similar to that used for extraction of oils from plant seeds. The extracted oil is then processed again using similar technologies to those employed in the vegetable oil industry.

One characteristic of SCOs that requires attention is the highly unsaturated nature of their constituent fatty acids. ARA- and DHA-rich SCOs each contain >40% of ARA (four double bonds) and DHA (six double bonds), respectively. Each of these double bonds is a potential site of oxidation, which would lead to rancidity and off-flavours. Generally, the more unsaturated a fatty acid the more unstable it is. Therefore these oils have to be treated very carefully during extraction/processing and even the microbial biomass must be handled with care prior to extraction in order to avoid fatty acid breakdown and the generation of off-flavours. In general, the precautions taken to stabilise the oil include: processing the oils rapidly, storing the biomass and oil at low temperature and under N_2 (to exclude O_2), and limiting heating during processing. During harvest of the microbial biomass a rapid heating (pasteurisation) step is often employed. This has two benefits: it avoids bacterial contamination during the harvesting steps and it kills the production organism. The latter is important because if the production organism remained alive and active after harvest there is a possibility that the biomass would start to break down its internal storage reserves (the valuable oil) after the C source is removed during washing. Endogenous breakdown of the fungal TAG by β-oxidation would not only decrease the oil yield but also seriously impact on the oil quality and significantly increase losses during processing.

ARA-rich SCO

An ARA-rich oil has been a target for biotechnologists for many years, and pre-dates the recognition of ARA's importance in neonate nutrition. Over 40 years ago, work began at Unilever (UK) to identify a microbial source of ARA-rich oil in the belief (mistakenly as it turned out) that ARA was a chicken-flavour precursor. ARA-rich oil production from a microbial source was also instigated in Japan, by Lion Corp., as a cosmetic ingredient. Neither of these processes were successful, but laid the ground work for future development once a worthwhile application for ARA-rich oil was identified. Several filamentous fungi have been shown to produce ARA and a survey of these identified *Mortierella alpina* as the most promising production organism. There are currently at least three separate processes utilising this fungus in operation: two are in the Far East (one in Japan is run by Suntory Co. Ltd and the other in China by Wuhan Alking Bioengineering Co. Ltd) and one in Western Europe and Northern America (run by DSM Food Specialities in Italy and then sold into the USA under an exclusive contract with Martek Biosciences). Of these processes, that operated by DSM is by far the most significant, producing over 95% of the ARA-rich SCO produced annually.

A proprietary strain of *Mortierella alpina* (obtained using classical selection methods for desirable growth and lipid accumulation characteristics, i.e. not obtained using any form of genetic engineering – all current SCOs are non-GMO) is cultivated in successively large fermentation vessels to a final volume in excess of 50 000 litres. To achieve the highest possible cell density, both nitrogen and carbon are fed into the fermenter during the fermentation. Once a high cell density is obtained the N feed is discontinued, but the C feed is maintained. Under these N-limited conditions, the fungus can no longer grow but continues to assimilate the C source supplied, converting it into storage lipid (the desired product) – see also Fig. 16.14.

Once sufficient lipid has accumulated in the fungal biomass, the culture broth is harvested, using either a continuous centrifuge or a filter press, and is then dried. The dry biomass is pelleted to aid lipid extraction and is extracted using hexane. Extracted lipid is steam stripped to remove the hexane, which is then processed using essentially the same technology as for vegetable oils. Oil processing is usually described by the acronym RBD standing for refining, bleaching and deodourising. These three processes remove the small amounts of other cellular components extracted along with the TAG.

The resulting oil is a yellow (due to some carotenoids remaining even after RBD) brilliant oil that has a characteristic, but not unpleasant, taste and odour. Although the fungal oil is remarkably resilient to oxidation, due to the presence in the oil of endogenous antioxidant compounds, additional antioxidants (vitamin E) are added during processing to ensure complete protection against oxidation.

DHA-rich SCO

Although DHA-containing oils are available from fish (Table 16.3) and, therefore, would ordinarily preclude the necessity to develop a SCO process (see above), the fact that fish oil also inevitably contains EPA means that fish oil is not appropriate for addition to infant formula. Therefore commercial production of an SCO very rich in DHA but devoid of EPA represents a unique opportunity that has been exploited. Marine micro-organisms are known that produce DHA, some of them without EPA. Synthesis of these two VLC PUFA appears to be linked strongly, though not causally, to cold marine (i.e. high-salinity) environments.

Many of the marine microbes that produce DHA could be excluded from commercial development because they were either bacteria (which do not accumulate significant amounts of TAG) or were obligate photosynthetic organisms (see above). Two heterotrophic eukaryotes were identified (by separate US-based companies) and developed as production organisms for DHA-rich SCO (see Table 16.3 for their fatty acid compositions). Both are microalgae: one (*Cryptheco-dinium cohnii*, developed by Martek Biosciences, Columbia, MD) being a dinoflagellate and the other (*Schizochytrium*, developed by OmegaTech Inc., Boulder, CO) belonging to the order thraustochytriales. Both of these produce oils rich in DHA; however, the *Schiozochytrium* oil also contains another very long chain PUFA docosapentaenoic acid (DPAn-6, 20:5n-6). In 2001, Martek acquired OmegaTech in order to consolidate the expertise and intellectual property of these two companies.

The SCO from *C. cohnii* is the SCO (DHASCO) used for neonatal nutritional supplementation. It constitutes greater than 95% of the global market for DHA-rich SCO. *C. cohnii* is cultivated essentially as outlined in Fig. 16.17, the key feature of this process is the requirement for saline culture medium to grow this marine microbe. The salinity of seawater, the natural habitat for *C. cohnii*, is far too high for steel fermentation vessels used on a large scale. Therefore low-chloride media and adapted strains have been developed (again using classical strain development techniques) to allow the commercial process to operate at chloride concentrations below the corrosion limits of the cultivation tanks.

As with ARA-SCO, once the biomass and oil levels in the fermenter are sufficient the biomass is separated from the culture broth before being dried and subsequently extracted with hexane. The DHASCO is an orange oil with, again, a distinctive but not unpleasant flavour. It certainly lacks the undesirable fishy taste of fish oils.

16.3.6   Safety of SCOs

Due to their novel nature, and as they are derived from microbial sources, the safety of SCOs had to be carefully evaluated before being released onto the market, particularly as an additive for infant formula! As a result these oils are possibly the most thoroughly tested *food* oils currently available. Numerous clinical and safety studies involving animal models and human volunteers have been completed; these have even tested the effects of large single doses (acute toxicity studies) and multiple smaller doses (chronic toxicity studies) in human volunteers. No adverse effects have been noted more serious than diarrhoea and or *fishy burps* after administration of extremely large doses (equivalent to about 100 g person^{-1}).

16.3.7   Future of SCOs

Currently all SCOs are oils containing either DHA and/or ARA, and the vast majority of the production is targeted to infant formula. Indeed, the take-up of the DHA/ARA mixture by infant formula companies means that, at the time of writing (2005), the market is supply- rather than demand-limited. In order to rectify this situation, new plants for the production of both DHASCO and ARASCO are being built in the USA. Clinical studies have demonstrated the efficacy of DHA against a range of clinical indications from high-blood triglyceride (a marker for increased risk of heart attacks) and in mental deterioration in the elderly. It is assumed that these areas will provide future growth for DHA-rich SCOs once the present demand has been met and exceeded.

Other very long chain PUFAs could also be developed commercially if suitable production organisms can be identified. The most likely to be developed in the short to medium future is EPA. This fatty acid appears to have anti-inflammatory activity and could be used to treat autoimmune diseases such as arthritis. Also the anti-inflammatory activity of EPA appears to act as a cardio-protectant reducing the risk of heart disease. Another exciting application of EPA is in the treatment of various cancers and for cachexia, the chronic wastage that sometimes is associated with cancer and which seriously decreases the chances of survival. In all these cases, however, the challenge to the biotechnologist will be demonstrating the advantage of a high cost SCO containing EPA over low cost fish oil which also contains EPA, but the simultaneous occurrence of DHA in fish oil is unlikely to be a disadvantage when giving such oils to adults.

The biggest potential threat to SCO production could be the production of cheap oils containing very long chain PUFA from plant sources derived by genetic engineering. All the genes required for VLC PUFA have now been cloned from various microbial sources and although the technical issues with re-assembling the VLC PUFA biosynthetic machinery in a plant usually capable only of synthesising C18 PUFA are considerable, it must be assumed that these will be overcome.

Even when crop plants synthesising VLC PUFA are available there may still be environmental and consumer resistance (especially in Europe) to the cultivation of these genetically engineered plants and/or to the eating of their products. The considerable cost of the development of these transgenic crop plants making VLC PUFA must also be recovered by the companies carrying out the work, via a premium price on the engineered plant oil. In short, it has taken a considerable time for SCO to become a commercial reality and continual efforts are required to maintain the market position of these oils; however, for the immediate and foreseeable future, at least, the success of SCOs looks secure.

16.4 | Further reading

Arterburn, L. M., Boswell, K. D., Lawlor, T., et al. In vitro genotoxicity testing of ARASCO and DHASCO oils. *Food and Chemical Toxicology* **38**: 971–976, 2000.

Cohen, Z. and Ratledge, C., eds. *Single Cell Oils*. Champaign, IL: American Oil Chemists' Society, 2005.

Knapp, H. R., Salem, N. and Cunnane, S. Dietary fats and health. *Lipids* **38**: 297–496, 2003. A collection of key papers and reviews presented at the 5th Congress of the International Society for the Study of Fatty Acids and Lipids.

Ratledge, C. and Wynn, J. P. The biochemistry and molecular biology of lipid accumulation in oleaginous microorganisms. *Advances in Applied Microbiology* **51**: 1–51, 2002.

Sorger, D. and Daum, G. Triacylglycerol biosynthesis in yeast. *Applied Microbiology and Biotechnology* **61**: 289–299, 2003.

Sutherland, I. W. Biotechnology of microbial polysaccharides in food. In *Food Biotechnology*, 2nd edition. (K. Shetty, G. Paliyath, A. Pometto and R. E. Levin, eds), pp. 193–220. Taylor & Francis, Boca Raton, FL, USA.

Tombs, M. and Harding, S. E. *An Introduction to Polysaccharide Biotechnology*. London: Taylor & Francis, 1998.

Chapter 17

Environmental applications

Philippe Vandevivere
Seawater Foundation, Tucson, USA

Willy Verstraete
Ghent University, Belgium

17.1 Introduction

Until recently, *sanitary engineering* monopolised environmental-related industrial activities. Because sanitary engineering gradually developed as an off-shoot of civil engineering during the past century, emphasis has been on conventional engineering techniques in which the *bio* component is largely ignored and dealt with stochastically rather than mechanistically. Sanitary engineering is well established for:

- the catchment, treatment and distribution of drinking water;
- the treatment of wastewater;
- the treatment and disposal of solid wastes, e.g. municipal;
- the treatment of industrial off-gases.

Many of the conventional technologies used in sanitary engineering are, however, perfect illustrations of Murphy's law in that they

Basic Biotechnology, third edition, eds. Colin Ratledge and Bjørn Kristiansen.
Published by Cambridge University Press. © Cambridge University Press 2006.

transform one problem into another often more intractable one, as when water pollutants are stripped into the air or concentrated and dumped in the soil. Environmental strategies have to be conceived with respect to the *whole* of the environment in a long-term perspective. This integrated holistic approach requires a detailed knowledge of environmental biology and, more particularly, of the functioning of complex microbial communities. The new focus on the environment as a whole and on the detailed functioning of the *bio* component has led to the development of new industrial activities, referred to as *environmental biotechnologies*. These must address formidable environmental problems now facing the world:

- acid rain and ozone depletion;
- enrichment of ground and surface waters with nutrients and recalcitrant pesticides;
- recovery of reusable products and energy from wastes;
- soil remediation;
- disposal of animal manures.

While industrial biotechnologists use well-defined microorganisms to make products of predictable composition and quality such as lactic acid, beer or monosodium glutamate, environmental biotechnologists, on the other hand, start with poorly defined inocula and wait until desired phenomena occur. There is therefore a need to isolate, identify and characterise the microorganisms that exist and interact in soils, activated sludges, anaerobic granules, etc. Only when it becomes possible to re-assemble these microorganisms and their functions in a predictable way will environmental biotechnology become more generally accepted.

New developments are concerned with the introduction of organisms and genes in mixed cultures. Practical application of these new developments is somewhat impeded by poor survival of introduced microorganisms and regulatory constraints on deliberate introduction of modified organisms in the environment. The potential is, however, enormous as advances in molecular biology now make feasible the construction of novel genes and enzymes for the degradation of compounds that could not, until now, be biodegraded. These novel genes may become incorporated in the genomes of existing microbial communities, a process called *horizontal gene transfer*. For example, broad host range plasmids specialised in the degradation of synthetic chemicals, can be introduced into soil microbial communities, thereby enhancing their degradative capabilities.

17.2 Treatment of wastewater

17.2.1 Aerobic treatment by the activated sludge system

The most widely used process to purify wastewater is via aerobic biodegradation with the activated sludge system (see Box 17.1 for definitions). The wastewater flows through an aerated tank where the

Box 17.1 | Treatment of wastewater: definitions

BOD_5 Biological oxygen demand (after five days of incubation) is a parameter that quantifies the concentration of biodegradable organic matter present in wastewater. It is the amount of O_2 used by microorganisms to degrade the organic matter as determined in a standardised laboratory test.

Mixed liquor The suspension of microbial flocs (tiny aggregates of microorganisms) in the aeration tank of an activated sludge plant.

Sludge The microbial flocs in an activated sludge plant after these have been separated from the purified effluent via sedimentation in the settling tank.

Bulking sludge A sludge wherein overgrowth of filamentous microorganisms prevents the sedimentation of the *bulky* microbial flocs.

Nitrification The biochemical conversion of ammonium to nitrate carried out by autotrophic bacteria. It is an essential step during biological nitrogen removal in wastewater treatment plants, following the mineralisation of organic nitrogen to ammonium.

De-nitrification The biological reduction of nitrate to N_2. It occurs when O_2 is absent (anoxic conditions) and readily oxidisable organic compounds are present.

Anoxic A liquid wherein O_2 is absent but other oxidised species such as nitrate or ferric iron are present.

Anaerobic: A liquid wherein oxidised species are absent, the redox potential is below zero, and where biochemical reactions such as fermentations, sulphate reduction and methanogenesis take place.

dissolved organic matter is mineralised, i.e. oxidised to carbon dioxide, nitrate and phosphate:

$$\text{Dissolved organic matter} + O_2 \rightarrow \text{new biomass} + CO_2 + HNO_3 + H_3PO_4$$

This reaction is carried out mostly by bacteria, which are aggregated in flocs, about 0.1 mm in diameter. After a reaction time of several hours (municipal sewage) up to several days (more concentrated industrial effluents), the *mixed liquor* flows through a settling tank where the flocs are separated by gravity from the clean effluent (Fig. 17.1). The concentration of flocs in the aerated tank should not exceed 4 g l^{-1} in order to ensure proper settling. The settled flocs (called the *sludge*) are partly re-injected in the aerated tank and partly wasted. Good performance depends on the right choice of volumetric loading rate, which should lie in the range 0.5–1.5 g BOD_5 per litre mixed liquor per day in order to ensure proper floc formation and obtain +90% removal of dissolved organic matter. As one inhabitant equivalent produces 30 g BOD_5 per day on average, with peak values of 100 g per day, the aerated tanks are designed to have 100 litres of mixed liquor for each inhabitant equivalent.

The primary advantage of the activated sludge process, relative to other types of treatment, is a good effluent quality, with little BOD_5 (<20 mg l^{-1}) and little nutrients (<15 mg N l^{-1}) remaining after treatment. The process, however, suffers several drawbacks (Table 17.1).

Table 17.1 Comparison of different processes for the treatment of waste-water. Activated sludge systems provide good effluent quality but suffer several drawbacks. Membrane bioreactors achieve the same or better effluent quality in much smaller installations and produce much less waste sludge. UASB reactors offer the additional advantage of small energy expenditure (no aeration) but are less efficient in terms of nutrients and BOD_5 removal

	Aerobic treatment		Anaerobic
	Activated sludge	MBR[a]	UASB[b]
Residual BOD	Low	Very low	High
Residual N, P	Low	Low	High
Sludge production	High	Very low	Very low
Energy	High	High	Low
Floor area	Large	Very small	Very small
Reliability	Sludge bulking	Robust	Granule flotation

[a] MBR, membrane bio-reactor.
[b] UASB, upflow anaerobic sludge blanket reactor.

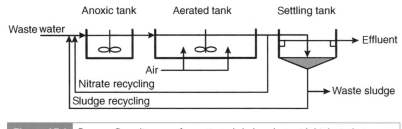
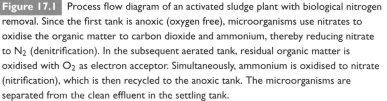

Figure 17.1 Process flow diagram of an activated sludge plant with biological nitrogen removal. Since the first tank is anoxic (oxygen free), microorganisms use nitrates to oxidise the organic matter to carbon dioxide and ammonium, thereby reducing nitrate to N_2 (denitrification). In the subsequent aerated tank, residual organic matter is oxidised with O_2 as electron acceptor. Simultaneously, ammonium is oxidised to nitrate (nitrification), which is then recycled to the anoxic tank. The microorganisms are separated from the clean effluent in the settling tank.

The biggest drawback is the large production of excess sludge since each kilogramme of BOD_5 produces about 0.3 kg of excess sludge solids. This excess sludge is usually stabilised in anaerobic digesters, dehydrated and, finally, disposed on agricultural land or landfilled. Disposal on land or in landfills is, however, becoming increasingly restricted in Europe and sludge disposal is becoming problematic.

Production of excess sludge can be somewhat lessened by including a carrier material in the aerated tank. In such reactors, the microorganisms will not form suspended flocs as in the activated sludge system but rather form a film on the surface of the carrier material. The latter can be stones, in which case the aerated tank is called a trickling filter, or fine suspended sand particles, as in fluidised bed reactors. These variants of the activated sludge process

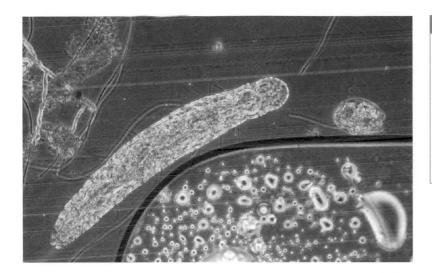

Figure 17.2 Floc of microorganisms as they occur in the mixed liquor of activated sludge tanks. Note the presence of a worm (*Nais elinguis*), which grazes the flocs actively. These worms could offer a very simple and elegant solution to the problem of sludge disposal (Photograph courtesy of Professor Eikelboom).

produce less excess sludge because the attached microorganisms remain longer in the aerated tank where autolysis takes place. Moreover, no settling tank is necessary. It was recently observed that excess sludge production in wastewater treatment plants does occasionally drop drastically during periods of a few weeks. These periods correspond to the sporadic growth of tiny worms (*Nais elinguis*) that graze on the sludge flocs (Fig. 17.2). If the current attempts to ensure the continuous presence of these worms in mixed liquors succeed, it would provide a very elegant and simple solution to the problem of sludge disposal.

An important breakthrough in terms of excess sludge production was the *membrane bioreactor (MBR)*. In MBR, the settling tank is replaced by a microfiltration unit that separates the microorganisms from the treated effluent. In such a system, separated sludge can be recirculated almost indefinitely in the aerated tank and, under these circumstances, sludge age is very long and excess sludge production very low (<0.1 kg kg^{-1} BODs removed). A second major advantage of MBR is that a very high sludge concentration is attained (up to 30 g l^{-1}), which allows much larger volumetric loading rates to be used than in the activated sludge system. As a consequence, very compact MBR installations can be built on a small fraction of the space required by an activated sludge plant. This small footprint is very attractive to industries producing concentrated wastewaters (BOD$_5$ > 2–3 g l^{-1}).

17.2.2 Anaerobic treatment of wastewater

Until recently, anaerobic digestion was only applied for the stabilisation of concentrated organic slurries such as animal manures and waste sewage sludge. The consensus was that anaerobic treatment was slow, did not remove much more than 50% of the organic load and, moreover, required high temperatures and was not reliable.

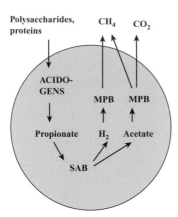

Figure 17.3 Sequence of biochemical reactions taking place in an anaerobic sludge granule, e.g. in an upflow anaerobic sludge blanket reactor treating wastewater. The sequence of reactions is thermodynamically favourable only in a narrow range of very low H_2 partial pressures. Growth closely together of acetogenic and methanogenic bacteria in a packed granule make the transfer of H_2 at low partial pressures much more efficient. SAB, syntrophic acetogenic bacteria; MPB, methane-producing bacteria.

This perception has changed drastically during the last two decades and anaerobic digestion is now an established-performance high-rate wastewater treatment technology. Through the use of anaerobic granular sludge, very high biomass concentrations (50 g l^{-1}) can be attained in reactors, allowing very high volumetric loading rates to be used (20 g BOD_5 l^{-1} reactor per day). New reactor designs that optimise the mass transfer of metabolites in the granular sludge now make it possible to treat wastewater of almost any composition (0.3--100 g BOD_5 l^{-1}) over a temperature range of 10–55 °C in a reliable manner.

Anaerobic conversion of organic compounds to biogas is a stepwise process wherein different groups of bacteria operating sequentially effect full degradation of the substrates:

- hydrolytic acidogens: cleave polymers into short chain fatty acids;
- syntrophic acetogens: degrade the fatty acids into acetate and H_2;
- methanogens: transform acetate and H_2 into CH_4 and CO_2 (biogas).

The last two groups are normally strictly dependent on one another (due to H_2 transfer) and are therefore referred to as the methanogenic association. Their metabolism is greatly enhanced by growing the anaerobic sludge in the form of densely packed granules that facilitate the transfer of H_2 and other intermediate degradation products (Fig. 17.3). The understanding of syntrophism, where several anaerobic microorganisms can share the energy available in the bioconversion of a molecule to CH_4 and CO_2 and thus can achieve intermediate reactions that are endergonic under standard conditions, has been essential in the rather striking development of anaerobic digestion during the last decades. It has been postulated that the minimum energy quantum for life is about -21 kJ mol^{-1} product formed or substrate converted. Applying the concept of minimal energy to the fermentation of propionate to methane suggests that both syntrophs have to operate in a very narrow region of H_2 partial pressure, pH_2 (Fig. 17.4). The conversion of one mole propionate yields >21 kJ only when $pH_2 < 10^{-5.4}$ atm; while the minimum pH_2 value allowing the production of one mol methane to generate -21 kJ is also in the range 10^{-5} atm. Thus only when pH_2 lies around 10^{-5} atm is the sequential conversion of propionate to acetate and acetate to methane possible. Similar conclusions can be drawn for the conversion of butyrate to methane and also with formate instead of H_2 as intermediate. The understanding of the nature of the *symbiosis* among syntrophic organisms is a challenging task and essential to the optimisation of anaerobic biotechnology.

Most anaerobic reactors treating wastewaters are *upflow anaerobic sludge blanket*, or UASB, reactors (Fig. 17.5). The wastewater enters the reactor at the bottom via a specially designed influent distribution system and subsequently flows through a sludge bed consisting of anaerobic bacteria growing in the form of granules, which settle very well (60–80 m h^{-1}). The mixture of sludge, biogas and water

Reaction A: propionate + 2H$_2$O
$\longrightarrow$ 3H$_2$ + acetate + CO$_2$
Reaction B. 4H$_2$ + CO$_2$
$\longrightarrow$ CH$_4$ + 2H$_2$O

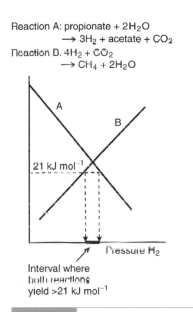

21 kJ mol^{-1}

Pressure H$_2$

Interval where
both reactions
yield >21 kJ mol^{-1}

Figure 17.4 Effect of H$_2$ partial pressure on the free energy of conversion of propionate by acetogens (reaction A) and of the subsequent transformation by methanogens of H$_2$ into methane (reaction B). Only in a very narrow range of H$_2$ partial pressure (around 10^{-5} atm) are both reactions thermodynamically favourable, i.e. they both yield >21 kJ mol^{-1} transformed.

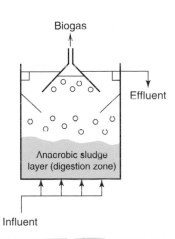

Biogas

Effluent

Anaerobic sludge
layer (digestion zone)

Influent

Figure 17.5 Schematic diagram of the upflow anaerobic sludge blanket reactor (UASB) used extensively for the treatment of concentrated wastewaters in temperate regions and also for the treatment of sewage (dilute wastewater) in tropical regions.

is separated in the three-phase separator situated in the top of the reactor.

The major advantages of anaerobic wastewater treatment over aerobic treatment are the small sludge production (0.1 kg kg^{-1} BOD$_5$); the low energy consumption, since no aeration is required; and the small floor area, typically 0.01 m^2 per inhabitant compared to 0.05 m^2 for activated sludge plants (Table 17.1). Moreover, energy is recovered in the form of biogas (0.35 l methane g^{-1} BOD$_5$).

The rate of BOD removal in anaerobic reactors drops markedly below 20 °C and the optimum temperature is about 35 °C. This explains why UASB reactors were first applied in tropical regions about 20 years ago. In temperate regions, UASB reactors have only been used to treat concentrated wastewater (>2 g BOD$_5$ l^{-1}) since the large production of biogas can be used to warm up the reactor. A new reactor design has recently been developed that permits sufficiently high rates to be attained even at 10 °C. This so-called *expanded granulated sludge blanket* (EGSB) reactor maximises mass transfer rates of nutrients with more intensive hydraulic mixing and makes it possible to treat sewage anaerobically even in temperate regions.

The major disadvantage of anaerobic digestion is that only negligible portions of the nutrients (N, P) are removed, due to the small excess sludge production. It is therefore necessary to apply a post-treatment step in order to remove these nutrients further, e.g. via the sequence nitrification/de-nitrification. The aerobic post-treatment step is also necessary to remove the residual BOD_5 remaining in the UASB effluent, because anaerobic bacteria do not easily scavenge substrates present at less than 50 mg l^{-1} while aerobic bacteria can easily lower BOD under 10 mg l^{-1}. The fact that nitrification requires costly aeration and that de-nitrification requires oxidisable organic matter (which is degraded in the prior anaerobic step!) has spurred the search for alternative types of post-treatments. A very interesting alternative, currently under development, uses the Anammox reaction (anaerobic ammonium oxidation). It was found that NH_4^+ was oxidised anaerobically to N_2 in the presence of NO_2^- according to:

$$NH_4^+ + NO_2^- \rightarrow N_2 + 2H_2O \qquad \Delta G^{\circ'} = -358 \text{ kJ per mol of } NH_4^+$$

Thus by splitting the ammonium-laden anaerobic effluent into two sub-streams, nitrifying partially one sub-stream to nitrite, and mixing again the two streams in a reactor where the Anammox reaction would occur, much less aeration would be required for the nitrification and no oxidisable organic matter would have to be added. The full-scale implementation of the Anammox reaction would open new doors for anaerobic digestion because it would enable a coherent sequence of organic carbon to methane and organic N via ammonium and nitrite to N_2. Using this scenario, even N-rich wastewater could be treated anaerobically at low cost.

Direct anaerobic treatment of domestic sewage, either in the sewer or in low-capital anaerobic–aerobic combined plants, will only attract the interest of the environmental industry provided it offers adequate profit margins. Hence, the challenge is to locate in anaerobic sewage treatment opportunities for high-tech added-value engineering. Two possibilities are discussed below.

Development of engineered anaerobic granulated sludges (biocatalyst)

Certain organic compounds produced by the chemical industry (xenobiotics) are not degraded in either aerobic or anaerobic digesters but are degraded in a sequential anaerobic/aerobic treatment. Examples are organic compounds with halo, nitro or azo substituents. It may take, however, several months and even up to a year in some cases before the sludge becomes adapted to these compounds. This time is needed for development or invasion of all species necessary to degrade the substrates completely, as complex xenobiotics often require more than one species to be completely mineralised. One option to accelerate the biodegradation of xenobiotics is to inoculate reactors with adequate bacterial strains. This was demonstrated with strains capable of dechlorinating chlorobenzoate or pentachlorophenol. The inocula were shown to have colonised the reactor in the long term and rapid breakdown of chlorobenzoate and pentachlorophenol could be obtained. Because adaptation of the association is probably also based on the proliferation of the correct plasmids, there is clearly a need for better insight in genetic evolution, plasmid transfer and species interaction in anaerobic communities dealing with xenobiotics. Another potential benefit associated with the large-scale availability of specialised microbial consortia is *biochemical re-routing,* i.e. the induction of desirable biochemical pathways, as for example the degradation of malodorous primary amines, anaerobic ammonium oxidation or homo-acetogenesis.

Development of performance-enhancing additives
Biomass retention through adequate granulation is of utmost importance in UASB technology, first in order to obtain a good effluent quality and, second, in order to ensure a minimal cell residence time of 7 to 12 days, that is required to avoid the wash-out of the slowest-growing anaerobic bacteria. One way to foster granular growth is to add polymers, clay or surfactants, which have a physico-chemical effect on granule formation. Another way is to provide the adequate nutrients, e.g. sugars, that stimulate the growth of microorganisms that cement anaerobic granules through the production of extracellular polymers. It appears therefore worthwhile, in order to make UASB technology more reliable, to develop biosupportive additives able to maintain the granular sludge in a proper state in periods of start-up or low-quality input wastewater.

17.2.3 Water recycling

In view of the steadily increasing shortage of water worldwide, the use of reclaimed wastewater will be an issue of growing concern in the next decade. Since two-thirds of the world water consumption is used to irrigate cropland, there are several instances in developing countries where raw domestic sewage of very large cities is directly re-used to irrigate food crops. Such a closed-loop system brings about the possibility of contaminating the food crops with pathogenic viruses or prions. It is a major challenge to work out cost-effective technologies to produce hygienically safe irrigation water without removing the fertilisers N and P. Anaerobic digestion might, in this respect, offer certain possibilities.

The second main consumer of water is industry, such as the food, metal, textile and paper sectors. These sectors are currently developing new treatment systems enabling them to recycle their wastewaters in a closed-loop system. Typically, a battery of modular processes are used that produce high-quality process water. The sequence usually combines biological treatments with final physico-chemical polishing treatments. For example, a potato chips factory uses a process train consisting of anaerobic and aerobic treatment, deep-bed filtration, disinfection with ozone gas and reverse osmosis. Such a complex treatment system is necessary to achieve complete removal of carbohydrates, antisprout herbicides and microorganisms.

The making of one tonne of steel requires 280 t of water. Efforts to recycle this water in coke plants via activated sludge treatment were confronted by rapid sludge intoxication when more than 50% of the process water was re-used. This was due to the accumulation of highly toxic organic compounds, indicating the need for careful

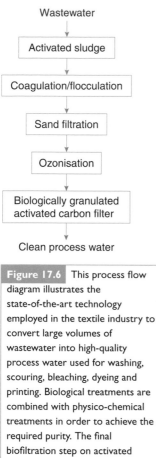

Wastewater

↓

Activated sludge

↓

Coagulation/flocculation

↓

Sand filtration

↓

Ozonisation

↓

Biologically granulated activated carbon filter

↓

Clean process water

Figure 17.6 This process flow diagram illustrates the state-of-the-art technology employed in the textile industry to convert large volumes of wastewater into high-quality process water used for washing, scouring, bleaching, dyeing and printing. Biological treatments are combined with physico-chemical treatments in order to achieve the required purity. The final biofiltration step on activated carbon, combining physical sorption with *in situ* biodegradation, is necessary to remove toxic compounds produced during the ozonisation step.

research on residual organics and even microbial products giving rise to abortive metabolism. A great many textile wet-processing plants are currently upgrading their wastewater treatment systems in order to recycle water. Because of the greatly variable chemical composition of the liquid effluents, depending on the types of fabrics and dyes being processed, no two textile factories apply the same treatment scheme to treat their effluent (Fig. 17.6).

17.2.4   Automatisation of wastewater treament plants

At present, most biological waste treatment systems, even multi-million dollar plants, generally are operated on the basis of a few rudimentary physical parameters such as pH, dissolved oxygen (DO) or redox potential. Dissolved oxygen probes are used in activated sludge plants to minimise energy expenditure to that just necessary to maintain a DO level around 2 mg l^{-1} in the aerated basin. Redox probes are used to monitor ammonium oxidation and nitrate removal in sequencing batch reactors. These control strategies fail, however, to ensure constant effluent quality because they do not detect variations in load, toxic shocks or process performance. The current control strategies must therefore be supplemented with dynamic mathematical models, i.e. models that can simulate and predict transient responses thus providing flexible automatic control strategies. The use of dynamic models requires the continuous input of data collected with on-line sensors.

On-line biomonitoring devices capable of quantifying the incoming load and effluent quality, and continuously transferring this information to the operation control system are currently being developed. One newly developed on-line biosensor measures the BOD of the incoming wastewater and its potential toxicity towards different groups of microorganisms present in the activated sludge (Fig. 17.7).

The development of other types of biosensors would help to ensure a more stable biological activity and therefore a more reliable treatment. For example, it was mentioned above that the occasional appearance of small worms in activated sludge plants was very beneficial to decrease sludge production (Fig. 17.2). These worms do, however, disappear as inexplicably as they appear and very variable process performance ensues. On-line biosensors capable of following and predicting the population size of these worms may help to maintain their profitable activity. The same strategy could be employed to stabilise the populations of other very valuable microorganisms, such as bactivorous protozoa, which are essential to obtain good-quality effluents, or to show the development of detrimental microorganisms, such as the filamentous bacteria that cause sludge bulking.

17.3 | Digestion of organic slurries

Production of organic slurries, e.g. sewage sludge or animal manures, is increasing in many parts of the world causing the traditional

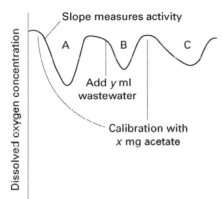

Figure 17.7 Respirogram obtained with a biosensor used to measure on-line the BOD and potential toxicity of wastewater before it enters a treatment plant. The addition of acetate to an aerated vessel containing activated sludge causes a temporary drop in the O_2 concentration (trough A). The initial slope of O_2 decline is an indication of the activity of acetate-utilising microorganisms, while the surface area of trough A reflects the amount of BOD added. The latter can be used to measure the BOD_5 and the total BOD of a wastewater sample by comparing the surface areas of troughs A and B. The BOD measurement is then used to adjust the flow rate to the plant. Trough C, obtained with a second pulse of acetate, indicates that the activity of acetate-utilising microorganisms has decreased (smaller slope) due to the presence of a toxic compound in the wastewater sample added in B. Possible remedial actions are: (i) the addition of toxicant-neutralising additives in the main flow to the plant, e.g. powder activated carbon; (ii) the buffering and dilution of the toxic wastewater with non-toxic effluent; or (iii) the addition of stored sludge in order to boost the microbial activity. Use of ammonium, or other substrates, in place of acetate allows the activity of other types of microorganisms to be followed.

disposal schemes, such as their application onto agricultural land, to become saturated. An increasing number of countries are even banning these disposal schemes due to contamination of groundwater. More environmentally friendly treatment processes for organic slurries suffer high cost and/or poor efficiency.

A well-known treatment process for sewage sludge and animal manures is anaerobic digestion in completely mixed anaerobic reactors. During this process, about 50% of the solids are converted to biogas, while the remainder is more or less stabilised. The performance, profitability and biogas output of anaerobic digesters can be increased by co-digesting animal manure or waste sewage sludge with 10–20% solid wastes from the agro and food industry, such as slaughterhouse, pharmaceutical, kitchen, fermentation or municipal wastes. Many full-scale installations using this co-digestion approach have recently been built in several European countries.

The completely mixed reactors treating organic slurries are operated at low volumetric loading rates, i.e. 2–5 kg organics m^{-3} day^{-1} because the particulate organics must be solubilised before they can be subjected to anaerobic conversions (Table 17.2). The rate of

Table 17.2 Design parameters for various types of anaerobic reactors. The loading rate, a measure of the process efficiency, is high with UASB reactors due to biomass retention in sludge granules and high in solid--state reactors due to high biomass concentration. Completely mixed reactors share none of these advantages and are therefore less efficient (small loading rate and long hydraulic retention times)

	UASB[a] reactor	Completely mixed reactor	Solid-state reactor
Effluent treated	Wastewater	Organic slurry	Solid wastes
Solid concentration in reactor, g l^{-1}	<50	50–100	200–400
Loading rate, kg organics m^{-3} day^{-1}	10–30	2–5	20–40
Hydraulic retention time, days	0.3–1	20–40	10–20
Solid retention time, days	>20	20–40	10–20

[a] UASB, upflow anaerobic sludge blanket.

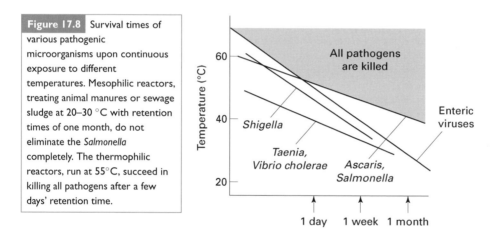

Figure 17.8 Survival times of various pathogenic microorganisms upon continuous exposure to different temperatures. Mesophilic reactors, treating animal manures or sewage sludge at 20–30 °C with retention times of one month, do not eliminate the *Salmonella* completely. The thermophilic reactors, run at 55°C, succeed in killing all pathogens after a few days' retention time.

solubilisation of particulate organics may be rather slow as in the case of waste activated sludge, which takes 15 days to reach 90% hydrolysis. As a consequence, retention times of at least 20 days and up to 60 days or longer are used. Several new developments increase the performance of anaerobic digesters. For example, the hydraulic retention time in the reactor can be uncoupled from the solid retention time by filtering the treated effluent and re-injecting the solids in the reactor until the hydrolysis products pass through the membrane. This reactor design removes a greater proportion of solids due to the longer solid retention time and achieves this in a smaller (cheaper) reactor due to the smaller hydraulic retention time.

Improved performance can also be obtained by running the digestion at higher temperatures since the rate of hydrolysis of particulate matter increases with temperature. New insights in thermophilic digestion resulted in the construction in Denmark of several large-scale thermophilic digestors to treat farm manure. Being run at higher temperatures, these reactors yield a pathogen-free effluent, unlike the mesophilic digesters that often fail to meet the regulations in terms of faecal pathogens (Fig. 17.8). Several drawbacks have, in the past, kept thermophilic digestion from becoming popular, for example the difficulty of start-up and the sensitivity to certain stress factors such as NH_3 and H_2S. Bentonite clay can be used to remove NH_3 inhibition. H_2S, on the other hand, can be destroyed by injecting electron acceptors, e.g. oxygen or nitrate, in the reactor.

Perhaps the major problem, at least for sewage sludge digesters, is to minimise the mass of N and P being recycled to the main plant flow via the so-called *sludge water*. Indeed, more than 50% of the sludge N is hydrolysed during digestion and the resulting recycle load contains typically about 1 g NH_4^+ l^{-1} and may contribute 20% of the influent N load.

This extra nutrient load may cause problems in view of the new, more stringent, standards concerning the nutrient content of discharged effluents. This may also be the case for P as some investigators have found that up to 60% of the sludge-bound P may be released during anaerobic digestion. Various treatments have in the past been optimised to precipitate P chemically. The cost of these treatments have, however, prevented them from being used in practice. The pH-controlled precipitation with lime seems attractive because the high pH may also serve to remove the ammonium by stripping. The cost associated with the lime addition can be greatly reduced by pre-aerating the effluent in order to remove the buffering capacity associated with the alkalinity. This method can also be combined with the addition of Al or Fe salts, preferably from a cheap source such as Al/Fe-rich sludge from drinking water production plants. Still another method is to optimise the conditions for struvite ($MgNH_4PO_4$) precipitation through cooling and CO_2 stripping.

Current technologies such as aerobic or anaerobic stabilisation, land disposal and incineration of organic slurries could become much less costly provided more efficient and cheaper methods of de-watering sludges from 2–5% to 25–40% dry matter could be developed. A major challenge to environmental biotechnologists is to develop enzymes, products and treatments that will permit more satisfactory de-watering of surplus sludge microbial biomass. New developments are being applied commercially that rely on the heat production during aerobic post-treatment to evaporate the excess water. This *biological drying* process requires less energy than the thermal drying techniques. One very sensitive problem, however, is the generation of bad odours, which have caused the shut-down of several plants.

17.4 | Treatment of solid wastes

Solid waste treatment is at present dominated by landfilling and incineration. Landfills are becoming less and less viewed as an option because they prevent the recycling of reusable products (plastics, paper, construction materials, etc) and they are inefficient in terms of energy (biogas) recovery. Moreover, landfill leachates and gas emissions pollute the environment. Likewise, incinerators do not allow

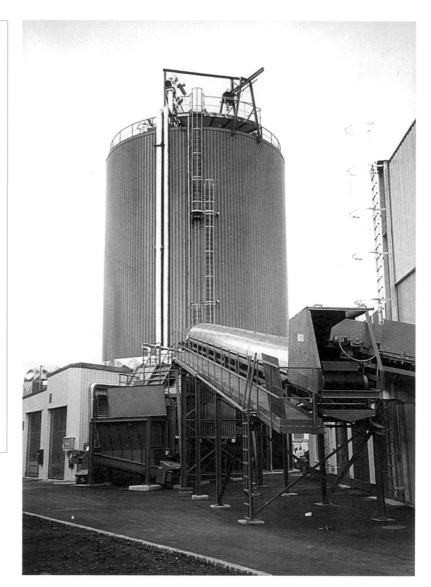

Figure 17.9 Closed reactor used for the anaerobic biological conversion of biowastes into biogas (mixture of methane and carbon dioxide). Biogas is then converted into electrical power, which is sold to the network. The picture illustrates a plant in Salzburg, Austria, treating 20 000 t biowaste annually with a single-phase thermophilic solid-state fermentation process. The conveyor belt in the foreground transports the shredded and screened (40 mm) biowaste to a dosing unit. After thorough mixing with digested waste (to ensure inoculation) and heating up to 55°C via steam injection, the hot mixture is pumped to the top of the reactor via the left pipe, while the pipe at the right-hand side transports the biogas from the top of the reactor to gas motors. Each tonne of wet waste produces about 135 m^3 biogas (250 kW h) after a retention time of 16 days (9 m^3 biogas m^{-3} day^{-1}).

material recovery though they may be designed to recover energy from waste. Incinerators suffer the drawbacks of high costs ($\sim$100–250 € t^{-1} municipal waste incinerated) and, moreover, require very sophisticated and costly flue gas purification systems to avoid environmental harm.

An elegant alternative for the treatment of municipal and industrial solid waste is currently making its way to the market place, the so-called *separation and composting plant*. These are very large and sophisticated plants, working at high capacities (100 000 to 300 000 t a^{-1} of waste), and wherein a battery of physical separation units recover the following materials from rubbish:

* *sand* and *gravel*, sold as construction material;
* *iron*, sold to metallurgic industry;

Table 17.3 Comparison of aerobic and anaerobic composting. While aerobic composting is slightly cheaper and has often been preferred in the past, recent developments in anaerobic composting technology make this new technology more attractive. Because it is carried out in closed reactors, anaerobic composting requires less space, produces less odours and kills pathogens more efficiently than aerobic composting

	Aerobic composting	Anaerobic composting
Cost	60 € t^{-1} wet	75 € t^{-1} wet
Floor area	Large	Small
Energy balance	Consumes energy	Produces energy[a]
Odours	Problem	No problem
Quality final compost		
Salt content	High (toxic)	Low
Pathogens	Present	Absent

[a] 600 kW h energy is produced in the form of bio-gas per tonne wet biowaste; upon combustion in a gas motor with 33% electrical conversion, it produces 200 kW h electricity.

- *aluminium* and other non-ferrous metals with high re-sale value;
- *cardboard* and *paper*, sold to paper industry;
- hard and soft *plastics*, re-used or incinerated;
- biodegradable organics, transformed into *compost* and *biogas*.

The philosophy of this new type of municipal waste treatment plant, of which the first are being operated in Germany, The Netherlands and Belgium, is to minimise the non-reusable residual fractions that have to be landfilled or incinerated (Fig. 17.9). Since the biodegradable organics constitute ~60% of municipal solid wastes, the last item in the above list deserves special attention. The composting of these biodegradable organics is already widely applied in regions where this waste fraction (the vegetable, fruit and garden waste or biowaste) is selectively collected.

The organic fraction of municipal solid waste is composted either aerobically or anaerobically. While aerobic composting is a well-known technology and has traditionally been applied, recent developments in anaerobic composting are conferring several advantages to this new technology, making it increasingly attractive and increasing steadily its market share (Table 17.3).

Different environmental companies commercialise various designs of anaerobic digesters of solid waste, differing in terms of:

- solids concentration in the reactor (from 50 to 400 g l^{-1});
- temperature (from mesophilic, at 35 °C, to thermophilic, at 55 °C);
- number of stages (one or two).

One such design, the DRANCO (*dry anaerobic composting*) process, uses thermophilic temperature (55 °C) at high solid concentration (200–400 g l^{-1}) in a one-stage fermentation. It is in fact a similar process to

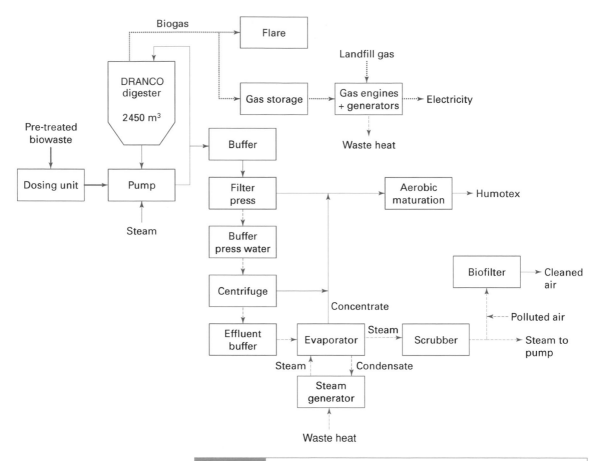

Figure 17.10 Process flow diagram of the anaerobic composting plant treating 20 000 t a^{-1} biowaste in Kaiserslautern, Austria. The waste is directly fed in *solid-state* (300 g solids l^{-1}) one-stage anaerobic digester, maintained at 55°C, wherein each tonne of wet waste produces ~150 m^3 biogas (60% methane). The biogas is converted to steam to warm up the digester and to electricity in a gas engine. Waste heat from the motors is reused to evaporate the wastewater generated during the mechanical dewatering of the digested paste. Dewatered paste (500 g solids l^{-1}) is subjected to a short (1–2 weeks) aerobic post-treatment yielding a humus-like material. The various points where odours are produced, e.g. the aerobic post-composting, are ventilated and the waste air is treated in a biofilter where volatile organic compounds are removed.

that taking place in landfills, with the difference that it is carried out in a closed reactor under well-controlled conditions and at a much greater reaction rate. The very high reaction rates attained make it possible to complete the digestion process in two weeks (Table 17.2) instead of 20 years as in landfills. Key to the process is the high temperature and intense mixing through recirculation allowing much higher reaction rates and the feeding of the solids directly in the reactor without addition of dilution water (Fig. 17.10). Wet processes, on the other hand, require dilution water in order to feed a slurry in the reactor. This has the drawbacks of higher water usage and much larger reactor volumes. Because mechanical agitation is not possible in the dry process, the output of the reactor is recycled several times, with addition of fresh feed material at each passage (Fig. 17.10). This recycle loop ensures adequate mixing and inoculation of the feed material.

The humus end-product has proven an excellent soil conditioner, superior to conventional aerobic composts in terms of plant germination and yield. The reason is that aerobic composts may be phytotoxic due to their high salt content, while anaerobic composts contain much less salts due to the fact that about half of these are eliminated with the water in the filter press (Fig. 17.10). Moreover, anaerobic composts contain far fewer weed seeds and microbial pathogens compared to aerobic composts. The market value of composts is, however, low and special post-treatments should be sought for targeted applications. The latter can be achieved by adding beneficial microorganisms such as N-fixing and plant-growth-promoting bacteria, mycorrhizae or biocontrol microorganisms. The restoration of polluted soils can also benefit from compost addition as this can serve either as a source of inoculum and nutrients for the degradation of xenobiotic compounds or as an organic matrix promoting the binding of xenobiotics.

17.5 | Treatment of waste gases

Waste gases polluted with a wide variety of organics – most of them at the $\mu g\ m^{-3}$ level or below – are inherent to domestic and industrial activities. In the coming years, air pollution control, in general, and odour abatement, in particular, will become of increasing importance. Biotechnological cleanup of waste gases, of odours and of in-house air is an area undergoing full development. The focal point of this technology is the possibility of growing and maintaining organisms capable of removing a wide spectrum of pollutants even at the extremely low concentrations at which they occur in the gas phase.

17.5.1 Removal of volatile organic compounds (VOCs)

Conventional physico-chemical treatment of polluted industrial waste gases, such as combustion or adsorption on activated coal filters, tend to waste a lot of energy and create secondary pollution. Pollutant concentrations in industrial emissions, for example, are of the order of 100 ml m^{-3}. To burn these gases in an incinerator, at least 50 l of methane need to be added per cubic metre in order to ensure complete destruction. A bioreactor may, in most cases, achieve the same oxidation provided the VOCs are brought in close contact with degradative microbes, O_2, H_2O and nutrients. Biodegradation rates vary with the pollutant being degraded:

- quickly biodegraded: alcohols, ketones, aldehydes, organic acids, organo-N;
- slowly biodegraded: phenols, hydrocarbons, solvents (e.g. chloroethene);
- very slowly biodegraded: polyhalogenated and polyaromatic hydrocarbons.

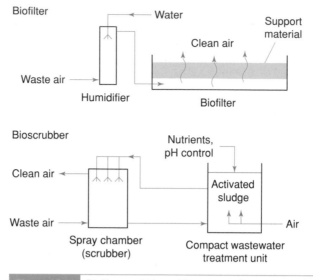

Figure 17.11 Biofilters and bioscrubbers are used to remove volatile organic compounds (VOCs) from waste gases via biological means. Biofilters are simple, robust and cheap, but require a large floor area. Bioscrubbers rely on classical wastewater treatment processes (activated sludge or trickling filter) after having transferred the pollutants from a gaseous stream to an aqueous phase in a scrubber. Bioscrubbers are more amenable to process optimisation and require less floor area than biofilters. They are, however, more costly and are less efficient at removing poorly soluble VOCs, e.g. hydrocarbons.

Despite the broad spectrum of air pollutants amenable to biofilter treatment, the introduction of this new technology is slow, perhaps because its low cost does not ensure high profit margins and because the physico-chemical air pollution control industry is well entrenched.

Various types of reactor designs are used to treat air biologically (Fig. 17.11). In *biofilters*, contaminated air flows slowly through a wet porous medium – compost, peat or wood chips – that supports a degradative microbial population living in the thin water film coating the solid support material. The superficial gas flow varies from 1 to 15 cm s^{-1}. This yields a contact time, for a typical bed height of 1–3 m, of 10–100 s. For normally biodegradable compounds, removal efficiencies of 90% can be expected at volumetric loading rates of 0.1–0.25 kg organics m^{-3} reactor day^{-1}. The advantages of biofilters are:

- simple and cheap design (support material replaced every 2–4 years);
- high internal surface area makes biofilters ideally suited to remove poorly soluble pollutants, e.g. hydrocarbons;
- possibility to inoculate with bacteria especially adapted for the breakdown of xenobiotic compounds, e.g. chloromethane.

The most difficult problem is the control of the pH in the biofilter since H_2S is oxidised to H_2SO_4, NH_3 to HNO_3, and chloroorganics to HCl. For example, the removal efficiency of dimethyl sulphide in a compost biofilter seeded with the bacterium *Hyphomicrobium* dropped within two months of operation, from 1 to 0.1 g m^{-3} day^{-1} due to a pH drop to 4. Repeated dosing of 25 kg limestone powder (CaCO$_3$) per cubic metre of compost carrier eliminated the inhibition for a two-month period. The biggest disadvantages of biofilters are:

- large floor space necessary;
- not possible to control the process conditions, e.g. pH;
- support materials, such as compost, themselves generate odours.

The disadvantages of the biofilter can be avoided in a *bioscrubber* (Fig. 17.11). A conventional scrubber transfers a substance present in a gaseous stream to a liquid stream by spraying a liquid in a chamber through which the gas is passed. In a bioscrubber, the sprayed liquid is a suspension of micro-organisms, which cycles back and forth between the spray chamber and a wastewater treatment unit where biodegradation takes place. The process parameters such as adequate nutrient supply and pH are much more easily controlled (in the circulating liquid) than in a biofilter, leading to fast reaction rates. While biofilters require a large footprint since their height preferably should not exceed 1 m in order to avoid clogging, bioscrubbers require much less space because the tank where biodegradation takes place can be several metres high.

Bioscrubbers appear best suited for large air flows because of their low back pressure and small size. They can, however, only be employed for the removal of gases that are sufficiently soluble because the mass transfer rate in a spray chamber is less than that attainable in a biofilter unit. In case the obtained contaminant concentration in the outlet gas is too high, a second bioscrubber inoculated with micro-organisms capable of degrading lower contaminant concentrations must be installed. This aspect requires further development.

At present, considerable research is devoted to the design of a system that can combine the adsorption of the gas onto a solid surface (e.g. activated carbon) and biodegradation of the sorbed compound. *Biotrickle filters* are sheets of a plastic or other microbial support medium hung in the contaminated air stream. The sheets are bathed continuously by a re-circulating stream of water containing the nutrients required by the micro-organisms. Biotrickle filters hold promise where space utilisation is paramount. Biooxidation rates per unit volume are high so that these filters can be as small as physico-chemical units. Being operated at higher loading rates, they are, however, more sensitive to peak loads and nutritional requirements need to be monitored closely.

17.5.2 Biological removal of sulphur and nitrogen compounds from flue gases

Nitrogen oxides (NO$_x$) and sulphur dioxide (SO$_2$) are major air pollutants formed during the combustion of coal and oil and released in flue gases. There is considerable interest in the development of an efficient and low-cost biotechnology for the simultaneous removal

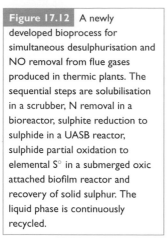

Figure 17.12 A newly developed bioprocess for simultaneous desulphurisation and NO removal from flue gases produced in thermic plants. The sequential steps are solubilisation in a scrubber, N removal in a bioreactor, sulphite reduction to sulphide in a UASB reactor, sulphide partial oxidation to elemental S° in a submerged oxic attached biofilm reactor and recovery of solid sulphur. The liquid phase is continuously recycled.

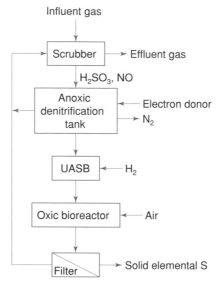

of these air pollutants, since conventional physico-chemical technologies are either very expensive or inefficient. A new system is currently being proposed in which the flue gas is led through a scrubber in which >95% SO_2 and >80% NO_x dissolve in a solution of $NaHCO_3$ and Fe(II)-EDTA (the latter compound seems to raise the solubility of NO_x, the bottle-neck of the process). The S- and N-laden solution is regenerated in three sequential biological steps (Fig. 17.12). The first step consists of an anoxic reactor wherein NO is converted to inert N_2 gas via biological denitrification:

$$2\,Fe^{II}(EDTA)(NO) + \text{electron donor}$$
$$\rightarrow 2\,Fe^{II}(EDTA) + N_2 + CO_2 + H_2O$$

An electron donor, e.g. methanol or ethanol, needs to be added in order to sustain the reaction. In the two following steps, H_2SO_3 is sequentially reduced biologically to H_2S and, finally, partially re-oxidised to solid elemental sulphur:

$$H_2SO_3 + 3\,H_2 \rightarrow H_2S + 3\,H_2O$$
$$H_2S + \tfrac{1}{2}O_2 \rightarrow S° + H_2O$$

The reduction of H_2SO_3 takes place in a UASB reactor (Fig. 17.5) seeded with sulphate-reducing bacteria. Flocculant polymers are added, together with the necessary nutrients and reducing equivalents (ethanol or H_2) to adjust the (BOD/H_2SO_3) molar ratio at a value of one. In the third bioreactor, aerobic bacteria oxidise sulphide back to solid S° (end-product). The further oxidation of S° to H_2SO_3 and H_2SO_4 is prevented by dosing limiting amounts of O_2. The overall process is fully automated with about 120 parameters being continuously analysed, most of them on-line. The water is continuously recycled.

This process of biodesulphurisation will undoubtedly also be applied in the future to treat other waste streams. There is a growing interest in depolluting wastewaters through the activity of sulphate-reducing bacteria in sulphidogenic UASB reactors. Sulphate concentrations reach very high levels in effluents from the paper board industries ($2 \, g \, l^{-1}$), in molasses-based fermentation industries (2–$9 \, g \, l^{-1}$) and in edible oil refineries (up to $50 \, g \, l^{-1}$). Very large amounts of sulphate are also present in acidic mine drainage where pyrite rock is being processed. When heavy metals are present, these can be very efficiently removed (>99%) via sulphide precipitation.

17.6 | Soil remediation

One of the major problems facing the industrialised world today is the contamination of soils, groundwater and sediments. The total world hazardous waste remediation market is approximately US$16 billion per year. There are at least 350 000 contaminated sites in Western Europe alone and it may cost as much as 100 billion € to clean just the riskiest of these sites over the next 20–25 years. The most common contaminants are chlorinated solvents, hydrocarbons, polychlorobiphenyls and metals. *Bioremediation*, i.e. the use of microorganisms to degrade or detoxify pollutants, is becoming increasingly used mostly in cases of hydrocarbon pollution. However, bioremediation is not yet universally understood or trusted by those who must approve of its use and its success is still an intensively debated issue. One reason is the lack of predictability of bioremediation, due to insufficient information on:

- *bioavailability*, i.e. how to obtain good contact between contaminant molecules and microorganisms (see Box 17.2);
- *biostimulation*, i.e. how to supply the microbes with stimulating agents;
- *bioaugmentation*, i.e. how introduced microbes behave in the field.

17.6.1 Biostimulation and bioaugmentation

The microorganisms capable of biodegrading pollutants are usually already present in contaminated soils and groundwater. Thus, in the vast majority of cases, bioremediation of soils or groundwater will occur satisfactorily by stimulating the microorganisms already in place with the required nutrients or other factors (*biostimulation*). Thus, oil spills at sea or hydrocarbon leakages in groundwater are remedied by *fertilising* the sea or ground with nitrogenous and other nutritious compounds (Table 17.4). Surfactants may also be added in order to facilitate the mass transfer of poorly soluble hydrocarbons into the water phase where the microorganisms live. Another example of biostimulation is the injection of methane in aquifers polluted with certain chlorinated solvents or benzoic acid in aquifers polluted with certain polychlorobiphenyls (PCBs). The injected carbon sources,

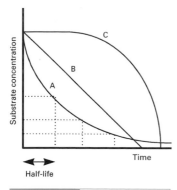

Figure 17.13 The kinetics of biodegradation of pollutants in soil systems are usually first order, which means that the rate of substrate disappearance is proportional to the substrate concentration (curve A). With first-order kinetics, the half-life defines the time during which half of the substrate is degraded. First-order kinetics occur when the substrate concentration is low (smaller than the affinity constant K_s) as is often the case in soils. Zero order refers to a constant reaction rate which is independent of the substrate concentration and which typically occurs during co-metabolism (curve B). In cases of high pollutant concentrations, microbial growth can occur resulting in increasing rates with time and the curve C is typically observed.

Box 17.2 | Bioavailability of pollutants

Under *in situ* soil conditions, contaminant removal is often exceedingly slow due to poor availability to microorganisms that bring about their degradation. Compounds that tend to sorb onto solid particles, such as clay and humus, are less easily taken up by microorganisms. This tendency is quantified by the Freundlich equation:

$$S_{eq} = (OM)K_{oc} C_{eq}^{1/n}$$

where S_{eq} is the concentration of the pollutant on the sorbent phase (mg g^{-1}), OM is the % organic matter in the soil, K_{oc} is the partition coefficient, C_{eq} is the concentration in the aqueous phase (mg l^{-1}), and n is a constant related to the sorbent. Compounds with $K_{oc} < 100$ are little sorbed and therefore readily available (e.g. benzene; $K_{oc} = 10^{1.9}$), whereas compounds with $K_{oc} > 1000$ are quite well sorbed (e.g. phenanthrene; $K_{oc} = 10^{4.4}$). The K_{oc} is easily estimated in the laboratory from a measurement of the octanol/water partition coefficient (K_{ow}), i.e. the ratio of compound concentration in n-octanol and in water. The K_{ow} value of hydrocarbons can be used to estimate their half-life in soils. Half-life is an indication of disappearance rate of substrates which are degraded according to first-order kinetics (Fig. 17.13).

These concepts do not, however, explain the observation that certain pollutants in soil cannot be removed below a certain level. This phenomenon, common with pesticides, has been called *aging*. It is thought that aging results from the diffusion of the pollutant molecules through the interstitial micropores of aggregates and through the three-dimensional matrix of natural organic matter. As this process is not reversible, the Freundlich equation is no longer valid and different molecules of the same compound have different half-life values. Pesticides may persist in soil at non-removable residual levels as a result of this phenomenon.

methane and benzoic acid, promote the growth of specific microorganisms that possess enzymes that will degrade both the injected substrate and the pollutant already present. As the microorganisms do not seem to draw any advantage from the breakdown of the pollutant, this reaction is called *co-metabolism*.

Inoculation with specific populations of microorganisms (*bioaugmentation*) may be advantageous in certain polluted sites, for example when the pollutant is a complex molecule that can be broken down only by a particular combination of very specific microorganisms (called a consortium). Such pollutants include polyaromatic hydrocarbons (PAHs), halogenated organic compounds, certain pesticides, explosives such as trinitrotoluene (TNT), polychlorobiphenyls (PCBs), etc. Proper conditions and appropriate microbial strains have been found that affect biodegradation of these compounds in laboratory setups. For example, the degradation of simple chlorinated aromatics in soils and wastewater treatment plants can be accelerated by inoculating pure cultures of microorganisms selected in the laboratory. More complex pollutants, e.g. PCB, may require the concerted action of several microbial strains. For this particular case, dechlorinating

Table 17.4 Different possible strategies to induce bioremediation of soils and groundwater. While biostimulation relies on autochthonous microorganisms, i.e. those already present in the contaminated site, bioaugmentation makes use of laboratory-grown bacteria, fungi or pre-adapted consortia

Action	Mechanism	Example
Bio-stimulation, i.e. to stimulate the microorganisms already present		
Add nutrients N, P	Optimise the chemical make-up for balanced growth	*Fertilise* oil slicks at sea (Exxon Valdez spill in Alaska)
Add co-substrates	Pollutant is degraded by an enzyme intended to process the co-substrate	Inject methane to degrade trichloroethylene in aquifers
Add electron acceptors	Oxidation of organics in groundwater typically limited by poor solubility of O_2	Bioventing of aquifers (air injection) or addition of nitrate
Add surfactants	Hydrocarbons and non-aqueous phase liquids (NAPLs) are not available to microorganisms	Adding surfactants will disperse the hydrophobic compounds in the water phase
Bio-augmentation, i.e. to (re)introduce microbial cultures grown in the laboratory		
Add a pre-adapted strain	Certain sites may not contain adequate microorganisms to degrade pollutants	Inoculation of soils and wastewater treatment plants with chloroaromatic degraders
Add pre-adapted consortia	The presence of the right combination of microorganisms is ensured	Seed sediments with PCB-dechlorinating enrichment cultures
Add genetically optimised strains	Existing degradation pathways may release dead-end or toxic intermediates	Construction of strains effecting complete simultaneous oxidation of chloro- and methylaromatics
Add genes packaged in a vector	Genes encoding for desirable functions are transferred into microorganisms already present	Degradation of PCBs or pesticides

consortia developed from contaminated sediments have been mass cultured in granular form in methanogenic UASB reactors. These granules have been shown to accelerate the degradation of PCB *in situ* in soils and sediments.

For specific applications, bioaugmentation can be carried out with genetically engineered microorganisms (GEMs). GEMs may be particularly useful to avoid the misrouting of degradation intermediates into unproductive dead-end pathways as may occur during the degradation of mixtures of chloro- and methylaromatics. GEMs may also help to prevent the formation of toxic intermediate products that may destabilise the community and inhibit biodegradative processes. One example is PCB degradation during which a first group of microorganisms release chlorobenzoates, which are further attacked by a second group of microorganisms. PCB degradation is normally blocked by a by-product of chlorobenzoate degradation. GEMs have been constructed which do not produce the toxic intermediates, hence giving better survival of the PCB degraders. The greatest challenge is indeed to increase the chances of survival of inoculated strains, i.e. to make them ecologically competent. In this respect, chances of survival are usually greater when the inoculated strain was originally isolated from the site which is to be bioaugmented.

17.6.2 Soil remediation techniques

A great variety of biotechnologies are being used to treat polluted soil. In increasing degree of complexity and cost, the most commonly used techniques include:

- *in situ* bioremediation;
- landfarming;
- slurry-phase bioreactors.

In situ bioremediation relies on biological clean-up without excavation. It is usually applied in situations where contamination is deep in the sub-surface or under buildings, roadways, etc. *In situ* biorestoration of pollutants is gaining interest since it avoids excavation costs and produces no toxic by-products as is the case with *ex situ* physico-chemical treatment. Water is cycled through the sub-surface using a series of recovery and recharge trenches or wells. Water may be oxygenated by sparging with air or via addition of H_2O_2. Microbial clean-up by enhancement of anaerobic degradative activity *in situ* has received less study. The obvious drawback of *in situ* bioremediation is that it is difficult to stimulate microbial activity throughout the contaminated soil volume because the injected water carrying the necessary nutrients and microorganisms tends to flow through larger soil interstices, leaving substantial amounts of residual contaminant within more impermeable layers. It may take years for the contaminants to diffuse to the bioactive zones where biodegradation is occurring.

One specific type of *in situ* soil bioremediation, called *bioventing*, has emerged recently as one of the most cost-effective and efficient technologies available for the remediation of the vadose zone (unsaturated zone above the groundwater table) of petroleum-contaminated sites. Bioventing consists of stimulating aerobic biodegradation by circulating air through the sub-surface. High removal efficiencies ($>97\%$) can be obtained for soluble paraffins ($<C_{16}$) and polyaromatic hydrocarbons (PAHs) after several years operation. Bioventing is, however, limited to homogeneous sub-surface formations since heterogeneities would cause the air to move through the most permeable areas causing treatment to occur only in limited areas.

Another success story of *in situ* soil bioremediation is *phytoremediation*. Here specific plants are cultivated that accumulate heavy metals in the above-ground plant tissue or stimulate organic breakdown in their rhizosphere (the zone immediately adjacent to the roots). While phytoremediation is elegant, *clean* and cheap, its main drawbacks are that only the surface layer of soil (0–50 cm) can be treated and that the treatment takes several years and leaves substantial residual levels of contaminants in the soil. Phytoremediation is, however, undergoing full development at present.

Removal of oil slicks by so-called *landfarming* is an established method based on microbial degradation (Fig 17.14). Given half-lives of the order of one year, it would take about 7 years of treatment to remove 6.4 g hydrocarbon kg^{-1} soil down to the clean-up goal of 50 mg kg^{-1}. This low-tech method can be somewhat upgraded by mixing the soil with fresh organic residues (compost). Elevated temperatures and increased microbial diversity and activity increase reaction rates. Moreover specific co-substrates favour co-metabolism. Landfarming systems can be upgraded by including anaerobic pre-treatment. For example, anaerobic tunnels are used to reduce compounds such as trinitrotoluene by adding nutrients and co-substrates for the indigenous bacteria. In a second aerobic stage, the reduced metabolites are either completely mineralised or polymerised and irreversibly immobilised in the soil matrix. This approach has also been used successfully to decontaminate soils polluted with chloroethene and BTX (mixtures of benzene, toluene and xylene) aromatics.

Slurry-phase bioreactors may achieve the same clean-up levels in considerably less time. In this case, excavated polluted soil is treated under controlled optimal conditions, ensuring effective contact between contaminant and microorganisms. The latter are, in most cases, specific cultures of adapted microorganisms. With overall degradation rates in the range of 0.2–2 g oil kg^{-1} soil day^{-1}, solid residence times of 30 days, in place of several years, are sufficient to meet the clean-up levels. Treatment costs increase accordingly and can be up to 200 € t^{-1} of soil.

17.7 | Treatment of groundwater

17.7.1 Active remediation

The predominant groundwater remediation strategy in the USA and Europe has been the application of the so-called *pump-and-treat* technology. This approach uses mainly physico-chemical techniques to remove the pollutants in the above-ground treatment units, via for example air stripping and activated carbon, while biological reactors are used in fewer than 10% of cases (Fig. 17.15). The limited use of biological treatment may be due to limited experience and demonstration data, limited acceptance of the technology, but also failures to achieve the clean-up levels required. To date, probably most experience with full-scale *ex situ* and *in situ* applications of bioremediation has been acquired for the biodegradation of petroleum hydrocarbons, comprising straight and branched chain, saturated, unsaturated and cyclic aliphatics to mono-, di and polyaromatic hydrocarbons. Recently, however, new types of bioreactor designs have been developed that eliminate polychlorinated solvents and aromatics as well. For example, UASB reactors seeded with granular methanogenic sludge have been shown to completely (>99%)

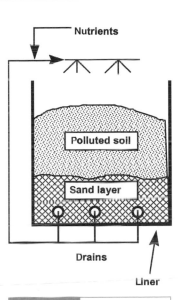

Figure 17.14 Cross-sectional view of a solid-phase soil *reactor*, or landfarming system. The soil is excavated, mixed with nutrients and microorganisms, and evenly spread out on a liner. With regular ploughing to favour mixing and aeration, mineralisation of petroleum hydrocarbons present at initial concentrations of tens of g kg^{-1} follows first-order kinetics with a half-life of ~2 years. Landfarming is an established technique for the remediation of hydrocarbon-contaminated soil.

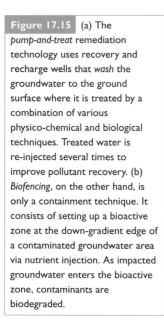

Figure 17.15 (a) The *pump-and-treat* remediation technology uses recovery and recharge wells that *wash* the groundwater to the ground surface where it is treated by a combination of various physico-chemical and biological techniques. Treated water is re-injected several times to improve pollutant recovery. (b) *Biofencing*, on the other hand, is only a containment technique. It consists of setting up a bioactive zone at the down-gradient edge of a contaminated groundwater area via nutrient injection. As impacted groundwater enters the bioactive zone, contaminants are biodegraded.

(a) Pump-and-treat

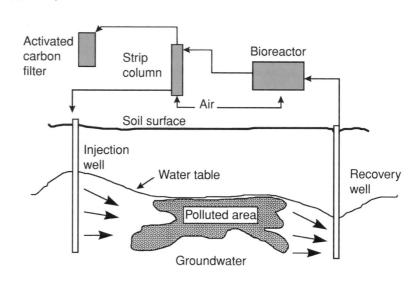

(b) Biofencing

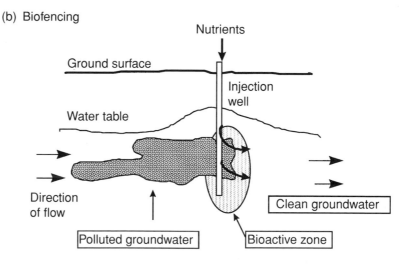

dechlorinate tetrachloroethylene present at 4 mg l^{-1} in polluted groundwater. Acetate was used as carbon source and electron donor and process costs were competitive (US$1.2 m^{-3} treated). The UASB reactor technology is also being upgraded with granular sludge combining both anaerobic and aerobic bacteria.

The *pump-and-treat* strategy fails, however, to achieve clean-up targets in most cases and, moreover, requires long clean-up times. Of the 77 pump-and-treat sites recently evaluated by a committee under the auspices of the US National Research Council (NRC), only eight had reached the clean-up goals, which in all cases were the maximum contaminant levels for constituents regulated under the Safe Drinking Water Act. Of the eight successful sites, six were polluted with petroleum hydrocarbons which would also have been eliminated via natural attenuation. Today (2005), pump-and-treat is most frequently used for remediation of methyl *tert.*-butyl ether found whenever petrol has been stored in underground tanks. The US NRC Committee concluded that pump-and-treat methods often failed in their ability to remove contaminant mass from the sub-surface because of sub-surface heterogeneities, presence of fractures, low-permeability layers, strongly adsorbed compounds and slow mass transfer in the sub-surface. Even with the best extraction methods, very often only a small fraction of soil-bound contaminants can be mobilised, leaving a large residual fraction in the soil. As a result of this failure, remediation policy and technical developments are shifting towards increased use of *in situ* containment practices, e.g. *biofencing* (Fig. 17.15), rather than full-treatment scenarios. In cases where full treatment is necessary, less stringent clean-up goals are set, based on risk assessment taking into account type of land use.

Aside from the much-studied generic compounds discussed above in this chapter, there is a host of toxic compounds usually present at trace level and whose fate remains poorly studied. One example are the polychlorinated dioxins and furans which are formed as by-products of chemical synthesis processes. They are also produced by combustion of garbage, waste oils, soils polluted with oils, chemical wastes containing PCBs, and by various other high-temperature processes. Because of the high toxicity of some dioxins and furans, these compounds are of major ecotoxicological concern. Ongoing research and development has attempted to minimise their formation in incinerators and emission via fly ashes. Yet, the biological breakdown of these compounds in the environment is of considerable importance. Indeed, they are often present in wastes that are extremely difficult to treat properly by incineration (e.g. polluted soils and river sediments). They are also present in fly ashes of incinerators, which are deposited in landfills and, notwithstanding all precautions, can contaminate landfill leachates.

17.7.2 Natural attenuation and monitoring

Several factors have recently generated a lot of interest in new monitoring techniques. One such factor is the fact that remediation technologies are often insufficient to meet stringent clean-up targets. This limitation is making legislators reassess the target pollutant levels and making them consider the use of risk-based end-points in place of absolute end-point values. The new concept of risk-based end-points requires the development of new analytical tools that assess the bioavailable rather than the total pollutant concentration. These new tools typically rely on bioassays because the traditional analytical methods cannot distinguish pollutants that are available to biological systems from those that exist in inert, or complexed, unavailable forms. Subjecting a polluted soil to a period of intensive microbial activity can reduce the toxicity by a factor of 5 to 10. This ecotoxicological information can be easily deduced by running a simple bioassay with soil leachates. One type of bioassay is based on the inhibition of the natural bioluminescence of the marine organism *Photobacterium phosphoreum*, which is used, for example, in the Microtox, Lumistox and Biotox tests. These assays are, however, not specific, since light inhibition will occur upon exposure to any toxicant. This limitation is circumvented in a new class of bacterial biosensors that are specific to certain types of toxicants. For example, biosensors able to detect bioavailable metals were constructed by placing *lux* genes of *Vibrio fischeri* as reporter genes under the control of genes involved in the regulation of heavy metal resistance in the bacterium *Alcaligenes eutrophus*. The recombinant strains, upon mixing with metal-polluted soils or water, emit light in proportion to the concentration of specific bioavailable metals. Light emission is easily measured spectrophotometrically.

Another factor responsible for the recent interest in new monitoring tools is the high cost and slow pace of remediation technologies. A more pragmatic remediation approach, termed natural attenuation (or *intrinsic bioremediation*), is being advocated by the US Environmental Protection Agency. Intrinsic bioremediation relies on natural processes to remove, sequester or detoxify pollutants without human intervention. Intrinsic bioremediation has been observed most frequently with groundwater contaminated with hydrocarbons. If evidence suggests that a site is improving due to intrinsic bioremediation, and that the pollution does not pose a threat to human health, the environmental regulating agency may grant that site *monitoring only* status. This strategy simply requires remote monitoring in order to follow sub-surface contaminant concentrations *in situ*. Remote monitoring can be carried out with a ground-penetrating radar, which monitors contaminant breakdown in the sub-surface based on the increase of solution conductance that accompanies the breakdown of hydrocarbons or chlorinated solvents. Another technique employed in remote monitoring uses genetically engineered microorganisms that produce light in response to the presence of specific contaminants. As these microorganisms are attached on a photocell connected to a radio chip, the light signals are converted into radio waves, which are detected at a distance. These sensors can be scattered throughout polluted sites to monitor the progress of pollutant breakdown.

17.8 | Further reading

Baveye, Ph., Block, J.-C. and Goncharuk, V. V. *Bioavailability of Organic Xenobiotics in the Environment: Practical Consequences for the Environment.* Dordrecht: Kluwer Academic, 1999.

Boon, N., Goris, J., de Vos, P., Verstraete, W. and Top, E. M. Bioaugmentation of activated sludge by an indigenous 3-chloroaniline-degrading *Comamonas testosteroni* strain, 12gfp. *Applied and Environmental Microbiology* **66**: 2906–2913, 2000.

Devinny, J. S. Biological treatment of contaminated air: theory, practice, and everything in-between. *Environmental Progress* **22**(2): J18–J19, 2003.

Farre, M. and Barcelo, D. Toxicity testing of wastewater and sewage sludge by biosensors, bioassays and chemical analysis. *Trac-Trends in Analytical Chemistry* **22**(5): 299–310, 2003.

Grady, L. C. P., Daigger, G. T. and Lim, H. C. *Biological Wastewater Treatment*, second edition. New York: Marcel Dekker, 1999.

Lendvay, J. M., Loffer, F. E., Dollhopf, M., *et al.* Bioreactive barriers: a comparison of bioaugmentation and biostimulation for chlorinated solvent remediation. *Environmental Science and Technology* **37**(7): 1422–1431, 2003.

Nivens, D. E., McKnight, T. E., Moser, S. A., *et al.* Bioluminescent bioreporter integrated circuits: potentially small, rugged and inexpensive whole-cell biosensors for remote environmental monitoring. *Journal of Applied Microbiology* **96**(1): 33–46, 2004.

Sayler, G. S., Sanseverino, J. and Davis, K. L. *Biotechnology in the Sustainable Environment*. New York: Plenum Press, 1997.

Schmidt, I., Sliekers, O., Schmidt, M. *et al.* New concepts of microbial treatment processes for the nitrogen removal in wastewater. *FEMS Microbiology Reviews* **27**(4): 481–492, 2003.

Verstraete, W. Environmental biotechnology for sustainability. *Journal of Biotechnology* **94**(1): 93–100, 2002.

Chapter 18

Production of antibiotics by fermentation

Derek J. Hook

3M Pharmaceuticals, USA

18.1 | Introduction

Production of antibiotics by fermentation, either for use directly in human therapy or to act as feedstock for the synthesis of chemically modified derivatives of the core antibiotic structure, still make up the majority contribution of antibiotic agents in the treatment of human disease. Only two classes of chemically synthetic agents have significant market share as antibiotic agents: the sulphonamides and the fluoroquinolones. A novel chemical class, the oxazolidinones, recently entered the marketplace but still does not have significant market penetration, and is carefully managed as a reserve antibiotic. Also, in the current reimbursement environment, it is clear that it will be extremely difficult for any new antibiotic to compete economically with generic β-lactams, macrolides and tetracyclines unless they have a distinct clinical advantage and improved cost of care.

The continued development of antibiotic-resistant organisms has started to reveal weaknesses in the armoury of drugs available to treat serious hospital and community acquired infections. Thus the focus in drug discovery has shifted away from the identification of broad spectrum antibiotics to new entities that target the resistant

Basic Biotechnology, third edition, eds. Colin Ratledge and Bjørn Kristiansen.
Published by Cambridge University Press. © Cambridge University Press 2006.

organisms. A focus on this market niche, however, reduces the potential market for these new narrow-spectrum agents and has an impact on business decisions whether or not to proceed with discovery efforts. In addition, the emphasis on cost savings by the health-care industry continues to drive the expansion of use of generic broad spectrum antibiotics where they are effective. This has led to a dilemma for the pharmaceutical industry as to whether or not it is cost effective to proceed with such drug discovery efforts, with the prospect of minimal return on investment. This has led some major pharmaceutical companies to abandon antibiotic drug discovery completely but, conversely, has opened up niches for biotechnology companies that might be more willing to take risks and accept smaller market sizes. A recent example was the decision by Bristol-Myers Squibb in late 2004 to shut down antibiotic production at its Syracuse, NY, facility citing economic reasons.

18.2 | Overview of antibiotic classes

Worldwide sales of antibiotics and antifungals for human therapy were estimated to be approaching US$26 billion in 2001, of which oral antibiotics accounted for about US$19 billion. In spite of the patent expiry of the top 20 antibiotics in sales, the world market for antibiotics continues to expand, driven primarily by increased use in India and Asia. However, a far larger quantity (tonnage) of antibiotics is still used as non-therapeutic agents in agriculture. Exact figures are difficult to come by, but it seems that about 7500–12 500 tonnes of antibiotics are used in the USA alone for non-therapeutic agricultural use, especially for growth promotion in chickens, pigs and cows. Some of this is made up of classes of agents that are little used in human therapy. The situation in Europe has changed, with EU policies banning the use of many antibiotics used for human therapy as growth promotion agents, and sales have declined, despite continued use of many antibiotics for veterinary purposes.

The market for antibacterial drugs is split about 50 : 50 between beta-lactam antibiotics and other classes. The beta-lactam market is split between cephalosporins (30%), penicillins (7%) and other beta-lactams (15%). Fluoroquinolones accounted for about 24% of the market, and macrolides about 20%. Oxazolidinones, streptogramins, tetracyclines, aminoglycosides and carbapenems make up the remaining 4%. The following presentation will cover all major classes of antibiotics. However, the history of the use of antibiotics, their production methods and the biotechnology used to improve production and the approaches used to address the emergence of bacterial resistance are illustrated clearly through the history of the development of penicillins and cephalosporins as therapeutic agents. Indeed, these agents are still significant therapies for bacterial infections because of the development of wide-spectrum, oral and cheap generic versions of the major second and third versions of these antibiotics.

In general, antibiotics that are commercially useful can be divided into a few major classes. This is normally based on their biosynthetic routes and precursors used by the organism to make these compounds, often followed by specific and unique biosynthetic modifications. The main classes include:

- antibiotics derived from amino acid precursors either made through a non-ribosome synthetic pathway (beta-lactams, cyclic peptides, lipopeptides) or those based on a normal ribosome-based synthetic route (nisins);
- antibiotics manufactured from sugars (aminoglycosides);
- antibiotics derived from fatty acid precursors (polyketide antibiotics) such as the tetracyclines, macrolides and polyenes.

Often these biosynthetic routes converge to produce hybrid classes, for example the glycopeptides, which consist of a modified peptide backbone with the addition of critical sugar residues.

18.2.1 Overview of β-lactam antibiotics

There are two major classes of microbially produced beta-lactam antibiotics that are still manufactured in quantity, the penicillins and cephalosporins. β-Lactam antibiotics (penicillin, ampicillin, cephalosporins, etc.) are narrow- and moderate-spectrum antibiotics because some members are only effective against Gram-positive organisms while other members can also kill certain Gram-negative bacteria. Despite these limitations, their use is widespread because of their general safety and the development of the later generations of beta-lactams with increased spectrum of antimicrobial activities. The development of the large range of penicillins and cephalosporins in clinical use has been dependent upon the subsequent chemical manipulation of the core nuclei of these antibiotics. Two major biological processes were involved in industrial production of these penicillin and cephalosporin variants:

- The development of strain-improvement programmes leading to modified industrial production strains of producing organisms that can economically produce the tonnes of antibiotics needed for the subsequent chemical manipulation of the bulk antibiotics.
- The development of efficient and economical industrial-scale enzymatic cleavage methods to remove the unwanted side chains of the bulk materials, yielding the core nucleus for subsequent chemical manipulation. These enzymatic methods have significantly reduced the use of industrial solvents and so have contributed to a major reduction in costs for treatment of waste streams from the production plants.

18.2.2 Penicillins

The first microbially produced antibiotics to be discovered were the penicillins. To meet the demand, especially during and after the Second World War, a submerged fermentation process was developed

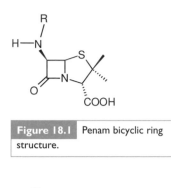

Figure 18.1 Penam bicyclic ring structure.

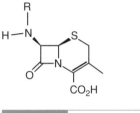

Figure 18.2 Cephem bicyclic ring structure.

for the two major antibiotics of the class, penicillin G and penicillin V. Penicillin G and V share a common bicyclic ring structure, with the beta-lactam portion of the molecule being responsible for the biological activity. Variations in the R group of the side chain are responsible for the differing antimicrobial spectrum of activity and also pharmacokinetic properties. For example, penicillin G is acid labile and cannot be given orally since it is destroyed by the acid pH of the stomach, and needs to be delivered by injection. Penicillin V, however, is acid stable and thus has the advantage that it can be delivered orally.

It was early established that variations in the fermentation media components could direct the biosynthesis of the producing organism to make penicillins with differing side chains. The bulk of the penicillin G and V is produced by feeding either phenylacetic or phenoxyacetic acid, respectively, during the fermentation process and the amide that is generated on the beta-lactam ring gives the penicillin its characteristic structure. However, this approach is restricted to a limited range of organic acids and there are limitations in the ability of the producing organism to substitute desirably more complex precursors into this portion of the penicillin molecule. This is due to the inability of the acylating enzyme to accept these donors.

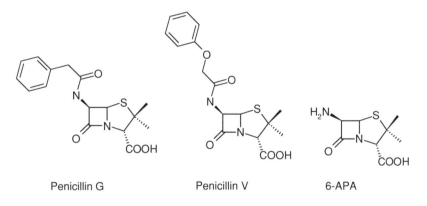

Penicillin G   Penicillin V   6-APA

In order to overcome these limitations of the fermentation process a different, semisynthetic approach has been developed to produce penicillins with both an extended biological spectrum and biological and chemical stability.

The core biological activity of the penicillins resides in the bicyclic chemical substructure shown in Fig. 18.1. This sub-structure is referred to as the 'penam' nucleus. New penicillins are made by taking this basic nucleus in the form of 6-aminopenicillanic acid (6-APA) and chemically conjugating new novel side chains (= R in Fig. 18.1) on to the nucleus at the free amino group of 6-APA. Similarly, the core biological activity of the cephalosporins resides in the bi-cyclic chemical sub-structure shown in Fig. 18.2. This substructure is referred to as the 'cephem' nucleus. In an identical fashion, new cephalosporins are made by taking this basic nucleus in the form of 7-amino-desacetoxycephalonsporic acid (7-ADCA, R = H) and chemically conjugating new novel side chains (= R in Fig. 18.2) onto the nucleus at the free amino group of 7-ADCA. These substructures that contain the core biological activity of a molecule are also referred to as 'pharmacophores'. This allowed new penicillins to be developed that had expanded biological spectrum, including coverage of both Gram-negative and Gram-positive activity, and also resistance to the bacterial enzymes, called beta-lactamases, which destroy the antibiotics before they are effective in killing bacteria. Two of the earliest second-generation penicillins were ampicillin and amoxacillin. These antibiotics not only had activity against Gram-positive bacteria, but showed significant activity against Gram-negative species that are clinically important, such as *Haemophilus influenzae*, *Escherichia coli* and *Proteus mirabilis*.

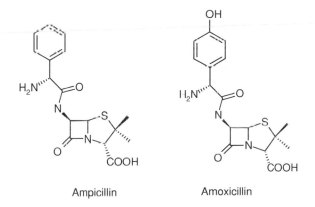

Ampicillin   Amoxicillin

Another example of the synergy between a fermentation product and a chemical process is the use of 6-APA as a feedstock not only for semisynthetic penicillins, but for the corresponding production of the 7-ADCA nucleus of the cephalosporins through a chemical ring expansion of the 5-member 'penam' nucleus to the 6-member 'cephem' (see above, Figs. 18.1 and 18.2). Addition of various side chains to the amino group of the cephalosporin ring system leads to a large number of second- and third-generation cephalosporins.

18.2.3 Cephalosporins

The cephalosporin class of beta-lactam antibiotics was discovered by chance from a sewage outlet in Sardinia, Italy. The producer microorganism (originally classified as *Cephalosporium*, but reclassified as *Acremonium chrysogenum*) produced two hydrophilic beta-lactam components, one of which was penicillin N, and the other was cephalosporin C. They expressed rather weak activity, albeit with both Gram-positive and Gram-negative activity. The discovery of a new related beta-lactam class of antibiotics opened up the possibilities of creating semisynthetic cephalosporins as indicated above. Cephalosporin C is more stable than penicillin N and this allowed industrial strain-improvement programmes to develop strains of *Cephalosporium* that produce very high titres of cephalosporin C.

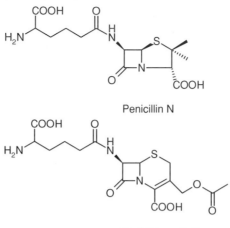

Penicillin N

Cephalosporin C

Once the parent molecule cephalosporin C has been obtained in quantity, it is then necessary to develop technology to remove the side chain. Two approaches are taken for the production of the cephalosporin nucleus:

- Enzymatic de-amidation of the amino-adipic acid side chain yielding glutarylcephalosprins, which are subsequently de-acylated to 7-ACA.
- Chemical ring expansion of the penicillin ring to the cephalosporin ring through a sulfoxide intermediate to 7-ADCA. This can be subsequently acylated in a manner to that for producing semisynthetic penicillins.

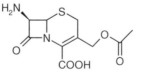   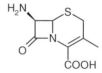

7-Aminocephalosporanic acid   7-Aminodesacetoxycephosporanic acid
(7-ACA)   (7-ADCA)

The cephalosporins are classified into generations based on their general features of antimicrobial activity. First-generation cephalosporins include agents with good activity against Gram-positive bacteria (*S. aureus*, group A streptococci, *Streptococcus pneumoniae*) and relatively modest coverage for Gram-negative organisms. Second-generation antimicrobials have increased activity against certain Gram-negative pathogens, including *Haemophilus influenzae*, *Neisseria meningitidis* and *Moraxella catarrhalis*. Third-generation cephalosporins are somewhat less active against Gram-positive cocci, but much more active against enteric Gram-negative organisms.

18.2.4 Other beta-lactam classes

Wide-scale screening over the last 50 years has led to the discovery of a number of major different classes of lactam antibiotics, all of which show unique antimicrobial spectra and physicochemical characteristics. Most of this effort has been driven by the continuous need to out-smart the evolution of resistance mechanisms by disease bacteria. The major core structures of the beta-lactam classes are shown below.

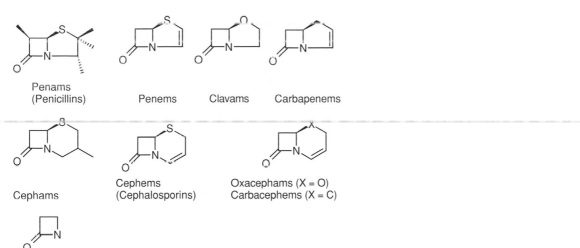

Penams (Penicillins)   Penems   Clavams   Carbapenems

Cephams   Cephems (Cephalosporins)   Oxacephams (X = O) Carbacephems (X = C)

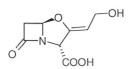

Monobactams

18.2.5 β-Lactamase inhibitors

An approach has been taken to enhance the activity of penicillins that otherwise had lost their effectiveness because of the production of beta-lactamase enzymes by previously susceptible bacteria. These enzymes destroy the beta-lactam ring before the antibiotics reach the cell-wall target enzymes and render them ineffective. One strategy around this problem was the screening for, and identification of, compounds that inhibited the action of the beta-lactamases, but themselves did not show significant antibacterial activity. The compound that was finally identified as being an effective agent for this purpose was clavulanic acid.

Clavulanic acid

Fortunately, the compound was found to be safe for human use, and is used in combination with amoxicillin under the trade name Augmentin™. It is used to treat different types of bacterial infections such as sinusitis, pneumonia, ear infections, bronchitis, urinary tract infections and infections of the skin. As can be seen from the structure of the molecule, it has a core bi-cyclic ring structure very similar to that of penicillin. The use of this combination therapy pioneered the way for use of specifically directed combination therapy. It is of interest that many cephalosporins are also subjected to degradation by beta-lactamases (penicillinases and cephalosporinases) by resistant organisms, but a similar cephalosporinase inhibitor has not been developed for this class of antibiotics, leaving a challenge for future biotechnologists to extend the life of these antibiotics.

18.2.6 Tetracyclines

These are an important class of broad-spectrum antibiotics, and are used widely to treat human infections and in agricultural and veterinary practice. They are effective against many Gram-positive and Gram-negative bacterial infections and are suitable for treating rickettsial, chlamydial, mycoplasmal and some fungal infections. As they have such a wide spectrum of activity, they also destroy the normal intestinal microbiota and often produce severe gastrointestinal disorders. Oxytetracycline, in particular, is used both to treat infections in animals and as a growth promotion agent. It has also been used in plant protection. Recently this group of antibiotics was recommended as one of the treatments for anthrax, as well as for use in the treatment of stomach ulcers, because they exhibit activity against *Helicobacter pylori*. Because of the issues of development of antibiotic resistance in human pathogens, there have been moves to restrict the use of tetracyclines for animal growth promotion and plant protection, especially in Europe.

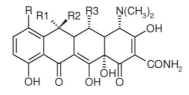

Tetracycline nucleus

Antibiotic	R	RI	R2	R3
Chlorotetracycline	Cl	CH$_3$	OH	H
Oxytetracycline	H	CH$_3$	OH	OH
Tetracycline	H	CH$_3$	OH	H
Doxycycline	H	CH$_3$	H	OH
Minocycline	N(CH$_3$)$_2$	H	H	H

These antibiotics are formed through the polyketide biosynthetic pathway. Chlorotetracycline contains a chlorine atom in its structure and the amount of this component can be increased by directed fermentation by including chloride ions in the medium. The producing organism can be directed to produce solely tetracycline by the deletion of the chlorination gene, while doxycycline and minocycline are produced by chemical modifications of chlorotetracycline, oxy-tetracycline or tetracycline.

18.2.7 Macrolides

The macrolides are another important group of antibiotics and are formed by a combination of a polyketide biosynthetic pathway with the addition of unusual sugars. This group of antibiotics is also very amenable to genetic manipulation of the producing organisms, both by traditional methods to improve yield and more recently to the application of the knowledge of the polyketide synthetic gene cassettes and how the biosynthesis is regulated by the resulting multi-enzyme complexes. The macrolides that are used most commonly in human therapy have 12, 14 or 16 carbon macrocyclic lactone rings. They are effective against Gram-positive bacteria, *Mycoplasma* and *Legionella*. The original members of the class, such as erythromycin, clarithromycin and azithromycin (zithromax), which are produced by chemical modification of the core erythromycin macrolide nucleus, have now been augmented in medical practice by more effective, wider spectrum ketolides (14-membered ring macrolide derivatives characterised by a keto group at the C-3 position), such as telithromycin.

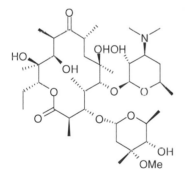

Erythromycin

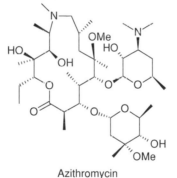

Azithromycin

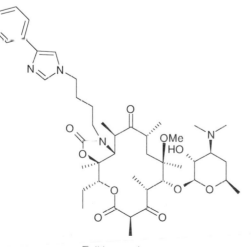

Telithromycin

Tylosin is a 16-membered macrolide that is widely used in animals for veterinary treatment and growth promotion, but is also used in crop protection. Again, the issue of whether or not the reservoir of macrolide-resistant strains of human pathogens is due to the use of this closely related macrolide to molecules used in human therapy, or whether this reservoir exists because of poor medical practice in use of the macrolides that are approved for human therapy is one that has not been answered satisfactorily.

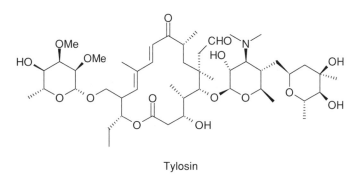

Tylosin

18.2.8 Aminoglycosides

Aminoglycosides were among the first of the antibiotic classes to be discovered after Fleming's initial discovery of penicillin in 1927. Waksman initiated a screening programme from soil extracts in the mid to late 1930s and discovered streptomycin, one of a new class of antibiotics that consisted of unusual sugar molecules joined together. The major disadvantage to this group, despite their extended spectrum of antimicrobial activity against Gram-negative organisms is the fact that they are not orally bioavailable, and must be administered by injection. In addition, the compounds exhibit a narrow therapeutic index with adverse effects being seen close to the therapeutic dose. Despite this they were, until recently, considered last line therapy against resistant organisms. Due to the structural complexity of these molecules they are exclusively produced by fermentation, although semisynthetic versions of the original antibiotics have been produced to overcome bacterial enzymatic resistance mechanisms by acetylation of the numerous amino groups, or by phosphorylation on the sugar portions of these molecules. This issue is resolved in the semisynthetic derivative, Amikacin. This molecule is obtained from kanamycin B.

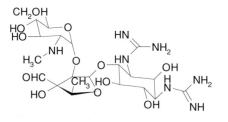

Streptomycin

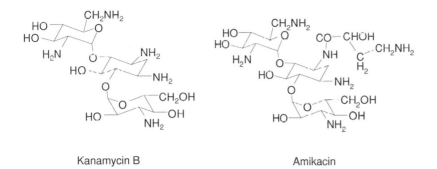

Kanamycin B   Amikacin

18.2.9   Glycopeptides

This important class of antibiotics consist of an aminoglycoside core that is derived from the condensation of seven modified, or unusual, aromatic amino acids or from a mixture of aliphatic and aromatic amino acids with the additional substitution of amino sugars yielding the parent antibiotics. While several hundred compounds are in this class, the most important is vancomycin. Until recently the glycopeptides were the last line of defence against drug resistant microbes. Now glycopeptide-resistant organisms are appearing in clinical settings. As in the case of beta-lactams and macrolides, the use of a glycopeptide in animals that is related to those used in human therapy, apovaricin, has led to the suspicion that glycopeptide-resistant organisms generated by exposure to avoparicin are transferring their resistance mechanisms to clinical settings. The organism used for commercial production is *Amycolotopis orientalis*, and the parent glycopeptides are used as such or as semisynthetic modified derivatives.

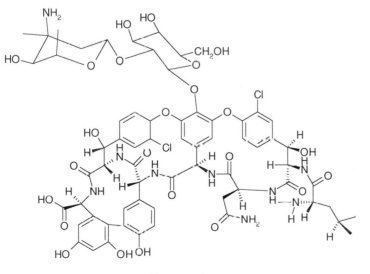

Vancomycin

18.2.10   Streptogramins

The streptogramins, one of the two new microbially produced classes of antibiotics to appear on the market in the last few years, are unusual in that the therapeutically administered material (Synercid™) is a combination of two streptogramins, A and B, which have quite different structures. Streptogramin A is a polyunsaturated cyclic macrolactone and streptogram B is a cyclic depsipeptide. Individually, the antibiotics are bacteriostatic, but when combined, exhibit bactericidal activity. The antibiotic is administered intravenously and is active against Gram-positive bacteria especially vancomycin-resistant *Enterococcus faecium* and methicillin-resistant *Staphylococcus aureus*. Resistance has been detected and seems to be exacerbated by the use or virginamycin in animal feeds.

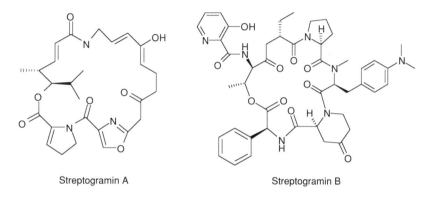

Streptogramin A   Streptogramin B

18.2.11   New lipopeptides

Daptomycin is a member of the lipopetide group of antibiotics that has recently been approved for use for the treatment of complicated skin and skin structure infections caused by susceptible strains including *Staphylococcus aureus* (including methicillin-resistant strains), *Streptococcus pyogenes* and vancomycin-susceptible strains of *Enterococcus faecalis*. It is administered intravenously. Members of this class are examples of antibiotics resurrected for use as narrow-spectrum antibiotics for special situations such as against vancomycin- and methicillin-resistant organisms. Originally they were not considered for therapeutic use because of their restricted spectrum of activity when the focus of screening programmes was on identifying antibiotics with a broad spectrum of activities and compounds that were developable as oral agents. With the success of daptomycin, other class members are also being investigated for possible use against antibiotic-resistant organisms. The activity of these antibiotics is mainly due to disrupting multiple aspects of bacterial membrane function. The structure of these antibiotics consist of a common cyclic peptide nucleus with various lipid acyl chains at the *N*-terminus of the peptide.

18.2.12   Bacitracin and other peptide antibiotics

Bacitracin and tyrocidins belong to another class of small cyclic peptide antibiotics that are primarily used in human therapy as topical antimicrobial agents. These molecules lack the lipid side chain that are present in the lipopeptides exemplified by daptomycin described above. They were discovered early in the search for antibiotics and all are off-patent and are sold as over-the-counter agents, either singly or in combination. They are made by a non-ribosomal synthetic mechanism by *Bacillus* species and have poor pharmacokinetic and safety properties as oral agents, but continue to have a significant therapeutic niche since they are bactericidal and there is little evidence that bacterial resistance has developed despite widespread and uncontrolled use.

18.2.13 Bacteriocins

These antimicrobial agents, although they are not classified as antibiotics for human use, are classified as food additives with use for food preservation. The bacteriocins deserve mention as a small, but industrially significant, set of compounds that are produced microbially and have an inherent antimicrobial activity. The class example is nisin. This is a ribosomally produced small peptide/protein that contains post-translational modification to introduce novel amino acids (lanthionines) into the molecule. It thus differs from the penicillins/cephalosporins and from the bacitracin/tyrocidin class of antibiotics that are produced by non-ribosomal enzyme complexes. Nisin is used widely to preserve cheese, clotted cream and some canned vegetables. It is classified as a generally recognized as safe (GRAS) substance in the USA, EU and Japan.

18.2.14 Polyenes

Another group of polyketide antibiotics are the large polyenes, chiefly used for antifungal therapy rather than for antibacterial use. The agents disrupt the sterol membranes of fungi and kill the organism. The class examples are amphotericin B and nystatin. Both are quite toxic, but amphotericin B is often used as a last choice when therapy with fungiostatic agents, such as with the azoles, fail. Amphotericin B has to be administered intravenously and is not very soluble. Both colloidal suspensions and liposomal formulations have been used to achieve greater exposure levels. Generally speaking, amphotericin B has a very broad range of activity and is active against most pathogenic fungi.

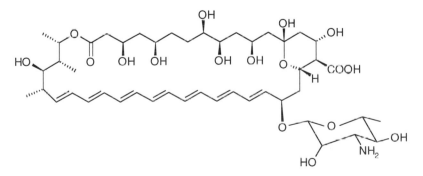

Amphotericin B

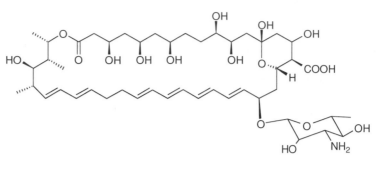

Nystatin A

18.2.15 Griseofulvin

Griseofulvin is an antifungal agent first isolated from a *Penicillium* spp. in 1939. The compound is insoluble in water. It is effective orally. It is deposited primarily in keratin precursor cells and is mainly effective on *dermatophytes*. It acts by interfering with the microtubular structure of cell division so that fungal cells cannot reproduce. The infection is then eliminated by the host's immune system. Griseofulvin has been the first-line drug for treatment of dermatophytosis for many years and adverse reactions are uncommon. However, following the emergence of alternatives such as itraconazole and terbinafine, its use has been limited.

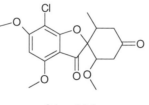

Griseofulvin

18.2.16 Bacteriophages

Although not in widespread use, this class of agents has been used for human therapy, especially in the former Soviet Union, and the concept is attracting attention as a method of treatment of resistant strains of bacteria. These agents are very specific to species and particular strains of bacteria, but generally are benign as regards to the human host during infections. Bacteriophages are viruses that reproduce and ultimately kill the host bacteria by lysis. While they are produced by fermentation technology similar to the antibiotics, their use therapeutically is challenging. Bacteriophages are host specific, even down to sub-strains of bacteria, so for them to be useful therapeutically two requirements must be met: first, good and rapid diagnostics are essential to identify the host strain; and, second, the bacteriophage for that strain must be immediately available. This is more challenging than the availability of wide-spectrum antibiotics. Side effects are minimal and they are subjected to phagocytosis (clearance by engulfment and destruction by white blood cells) within the host, so clearance is rapid. There may be some immunological response from the host. Thus, repeat use can be a problem, but they seem to be non-toxic to humans. They have been used topically in cases of sepsis resulting from burn injury. The most promising application seems to be in agriculture, where they may be able to replace anti-biotics that are used as growth promoters. This class of agents offers a challenge to the industrial biotechnologist to find the best way of producing a wide range of off-the-shelf agents for therapeutic use and in an economically viable model.

18.3 | Strain improvement

There are three major applications of genetic engineering technology to antibiotic production;

- strain improvement programs;
- introduction of genes to produce novel antibiotics; and
- the engineering of microbial strains and enzymes involved in the production process.

The growing wealth of knowledge of biosynthetic pathways is allowing a more rational approach to the genetic manipulation of the producing organisms, and is also suggesting new approaches to combining biosynthetic pathways from different organisms either to optimise the production of known antibiotics or to propose construction of hybrid molecules with potentially improved or novel characteristics. In addition, there continues to be a hope that some of the chemical manipulations carried out on core molecular structures can be replaced by new enzymatic approaches to production of these desirable products.

18.3.1 Conventional strain improvement

Strain improvement programmes have been either empirical in nature, i.e. mutation and selection of organisms for improved production of an antibiotic, or more recently have been directed by knowledge of the pathways involved in the biosynthetic process. The challenges in such strain improvement programmes include:

- work to enhance production from already engineered strains that are close to the limits of their biosynthetic capacity;
- maintenance of these production levels in an industrial processing environment, where reversion to low levels of production frequently occurs; and
- adaptation to cheaper sources of raw materials.

In these programmes, spores of the producing organism are exposed to a variety of mutagenic agents such as those given in Table 18.1, either individually or in combination.

After treatment, the spores are allowed to germinate and give rise to single colonies. These are then tested for antibiotic production and

Table 18.1	Common mutating agents
Physical agents	UV-irradiation
	X-rays
	γ-rays
Chemical agents	Nitrogen mustards
	N-methyl-N′-nitro-N-nitroso guanidine

selected on the basis of this and other parameters, such as reduced pigment formation. In addition, the isolates are tested for growth and sporulation ability. Isolates exhibiting poor characteristics are discarded. This process requires that a large number of single colony isolates are tested and suitable screening and analytical methods have to be developed to allow a robust judgement to be made about strains selected to go forward for testing on a larger scale and with the media components used in the production process (see Chapter 12). Also, it is possible to generate desirable characteristics by back crossing different strains and repeating the selection process. Some of the improved strain characteristics that have been selected for by strain improvement programs include:

- cultures that grow as pellets rather than filaments,
- cultures that have lost pigmentation, and
- elimination of side products.

18.3.2 Genetic engineering

A more rational approach has been taken in the manipulation of antibiotic-producing stains with the sequencing of the genomes of antibiotic producers or at least the sequencing of the gene clusters responsible for antibiotic biosynthesis. With the discovery that many of the biosynthetic genes for a number of different antibiotic families are clustered on the chromosomes of the producing organisms, and are regulated together, it has become clear that manipulating these genes in a systematic way might lead to both production improvements and to the production of novel antibiotics. This is clearly the case with the polyketide gene clusters responsible for macrolide production. The oxidation and dehydration processes that occur stepwise in the biosynthesis of these molecules can be manipulated by the appropriate deletion or insertion of genes into the biosynthetic cassettes. A number of companies are actively working to achieve the goal of producing novel antibiotics or core molecules that can be used in the semisynthetic manipulation of their final structure. In addition, genetic analysis of the higher yielding penicillin and cephalosporin strains has shown that part of the productivity increase can be explained by duplication of gene cluster on the same or different chromosomes of the original low-yielding strains.

A challenging area for future exploitation is the creation of hybrid antibiotics by inserting genes from different organisms. A few simple examples have been reported in the anthracycline antibiotic series, but the challenge is much greater because of the existing, and difficult to change, substrate specificity of the biosynthetic enzymes. To engineer a strain directly capable of making solvent extractable cephalosporins, such as cephalosporin G or V, by adding aromatic acetic acids, such as phenylacetic or phenoxyacetic acid, onto the cephalosporin nucleus using a combination of the enzymes from the penicillin V and the cephalosporin C biosynthetic pathway, has long been the holy grail. Despite considerable effort this has not yet been accomplished. Another challenge that still has to be met is the alternative of introducing the expandase enzyme from *Cephalosporium* into *Penicillium*, again leading to direct production of solvent extractable cephalosporins.

18.4 | Production processes

The industrial production of antibiotics involves many processing steps, each of which have changed since the early days of production in the 1940s and 1950s, to efficient computer-controlled manufacturing processes in use today. This trend has resulted from the constant demand to increase yield and decrease production costs. The process consists of a number of steps, including:

- culture preservation and preparation for scale-up,
- scale up of inocula for production,
- the production fermentation, and
- the recovery and post-processing steps.

In addition, off-line from these manufacturing processes are the

- processes to manipulate the production strains to continue to generate new strains with desirable characteristics,
- improvements of the physical characteristics for the fermentation, and
- work on strains that can utilise cheaper raw materials.

In the following sections, each of these aspects will be touched on to illustrate that modern biotechnological processes for antibiotic production have become more complex and sophisticated.

18.5 | The fermentation process

The process of the production for penicillins can be used as an example of the process flow involved in the large-scale industrial production of antibiotics and some of the process changes that have occurred over the last 30 years. Penicillin production in the 1950s typically involved a batch process. Not only was the fermentation process itself a single batch process, the process of media sterilisation was also an *in situ* process in the fermenter. The media consisted of lactose, cycle times were about 120 hours and minimal process control was used. The morphology of the organism was filamentous. Removal of the mycelium was by batch filtration and there were many subsequent extraction stages. Tank volumes were 50–100 m^3, titres were 0.5–1.0 g l^{-1}, process efficiency was 70–80% and costs were US$275–350 kg^{-1}.

In contrast, modern fermentations are highly efficient processes. Cheaper and more readily available carbons sources such as glucose/sucrose mixtures are fed continuously to the fermentation in a controlled manner, first to promote growth and then to sustain maximum production phases. The media are sterilised continuously and the operational mode is semicontinuous, with part of the fermentation broth being drawn off and continuously processed. Fermentation variables such as pH and aeration are computer controlled. Growth is now in the form of pellets, and downstream processing is based on whole broth recovery (no removal of the biomass) and continuous extraction with recovery of solvents and precursor after splitting. Fermentation tank volumes are larger (100–200 m^3) and titres are now >40 g l^{-1}. Efficiencies are over 90%. These factors have decreased costs to US$15–20 kg^{-1}. Similar improvements have been made in other antibiotic fermentations, with consequent improvements in the scale of production and reduction of cost of bulk antibiotics and precursors to semisynthetic derivatives

18.5.1 The growth medium

Media for cell-mass build-up are designed to provide fast growth in a batch mode with minimal changes in pH. Individual medium components do not have to be greater than 3–5% and provide a readily available carbohydrate, such as glucose or sucrose, and a soluble form of nitrogen, such as corn steep liquor or yeast extract. Calcium carbonate or phosphates can be added if buffering is required, which is often the case due to organic acids that can be produced by the rapid metabolism of sugars. Ammonium sulphate can be used to provide additional nitrogen.

18.5.2 The production media

These are proprietary and have been developed and fine tuned over the years. Invariably they are a compromise between cost and performance. The most suitable media are those that use inexpensive raw materials in combinations that can lead to maximal productivity. The production stage fermentations are fed-batch, which provides the chance to optimise the fermentation to provide the fine balance between controlled cell growth and maximum biosynthesis. Raw materials for use in the initial batch phase have to provide both immediate utilisable soluble nutrients as well as longer lasting and, therefore, less-soluble sources. Initial carbon sources are the least critical as they are easily added in a soluble form during the fermentation. Nitrogen sources are more critical as they serve as a main nutrient source throughout the fermentation. Ideal nitrogen sources are derived from agricultural origins, however questions of quality and variability can arise both within seasons and between seasons. This represents an on-going concern for maintaining reproducible fermentations. To alleviate this situation, several different raw materials can be used to prevent excess variation.

In some of today's highly productive fermentations there is no clear separation of the primary (tropophasic) and secondary (idiophasic) stages. To obtain maximum production rates, conditions are created that can provide rapid and early antibiotic production with continued cell growth, and these are the most common fermentation conditions employed in a modern antibiotic production plant. Supplemented raw materials are soluble and rapidly utilised. Suitable carbohydrates are sucrose, glucose or enzyme-hydrolysed corn syrups. Other carbon sources can be used. If necessary they can be supplemented with soluble nitrogen from corn steep liquor. The diligent feeding of a soluble, readily utilised carbohydrate such as glucose can prevent catabolic repression, as the concentration of the sugar will always be very low.

18.5.3 Foam control

The metabolism of the proteinaceous nutrients from the complex raw materials invariably create foaming, and thus control of the level of foam forming on top of the fermentation broth is essential. Oils, such as triacylglycerol, lard oil or soy oil, palm oil, peanut oil or rape seed oil are commonly used as antifoam agents, the final choice being dictated by local availability. These oils have the supplemental effect of acting as an alternative carbon source stimulating product formation. Other antifoam agents, such as silicone-based products or polypropylene glycol, are also used to supplement or replace oil. As foaming often occurs at unpredicted times, it is important to have automated feed-back for effective antifoam addition, to provide sufficient control without excess usage of these agents. Antifoam should be available on an as-needed basis and not simply batched into the starting medium due to the toxic nature of some antifoams as well as the resulting reduction in air hold-up at excessive antifoam levels (see Chapter 8). Excess use can also cause processing difficulties on downstream recovery.

18.5.4 Fed-batch feeding

The added volume of soluble nutrient feed can vary depending upon its concentration (typically 30–65%). At lower sugar concentrations, early partial harvests may be necessary to decrease the increase in broth volume caused by the high volume of feed addition. This addition of dilute solutions has the added benefit of lowering the viscosity of the broth, typically a problem with filamentous cultures. Early partial harvests produce large volumes of dilute antibiotic for product recovery. With correct handling, however, such protocols can be very productive as the maximum production rate of the fermentation can be maintained for long periods.

18.5.5   pH

The pH of the broth can be controlled to within 0.1 pH units by the addition of acid (sulphuric) or base (caustic or ammonia gas added through the air input). The pH can also be controlled by using the culture's own metabolism of sugar. Excess feeding of sugar in some conditions will produce acetic acid, which will lower the pH. Conversely, a cut-back in the sugar feed-rate can raise the pH.

18.5.6   Dissolved oxygen

Dissolved oxygen (DO) levels are critical for maintaining the maximum rate of antibiotic production and culture viability. As the use of pure oxygen is too costly, as well as being a safety concern, ambient air is used as the source of oxygen. A fine balance has to be established between aeration and the agitation necessary to distribute the oxygen into the liquid phase, the back pressure in the tank to increase oxygen solubility, the volume expansion of the fermentation broth, and the compounding of several of these effects on the dissolved carbon dioxide levels (see also Chapter 8). Dissolved oxygen levels should be maintained higher than 20% saturation at 1.5–2 atm. pressure throughout the fermentation and at air flow rates high enough to sweep out as much carbon dioxide as possible. A build-up of carbon dioxide can affect the microorganism adversely.

18.5.7   Culture preservation and aseptic propagation

Attention has to be given to the correct preservation and consistent propagation of high producing strains. Today's cultures with their long mutation history, increased copy number of certain genes and possible recombinant status do have questionable stability. Repeated slant-to-slant transfer of high yielding strains can produce subpopulations with lower productivity with the appearance of wild-type morphology. Storage in liquid N_2 is the most convenient way of long-term culture preservation. Stock cultures are typically maintained through a master cell bank hierarchy, where each master frozen culture, from a stock of many such cultures, is used to make a large number of working stock cultures. In this way, there is always a common lineage from which to start cellular propagation.

Preparation of a new master cell line is carried out through single cell or spore re-isolation and each lot rigorously evaluated both in shake-flask and pilot-plant fermentations to confirm superiority and stability before the culture is used in large-scale manufacturing. Considerable care is taken to maintain aseptic conditions throughout the build-up of culture volumes. This is especially critical at the seed stage where the cultures are growing fast and scheduled tank transfers occur before full status of asepsis is known.

18.5.8   Scaling up

For evaluation of new strain performance, shake-flask media and conditions are selected to provide environments as close as possible to the stirred-tank large-scale fermentations. This is not always possible and many compromises have to be taken. A good relationship between shake-flask performance, pilot-plant and large-scale fermentations can only be established after years of careful comparison. Potential titre increases of 5% or less are not only difficult to assess in shake-flask experiments but also difficult to assess at the pilot-plant stage where resources are limited and evaluations expensive. It is always desirable to have new cultures that easily fit into the existing fermentation protocols without further development work. However, new cultures often have properties that need further development to express their full potential. Here the interdisciplinary skills of the bioengineers, microbiologists and biochemists can prove to be rewarding.

For the actual process of scaling up culture seed from shake flask to production tank, the initial master stock culture is first expanded through a train of smaller vessels, which allow for rapid build-up of cell mass, usually in 1–3 day fermentations, until enough cell mass is obtained to allow for a 5–10% v/v inoculum into the production fermenter.

18.6 | Recovery and post-recovery processing

A comprehensive review of the possible recovery and post-processing procedures is given in Chapter 9. For the antibiotics described above, the downstream recovery needs to be tailored to the specific compounds. For example, aminoglycosides are extremely polar compounds and solvent extraction is not an option for these molecules, and ion exchange is used instead. Solvent recovery, however, is the preferred option for compounds like penicillin G and V. Either the whole broth is acidified and the antibiotic extracted with organic solvents, followed by a clean-up process and then precipitation as the sodium or potassium salt, or penicillin V can be directly precipitated at pH 2 from clear filtrates with subsequent clean up. In addition, modern processes that use penicillin to make the 6-APA ring nucleus, employ back-extraction from the solvent into an aqueous phase, which is used as the mother liquor for the enzymatic process that converts the penicillin to 6-APA. This process of conversion of the penicillin feed-stock for the generation of the core 6-APA intermediate was prompted by the need to produce the expanded new generations of penicillin antibiotics, although even with these molecules, direct precipitation from the clarified broth is one engineering process option used. It has to be realised that recovery and post-processing of the antibiotic is a method that often has considerable associated production costs: those directly associated with the recovery of the antibiotic, as well as environmental costs associated with the techniques used. For example, improved solvent and precursor recovery have reduced the cost of producing penicillin and cephalosporins, and the regeneration and recycling of resins utilised in other antibiotic recovery processes have improved economics for production of these compounds.

Figure 18.3 shows the recovery and purification of penicillin. The key step is organic solvent extraction. To obtain active, high-purity

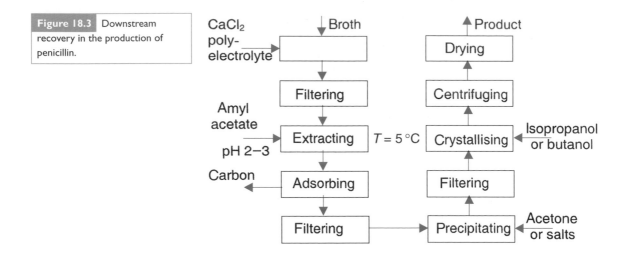

penicillin, the extraction uses a Podbielniak: a special centrifugal extractor. This allows a short extraction time with little penicillin degradation in the organic solvent. Moulds are used to manufacture penicillin, and mould colonies (mycelia) can be separated with a rotary vacuum filter. First, calcium chloride and a polyelectrolyte are added to the mycelium to form large particles (flocs). The penicillin is extracted from the filtrate into an organic solvent (usually amyl acetate). The penicillin is then transferred from the solvent into a pH-neutral aqueous solution. These steps increase the penicillin concentration about one hundred times. To remove impurities, activated carbon is used after the extraction. Filtration removes this carbon and prepares the penicillin for precipitation as a sodium or potassium salt. Precipitation is induced by acetone and followed by washing with an alcohol to remove remaining impurities. Because three different solvents are used, the economics of the process are governed by recovery of the solvents.

18.7 | Future prospects for fermentation-based antibiotics

There will be a continued need to develop both new broad-spectrum and narrow-spectrum antibiotics. Some of these will come from screening synthetic chemical compounds and chemical combinatorial libraries against bacterial or novel bacterial targets in traditional screening paradigms. However, there is a significant likelihood that new agents will emerge from a rescreening of natural products as sources of novel chemical diversity. Some of these natural products will be complex enough that either the agent will need (1) to be produced by traditional fermentation and biotechnology methods to be used as such, or (2) to be used to produce a core pharamcophore that can be chemically modified to produce a hybrid antibiotic in the tradition of the penicillins, cephalosporin and aminoglycosides.

Despite the fact that most major pharmaceutical companies have dropped out of the search for antibiotics and have abandoned their natural product drug discovery programmes for the development of new completely synthetic molecules, the smaller biotechnology companies have discovered that natural product screening can be a niche in which they can compete and offer added value.

The search for new antibiotics from natural products is proceeding on two fronts. The first is to re-discover antibiotics that may have been dropped (1) during research programme prioritisation by the larger pharmaceutical companies, or (2) for business reasons that the estimate of market sizes was too low to continue development and get an adequate return on investment. The market size and return may be appropriate for smaller companies. The second front is to search for narrow-spectrum antibiotics, either *de novo* or from historical data from the 'fallen angels' of research programmes. Such is the case with the streptogramins, which have a narrow spectrum of antimicrobial activity, and have only a small, albeit a significant, market penetration. However, there may be some novel issues to be tackled in the search for antibiotics against the new 'super-bugs' whether these agents be broad spectrum or narrow spectrum. In order to determine the effectiveness of new agents against resistant organisms in an efficient manner, it may become necessary to use these highly resistant organisms directly as the primary screening target. To do this it will be necessary to employ very stringent safety and security precautions (such as level P3 and P4 laboratories): it will not be able to carry these out in the traditional 'open-lab' environment of current industrial or academic screening laboratories. Just as there are very few facilities that are capable of screening agents against HIV or SARS, there will likely be few facilities that can be used to screen for agents active against these very resistant strains.

18.8 | Further reading

Andersson, I., Terwisscha van Scheltinga, A. C and Valegård, K. Towards new β-lactam antibiotics. *Cellular and Molecular Life Sciences* **58**: 1897–1906, 2001.

Bhal, V. Antibiotics. In *Biotechnology Annual Review*, Vol. 8, ed. M. R. El-Gewely. London: Elsevier Science, pp. 227–265, 2002.

Demain, A. L. and Elander, R. P. The β-lactam antibiotics: past, present and future. *Antonie van Leeuwenhoek* **75**: 5–19, 1999.

Elander, R. P. Industrial production of β-lactam antibiotics. *Applied Microbiology and Biotechnology* **61**: 385–392, 2003.

Liu, J., Dehbi, M., Moeck, G., et. al. Antimicrobial drug discovery through bacteriophage genomics. *Nature Biotechnology* **22**: 185–191, 2004.

Ohno, M., Otsuka, M., Yagisawa, M., et. al. Antibiotics. *Ullman's Encyclopedia of Industrial Chemistry*, Vol. A3. Weinheim: Wiley-VCH, pp. 341–440, 2004.

Service, R. F. Orphan drugs of the future? *Science* **303**: 1798, 2004.

Chapter 19

Strategies of cultivation

Sven-Olof Enfors

Royal Institute of Technology, Sweden

Nomenclature

C_S	carbon concentration in the substrate (mole C g^{-1})
C_X	carbon concentration in the cells (mole C g^{-1})
C	dissolved oxygen concentration (kg m^{-3})
C^*	dissolved oxygen concentration in equilibrium with the gas phase (kg m^{-3})
D	dilution rate (h^{-1})
D_{crit}	critical dilution rate (h^{-1})
DOT	dissolved oxygen tension (% air sat.)
DOT^*	dissolved oxygen tension in equilibrium with the gas phase (% air sat.)
F	medium flow rate (m^3 h^{-1})
GTR	gas transfer rate (kg m^{-3} h^{-1})
H	conversion constant (% l g^{-1})
k_d	specific death rate constant (h^{-1})
$K_L a$	oxygen transfer coefficient (h^{-1})
K_s	saturation constant (kg m^{-3})
N	cell number
OTR	oxygen transfer rate (kg m^{-3} h^{-1})
P	product concentration (kg m^{-3})

Basic Biotechnology, third edition, eds. Colin Ratledge and Bjørn Kristiansen.
Published by Cambridge University Press. © Cambridge University Press 2006.

Q	air flow rate ($m^3\,h^{-1}$)
q	specific reaction rate ($kg\,kg^{-1}\,h^{-1}$)
q_O	specific oxygen consumption rate ($kg\,kg^{-1}\,h^{-1}$)
q_P	specific product formation rate ($kg\,kg^{-1}\,h^{-1}$)
q_S	specific consumption rate of limiting substrate ($kg\,kg^{-1}\,h^{-1}$)
q_{S2}	specific consumption rate of non-limiting substrate ($kg\,kg^{-1}\,h^{-1}$)
q_m	specific substrate consumption for maintenance, see Fig. 19.4 ($kg\,kg^{-1}\,h^{-1}$)
$q_{S,an}$	specific substrate consumption for anabolism, see Fig. 19.4 ($kg\,kg^{-1}\,h^{-1}$)
$q_{S,en}$	specific substrate consumption for energy metabolism, see Fig. 19.4 ($kg\,kg^{-1}\,h^{-1}$)
$q_{S,en,growth}$	specific S-consumption in energy metabolism used for growth, see Fig. 19.4 ($kg\,kg^{-1}\,h^{-1}$)
r	volumetric reaction rate ($kg\,m^{-3}\,h^{-1}$)
S	limiting substrate concentration ($kg\,m^{-3}$)
$S2$	non-limiting substrate concentration ($kg\,m^{-3}$)
S_i	substrate concentration in inlet medium (limiting substrate) ($kg\,m^{-3}$)
$S2_i$	non-limiting substrate concentration in inlet medium ($kg\,m^{-3}$)
t	process time (h)
V	medium volume (m^3)
X	biomass concentration ($kg\,m^{-3}$)
X_d	concentration of dead cells ($kg\,m^{-3}$)
X_v	concentration of viable cells ($kg\,m^{-3}$)
y	concentration of arbitrary component in bioreactor ($kg\,m^{-3}$)
Y	yield coefficient ($kg\,kg^{-1}$)
Y_{em}	yield coefficient of biomass per substrate, exclusive maintenance ($kg\,kg^{-1}$)
$Y_{O/S}$	coefficient of oxygen consumed per substrate consumed ($kg\,kg^{-1}$)
$Y_{P/S}$	yield coefficient of product per substrate ($kg\,kg^{-1}$)
$Y_{X/S}$	yield coefficient of biomass per substrate, incl. maintenance ($kg\,kg^{-1}$)
$Y_{X/S2}$	yield coefficient for a non-limiting substrate ($kg\,kg^{-1}$)
δ	separation factor, defined in Fig. 19.1
μ	specific growth rate (h^{-1})

Subscripts

g	in gas phase
i	in inlet flow
max	maximum value
o	in outlet flow
y, s, x, O, p	refer parameter to non-specified compound, limiting substrate, biomass, oxygen and product

19.1 Introduction

There are two main principles of cultivation of suspended cells: *batch* and *continuous cultures*. The latter can, when correctly controlled, achieve steady state, which means that all concentrations in the bioreactor are constant with time. The cells are then expected to be constant with respect to composition and physiology, although mutation is a real possibility. The *batch* process is divided into true batch processes, to which no component except air and a pH titrating compound are added, and *fed-batch* processes to which a concentrated solution of one medium component, usually sugar, is also added. This chapter will describe the main characteristics of these types of cultivations.

19.2 Mass balance equations of the bioreactor

To simulate the performance of a bioreactor, whatever the mode of operation, we need expressions that show how the concentration of important medium components (*state variables*) are influenced by process conditions and in which way the state variables vary with time (*t*) in batch processes or with residence time in continuous processes (see Chapter 6). Let us designate an arbitrary state variable y. Important state variables in bioprocessing are concentrations of biomass (X), substrate components (S), products (P) and the dissolved oxygen tension (DOT). We may reach the goal by deriving differential equations of the type $dy/dt = \ldots$, which describe the rate of change of the variable y with time. The time dependence of this variable, $y(t)$, can then be simulated by numerical solution of the differential equation, starting from given initial conditions. For continuous processes, analytical solutions may be derived to describe how the residence time (or dilution rate, D) influences the state variable under steady-state conditions. The system is shown in Fig. 19.1.

A mass balance of an arbitrary component with concentration y in the reactor can be written:

$$\text{Change} = \text{input} - \text{output} + \text{reaction (kg h}^{-1})$$

$$\frac{d(Vy)}{dt} = F_i\,y_i + Q_i\,y_{gi} - F_o\,\delta y - Q_o\,y_{go} + Vr \tag{19.1}$$

where r is the *volumetric reaction rate* for production or consumption of the component with concentration y. Rearranging this equation we get a *general mass balance equation* that describes the change of y with time:

$$\frac{dy}{dt} = \frac{F_i}{V}\,(y_i - y) + \frac{F_o}{V}(y - \delta y) + r + \text{GTR} \tag{19.2}$$

where the gas transfer rate of the component is expressed by

$$\text{GTR} = \frac{Q_i}{V}\,y_{gi} - \frac{Q_o}{V}\,Y_{go} \tag{19.3}$$

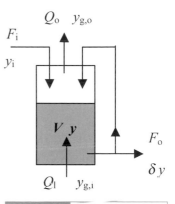

Figure 19.1 An ideally mixed reactor with medium volume V and the concentration y of a component in the reactor. Medium flow rates are designated F and gas flow rates Q. Concentrations in the gas phase are labelled with subscript g. Subscripts i and o refer to parameters of inlet and outlet flows, respectively. A separation factor, $\delta(0 \leq \delta \leq 1)$, specifies the concentration of y in the outlet medium.

The mode of process operation, i.e. batch, fed batch or continuous, is determined by the process operator by setting the values of F_i and F_o.

In a *continuous culture*, the inlet and outlet medium flow rates are $F_o = F_i = F$ and Eq. (19.2) becomes:

$$\frac{dy}{dt} = \frac{F}{V}(y_i - \delta y) + r + GTR \tag{19.4}$$

In a *fed-batch process* $F_o = 0$, the inlet feed rate is $F_i = F$ and Eq. (19.2) simplifies to:

$$\frac{dy}{dt} = \frac{F}{V}(y_i - y) + r + GTR \tag{19.5}$$

Mass balances of most components in the bioreactor do not involve any gas transfer and then the last term of Eqs. (19.4) and (19.5) disappears. Note that the general mass balance equations for a fed-batch culture, Eq. (19.5), and for a continuous culture, Eq. (19.4), become identical when no recirculation of the component is applied in the continuous culture, i.e. when $\delta = 1$. However, the physical meaning of the term $-F(y/V)$ is different in the two cases. In the continuous process (without recirculation), $-F(y/V)$ represents the rate of outflow of the component from the reactor, while in the fed-batch process this term represents the rate of dilution of the component caused by the inflow of medium. The general term y can now be replaced by X, S, P and DOT to represent the concentrations of biomass, substrate, product and the dissolved oxygen, respectively. Before we can apply the mass balance equations to study fed-batch and continuous processes, expressions for the biological reaction rates (r) and the gas transfer rate (GTR) must be inserted in the corresponding mass balance equation.

19.3 | Volumetric and specific rates

The *volumetric reaction rate, r*, is written:

$$r = qX \tag{19.6}$$

where q is *the specific reaction rate*, i.e. the rate per cell unit. An index is usually used to indicate which reaction the rate q refers to. The specific reaction rate for growth (q_x) is commonly expressed with μ and referred to as the specific growth rate.

19.3.1 The Monod model

The Monod model is one common model to describe how the growth rate depends on the concentration of a certain substrate component, S:

$$\mu = \mu_{max} \frac{S}{S + K_s} \tag{19.7}$$

It states that the higher the substrate concentration, the higher is the growth rate, up to a maximum growth rate, μ_{max}. The saturation

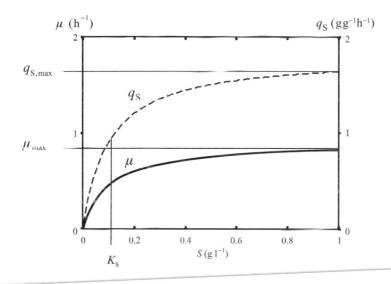

Figure 19.2 Graphical illustration of the Monod model. The specific growth rate (μ, solid line) and the specific uptake rate (q_S, dashed line) plotted against the limiting substrate concentration (S), assuming a constant biomass yield coefficient, $Y_{X/S} = 0.5$.

constant, K_s, is the concentration S when the growth rate is half the maximum. This is illustrated in Fig. 19.2, which also shows how the specific rate of uptake of the substrate (q_S) varies, assuming that the yield of biomass per substrate is constantly independent of the substrate concentration. This is seldom the case, however. The biomass produced per substrate often declines at very low growth rates (substrate concentrations) and therefore the Monod model is not useful for simulations of fed-batch cultures, thus a corresponding model for the specific substrate uptake rate is used:

$$q_S = q_{S,max} \frac{S}{S + K_s} \tag{19.8}$$

Note that the K_s values in these models are not always the same.

19.3.2 Cell yield and maintenance

The yield coefficient for a reaction is defined as the amount of product produced per consumed substrate, i.e.

$$Y_{P/S} = \frac{\Delta P}{-\Delta S} \tag{19.9}$$

More often it is defined as the ratio of the corresponding rates. The yield coefficient for cell growth on a substrate is then expressed as:

$$Y_{X/S} = \frac{\mu}{q_S} \tag{19.10}$$

However, this yield is usually not constant, and it declines when the specific growth rate becomes very low due to the maintenance demand. This can be illustrated by plotting the substrate uptake rate against the specific growth rate, as shown in Fig. 19.3.

According to Fig. 19.3, the substrate consumption rate can then be written in two ways, depending on whether the maintenance is

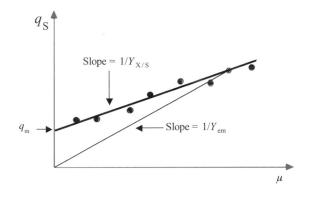

Figure 19.3 The maintenance concept. The specific substrate consumption rate (q_S) is plotted against the specific growth rate (μ). Extrapolation of the plots show the maintenance coefficient (q_m) as the intercept with the q_S-axis. The reciprocal slopes of the plots represent the yield coefficient exclusive maintenance (Y_{em}), while the reciprocal slope of a line drawn from an experimental point to the origin represents the observed yield coefficient ($Y_{X/S}$), which depends on the growth rate.

included or not:

$$\begin{cases} q_S = \dfrac{\mu}{Y_{X/S}} & (19.11a) \\[2ex] q_S = \dfrac{\mu}{Y_{em}} + q_m & (19.11b) \end{cases}$$

Thus, there are two types of yield coefficients for cell production from energy yielding substrates: net cell *yield exclusive maintenance*, here called Y_{em}, and the *observed yield of biomass* per consumed substrate, which includes the maintenance (here called $Y_{X/S}$). Rearrangement of (19.11a, b) shows that the observed yield depends on the specific growth rate:

$$Y_{X/S} = \frac{\mu Y_{em}}{\mu + q_m\,Y_{em}} \tag{19.12}$$

The consequences of the maintenance become evident in processes with high cell density, as will be discussed in the section on fed-batch cultures below.

19.3.3 Specific growth rate and uptake rate of non-limiting substrates

In fed-batch cultures, or during dynamic conditions in continuous cultures, the uptake rate of the limiting substrate (S) is first calculated from Eq. (19.8). Then the specific growth rate is obtained using Eq. (19.11b), which can be written

$$\mu = Y_{em}(q_S - q_m) \tag{19.13}$$

While the limiting substrate uptake rate is obtained according to the Monod model, other non-limiting substrates (here named S2) are

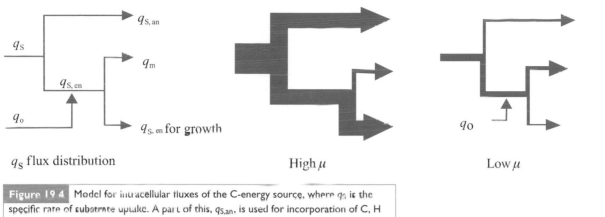

q_S flux distribution   High μ Low μ

Figure 19.4 Model for intracellular fluxes of the C-energy source, where q_S is the specific rate of substrate uptake. A part of this, $q_{S,an}$, is used for incorporation of C, H and O into the cells (anabolism); while the rest, $q_{S,en}$, is used for energy metabolism, which is further divided into the flux used for energy for maintenance (q_m) and the part used to provide energy for growth. When q_S declines, as in a fed-batch culture with constant feed rate, both $q_{S,an}$ and $q_{S,en}$ decline. However, the maintenance demand has a priority for the declining supply of energy and the consequence is that the ratio between the oxygen consuming fluxes ($q_{S,en}$) and the non-consuming flux ($q_{S,an}$) increases, as indicated by the relative width of the arrows. There are two main consequences of this when the specific growth rate declines: the biomass yield per energy substrate declines and the oxygen consumption per substrate unit increases.

usually calculated based on the growth rate and the yield constant for the reaction, i.e.

$$q_{S2} = \frac{\mu}{Y_{X/S2}} \tag{19.14}$$

19.3.4 Oxygen uptake rate

In continuous cultures, the uptake rate of oxygen may be adequately approximated by means of the growth rate and the yield coefficient according to Eq. (19.14); but in fed-batch cultures with constant feed, the specific rate of growth and the specific rate of substrate consumption decline gradually, and this must be accounted for in order to understand high cell density fed-batch cultures. The utilisation of the C-energy source can be divided into two metabolic fluxes corresponding to consumption for incorporation of the elements C, O and H into the biomass, i.e. the flux to anabolism ($q_{S,an}$) and the flux resulting in oxidation for energy production ($q_{S,en}$). The latter can be further split into a flux used for maintenance (q_m) and the rest used for energy for growth as depicted in Fig. 19.4. In reality there are no such separate fluxes in energy metabolism but the concept is useful for modelling.

$$q_S = q_{S,an} + q_{S,en} \tag{19.15}$$

Almost all consumption of molecular oxygen is used for respiration, unless the cells use oxygenases to attack the substrate (when growing on methanol, hydrocarbons or aromatic compounds). The cellular oxygen is mainly provided by the carbon source (e.g. glucose). Therefore, for growth on substrates like sugar, the oxygen consumption (q_O)

is proportional to the flux of substrate used for energy ($q_{S,en}$) with a stoichiometric coefficient called $R_{O/S}$:

$$q_O = q_{S,en} R_{O/S} \tag{19.16}$$

For respiration based on glucose, $R_{O/S}$ is 6 mol oxygen mol^{-1} glucose, or 1.067 g g^{-1}.

The flux to anabolism can be obtained from a mass balance on carbon, provided the yield exclusive maintenance and the carbon concentrations in the cells are known.

Flux of C to anabolism

$$C_S q_{S,an} \quad \text{(moles C g}^{-1}\text{cells h}^{-1}) \tag{19.17a}$$

Flux of C converted to biomass

$$C_X(q_S - q_m)Y_{em} \quad \text{(moles C g}^{-1}\text{cells h}^{-1}) \tag{19.17b}$$

where C_S and C_X are the carbon concentration in the substrate and cells, respectively. These C fluxes are equal and then $q_{S,an}$ can be solved from Eq. (19.17):

$$q_{S,an} = \frac{C_X}{C_S}(q_S - q_m)Y_{em} \tag{19.18}$$

and after insertion of this equation into Eq. (19.16) the specific rate of oxygen consumption is obtained:

$$q_O = \left[q_S - \frac{C_X}{C_S}(q_S - q_m)Y_{em} \right] R_{O/S} \tag{19.19}$$

The consequence of this is that the oxygen consumption rate in a fed-batch process gradually increases in spite of a constant feed of substrate. This is further illustrated in the section on fed-batch processes below.

19.3.5 Oxygen transfer rate

Only the oxygen dissolved in the medium is consumed in common microbial bioreactors. The solubility of oxygen in water in equilibrium with air is low, typically 6–8 mg L^{-1} or 0.19–0.25 mM (temperature- and medium-dependent value). This corresponds to production of about the same amounts of cells in sugar-based media. Thus, oxygen must continuously be supplied in an aerobic process, and the rate of transfer of oxygen from the air bubbles to dissolved oxygen in the medium (the oxygen transfer rate OTR, kg m^{-3} h^{-1} or, more commonly, mmol l^{-1} h^{-1}) is an important parameter since it determines the concentration of oxygen in the medium. If the outlet oxygen concentration and the air flow rates are known, the concentration of oxygen in the medium can be calculated according to Eq. (19.3). A common model to estimate the oxygen transfer rate is:

$$OTR = K_L a (C^* - C) \tag{19.20}$$

where $K_L a$ (h^{-1}) is the *volumetric oxygen transfer coefficient*, C (kg m^{-3}) is the dissolved oxygen concentration and C^* is the corresponding oxygen concentration in equilibrium with the gas phase, i.e. the oxygen concentration in the air bubbles of the reactor. However, the dissolved oxygen concentration, C, is difficult to monitor, while a related parameter, the dissolved oxygen tension (DOT), is available from steam sterilisable oxygen electrodes. The relationship between the dissolved oxygen concentration and the dissolved oxygen tension is given by a constant, H (% air sat. m^3 kg^{-1}), that is related to Henry's constant.

$$DOT = HC \qquad (19.21)$$

The value of H increases from 14 286 to 16 667 when the solubility of oxygen declines from 7 to 6 mg l^{-1}, which is the range of oxygen solubility in process media.

19.3.6 Specific mass balance equations

Based on the general mass balance equation, Eqs. (19.4) and (19.5), the specific rate equations for limiting substrate, growth and oxygen consumption, the following mass balance equations can be written and solved to obtain the concentrations of limiting substrate (S), viable biomass (X_v), and DOT. A first-order death rate constant (k_d) has been inserted in the biomass mass balance, Eq. (19.22), to account for cell death. The equations below represent a continuous culture, where the separation factor δ specifies possible recirculation of cells (see Fig. 19.1), but the same equations are also valid for fed-batch processes, if δ is omitted.

$$\frac{dX_v}{dt} = -\frac{F}{V}\delta X_v + \mu X_v - k_d X_v \qquad (19.22)$$

$$\frac{dS}{dt} = \frac{F}{V}(S_i - S) - q_S X_v \qquad (19.23)$$

$$\frac{dDOT}{dt} = K_L a(DOT^* - DOT) - q_O X_v H \qquad (19.24)$$

19.4 Continuous culture

Continuous processes operate with a constant flow of medium through the reactor. The inlet medium flow rate is controlled by one of several principles and the outlet medium flow rate is controlled by some device, for instance weight control, that keeps the quantity of the medium in the reactor constant. In the *turbidostat*, the inlet flow is determined by the optical density of the culture, i.e. it is controlled at a constant set point. In the *pH-auxostat* the flow is controlled to keep the pH constant. In the *chemostat* a constant inlet flow is applied. The chemostat is the most versatile variant of the continuous cultures and it permits growth of cells at any rate below μ_{max}, but it cannot be run close to μ_{max} due to instability problems. The pH-auxostat is complementary to the chemostat, since it permits growth at μ_{max}, while it becomes unstable below μ_{max}. Theory and properties of the chemostat are briefly presented here.

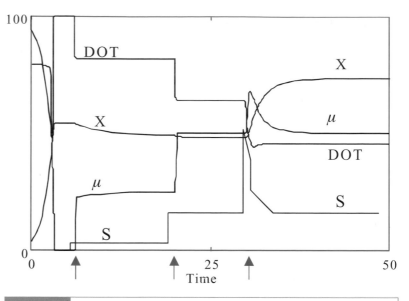

Figure 19.5 Start-up of a chemostat and control of growth rate and biomass concentration. The simulation of a 40-l process is based on numeric solution of mass balance equations (19.22) to (19.24). It includes an initial batch phase with exponential growth to increase the biomass concentration before the chemostat is started (at the first arrow). The substrate concentration is out of scale during the batch phase. At the first arrow, a medium flow of 10 l h⁻¹ with $S_i = 10$ g l⁻¹ was started. At the second arrow the flow rate was increased to 20 l h⁻¹. The third arrow indicates a change to a medium with a higher inlet concentration of limiting substrate ($S_i = 15$ g l⁻¹).

19.4.1 The chemostat

The chemostat must be limited with respect to one of the substrate components. In practice this is mostly the C/energy source but also other nutrient limitations may be utilised. The limitation is achieved if the inlet substrate feed rate does not exceed the maximum substrate consumption rate:

$$\frac{F}{V} S_i < q_{S,max} X \tag{19.25}$$

If the substrate concentration is not rate limiting, growth will continue at μ_{max} and X will increase until limitation is reached with one of the substrates. Figure 19.5 shows a dynamic simulation of the start-up of a chemostat and two steady-state conditions with different biomass concentrations and growth rates. Continuous processes are designed to work at steady state, and the variables are usually plotted against the *dilution rate*, $D = F/V$, which is the reciprocal of the *residence time*, $\tau = V/F$. The steady-state values of process variables X_v, X_d, S, $S2$, DOT and P can be obtained by analytical solutions of the relevant mass balance equations for steady-state conditions, i.e. when $dy/dt = 0$, as summarised in Table 19.1.

Note the order and from which equations the first three parameters (μ, S and X_v) are solved! The other parameters (X_d, DOT, $S2$ and P) are derived from their respective mass balance equations.

Table 19.1 Derivation of steady-state solutions for a chemostat

Model equation	Steady-state solution	Equation
MB on biomass $$\frac{dX}{dt} = -\frac{F}{V}\delta X_v + \mu X_v - k_d X_v$$	Specific growth rate $$\mu = \delta D + k_d$$	(19.26)
The Monod model $$\mu = \mu_{max}\frac{S}{S + K_s}$$	Limiting substrate conc. $$S = \frac{\mu K_s}{\mu_{max} - \mu}$$	(19.27)
MB on limiting substrate $$\frac{dS}{dt} = \frac{F}{V}(S_i - S) - q_s X_v$$	Biomass concentration $$X_v = \frac{D Y_{X/S}}{\mu}(S_i - S)$$	(19.28)
MB on DOT $$\frac{dDOT}{dt} = K_L a\,(DOT^* - DOT) - q_o X_v H$$	Dissolved oxygen $$DOT = DOT^* - \frac{\mu X_v / /}{Y_{x/o}K_L a}$$	(19.29)
MB on non-limiting substrate $$\frac{dS2}{dt} = \frac{F}{V}(S2_i - S2) - q_{S2}X_v$$	Non-limiting substrate conc. $$S2 = S2_i - \frac{\mu X_v}{Y_{X/S2} D}$$	(19.30)
MB on product $$\frac{dP}{dt} = -\frac{F}{V}P + q_P X_v$$	Product concentration $$P = \frac{q_P X_v}{D}$$	(19.31)

A simple algorithm for simulation of steady-state values in a chemostat with MATLAB (a well-know simulation programe) is shown in Table 19.2. This algorithm (with modified constants) can be used to illustrate the performance of a chemostat.

Enter this text in a MATLAB m-file (name it, for instance, chemostat.m) and run the simulation by entering the command "chemostat" in the Command Window of MATLAB. Note the transponation sign ('), the element-wise operation signs (./ and .*) and that text strings are embraced by single quotation signs ('   ')! Text after a % sign in the code are comments and they are neglected by MATLAB when the m-file is run. The simulation will demonstrate that:

- The limiting substrate concentration is close to zero over a wide range of dilution rates. Not until the dilution rate approaches a critical value at which the cells are washed out, is the limiting substrate concentration increasing substantially. The critical dilution rate is obtained from Eq. (19.26), since the cells cannot grow faster than with μ_{max}:

$$D_{crit} = \frac{\mu_{max} - k_d}{\delta} \tag{19.32}$$

- For a culture without cell death ($k_d = 0$) and without cell recirculation ($\delta = 1$), the critical dilution rate becomes equal to μ_{max}. In practice, the chemostat becomes instable when the dilution rate approaches the critical value.
- The limiting substrate concentration in the chemostat is determined by the K_s value. Thus, the lower the K_s, the lower is the

Table 19.2 | A MATLAB algorithm for simulation of steady-state in a chemostat

```
clear all
kd=0; delta=1;Mymax=0.8; Ks=0.01; Yem=0.5;
qm=0.04;Si=9;DOTstar=100;Yxo=1;H=14000;
KLa=800;S2i=0.5;Yxs2=10;alpha=0;beta=0;
% make an x-column vector
D=0.05:0.01:1;
D=D';
% y-vectors according to models:
My=delta*D+kd;
S=My*Ks ./(Mymax-My);
S(find(S<0))=Si;   % correction for boundary conditions
S(find(S>Si))=Si;   % correction for boundary conditions
Yxs=My*Yem . /(My+Yem*qm);
Xv=D ./My .*Yxs .*(Si-S);
Xd=kd*Xv . /(delta .*D);
DOT=DOTstar-My . /Yxo .*Xv*H/KLa;
S2=S2i-My . /Yxs2 .*Xv . /D;
rXv=My .*Xv;
qp=alpha*My+beta;   % Luedeking-Piret model
P=qp .*Xv./D;
% make matrix with y-variables in columns
y=[S, Xv,Xd,DOT,S2,rXv,P];
% enter scale max for each variable
ymax=[10,10,10,100,1,10,5];
% scale values to a 0–100 scale
for i=1:length(ymax)
    yscaled(:,i)=y(:,i)/ymax(i)*100;
end
% make plots and labels
yplot=plot(D,yscaled);
set(gca,'YLim',[0 100])
XLabel('D (/h)')
YLabel('rel. values')
title('Simulation of steady-state in a chemostat')
legend('S:0–10','Xv:0–10','Xd:0–10','DOT:0–100','S2:0–1','rXv:0–
    10','P:0–5')
```

substrate concentration; while the dilution rate has little effect until it approaches the critical dilution rate.

- The cell concentration is relatively constant over a broad range of dilution rates. At a high dilution rate, the cell concentration drops due to the high outlet concentration of the limiting substrate; but at a low dilution rate, the biomass concentration drops due to both cell death and the often observed low biomass yield on the energy substrate at low growth rates. If cell death is pronounced, dead cells accumulate more at lower dilution rates. Since the live cell concentration is reduced at low dilution rates, the viability $(X_v/(X_v + X_d))$ of a culture can be expected to increase with high dilution rate (provided the specific death rate, k_d, is constant).

- The productivity of cell mass, given by the product of biomass concentration and specific growth rate, increases approximately in proportion to the dilution rate. The higher the productivity of cells becomes, the higher is the oxygen consumption rate. If the oxygen transfer rate does not satisfy the oxygen demand, the chemostat is turned into an oxygen-limited chemostat.

- The concentration of the non-limiting substrate (except for DOT) is parallel to that of the limiting substrate, but located at a higher (non-limiting) concentration. If the inlet limiting substrate concentration (S_i alone) is increased in the inlet medium, this will result in reduced concentration of the non-limiting substrates and it may create a situation where the type of limitation is shifted. To test if the intended limiting substrate is the actual limiting substrate, a dose of this compound may be added to the culture. A transient response shown as increased cell concentration or reduced DOT would then confirm the limitation, while lack of such a response would indicate that some other substrate is limiting.

- The product concentration in the chemostat depends much on the type of product formation kinetics as described by the Luedeking–Piret model (included in the MATLAB code, Table 19.1). Growth-connected products are best suited for production in chemostats, since the concentration of non-growth connected products becomes diluted to low values at higher dilution rates. The high concentrations observed at a low dilution rate in the continuous culture are produced with low productivity and little advantage is then obtained compared to the fed-batch process, which gives the highest product concentration.

An important advantage of the chemostat is the high productivity compared to batch and fed-batch processes. Furthermore, since the cells are grown under constant conditions at a well-defined growth rate and cell density, the chemostat has become an important tool for microbial physiology research. The drawback that has hampered the industrial utilisation of the chemostat is mainly its genetic instability. The chemostat has a major limitation implicit in its metabolic control, namely the sensitivity to mutations. This is due to the fact that there is a balance between growth rate and substrate concentration. If an organism has been manipulated to overproduce large quantities of a product, it is likely that a mutation that eliminates or reduces the product formation confers a competitive advantage. Figure 19.6 shows an example with data from *Escherichia coli* W3110, which has a biomass yield coefficient of 0.46 g g^{-1} without plasmid. When a plasmid for production of protein ZZT2 was inserted, the yield coefficient dropped to 0.35 g g^{-1}. In the simulation, it was assumed that one plasmid-free cell appeared at the start of the simulation, and after

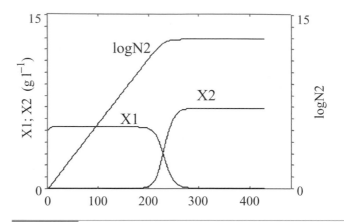

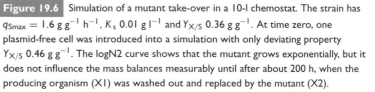

Figure 19.6 Simulation of a mutant take-over in a 10-l chemostat. The strain has $q_{Smax} = 1.6$ g g^{-1} h^{-1}, K_s 0.01 g l^{-1} and $Y_{X/S}$ 0.36 g g^{-1}. At time zero, one plasmid-free cell was introduced into a simulation with only deviating property $Y_{X/S}$ 0.46 g g^{-1}. The logN2 curve shows that the mutant grows exponentially, but it does not influence the mass balances measurably until after about 200 h, when the producing organism (X1) was washed out and replaced by the mutant (X2).

about 200 h this organism breaks through in the competition and eventually replaces the producing organism.

19.5 | Fed-batch cultures

Most industrial fermentation processes are so called fed-batch processes, which are batch processes fed with a substrate solution so that one substrate component is growth-rate limiting. The substrate feed is often a sugar rather than complete medium and it is common that the substrate concentration is as high as practically possible to reduce the volume increase. Sugar solutions with concentrations in the range 30–50% are often used. There are two main reasons for applying the fed-batch technique. The substrate limitation offers a tool for *reaction rate control* to avoid engineering limitations with respect to cooling and oxygen transfer. Substrate limitation also permits a sort of *metabolic control* by which catabolite repression and sugar over-flow metabolism can be avoided.

Fed-batch processes will not reach steady-state and therefore the solutions used for the continuous cultures cannot be used. Instead we have to solve the mass balance equations numerically from given initial values and plot the variables against time. As the general mass balance equation for a fed-batch process, Eq. (19.5), is identical to that of a chemostat without recirculation, Eq. (19.4) with $\delta = 1$, the mass balance equations of the left-hand side of Table 19.3 can be used also for fed-batch cultures. However, when calculating the specific growth rate (μ), Eq. (19.13) should be used to account for the declining biomass yield at increasing cell density (low growth rate). Furthermore, to account for the increasing oxygen demand per energy substrate unit

Table 19.3 MATLAB algorithms for a fed-batch simulation

File name: FBstart	Filename: FBmodel.m
`%FBstart; Initiation file for fed-batch simulation`	`function dydt=FBmodel(t,y)`
`% Requires a separate model file`	`% Model file to be initiated by FBstart.m`
`clear all`	`% extract variables from y-vector`
`global y2`	`global y2`
`y2=[];% for storage non-diff equation variables`	`X=y(1);`
`tspan=[0 50];%% time scale`	`S=y(2);`
`% enter initial values and locate in column vector`	`V=y(3);`
`X=0.5;`	`%Constants`
`S=0.1;`	`qSmax=1.6;`
`V=40;`	`Ks=0.1;`
`y=[X; S; V];`	`qm=0.04;`
`% call ODEsolver and the model file`	`Yem=0.5;`
`[t y]=ODE23s('FBmodel',tspan,y);`	`Si=500;`
`% option if non-diff eq. solutions are included`	`F0=0.03;`
`if isempty(y2)==0`	`SFR=0.3;`
`% eliminate duplicates`	`Fmax=0.8;`
`y2(find(diff(y2(:,1))<diff(tspan)/1000),:)=[];`	`%Algorithm`
`y2(find(diff(y2(:,1))<0),:)=[];`	`F=F0*exp(SFR*t);`
`%match to y-vector size`	`if F>Fmax`
`y2=interp1(y2(:,1),y2(:,2:length(y2(1,:))),t);`	`F=Fmax;`
`% merge with y-vector`	`end`
`y=[y,y2];`	`qS=qSmax*S/(S+Ks);`
`end`	`My=(qS-qm)*Yem;`
`% scale max values for scaling in graph`	`dXdt=-F/V*X+My*X;`
`ymax=[100,1,100,1,1];% X,S,V,F,My`	`dSdt=F/V*(Si-S)-qS*X;`
`% scale values to a 0–100 scale`	`dVdt=F;`
`for i=1:length(ymax)`	`% make a dydt-column vector`
`yscaled(:,i)=y(:,i)/ymax(i)*100;`	`dydt=[dXdt; dSdt; dVdt];`
`end`	`% store non-diff variables in y2`
`%plot and label`	`y2=[y2;[t,F,My]];`
`yplot=plot(t,yscaled);`	
`set(gca,'YLim',[0 100])`	
`legend('X: 0–100 g/L','S: 0–1 g/L','V: 0–100L', ...`	
`'F: 0–1 L/h','My: 0–1 /h')`	
`xlabel ('time (hrs)')`	
`title('Fed-batch with exponential/constant feed')`	
`figure(gcf)`	

at low growth rate the specific oxygen consumption rate (q_O), should be calculated on the basis of the partitioning between anabolism and energy metabolism, see Fig. 19.4 and Eq. (19.19).

Table 19.3 contains simple algorithms for simulation of a fed-batch culture, excluding over-flow metabolism and oxygen consumption. The *FBstart.m* file is used to give initial conditions and to call the differential equation solver ODE23S of MATLAB (on line 13 in

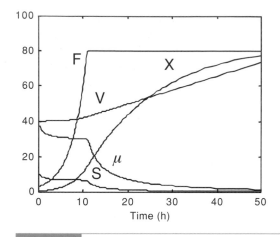

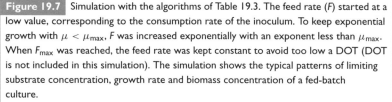

Figure 19.7 Simulation with the algorithms of Table 19.3. The feed rate (F) started at a low value, corresponding to the consumption rate of the inoculum. To keep exponential growth with $\mu < \mu_{max}$, F was increased exponentially with an exponent less than μ_{max}. When F_{max} was reached, the feed rate was kept constant to avoid too low a DOT (DOT is not included in this simulation). The simulation shows the typical patterns of limiting substrate concentration, growth rate and biomass concentration of a fed-batch culture.

the code). The model equations and constants are stored in the auxiliary *FBmodel.m* file. When all variables have been calculated they are packed in the y2-matrix in *FBmodel.m* and the program control returns to the *FBstart.m* file (on line 15) where the specifications for plotting are written. The result is shown in Fig. 19.7.

19.5.1 High cell density cultures

A specially interesting feature of the fed-batch technique, not offered by the other modes of operation, is the possibility to reach very high biomass concentrations. From the biomass concentration curve in Fig. 19.7 one might get the impression that the biomass concentration increases constantly in proportion to the feed rate, and one would just have to wait to reach a high cell density. However, the fed-batch technique is also limited with respect to the maximum cell density that can be reached. If the process is extended to very high cell densities, a number of effects may be encountered. If the feed contains only one substrate, e.g. sugar, other medium ingredients will sooner or later become exhausted. The first response to this would be to increase the initial concentrations of these components. The raw materials required for a certain biomass production can be calculated from the yield coefficients, which may be determined in batch experiments. Such supplementation must be done carefully, since too high an initial concentration of salts may be inhibitory or may result in precipitation. Another strategy would be to feed these components at a non-limiting rate in parallel with the feed of the limiting substrate.

For nitrogen source this is often achieved by using ammonia for pH control. Since the biomass concentration increases with time, the specific growth rate declines gradually during a fed-batch process with constant feed rate, as was shown in Fig. 19.7. This indicates that there is a theoretical maximum cell concentration when μ approaches the dilution rate in a fed-batch culture.

To reach a high cell quantity (kg), it is important to keep the maintenance as low as possible and to keep the feed rate as high as possible. To reach a high cell density (kg m^{-3}), the feed solution must also be as concentrated as possible to reduce the dilution caused by the feed. In industrial processes with complex raw materials, for instance when molasses is used in fed-batch processes, high concentrations of salts, and other inhibitory substances from the molasses that are not utilised by the cells, may accumulate in the reactor and increase the maintenance. Furthermore, the maximum feed rate is limited by the oxygen transfer capacity of the reactor.

19.5.2 Control of exponential growth in fed-batch cultures

There are two main reasons to apply the fed-batch technique: to avoid engineering limitations with respect to oxygen or heat transfer and to control the metabolism with respect to overflow metabolism or catabolite regulation. The engineering limitations are not encountered until the culture has reached a considerable biomass. If this is the only reason to apply the fed-batch technique, then the process can be run as a batch process with surplus of all medium ingredients until the limitation is approaching. However, if a metabolic restriction is required from the very beginning of the process, e.g. to avoid production of toxic by-products by overflow metabolism, then a constant feed rate corresponding to the initial low consumption rate of the culture would result in unnecessarily low productivity. The solution to this problem is to apply an initial phase of exponential growth at a specific growth rate, which is constant, but controlled so that the substrate concentration is kept below the critical value for the overflow metabolism. This is achieved by an exponentially increasing feed rate. Since this results in an exponentially increasing oxygen consumption rate, the oxygen transfer capacity will eventually be insufficient, as in an ordinary batch culture. The exponential feed then has to be switched to a constant feed. This is the typical feeding strategy used to combine high productivity with low ethanol formation in the production of baker's yeast, and it is a strategy also used for E. coli processes to avoid excessive acetate formation.

The principle is shown by the simulation in Fig. 19.8. To derive an expression for the time-dependent feed needed to achieve constant growth rate at $\mu < \mu_{max}$, we start from the mass balance on limiting substrate:

$$\frac{dS}{dt} = \frac{F}{V}(S_i - S) - q_s X = 0 \qquad (19.33)$$

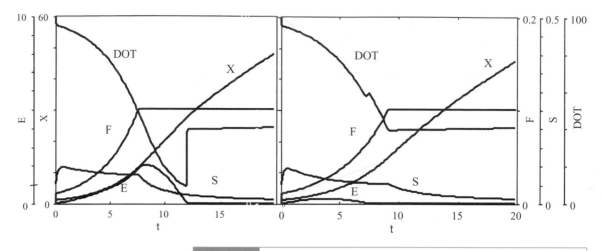

Since $S \ll S_i$ this equation can be simplified and solved for F:

$$F = \frac{q_S (XV)}{S_i} \qquad (19.34)$$

But since XV increases with time, F also should increase exponentially with time according to

$$(XV)_t = (XV)_0 \, e^{\mu t} \qquad (19.35)$$

where subscripts 0 and t denote the values initially and at time t, respectively. The time-dependent feed flow rate that enables the cells to grow at a specific growth rate μ is obtained by combining Eq. (19.34) and (19.35):

$$F(t) = \frac{q_S}{S_i}(XV)_0 \, e^{\mu t} \qquad (19.36)$$

which can be written as:

$$F(t) = F_0 \, e^{\mu t} \qquad (19.37)$$

where F_0 is the initial feed rate. An estimate of this feed rate is obtained from:

$$F_0 = \frac{\mu}{S_i Y_{X/S}}(XV)_0 \, e^{\mu t} \qquad (19.38)$$

The exponential feed technique is used primarily to control overflow metabolism in the initial phase of a fed-batch process as illustrated in Fig. 19.8. To the extent that the yield coefficient $Y_{X/S}$ is constant, application of this technique makes it possible to grow the cells at any constant growth rate below μ_{max}. For both E. coli and Saccharomyces cerevisiae the overflow metabolism is observed when $\mu =$ exceeds 0.3 h^{-1} and then the coefficient $Y_{X/S}$ is reduced considerably and the constant μ is not achieved. A typical fed batch strategy for E. coli and *S. cerevisiae* is to apply a fed-rate profile that results in some acetate or ethanol during the exponential feed and then to switch to a constant feed when DOT approaches about 20–30%. The substrate concentration then starts to decline and the acetate/ethanol is rapidly consumed. The constant feed is then maintained until the yield declines too much.

19.6 | Further reading

Anderson, L., Strandberg, L., Häggström, L. and Enfors, S.-O. Modelling of high cell density fed-batch cultures. *FEMS Microbiology Reviews* **14**: 39–44, 1994.

Pham, H., Larsson, G. and Enfors, S.-O. Growth and energy metabolism in aerobic fed-batch cultures of *Saccharomyces cerevisiae*: simulation and model verification. *Biotechnology and Bioengineering* **60**: 474–482, 1998.

Pham, H., Larsson, G. and Enfors, S.-O. Modelling of aerobic growth of *Saccharomyces cerevisiae* in a pH-auxostat. *Bioprocess Engineering* **20**: 544–573, 1999.

Xu, B., Jahic, M. and Enfors, S.-O. Modelling of overflow metabolism in batch and fed batch cultures of *Escherichia coli*. *Biotechnology Progress* **15**: 81–90, 1999.

Chapter 20

Enzyme biotechnology

Randy M. Berka
Novozymes Biotech, Inc., USA

Joel R. Cherry
Novozymes Biotech, Inc., USA

20.1 | Introduction

Society is facing a number of key socio-economic and environmental challenges: global warming, extinction of species in key ecosystems, malnutrition, shortages of water and other natural resources. All of these are human-made problems, and they require innovative solutions. While precious natural resources continue to dwindle, the number of consumers and polluters is growing. A major challenge for the future is development of products that are less hazardous, pollute less and require less energy. It is here that enzymes can make an impact on the future of society. In 1878, Kühne coined the term 'enzyme' from the Greek *enzumos*, which refers to the leavening of bread by yeast. However, the modern term refers to biological catalysts in the form of globular proteins that facilitate chemical reactions in the cells of all living organisms. Enzyme-catalysed reactions take place under relatively mild and ecologically friendly conditions, are highly specific and greatly accelerate the rates of the reactions in which they participate. Enzymes make better use of raw materials, save water and energy, and often replace toxic chemical processes.

Basic Biotechnology, third edition, eds. Colin Ratledge and Bjørn Kristiansen.
Published by Cambridge University Press. © Cambridge University Press 2006.

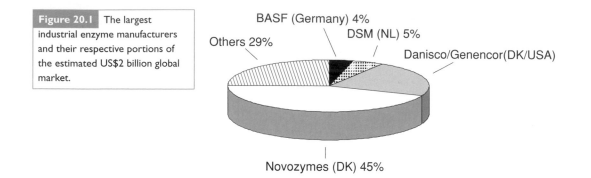

For example, the enzymes from bacteria and fungi in forest litter are primarily responsible for the breakdown of decaying plant biomass and, thus, they are critical in the recycling process we recognise as the global carbon cycle. These microbial enzymes may one day be harnessed to convert waste plant materials, such as corn stover, straw and grasses, into fuel and simple carbon compounds used for the synthesis of chemical and pharmaceutical intermediates, thereby decreasing our dependence on petroleum-based carbon.

Fermentation processes for brewing, baking and the production of alcohol have been used since prehistoric times. However, it was the widespread introduction of fermentation technology in the 1960s and the advent of genetic engineering two decades later that is behind the more recent expansion of the enzyme industry. Recombinant microorganisms are now the dominant source of enzymes for a wide variety of applications. This trend will likely intensify in the future due to the ease of genetic manipulation and the diversity of enzymes available from microorganisms found in disparate and extreme environments. The production of enzymes is an example of what is termed 'white biotechnology' for the application of nature's own toolset for various industrial processes. White biotechnology is differentiated from red (medical) and green (agricultural) biotechnology implementations. The benefits of white biotechnology include favourable impacts on both the environment and the economy. Energy efficiency is boosted, raw materials consumption is decreased, CO_2 emissions are significantly reduced and production costs are usually lowered.

20.1.1 Global market for enzymes

During the last five decades worldwide revenues from industrial enzymes have grown to more than US$2 billion, and they are anticipated to exceed US$3 billion by the year 2008. The volume of enzymes that is manufactured has increased by 12% annually over the last 10 years. Approximately 400 companies are currently involved in the manufacture of enzymes; however, Novozymes (Denmark), Danisco/Genencor (Denmark and USA), BASF (Germany) and DSM (The Netherlands) comprise the world's largest enzyme manufacturers with combined revenues encompassing 73% of the total (Fig. 20.1). Sixty per cent of enzyme production occurs in Europe, with 15% in the USA and 15% in Japan. However, the USA and Europe each consume 30% of world output.

The enzyme market is divided into three segments: technical, food and animal feed:

- Approximately 63% of all enzymes sold are intended for technical applications that include detergents, textiles, leather, pulp and paper, and fuels.
- Food enzymes represent the next largest category, accounting for 31% of total sales.
- Animal feed enzymes represent a small (6%), but rapidly growing, sector.

20.2 | Development of the producer strains

20.2.1 Screening from Nature's diversity

The diversity of microorganisms in nature is huge, but only a few organisms produce enzymes that are perfectly suited for a specific use. The challenge is to identify the best enzyme for each application from the plethora of candidates provided by our planet's biodiversity. The quest typically begins with the testing of thousands of samples from microorganisms that are collected from natural environments or various culture collections in order to identify those that produce the desired catalytic activity under conditions required for the intended application. For this purpose it is essential to develop an assay for the enzyme that is relevant to the intended application. For example, an ideal protease for cold-water laundry detergents might be one that has a high turnover number under alkaline conditions at temperatures of 5 to 10 °C in the presence of various detergent additives. Consequently, screening for such an enzyme might require an assay that measures removal of protein from stained fabric at low temperature, high pH and in the presence of detergent chemicals over a finite time interval corresponding to a wash cycle. A toolbox for enzyme screening typically comprises the following:

- *Culture collections:* Enzyme companies usually maintain large collections of microorganisms that have been assembled from various climates and environmental niches.
- *Enrichment techniques:* For identification of specific enzyme activities from nature, the principle of natural selection is applied on a microscale. Investigators employ culture conditions in which nutrients, temperature and pH are adjusted to favour the growth of one particular class of microorganism. An enrichment technique may involve inoculating these selective cultures with a mixed population of organisms (e.g. a soil sample), and ascertaining the predominant enzyme activities and corresponding organisms that are produced.
- *Assay technology:* An industry proverb states 'you get what you screen for,' thus proprietary and application-relevant assays are keys to finding the best enzyme candidates. This requires intimate

knowledge of the substrate, reaction parameters (temperature, pH, time) and customer preferences.

- *Gene libraries:* Enzyme companies generate diverse collections of ready-to-screen DNA and/or cDNA libraries from microorganisms. The genes represented in these libraries are usually introduced into surrogate host microorganisms that are easy to manipulate in the laboratory (e.g. *Saccharomyces cerevisiae, Escherichia coli*), and the resulting transformants are subsequently screened for the desired enzyme activities. This process is referred to as *expression cloning.*

- *Automation, robotics and data collection:* If it were done by hand, screening thousands of culture samples for specific enzymes would be an arduous assignment with endless repetitive tasks prone to human error. This type of work is best done with laboratory robots that are programmed to perform repetitive pipetting and biochemical assays in an automated fashion with data collection and analysis using sophisticated computer software (see Chapter 12).

- *Molecular screening:* DNA samples from gene libraries, isolated organisms, or field samples can be screened for nucleotide sequences encoding specific enzymes using molecular techniques such as PCR or DNA hybridisation, independently of functional assays.

- *Genome sequencing and bioinformatics:* The complete nucleotide sequences of many bacterial and fungal genomes have been generated and more are being completed each year. Most of these are publicly available, but a few are kept as proprietary information for the companies that generated them. Genomic sequence data can provide a rich reservoir for the discovery of novel enzymes using computer algorithms to identify the corresponding genes and/or functional domains within the proteins they encode.

Modern screening approaches are often divided into two phases, termed primary and secondary screens (Fig. 20.2). *Primary screening* involves a quick round of elimination, where the organisms that can produce the desired enzyme are sorted from those that cannot. This step usually tests thousands of organisms, as many as possible and practical, and utilises a very simple, quick and robust assay. In *secondary screening* the best hits selected during the primary screen are subjected to a rigorous process of elimination. In this phase, the microbial enzymes are tested under stringent application-relevant conditions employing assay technologies specifically developed for this purpose. Those enzymes that perform well are often purified and tested in small-scale models of the real application (see also Chapter 12).

The genes encoding the best candidates are usually cloned and expressed in one or more expression hosts to generate sufficient quantities of the enzymes for thorough characterisations, including providing customers with samples for testing under actual working conditions. As a routine part of this process, the complete nucleotide sequences of the cloned genes are determined. This yields valuable information for understanding the structures and specific functions

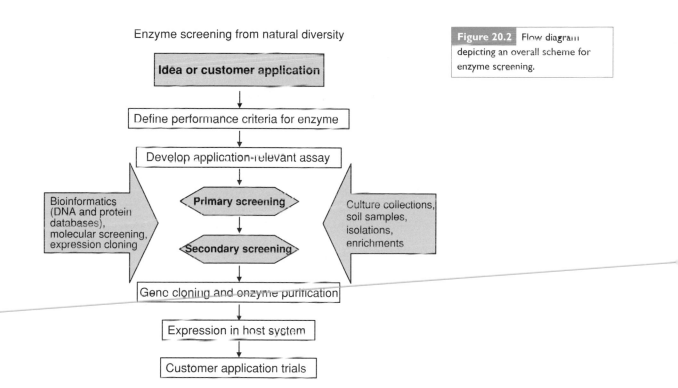

Enzyme screening from natural diversity

Figure 20.2 Flow diagram depicting an overall scheme for enzyme screening.

of the enzymes, allowing classification and comparison to similar enzymes. The DNA sequence information can be exploited with molecular genetics approaches to clone related genes quickly when more natural variation is desired. The screening is complete only when customers are provided with carefully selected enzymes for evaluation in their application, ensuring delivery of the right product tailored to customer needs.

20.2.2   Genetic engineering of production strains

No matter how an enzyme is discovered it must be produced at yields that are economically viable and at high purity. It is sometimes required to produce the enzyme at yields that are 1000 times higher than those obtained with its original source. These challenges are best addressed using gene technology. Accordingly, enzyme companies have developed several safe and environmentally friendly bacteria, yeasts and filamentous fungi that serve as production hosts to manufacture their products. The gene encoding a specific enzyme product is incorporated into the genetic material of these hosts so that it is stably maintained, transcribed and translated, as if it were a native constituent of the production cell. It is imperative that the host is free of unwanted side-activities, such as proteases, that may be deleterious to enzyme products. If post-translational modifications are required for enzyme activity and/or stability, it is important to choose a production host with a cellular machinery that will modify the protein so that its properties are similar to those of the enzyme produced by its original source. The production organisms used for large-scale enzyme fermentations were developed and improved over many years by selective mutation and breeding. Virtually all of the species employed for enzyme production have been used in industrial processes for more than 20 years and, consequently, companies have acquired considerable knowledge about fermentation and tools for genetic engineering. With few exceptions, industrial enzyme products are secreted by these selected production hosts. Secretion of the enzyme into the culture medium allows for rapid recovery and minimal purification. Lastly, a history of safe use is vital for host organisms. The Association of Manufacturers and Formulators of Enzyme Products (AMFEP, www.amfep.org) is an industry organisation that provides guidelines for the selection of host cells and many other environmental health and safety topics related to enzyme manufacturing.

20.2.3 Commonly used host organisms

The ability to express enzymes of any class from any source is fundamental to unlocking the practical potential of enzymes for the industry. While this is admittedly a lofty goal, enzyme companies employ multiple microbial hosts to offer alternatives for obtaining high enzyme yields. A general rule of thumb for selecting an appropriate host is that the best results are usually achieved by choosing one that is phylogenetically related to the organism that originally produced the enzyme. In other words, fungal enzymes are best produced by fungal host strains, bacterial enzymes by bacterial hosts and so on (see Table 20.1). In general, *Bacillus* species are used to produce extracellular bacterial enzymes such as proteases and amylases, whereas *Streptomyces* species are exploited primarily for the production of glucose isomerase, an enzyme deployed for production of high-fructose corn syrup. *Aspergillus* species and *Trichoderma* species are the most frequently used fungal hosts, due to their ability to secrete high levels of enzymes and their long history of safe use. A new fungal host, *Fusarium venenatum*, has recently been developed, owing to its history of safe use as a meat substitute for human consumption. Certain yeast species (e.g. *Saccharomyces cerevisiae, Kluyveromyces lactis*) are also used for production of specific enzymes, albeit less frequently than bacteria and filamentous fungi.

20.2.4 Expression vectors

In addition to an appropriate host strain, an optimized expression vector is required for an optimal production strain. Most expression vectors are plasmids, or DNA fragments from plasmids, that are integrated into the genome of the host organisms in one copy or in multiple copies. In principle, an expression vector harbours a selection marker (a gene that enables one to introduce and maintain the vector in a host cell), an expression cassette encoding the enzyme gene of interest and, for bacterial vectors, a region that allows propagation of the vector in a surrogate or intermediate host such as *E. coli*. The expression cassette also contains a strong promoter to direct

Table 20.1 Commonly used bacterial and fungal production hosts for some enzyme products and applications

Enzyme activity	Application/ industry	Host organism	Donor organism
Acetolactate decarboxylase	Brewing	*Bacillus subtilis*	*Bacillus* species
Amylase (fungal)	Baking, brewing, starch	*Aspergillus oryzae, A. niger*	*Aspergillus* species
Amylase (bacterial)	Starch	*Bacillus amyloliquefaciens, B. licheniformis, B. subtilis*	*Bacillus* species *Thermoactinomyces* species
Cellulase	Baking, brewing, detergents, textiles	*Trichoderma reesei, T. longibrachiatum*	*Trichoderma, Aspergillus, Humicola,* and *Thielavia* species
Glucoamylase	Starch	*Aspergillus niger, A. awamori*	*Aspergillus niger*
Glucose isomerase	Starch (high-fructose corn syrup)	*Streptomyces lividans, S. murinus, S. rubiginosus*	*Streptomyces* and *Actinoplanes* species
Lipase	Baking, dairy, fats and oils	*Aspergillus oryzae, A. niger*	*Thermomyces, Candida, Fusarium* and *Rhizomucor* species
Pectate lyase	Fruits and vegetables, textiles	*Bacillus licheniformis*	*Bacillus* species
Pectinase, polygalacturonase	Fruits and vegetables, beverages	*Aspergillus, Penicillium* and *Trichoderma* species	*Aspergillus* species
Pectin esterase	Fruits and vegetables, beverages	*Aspergillus oryzae, A. niger*	*Aspergillus* species
Phytase	Animal feed	*Aspergillus oryzae, A. niger*	*Aspergillus, Thermomyces* and *Peniophora* species
Protease (alkaline)	Detergents	*Bacillus subtilis, B. licheniformis, B. clausii*	*Bacillus* species
Protease (acidic)	Dairy (milk clotting)	*Aspergillus oryzae, A. niger, A. awamori*	Calf stomach, *Mucor, Rhizomucor* and *Cryphonectria* species
Pullulanase	Starch	*Bacillus subtilis, B. licheniformis*	*Bacillus* species
Xylanase (hemicellulase)	Pulp and paper, textiles	*Aspergillus niger, Bacillus subtilis, B. licheniformis, Trichoderma reesei*	*Actinomadura, Trichoderma* and *Bacillus* species

transcription of the gene that encodes the enzyme of choice and a transcriptional terminator (Fig. 20.3). The efficiency of the expression vector is largely determined by the amount of functional messenger RNA (mRNA) produced from the complex interplay between the promoter, the structural gene and the host strain.

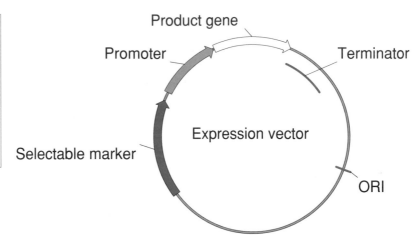

Figure 20.3 Generalised expression vector for production of industrial enzymes. A strong promoter from the production host is used to direct transcription of the product gene. The selectable marker gene is employed for selection of transformed cells that harbour the expression vector.

When the expression vector harbouring the enzyme gene has been assembled, it is transferred into the host strain by *transformation*. In this process, the host cells are chemically or enzymatically treated to render their cell walls permeable to the expression vector DNA. After incubating the cells in presence of the expression vector, the cells are allowed to regenerate their cell walls and placed onto selective growth medium that allows growth of only those cells that have incorporated the expression vector with its selection marker and provide for its stable replication. The resulting transformants can then be tested for their ability to produce the recombinant enzyme. In order to identify the strains with the highest expression levels, individual transformants are grown in small cultures (see Chapter 12) and the product yields are measured. The transformants are ultimately evaluated on the basis of fermentation yields, but additional parameters such as morphology may also be considered.

20.2.5 Improved enzyme production strains

When an optimal transformant is selected as described in the previous section, enzyme titres and other properties of the production strain can be improved by classical mutagenesis of the transformant. In this process the selected transformant is subjected to treatments that are intended to create random changes in its genome. The resulting population of mutant cells is then screened for individuals that exhibit yield increases or other improved characteristics in the same way as the transformants were originally screened. Creation of improved production strains is highly desirable because it improves the overall economy of the enzyme (higher yields translate to lower costs for the producer and the customer). Lower enzyme costs may allow for their use in new applications where the costs were previously too high. In addition, increased enzyme yields require less production capacity, thereby liberating fermenters for other products.

20.2.6 An alternative to DNA technology

For multi-component enzyme products like cellulases and pectinases, where the performance of the product depends on several enzyme activities, recombinant DNA technology is not always an easy way to obtain high-yielding strains, since a number of enzyme proteins have to be in the product, in precise ratios. For other products, the use of recombinant DNA technology is unwanted by the customers due to public concern about the use of genetically modified organisms (GMOs). In these cases, and when the performance of a recombinant production strain needs a further lift, traditional strain improvement is likely to be a solution. Traditional strain improvement through mutation and breeding has a long history of use. Glucoamylase production by *Aspergillus niger* and cellulase fermentation by *Trichoderma reesei* are examples of the power of this approach. Screening for improved strains is much like screening new enzymes from natural specimens in that it consists of a primary screen with a high capacity, so that 10 000 to 100 000 mutants can be tested using robotics and automated assays followed by a secondary screen, where the hits from the primary screen (e.g. 50 to 500 mutants) are re-tested for improvement in enzyme productivity. Finally, a sub-set of mutants from the secondary screen is analysed in laboratory-scale fermentations to choose the best candidates for further optimisation.

20.2.7 Protein engineering and directed evolution

Naturally occurring enzymes are the basis for all industrial enzyme products, but with new methods of protein design and directed molecular evolution, enzymes can be improved to meet any requirement a customer may have. By collecting enzymes and microorganisms from all over the world, researchers are able to find enzyme solutions for many industrial problems. Sometimes, though, even nature is unable to meet the extreme demands of modern commercial enzyme uses. The high temperatures, extreme pH values and harsh chemicals used in today's industrial processes may be too much for naturally occurring enzymes. However, by employing protein engineering strategies, these obstacles can be overcome. Enzyme producers and academic laboratories have together developed the technologies described in the following sections that can be used to improve the performance characteristics of enzymes by altering the genes that encode them.

20.2.8 Rational protein design: protein engineering

Protein engineering entails the selective replacement of specific amino acids within a protein to alter intentionally specific biochemical characteristics such as thermostability, pH optimum, or substrate specificity. In practice, this technology utilises site-directed mutagenesis to alter the gene encoding the protein. The engineering tasks are most often performed using a detailed three-dimensional model of the protein structure generated from the X-ray diffraction patterns of a crystallised sample of the protein. Based on years of research examining the relationship between enzyme structure and function, sophisticated predictive protein modelling software has been developed that helps protein engineers suggest amino acid substitutions. The structure of an enzyme can also be compared to other enzymes with similar three-dimensional structures, but different properties, for clues regarding the particular amino acids responsible for distinctive attributes. Similar strategies can be used even without knowledge of an enzyme's structure by amino acid sequence alignments. Comparing primary amino acid sequences among families of closely related enzymes with different functional properties can give important clues in identifying the amino acid residues that contribute to individual catalytic and thermodynamic behaviours.

20.2.9   Random mutagenesis and directed evolution

In many cases, a unique, isolated enzyme catalyses the desired reaction, but fails in an industrial application because it has the wrong pH optimum, temperature profile or is sensitive to chemicals (such as detergent components) that are present. In these cases, the enzyme is engineered using the relatively new method of directed evolution. This method mimics the process of natural evolution in that it involves gene mutation, selection and recombination, but is confined to a specific gene and occurs in a test tube rather than in a living organism. The gene encoding the targeted enzyme is first randomly mutagenised by making copies of the gene under conditions that introduce errors throughout the nucleotide sequence. The mutagenised genes are then cloned into plasmids and transformed into a unicellular expression host (usually a yeast, *E. coli* or *Bacillus* species) with each cell receiving a single copy of the mutagenised gene. The transformed cells are then screened for improved function in a high-throughput assay as described in Section 20.3 to identify those cells expressing the improved enzyme. Most often, a single round of mutagenesis identifies enzyme variants that are only marginally improved, so the genes encoding the improved variants are isolated and mutagenesis is carried out repeatedly in successive rounds of mutagenesis and screening. Not surprisingly, successive rounds of mutagenesis accumulate more and more mutations, and since it is much more likely to introduce mutations that negatively effect enzyme performance than improve it, it is often difficult to reach the desired level of improvement using only random mutagenesis. To avoid this conundrum, researchers now utilise recombination between improved enzyme genes to create gene libraries that contain genes with combinations of the mutations previously found in single isolated genes. This recombination can be carried out in vitro using a variety of techniques called *DNA shuffling* (Fig. 20.4) or directly in yeast using its natural homologous recombination system. DNA shuffling dramatically increases the speed with which improved enzymes can be generated since it increases the proportion of variants that are improved compared to successive rounds of random mutagenesis.

When a family of related enzyme genes is available, a technique known as *family shuffling* (Fig. 20.4) can be used. In this technique, the gene diversity introduced by random mutagenesis can be replaced by the diversity inherent in the naturally occurring genes. In family

Table 20.2 | Examples of protein engineered enzyme products

Enzyme	Mutation method	Advantages
Amylase	Protein engineering	Enhanced low calcium; and specific activity
Amylase	Protein engineering	Enhanced oxidation stability
Lipase	Directed evolution	Enhanced performance in first wash
Protease	Directed evolution	Enhanced performance
Phospholipase	Directed evolution	Altered substrate specificity
Peroxidase	Protein engineering and directed evolution	Increased thermostability and oxidation stability

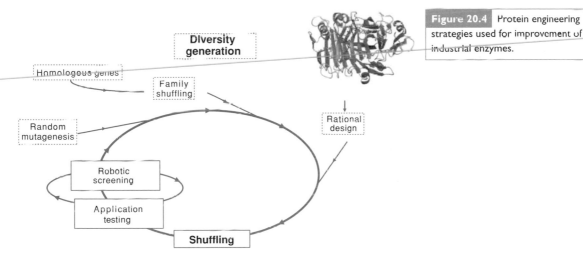

Figure 20.4 Protein engineering strategies used for improvement of industrial enzymes.

shuffling methods, the recombination step is performed directly with the related genes (usually having nucleotide sequence homology of greater than 70%), and results in a larger proportion of active recombinants since all the input genes encode active enzymes. In practice, both techniques – protein engineering and directed evolution – are used simultaneously to improve enzymes, as shown in Table 20.2.

20.3 | Large-scale production, recovery and formulation

In 1952, Novozymes introduced Thermozyme, the world's first enzyme produced by fermentation, and in doing so paved the way for large-scale production of enzymes. Since then enzyme producers have invested heavily in fermentation technology to harvest cheaper products with faster delivery times to the benefit of customers and consumers. Most industrial enzymes today are produced by submerged fermentation, a process involving cultivation of production strains in closed fermentation vessels that contain the nutrient medium for growth of the cells. As the cells metabolise the nutrients, the enzyme

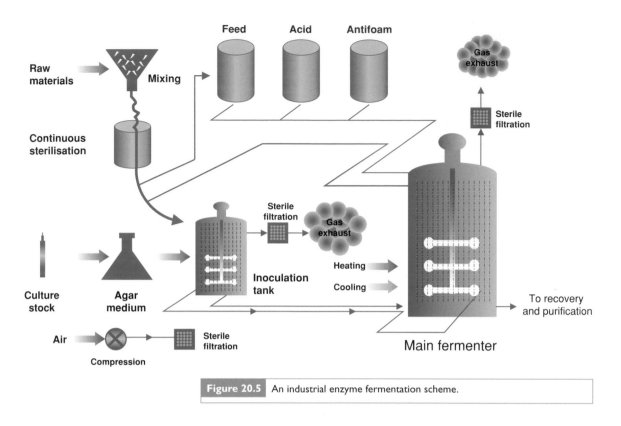

Figure 20.5 An industrial enzyme fermentation scheme.

product is released into the medium. Industrial fermenters can be as large as 1000 m^3.

20.3.1 Fermentation schemes

The fermentation medium comprises sterilised nutrients derived from renewable raw materials like cornstarch, sugars and soy protein. Three principal types of fermentation strategies are commonly employed. A *batch* fermentation protocol is the simplest scheme in which the inoculum is allowed to grow, and nothing is added after the initial charge of nutrients. In the so-called *fed-batch* process sterilised nutrients are added to the fermenter during the cell growth phase. In a *continuous fermentation* process sterilised nutrients are fed into the fermenter at the same rate as the spent broth is removed from the system, thereby achieving steady-state production. The continuous process can be maintained for long periods of time, theoretically for ever, but in practice up to several weeks. Temperature, pH and dissolved oxygen concentration can be monitored and controlled to maximize enzyme titres (Fig. 20.5).

After the fermentation process, the enzyme is separated from the cell biomass by means of filtration, flocculation, centrifugation or a combination of these. Following enzyme extraction, the enzyme is concentrated by means of semipermeable membranes or evaporation. If high enzyme purity is required, the downstream process often employs special steps to remove unwanted impurities. This may be done by selective precipitation, adsorption of the impurities or crystallisation techniques by which extremely pure enzyme products can be obtained. Finally, it is necessary to deliver the enzymes in a form that is desired by the customer. These may include various forms of dry and liquid formulation to immobilised enzymes. It should be noted that the behaviour of enzymes in various forms will vary slightly in their activity, stability and performance for various industrial uses. Regardless of the final formulation, enzyme products must satisfy three requirements:

- the enzyme activity must be stable,
- the physical form must be compatible with the intended use, and
- the product must be safe to use.

20.3.2 Liquid forms

Some industrial enzyme users prefer liquid enzyme formulations, because they are easy to handle. Typical formulation components include water and stabilisers such as glycerol, salt and sugar. Advanced forms of liquid products are also available such as the proprietary encapsulated enzyme product that Novozymes has recently developed, which offers improved stability and a delayed-release feature.

20.3.3 Solid forms

Solid enzyme products are typically free-flowing powders consisting of particles with a diameter between 0.1 and 1 mm. For some industrial applications, the dust from powdered formulations is undesirable and, therefore, most enzyme manufacturers produce granulated and immobilised products. Not surprisingly, there are several types of granulated preparations that are prepared using different compositions and coatings. For example, a low-dusting, reinforced core particle coated with a waxy material is predominantly used in powdered detergents. Other types of granulated formulations are intended for applications such as baking, and for immobilised enzymes, such as glucose isomerase, which is used in the conversion of glucose to fructose. Enzymes that are immobilised on solid supports can be re-used and are easily separated from their reaction products. Many support matrices are available including resins, glass beads, several modified cellulose polymers, gelatine, agarose, chitosans and other polysaccharides. Most of these supports require chemical activation prior to enzyme coupling. Other uses for immobilised enzymes include transesterification of fats and separation of chiral compounds. Enzyme granulates are often prepared in top-spray, fluid granulation towers (Fig. 20.6) in which enzyme droplets formulated with salt, cellulose and other ingredients are allowed to fall through a heated mist of polymer-coating material to produce agglomerated particles of about 0.5 mm in diameter. Granulates are a very efficient and safe way to deliver enzymes in a dust-free, dry form for many applications.

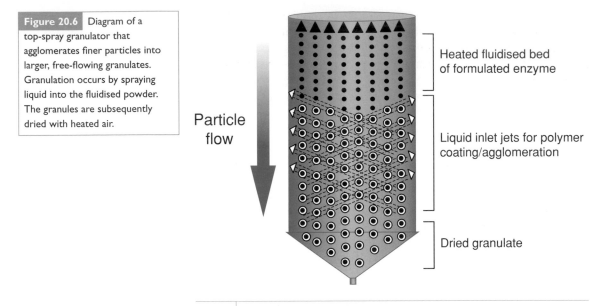

Figure 20.6 Diagram of a top-spray granulator that agglomerates finer particles into larger, free-flowing granulates. Granulation occurs by spraying liquid into the fluidised powder. The granules are subsequently dried with heated air.

Particle flow

Heated fluidised bed of formulated enzyme

Liquid inlet jets for polymer coating/agglomeration

Dried granulate

20.4 | Application of enzymes

Considering the multitude of benefits afforded by industrial enzymes it is not surprising that the number of commercial applications increases yearly. The following sections outline a few of the major applications for enzymes from the three principal markets: technical, food and animal feed.

20.4.1 Animal feed enzymes

Many feed ingredients are not fully digested or absorbed by livestock, effectively reducing the nutritional value of the feed and, consequently, the growth of the animals. However, by adding enzymes to the feed, the digestibility can be improved. Feed enzymes are now well-proven and successful tools that allow feed producers to extend the range of raw materials used in the feed and to improve the efficiency of existing formulations. A wide range of enzyme preparations is available to degrade substances such as phytic acid, cellulose, hemicelluloses, glucan, starch, protein, pectin-like polysaccharides, xylan, raffinose and stachyose. Enzymes are added to the feed, either directly or as a pre-mix, together with vitamins, minerals and other additives. The main benefits of supplementing feed with enzymes are faster growth of the animal, improved feed conversion ratio (i.e. better feed utilisation), more uniform production and better overall health.

The rearing of pigs and poultry can be significantly improved by supplementing their normal diet with enzymes, because the pig's digestive system does not produce enzymes capable of breaking down plant cell walls. The addition of commercial enzymes facilitates conversion of the feed into a form that the animals can absorb and utilise. For example, monogastric animals such as pigs and poultry are incapable of digesting phytic acid (inositol hexakisphosphate), the main phosphorus storage compound in legume plants such as soy beans. Supplementing feed with phytase has two advantages: First, it hydrolyses phytic acid, removing several of the phosphate groups, thereby making additional phosphate available as a nutrient. Second, by degrading phytic acid, detrimental effects on the environment caused by the release of organic phosphorus in animal manure are diminished.

20.4.2 Detergent enzymes

Modern households demand washing detergents that remove even the most difficult stains irrespective of wash temperature. Detergent enzymes are by far the widest application of enzymes today, with uses for household laundry, dishwashing and industrial and institutional detergents. The major benefits of enzymes in detergents include:

- better cleaning performance,
- shorter washing times,
- reduced energy consumption by lowering wash temperatures,
- reduced water consumption through higher cleaning efficiency,
- diminished environmental impact because enzymes are biodegradable,
- reduced environmental impact from addition of chemicals such as phosphates,
- rejuvenation of cotton fabric through the action of cellulases on fibres, and
- stain removal and improved whiteness.

The most widely used detergent enzymes are hydrolases, which remove stains composed of proteins, lipids and polysaccharides. Historically, proteases were the first to be used extensively in laundering. Today, proteases have been joined by lipases, amylases and cellulases in increasing the effectiveness of detergents, especially for household laundering at lower temperatures. Cellulases provide fabric care through selective reactions that contribute to cleaning and to overall fabric care by rejuvenating or maintaining the appearance of washed garments. Many detergent brands are based on a blend of two, three or even four different enzymes. A major challenge for the development of new enzymes or the modification of existing products for detergents is to make them more tolerant to detergent components like builders, surfactants and bleaching chemicals. The trend towards lower laundry wash temperatures, especially in Europe, has increased the need for adding enzymes. Starch and fat stains are easier to remove in very hot water, but the additional cleaning power provided by enzymes is required in cooler water.

20.4.3 Starch and fuel

Many valuable products are derived from starch. Corn starch is the most widespread raw material used in the starch processing industry, followed by wheat, tapioca and potatoes. Reaction efficiency, specific action and the ability to work under mild conditions all make

Figure 20.7 Major steps in the enzymatic processing of starch to various sweeteners.

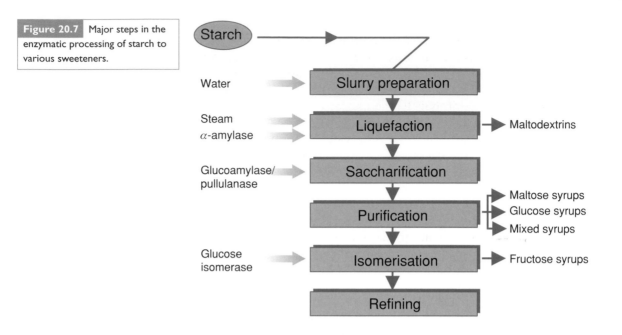

enzymes ideal catalysts for the starch processing industry. Additionally, the moderate temperatures and pH values used for enzyme reactions produce fewer by-products affecting flavour and colour than old processes involving acid hydrolysis. Furthermore, enzyme reactions are easily controlled and can be stopped when the desired degree of starch conversion is reached. The starch industry began using industrial enzymes for large-scale processing in the 1960s. Special types of syrup that could not be produced using conventional chemical hydrolysis were the first compounds made entirely by enzymatic processes. The first enzyme (glucoamylase) produced in the early 1960s was a major turning point for the food industry. This enzyme breaks down starch completely to glucose. Soon thereafter almost all glucose production changed from acid hydrolysis to enzymatic hydrolysis because of the clear product benefits of greater yields, higher degree of purity and easier crystallisation.

Heat-stable α-amylases are remarkable enzymes that were discovered in the early 1970s. These amylases can survive temperatures above boiling point, and they revolutionised industrial starch saccharification because they could be used in the large jet cookers that liquefy solid starch granules. Another significant breakthrough was achieved in 1973 with the development by Novozymes of immobilised glucose isomerase. This enzyme made the industrial production of high-fructose syrup feasible. It was a major achievement that led to the birth of a multi-billion dollar industry in the USA for the production of high-fructose syrups that are used as sweeteners in many types of food products.

An overview of the major steps used in starch processing is shown in Fig. 20.7. Maize (corn) starch is the most widely used raw material, but due to its insoluble and granular nature, raw starch must first be gelatinised and liquefied to make the starch susceptible to enzymatic attack. This is accomplished by heating the starch with steam and adding a temperature-stable α-amylase in stirred tank reactors or jet cookers. The α-amylase hydrolyses α-1,4-glycosidic bonds in the gelatinised starch, thereby lowering the viscosity and liberating maltodextrins. Further hydrolysis by the addition of glucoamylase, fungal α-amylase and pullulanase activities may yield a variety of syrups. Glucose may be isomerised to fructose using immobilised glucose isomerase. The immobilised enzyme product loses activity over time, and is typically replaced when activity falls to 10–15% of the initial value.

Enzymes are also used in the production of fuel ethanol from starch, a product that represents one of the most promising renewable sources of energy. In this process, starch is hydrolysed to glucose, which is subsequently converted to ethanol by yeast fermentation. Fuel ethanol can be produced from starch substrates found in renewable raw materials such as corn, wheat and rice. However, fuel ethanol is not only a renewable resource of energy; it also burns cleaner than gasoline and produces fewer harmful exhaust emissions. Environmentally friendly by nature, it also offers a biodegradable alternative to the gasoline oxygenate additive methyl tertiary butyl ether (MTBE) – a contaminant that has been found in drinking water in many parts of the world.

The demand for fuel ethanol is higher than ever. In the past few years, enzyme companies and the US Department of Energy have collaborated on developing new enzyme technologies (based on cellulases and hemicellulases) that will make it possible to produce fuel ethanol from cellulosic waste materials such as rice straw, wood chips and corn stalks. While starch is the preferred substrate today, the focus of the future will be on cellulose – the most abundant organic polymer on Earth. Glucose derived from starch and cellulose is also viewed as the raw material that will replace petroleum-based carbon for the synthesis of organic molecules and polymers of the future. Future facilities that integrate starch and cellulose conversion technologies to produce fuels, power and chemicals from renewable raw materials have been termed *biorefineries*. The biorefinery concept is analogous to today's petroleum refineries, which produce multiple fuels and products from petroleum.

20.4.4 Wine and beverages

The grape's own enzymes consist mainly of pectinesterase and polygalacturonase, but they are often insufficient to hydrolyse pectic substances, and they have little effect on complex polysaccharides found in the cell-wall. Since the introduction of pectinases into the wine industry in the 1970s, the development of specific cell-wall degrading enzymes offers winemakers the opportunity to improve wine quality and increase production flexibility. Enzyme preparations are used in the maceration (mash treatment) to release colour, aroma compounds and juice; clarification (must treatment) to speed up settling and wine maturation for aroma liberation, wine stabilisation and filtration:

- Glycosidases are known for their effect on aroma precursors. These enzymes can enhance the wine aroma of Muscat or similar grape varieties containing bound terpenes.
- Blends of pectinases and β-glucanase have been developed to hydrolyse the colloids formed in wine by the interaction of yeast glucans and grape pectins during fermentation, resulting in improvement of wine clarification, filtration and stabilisation after fermentation. This enzyme mixture accelerates the ageing process, resulting in reduced contact time and a faster clarification process.
- Preparations of β-glucanase are used for the treatment of wines produced from grapes affected by the fungus *Botrytis cinerea*. This fungus is referred to as 'noble rot' in the case of late harvest wines. The β-glucanase can be added near the end of the alcoholic fermentation or before the malolactic fermentation, whichever is preferred.

The production of fermented alcoholic drinks from starch-based raw materials (e.g. fruit, wine, sugar cane, potatoes and cereals) has been practised for centuries. Often the alcohol is distilled to create liquor with much higher alcohol content. Prior to the 1960s, starch hydrolysis was achieved by the addition of malt or koji (fermented rice), which provided the enzymes to convert the starch into fermentable sugars. Today, in most countries, addition of malt has been completely replaced by direct addition of selected commercial enzymes. A few litres of enzyme preparation can be used to replace 100 kg of malt. In terms of raw material costs, savings of 20–30% can be expected when switching to commercial enzymes. Furthermore, the enzymes are supplied with a uniform, standardised activity, so starch hydrolysis becomes more predictable, leading to improved consistency in the fermentation process. Finally, industrial enzymes perform better than those found in malt. Microbial amylases are available with better activity at the low pH values found in the mash. Extremely thermostable amylases are available that are able to liquefy starch at 100 °C, long after malt enzymes have been destroyed.

20.4.5   Brewing and baking

Beer is traditionally produced by mixing crushed barley malt and hot water in a large circular vessel called a mash copper. In addition to malted barley, grains such as maize, sorghum, rice or even pure starch may be added to the mash as adjuncts. The mash is subsequently filtered to produce a liquid known as sweet wort. The wort is boiled with added hops to enhance flavour, cooled, and transferred to fermentation tanks where it is mixed with yeast. After fermentation the 'green beer' is allowed to mature before filtration and bottling. In many large breweries, enzymes are used to increase efficiency, enhance control of the brewing process and produce beer of a consistently high quality. Auxiliary enzymes are often used to optimise adjunct liquefaction, produce low-carbohydrate beer ('light beer'), to shorten the beer maturation time and to produce beer from enhanced malts and cereals.

Enzymes have also become a major success in baking, where for decades fungal α-amylases have been used to degrade starch to maltodextrins for the yeast to act upon. A novel type of amylase can be used to modify a specific portion of the starch, producing an antistaling effect and thereby prolonging the shelf-life of bread. A number of exciting new advances have been made in the application of enzymes for baking. For example, oxidative enzymes can be used to replace potassium bromate, a chemical additive that has been banned in several countries. The gluten in flour is a combination of proteins that forms a large network during dough formation. The gluten network retains the carbon dioxide liberated during dough proofing and baking, and its strength is vital for the quality of yeast breads. Enzymes such as xylanases (hemicellulases), lipases and oxidases can increase the strength of the gluten network and thereby improve the quality of finished bread.

20.4.6　Fruits and vegetables

Over the past few decades, enzymes have played a major role in the development of new fruit processing technologies. Today, enzymes are indispensable tools for fruit juice producers, where they have a significant economic benefit by increasing the yields of juice. Special pectinolytic enzymes boost juice yields and processing capacity by a selective breakdown of pectin, which is a natural plant polysaccharide found in all fruit and is composed primarily of galacturonic acid. These acid groups may either be free, combined as a methyl ester, or as sodium, potassium, calcium or ammonium salts. Pectin acts as cell glue, giving structure to the fruit. In fruit mashes, pectin binds the water, thereby increasing the viscosity and making it difficult to release the juice from the crushed fruit. During later production stages, pectin must be hydrolysed to allow for rapid clarification and filtering of the final juice product. Fruit juice processors often filter the juice with special ultrafiltration equipment; but without using enzymes to degrade the pectin, the juice filtration process would be far too slow and costly.

A special application is the use of pectin esterase to keep fruit pieces for fruit preparations intact. This is desirable for canned and frozen fruit to prevent fruit pieces from becoming too soft. Pectin esterase is also used to maintain the firmness of pieces of processed vegetables.

20.4.7　Forest products

Enzymes offer significant benefits for the forestry industry, most notably environmental protection. Specific xylanases were introduced in the 1990s to reduce the amount of chemicals, such as chlorine and chlorine dioxide, that are used to de-colourise wood pulp. Use of xylanases as an alternative to harsh bleaching chemicals gives corresponding reductions in the amount of harmful chlorinated organic compounds that are released into the environment. There is a general trend around the world to cut the amount of chlorine used for bleaching pulp, and environmental regulations are becoming tougher accompanied by an increasing demand for totally chlorine-free paper.

The recycling of paper is another growing trend. For example, about 30% of the paper consumed in the USA is recycled. Processes for de-inking of mixed office waste paper have been developed using special cellulase blends that considerably reduce the use of harsh chemicals. Enzymes also help to keep high-speed paper machines running smoothly by removing pitch or slime. Pitch is a resinous substance, while slime is the general term for deposits of a microbial origin. Both of these undesirable materials can be removed enzymatically from paper-making equipment, replacing hazardous caustic soda and minimising down time.

20.4.8 Dairy

The application of enzymes in the processing of milk products dates from the earliest times of recorded history. In ancient times, calf stomach extracts, which contain the enzyme chymosin, were used to coagulate milk for cheese production. Nowadays bovine chymosin is produced in recombinant microorganisms, and there are several microbial proteases sold as chymosin substitutes. Fresh cheese curds are composed of milk protein (casein), lipids, carbohydrates and minerals. These compounds have a very mild taste, but the distinctive flavours of ripened cheese develop as a result of progressive enzymatic hydrolysis of the proteins and lipids. Traditionally, cheese ripening requires long-term storage, space, and controlled temperature and humidity. Consequently, it is a very expensive process. Accelerating the ripening process by addition of specific enzymes can save costs, especially with the low-moisture, slow-ripening cheese varieties. Much of the research on cheese ripening has focused on limited proteolysis that occurs in cheddar cheese. This process involves the formation of amino acids and short peptides by endo- and exo-peptidases to accelerate the development of characteristic cheddar aroma and taste. Lipases are becoming established as a substitute for rennet paste, a stomach extract from suckling calves or lambs. Rennet pastes serve as a source of lipases to enhance the piquancy of Italian and blue cheeses. Several microbial lipases can produce profiles of short chain fatty acids that are similar to those of rennet paste. In addition, because of possible health risks, rennet pastes are prohibited in some countries.

20.5 Regulatory and safety aspects

Safety and quality are extremely important in all production processes. This is equally true when using nature's own technology – enzymes – in industrial processes. Although enzymes are natural products and their past use in food processing illustrates their safety, responsible companies strive to ensure that their products pose no risks to customers and consumers. In most countries, the regulatory status, classification and labelling of technical enzymes are governed by existing laws concerning chemicals. Most are listed in chemical inventories such as the European Inventory of Existing Commercial Substances (EINECS) in the EU and the Toxic Substances Control Act (TSCA) in the USA. Because they are considered natural products, some enzymes are exempt from listing, but in other cases they are regulated by specific legislation covering biotechnology products.

The application of enzymes in food processing is regulated by government agencies that administrate food purity and safety laws. Within the EU, member states have harmonised their respective directives and regulations. The Joint FAO/WHO Expert Committee on Food Additives (JECFA) and the Food Chemicals Codex (FCC) have established guidelines for the use of enzymes as food additives. Agencies such as AMFEP (Europe) and the Enzyme Technical Association (USA) standardise regulations internationally. AMFEP has also delineated a *good manufacturing practice* (GMP) standard for microbial food enzymes. Its members ensure that enzymes used in food processing are obtained from non-pathogenic and non-toxicogenic microorganisms. For production strains that contain recombinant DNA (GMOs), the characteristics and safety record of all donor organisms contributing genetic material to the production strain are assessed.

Based on government safety standards all over the world, enzyme companies must ensure that their products cannot harm people or the environment, for example by causing allergies. An important part of the process is the collection of toxicity data to satisfy requirements from regulatory agencies such as the US Food and Drug Administration or Environmental Protection Agency. Wherever possible enzyme manufacturers are encouraged to use in-vitro or alternative tests that do not involve live animals, but cell cultures, bacteria or organs obtained from slaughterhouses. Since the late 1960s it has been known that enzymes may induce allergic reactions in some people if inhaled as dust or aerosols. The effect is comparable to inhalation of pollen, animal dander or dust mites. Enzyme allergy is solely an occupational health hazard, and no cases of health effects to enzymes among consumers have been reported for almost 30 years. Occupational allergies can be prevented by simply eliminating airborne dust or aerosols through the use of liquid and granulated formulations.

20.6 | Further reading

Alberghina, L. (ed.). *Protein Engineering in Industrial Biotechnology*. Amsterdam: Hardwood Academic, 2000.

Flickinger, M. C. and Drew, S. W. (eds.). *The Encyclopedia of Bioprocess Technology: Fermentation, Biocatalysis and Bioseparation*. New York: John Wiley & Sons, 1999.

Godfrey, T. and West, S. (eds.). *Industrial Enzymology*, second edition, New York: Stockton Press, and London: Macmillan, 1996.

Kearlsley, M. W. and Dziedzic, S. Z. (eds.). *Handbook of Starch Hydrolysis Products and Their Derivatives*. Glasgow: Blackie Academic and Professional, 1995.

Kirk, O., Borchert, T. V. and Fuglsang, C. C. Industrial enzyme applications. *Current Opinions in Biotechnology* **13**: 345–351, 2002.

Panke, S. and Wubbolts, M. G. Enzyme technology and bioprocess engineering. *Current Opinions in Biotechnology* **13**, 111–116, 2002.

Uhlig, H. (ed.). *Industrial Enzymes and Their Applications*. New York: John Wiley & Sons, 1998.

Van Beilen, J. B. and Li, Z. Enzyme technology: an overview. *Current Opinions in Biotechnology* **13**: 338–344, 2002.

Chapter 21

Recombinant proteins of high value

Georg-B. Kresse

Roche Diagnostics GmbH, Germany

21.1 | Applications of high-value proteins

Proteins used in industrial enzyme technology, e.g. detergent proteinases or enzymes applied in the food industry, are in most cases rather crude preparations and usually mixtures of different enzymes. In contrast, there are a number of commercial applications where highly purified (and therefore high-value) proteins are needed. Examples are:

- *Analytical enzymes and antibodies:* Used in medical diagnostics, food analysis, as well as biochemical and molecular biological analysis (see Section 21.2).
- *Enzymes used as tools in genetic engineering technology:* Gene technology has become possible through the availability of highly purified restriction endonucleases, DNA and RNA polymerases, nucleases and modifying enzymes (see Chapters 4 and 5). Similarly, glycohydrolases and glycosyl transferases are used increasingly in glycobiotechnology in order to modify the sugar residues of glycoproteins.
- *Therapeutic proteins:* Growth factors, antibodies and enzymes are used as the active drug ingredients for the treatment of diseases (see Section 21.3).

Basic Biotechnology, third edition, eds. Colin Ratledge and Bjørn Kristiansen.
Published by Cambridge University Press. © Cambridge University Press 2006.

Furthermore, proteins with proven or supposed biological relevance in pathomechanisms are needed as targets for the search of new ligands (agonists or antagonists) or inhibitors and for X-ray or nuclear magnetic resonance (NMR) structural analysis in order to design novel interacting compounds by structure-based molecular modelling. This requires the production of these proteins on a relatively small scale (10 to 100 mg), but often with high purity depending on the intended use.

21.2 | Analytical enzymes

Enzymes are highly specific both in the reaction catalysed as well as in their choice of substrates. Indeed, enzymes are, besides antibodies, the most specific reagents known. The use of enzymes in analysis, especially in medical diagnostics and in food analysis, therefore offers a number of advantages compared to chemical reagents. The reactants may either become chemically transformed in the presence of an enzyme (if they are substrates), or they may modulate the enzymatic activity in a manner related to their concentration (if they act as activators or inhibitors). Enzymes also serve as 'markers' in assay techniques based on non-enzymatic interactions, such as antigen–antibody binding (see Chapter 25) or DNA–oligonucleotide hybridisation.

Recombinant DNA technology has made it possible to clone any gene of interest and to manipulate bacterial, fungal, insect or mammalian cells to overproduce the desired protein. Many enzymes have been expressed in recombinant microorganisms at levels 10 to 100 times higher than in the natural host cell. This has allowed not only better economics in enzyme production, but also significant reductions of the environmental burden because of the decrease in fermentation volumes (and, thereby, in waste formation). Furthermore, the techniques of site-directed mutagenesis have opened the way to improve relevant properties of enzymes for analytical applications, e.g. stability under the assay conditions, pH optimum or solubility.

21.2.1 Enzymes in diagnostic assays

In *end-point assays*, the compound whose concentration is to be determined (the *analyte*) takes part as the substrate in an enzyme-catalysed reaction and is converted with the simultaneous and stoichiometric production of a detectable signal (e.g. a positive or negative change in absorbance), which may result either from the analyte conversion itself or from a stoichiometrically linked conversion of a co-substrate or co-factor (such as NADH formation in dehydrogenase-catalysed reactions). The reaction is allowed to proceed until completion and the result can easily be calculated from known physical constants; e.g. the molar absorption coefficient in the case of light-absorbing substances. The specificity of the assay system depends on the substrate specificity

Table 21.1 Examples of enzymes important in diagnostics

Enzyme	Source (original)	Used for the assay of
Cholesterol oxidase	*Nocardia erythropolis* or *Brevibacterium* sp.	Cholesterol
Creatinase	*Pseudomonas* sp.	Creatine, creatinine
Creatininase	*Pseudomonas* sp.	Creatinine
β-Galactosidase	*Escherichia coli*	Sodium ions; immunoassay marker enzyme
Glucose oxidase	*Aspergillus niger*	Glucose
Glucose 6-phosphate dehydrogenase	*Leuconostoc mesenteroides*	Glucose (indicator enzyme)
α-Glucosidase	Yeast or *Bacillus* sp.	α-Amylase activity
Glycerol-3-phosphate oxidase	*Aerococcus viridans*	Triglycerides
Hexokinase	Yeast	Glucose and other hexoses
Peroxidase	Horseradish	Indicator enzyme and immunoassay marker enzyme
Pyruvate oxidase	*Pediococcus* sp.	Pyruvate; transaminase activity
Sarcosine oxidase	*Pseudomonas* sp., *Bacillus* sp.	Creatinine
Urate oxidase (uricase)	*Arthrobacter protophormiae*	Uric acid
Urease	*Klebsiella aerogenes*	Urea

[a] All listed enzymes are manufactured from recombinant expression systems and are commercially available.

of the enzyme employed. An overview of important enzymes used in diagnostic assays is given in Table 21.1. Most of the enzymes used in enzymatic analysis are derived from bacteria or yeast, and are produced using microbial (mostly *E. coli* or yeast) expression systems due to the lower production costs.

If none of the reactants or products of an enzymatic reaction produces a detectable signal on conversion, the primary (called 'auxiliary') reaction can be coupled to a stoichiometrically linked 'indicator' reaction (usually also enzyme catalysed), with one of the products of this second reaction being easily detectable. In practice, general (i.e. unspecific) indicator reactions can often be coupled without individual optimisation to various specific auxiliary reactions. Horseradish peroxidase is a well-known example of an indicator enzyme used in a large number of commercial oxidase-based coupled assays. An example of a coupled glucose assay that uses recombinant enzymes as the indicator enzyme is shown in Fig. 21.1. Similarly, enzymes (e.g. peroxidase, alkaline phosphatase) are used for signal generation in enzyme-linked immunoassays known as ELISAs (see Chapter 25).

Under conditions where the substrate concentration is much smaller than the Michaelis–Menten constant, the K_m value, of an enzyme, substrate concentrations can be derived from measurement of the reaction kinetics (*kinetic assay*) because the observed reaction rate then becomes linearly proportional to substrate concentration. Kinetic assays allow a drastic reduction of the time required for analysis and are less sensitive to interferences than end-point assays. In

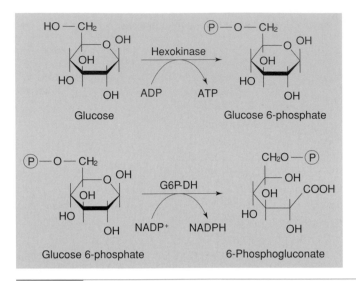

Figure 21.1 An example of a coupled enzymatic assay system using an indicator enzyme: glucose assay with hexokinase and glucose 6-phosphate dehydrogenase. The determination of glucose comprises its phosphorylation catalysed by yeast hexokinase as an auxiliary reaction which cannot be detected directly. This is coupled to the oxidation of glucose 6-phosphate to 6-phosphogluconate catalysed by glucose 6-phosphate dehydrogenase (G6PDH). In this second 'indicator' reaction, 1 mol of $NADP^+$ is reduced per mol of glucose 6-phosphate, which in turn is stoichiometrically equivalent to the glucose present in the original sample, to give NADPH, which can be determined spectrophotometrically at 340 nm. Hexokinase is an unspecific enzyme that would phosphorylate many hexoses. Since, however, G6PDH is strictly specific for glucose 6-phosphate and would not accept other sugar phosphates, the reaction system is specific for the assay of glucose also in the presence of other carbohydrates.

these cases, and in contrast to end-point assays, enzymes with high K_m values (i.e. low substrate affinity) are used to increase the dynamic concentration range of the assay. In order to facilitate handling of the reagents, immobilised enzymes are often used for analytical purposes. An early and still useful approach is to bind the enzyme non-covalently to paper, which is widely used in the design of the *test strips* for assays in biological samples such as urine or blood. In *biosensors*, the enzyme (usually an oxidoreductase) serves as the 'specifier' mediating analyte recognition. This biological interaction is then transformed through a 'transducer' component into an electrical signal which can be amplified and processed electronically (see Fig. 21.2). A number of commercial test strip and biosensor systems for use in clinical chemistry have been developed, especially for glucose measurement in diabetic patients.

21.2.2 Enzymes as tools in biochemical analysis

Purified enzymes are widely used for analytical problems outside medical diagnostics and food analysis, e.g. in molecular biology and gene technology, and in protein and glycoconjugate analysis.

Table 21.2 Some enzymes used in biochemical analysis

Enzyme (source)	Use

Proteases
  Trypsin (bovine)
  Chymotrypsin (bovine)
  Endoproteinase Lys-C from *Lysobacter*
    enzymogenes
  Endoproteinase Glu-C (V-8 protease)
    from *Staphylococcus aureus* V8
	Protein fragmentation for sequence analysis, peptide fingerprinting, limited proteolysis of enzymes or receptors to study structure–function relationships

Carboxypeptidases A, B, C, Y	C-terminal protein sequencing

Restriction proteases
  Factor Xa (bovine or human)
  Enterokinase (bovine)
  IgA protease from *Neisseria gonorrhoea*
	Processing of recombinant fusion proteins

Glycosidases
  Endoglycosidase D and *O*-Glycosidase
    from *Diplococcus pneumoniae*
  Endoglycosidase F and *N*-Glycosidase F
    from *Flavobacterium meningosepticum*
  Endoglycosidase H from *Streptomyces*
    plicatus
  Many exoglycosidases
	Carbohydrate and glycoprotein analysis

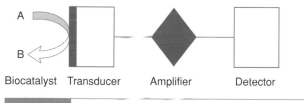

Biocatalyst   Transducer   Amplifier   Detector

Figure 21.2 The general concept of a biosensor. The biocatalyst converts the substrate into product with a concurrent change in a physicochemical parameter (e.g. heat, electron transfer, light, ion or proton flow, etc.) which is concerted into an electrical signal by the transducer, amplified and processed by a detector.

In *molecular biology*, enzymes serve as tools for molecular analysis of chromosome and genome structure, for the characterisation of genetic defects on the DNA level, for taxonomy of viruses and other organisms by correlation of characteristic fragment patterns, as well as for elucidating phylogenetic relationships. In addition, DNA and RNA modifying enzymes as well as polymerases (e.g. recombinant Taq DNA polymerase) are essential tools for all cloning techniques as described in Chapters 4 and 5.

Highly purified enzymes are also important tools in *analysis of protein structure and modification*. Specific proteases are used for protein fragmentation and fingerprinting as well as for C-terminal protein sequencing. Similarly, a set of glycohydrolases is used to analyse, or modify, the carbohydrate residue structures of glycoproteins. A number of enzymes used for this purpose are listed in Table 21.2.

21.2.3 Special requirements for analytical enzymes

Enzymes to be used for analytical applications have to satisfy a number of quality criteria concerning:

- *specificity*: absence of side activities towards other substances which may be present in the sample or the reaction mixture;
- *purity*: absence of contaminating activities or other contaminants interfering with the analytical and detection systems (but, depending on the intended use, not necessarily purity with respect to the absence of other inactive proteins);
- *stability*: in the reaction mixture during the reaction, as well as in long-term storage;
- *kinetic properties*: suitable K_m and k_{cat} values and no inhibition by substances present in the sample;
- *pH optimum*: suitable for the required experimental conditions;
- *solubility and surface properties*: no interference by adsorption or aggregation effects;
- *cost*.

These criteria are dependent on each other. Therefore the choice and quality of an enzyme must be optimised in each case with regard to the particular analytical application.

21.3 | Therapeutic proteins

Proteins are part of numerous traditional medicines, such as snake and bee venom and enzyme preparations; but, in most cases, these are ill-defined mixtures. Furthermore, naturally occurring proteins obtained from animals, plants or microorganisms, as well as from the human body (blood, urine, placenta or adenohypophysis), have long been used as drug ingredients. Typical examples are porcine insulin, blood coagulation factors VIII and IX from human blood fractionation, pancreatin as a digestive aid, or the Ancrod and Batroxobin proteases obtained from snake venoms. However, foreign proteins are immunogenic for humans. This may lead to rapid inactivation and prevent repeated application of the protein drug if applied parenterally. Furthermore, the isolation of therapeutic proteins from human (and animal) fluids and tissues poses a potential risk of viral contamination leading to the risk of infection of patients with other diseases, for example with human immunodeficiency virus (HIV).

The concentration of physiologically active proteins in human body fluids or organs is very low, necessitating the processing of much material for low amounts of product. Chemical synthesis of proteins, although feasible in principle, is not normally an economically viable production method for protein drugs. So, only through gene technology has it become possible to produce human proteins in large amounts and high purity. In many cases, recombinant human proteins have allowed, for the first time, a rational therapy with the body's own substances based on knowledge of the causes of disease and pathobiological mechanisms. Therapeutic proteins such as hormones, growth and differentiation factors, act in signalling; while others function as biocatalysts (enzymes) or inhibitors or effectors of the immune system (antibodies). Thus, they are used for substitution, amplification or inhibition of physiological processes.

At present, more than 100 recombinant proteins are used in therapy (a selection is given in Table 21.3), and more than 500 others are in different stages of development. Erythropoietin (EPO), insulin, somatotropin (human growth hormone), granulocyte-colony stimulating factor (G-CSF), interferon-α and several monoclonal antibodies are among the most successful drugs and are placed in the 'top twenty' on the list of worldwide sales of pharmaceuticals. The global market for pharmaceuticals based on gene technology is still growing at a rapid rate.

21.3.1 Choice of expression system

Bacteria, yeast, insect and mammalian cells are the most commonly used hosts for heterologous protein expression. A brief overview of the main advantages and disadvantages of the various host systems, referring especially to the use of the expression systems for therapeutic proteins, is given below.

Mammalian cells

In mammalian host cells, such as Chinese hamster ovary (CHO), baby hamster kidney (BHK) or mouse myeloma (NS0, SP/0) cells, high-level expression (up to than 100 pg day^{-1} cell^{-1}) of recombinant proteins can be achieved (see Chapter 22). Usually, the proteins are secreted into the fermentation medium in a properly folded, active form and, in most cases, glycosylation and other post-translational modifications occur in a more or less 'human-like' manner, although minor differences may exist that can influence the immunogenicity of the protein. However, development of a stable cell line that expresses the therapeutic protein at a high level may require several rounds of amplification and take many months, and the manufacturing costs are high. Cell fermentation technology using mammalian host cells is used for the large part of presently approved biopharmaceuticals and is the system of choice for large-scale production of modified, e.g. glycosylated, therapeutic proteins, especially if correct protein modification is crucial for the therapeutic effect.

Human cells

One way to ensure the identity of the recombinant protein product with the original human protein is to use human cell lines as the expression system. Instead of cloning a gene or DNA sequence coding for the desired protein into the host cell, it is an interesting alternative to manipulate not the gene itself, but its promoter, in order

Table 21.3 A selection of recombinant protein[a],[b] drugs

Cytokines and antagonists	Hormones and peptides	Coagulation factors and inhibitors	Enzymes	Vaccines	Fusion proteins
Interferon alpha-2a	Insulin	Eptacog alpha	Alteplase (t-PA)	Hepatitis vaccine	**Denileukin diftitox**
Interferon alpha-2b	**Insulin lispro**	**Antihemophilic factor**	**Reteplase (t-PA mutein)**	Lyme disease vaccine	Etanercept
Interferon alfacon-1	**Insulin aspart**	**Moroctocog alpha (FVIII mutein)**	**Tenecteplase (t-PA mutein)**	Diphtheria/tetanus/pertussis vaccine	Alefacept
Peginterferon alfa-2a	**Insulin glargine**	Nonacog alpha	**Monteplase (t-PA mutein)**	Rotavirus vaccine	
Peginterferon alfa-2b	Epoetin-alpha	Desirudin	Dornase-alpha (RNase)		
Interferon beta-1a	Epoetin-beta	**Lepirudin**	**Imiglucerase**		
Interferon beta-1b	Epoetin-delta	Drotrecogin-alfa (Protein C activated)	Agalsidase alpha		
		α₁-Proteinase Inhibitor	Agalsidase beta		
Interferon gamma-1b	**Darbepoetin-alpha**		Rasburicase		
Aldesleukin (IL-2)	Follitropin alpha		Laronidase		
Filgrastim (G-CSF)	Follitropin beta				
Pegfilgrastim	Glucagon				
Lenograstim (G-CSF)	Somatropin				
Molgramostim (GM-CSF)	Lutropin-alpha				
Sargramostim (GM-CSF)	**Teriparatide (PTH 1-34)**				
Tasonermin (TNF-α)	Salmon calcitonin				
Becaplermin (PDGF-BB)	Thyrotropin-alpha				
Oprevelkin (IL-11)	Choriogonadotropin A2				
Anakinra (IL-1RA)	Osteogenic Protein-1				
	Dibotermin alpha (BMP-2)				
	Pegvisomant (hGH antagonist)				
	Nesiritide (natriuretic peptide)				

[a] Proteins that are used in a modified form (as compared to the original human protein) are marked in bold.

[b] Several of the proteins listed are commercialised as various brands by the same or different pharmaceutical companies. For details concerning the individual protein drugs, see the manufacturers websites.

to activate expression of the endogenous human gene. This 'gene activation' technology may eventually become a commercially advantageous way for the production of therapeutic proteins.

Insect cells

The gene coding for a recombinant protein can be inserted into the genome of a baculovirus that infects insect cells very efficiently (see Chapter 22) and uses their protein synthesis machinery to produce large amounts of protein (up to 500 mg of protein per litre of culture medium) transiently within two to three days after infection. Therefore, this system is very suitable to obtain small amounts of protein rapidly for pre-clinical studies. However, post-translational processing differs from the mammalian systems and the system is not suitable for scaling-up.

Yeast

Yeast and other fungi (e.g. *Saccharomyces cerevisiae, Pichia pastoris*) are eukaryotic microorganisms that are routinely cultivated on a large scale. Recombinant proteins are usually located inside the yeast cell; however, it is also possible to attach a leader sequence in order to induce protein secretion (see Chapter 5). Whereas intracellular heterologous proteins may accumulate to the g l^{-1} level, secreted proteins usually reach titres of only about 10 to 100 mg l^{-1}. Human proteins expressed in yeast are correctly folded and disulphide-bridged, but glycosylation differs significantly from the mammalian pattern. At present, only one marketed therapeutic protein (insulin) is produced from yeast.

Bacteria

Bacterial host systems offer fast development, high efficiency and relatively inexpensive production as the main advantages. Recombinant proteins can be accumulated intracellularly or secreted into the periplasmic space (*Escherichia coli*) or into the fermentation medium (*Bacillus* species). However, post-translational processing of complex eukaryotic proteins, such as glycosylation or disulphide bond formation, does not occur in the bacterial cell. Protein expressed in bacteria may also differ from their natural form concerning their amino terminus where an N-formylmethionine residue may be present. To obtain a correct N-terminus, the recombinant protein can be expressed as a fusion construct with an N-terminal extension which is then cleaved off with a suitable protease. In many cases, the sequence of this fusion tail is chosen so that it can be exploited to facilitate purification. For example, tails of a sequence of histidine residues – usually six are used and are known as *poly(His) tails* – are attached to the protein of interest so that it can then bind specifically to metal chelate chromatography materials. The histidine residues are added by adding six codons for histidine to the DNA next to the gene sequence that is coding for the protein itself; it is therefore the cell itself that makes the modified protein.

In addition, upon high-level expression in bacterial cells, whether cytosolic or periplasmic, many eukaryotic proteins are accumulated as mis-folded, aggregated and insoluble particles (termed *inclusion bodies*) that have to be re-folded in vitro into their native conformations (see also Section 21.3.2). If this re-folding process can be designed to offer a fair yield and good economics, the bacterial (especially *E. coli*) host system is very well suited for the production of all those therapeutic proteins that do not require post-translational processing for in-vivo bioactivity.

Transgenic animals and plants

Transgenic manipulation means that a gene from one species (*the transgene*) is introduced into the germ line of another species, either plant or animal, so that all progeny from the animal or plant will now make the new protein. Milk and blood, as well as urine, have been proposed for transgenic protein production, and a number of different proteins have already been produced in this way; some proteins, e.g. milk-produced antithrombin-III and α_1-antitrypsin, are currently in clinical trials. Expression levels up to 35 g l^{-1} milk have been reported, suggesting that transgenic dairy animals may provide a cost-effective route to the large-scale manufacture of biotherapeutics. However, development times are long because the gestation period and the onset of sexual maturity of the animal are rate limiting, and there are still a number of concerns with respect to the consistency of protein production from different animals. Nevertheless, transgenic technology represents a real challenge for biotechnology.

Production from transgenic plants is potentially a more economically attractive system for large-scale production of recombinant proteins, offering advantages in the low cost of growing plants on large acreage, the availability of natural protein-storage organs, and the established practices for harvesting, transporting, storing and processing. At present, the main disadvantages are low accumulation levels of recombinant proteins, insufficient information on post-translational events and limited knowledge of relevant downstream processing technology.

21.3.2 Protein folding from inclusion bodies

Protein folding in vitro has often been compared to the task of unboiling an egg – to reform the biologically active, native protein conformation from insoluble and inactive aggregates. This *naturation* process is usually done in several steps, as shown in Fig. 21.3. In unfolded proteins, hydrophobic regions that would be buried within the native globular protein structure are exposed. These parts of the polypeptide chain tend to induce non-specific aggregation, thereby decreasing the refolding yield.

Aggregation is a bimolecular reaction and is therefore concentration dependent. As a consequence, protein naturation usually has to be performed at high dilution, and the resulting low protein concentrations and large reaction volumes lead to unfavourable economics

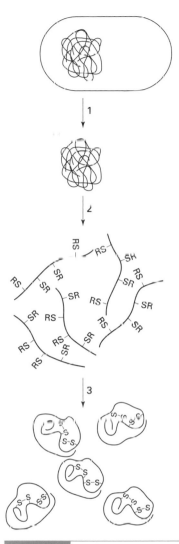

Figure 21.3 Protein 'naturation' from inclusion bodies. Recombinant proteins overexpressed in bacterial cells often are formed as insoluble and misfolded 'inclusion bodies' (1). After cell lysis, the inclusion bodies are collected by centrifugation, washed with buffer to remove soluble cell components (which may already lead to $\geq 90\%$ purity of the desired protein) and are then dissolved in a concentrated solution of a strong denaturant, e.g. 6–8 mol urea l^{-1} or 5–6 mol guanidinium.HCl l^{-1} (2). If the recombinant protein contains cysteine residues, a redox buffer system, such as a mixture of reduced and oxidised glutathione (GSH/GSSG) at a slightly alkaline pH, is added. In some cases, it has proven advantageous to modify the sulphydryl groups reversibly, e.g. by formation of mixed disulphides with glutathione, to increase solubility of the denatured polypeptide chain (R). The protein is then allowed to refold by slow removal of the denaturing agent, usually by dilution or dialysis, with concomitant formation of the correct disulphide bonds (3). Often, the addition of additives such as arginine, tris(hydroxymethyl)amino methane or alkylurea derivatives has been shown to improve the refolding yields considerably. (Figure modified with permission from Marston, F. A. O., 1986. The purification of eukaryotic polypeptides synthesized in *Escherichia coli. Biochemistry Journal* **240**: 1–12. © The Biochemical Society.)

for large-scale production. However, it has been demonstrated that a correctly folded (thus, hydrophilic) protein does not interfere with folding of further portions of the same, still unfolded protein. Therefore, if one starts refolding at a low protein concentration and adds further portions of unfolded protein continuously or discontinuously to the same mixture only after the initial amount has already found its correct conformation, the total protein concentration can be increased stepwise up to attractive economic levels. This process of 'pulse naturation' is commercially used in the production of a plasminogen activator mutein (see Section 21.3.4).

21.3.3 Application, delivery and targeting of therapeutic proteins

Because of their typical properties, proteins generally would by no means be considered 'ideal' therapeutic agents for reasons related to their stability, application and potential immunogenicity.

Stability

Proteins are polypeptides and, therefore, are labile when heated or exposed to extreme pH values. They can also readily undergo biological degradation. This may lead to limited shelf-life as well as to short half-lives in the human body, e.g. due to proteolysis in the stomach and intestine and to receptor-mediated clearance from the blood followed by *proteolytic* degradation in the liver. In addition to the risk of proteolytic cleavage of the polypeptide chain, amino acid side chains of proteins may also be modified during storage, e.g. by oxidation or isopeptide bond formation. Whereas shelf-life can be improved by suitable formulation additives such as sugars or amino acids, attempts to prolong the biological in-vivo half-life of protein drugs have met limited success until now, the most successful being chemical modification by coupling to poly(ethylene glycol). Microencapsulation into biodegradable polymers, mostly polylactide-polyglycolide co-polymers, appears to offer an interesting novel approach in this respect. Proteolytic degradation in the stomach can be prevented by encapsulation, giving the protein resistance against the acid pH and proteases in the digestive system.

Ways of application

The molecular surface of soluble proteins is hydrophilic. Therefore, as a rule, proteins cannot pass through biological membranes and will not enter into tissue through the intestinal wall or into human cells from the bloodstream. Oral application of protein drugs, therefore, would not result in sufficient bioavailability unless the protein is intended to act in the oral cavity itself (as, for example, lysozyme, which is used to inhibit bacterial infections in the mouth) or in the gastrointestinal tract (e.g. lipases and amylases, used to support food digestion). Protein therapeutics, therefore, cannot be given orally but have to be injected or infused into the bloodstream. However, recent approaches to deliver protein drugs (e.g. insulin) via the pulmonal route (that is by direct inhalation into the lung) appear to be promising.

Immunogenicity of foreign proteins

Proteins that are foreign to the human body are immunogenic. When injected into the bloodstream, they may induce the formation of antibodies and cellular immune response. Furthermore, proteins obtained from natural sources may contain immunogenic contaminants. This may prevent repeated or prolonged application of the same protein drug. (On the other hand, immunogenicity is desired when proteins are used as vaccines.)

One way to decrease immunogenicity of proteins (and simultaneously prolong their in-vivo half life) is chemical coupling to water-soluble polymers, especially poly(ethylene glycol) (PEG). Such 'pegylated' proteins are in use as therapeutics; e.g. PEG-adenosine deaminase (PEG-ADA) for treatment of ADA deficiency by substitution of the missing enzyme, PEG-interferon-α for treatment of viral infections and pegfilgrastim (pegylated G-CSF) used in leukopenia.

21.3.4 Examples of therapeutic proteins

The 'first generation' of recombinant therapeutic proteins are protein drugs made with the aid of gene technology whose amino acid sequence is identical to natural human proteins. However, DNA sequences coding for proteins can nowadays be modified by site directed mutagenesis so that the primary structure of recombinant proteins can be designed as desired. This is known as *protein engineering*. Mutated proteins obtained in this way are called *muteins*. The changes may be restricted to isolated amino acid residues (point mutations), but may also involve the deletion or insertion of larger sequences, or may connect amino acid residues in two separate proteins (known as *protein fusions*). These technologies offer a strategic approach to modify protein properties in a rational way, such as stability, solubility, substrate or receptor-binding specificity, effector functions, or pharmacokinetics. Muteins obtained by rational design have been described as the 'second generation' of therapeutic proteins.

Present knowledge of structure–function relationships in proteins is still far from complete, and only in some simple cases has it been possible to predict the effects of sequence changes on observable protein properties. Nevertheless, in many cases recombinant proteins have been successfully designed for use as therapeutic agents, and about half of the biopharmaceuticals marketed presently contain engineered proteins as the active pharmaceutical ingredient.

Some examples of 'first-generation' and 'second-generation' protein drugs are given here.

Insulin

Insulin is a pancreatic hormone that has been used for treatment of type I diabetes since 1922 because of its effect in lowering blood glucose levels. Insulin consists of two polypeptide chains connected

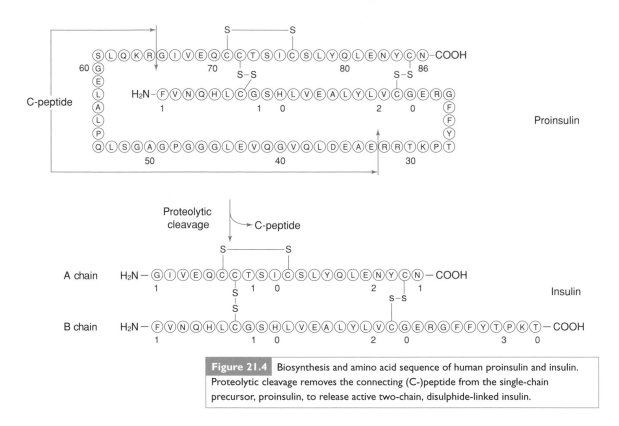

Figure 21.4 Biosynthesis and amino acid sequence of human proinsulin and insulin. Proteolytic cleavage removes the connecting (C-)peptide from the single-chain precursor, proinsulin, to release active two-chain, disulphide-linked insulin.

by disulphide bonds. The A chain has 21 amino acid residues and the B chain has 30 amino acid residues. Insulin biosynthesis involves proteolytic processing from the single-chain precursor molecule, proinsulin, with release of a connecting (C-) peptide, as illustrated in Fig. 21.4.

During the first decades of insulin therapy, bovine or porcine insulin were used. In these animal proteins, there are some differences in amino acid sequence from human insulin that may lead to formation of insulin antibodies during long-term application. In the 1970s, it became possible to replace the alanine residue at position 30 on the B chain of porcine insulin with a threonine residue by protease-catalysed semi synthesis and, thus, insulin identical to the human molecule could now be produced. However, due to the growing population of patients needing insulin (about 1 in 1000), there were concerns that the supply of porcine insulin might become limited. Porcine and also the semisynthetic human material derived from it have now largely been replaced by recombinant production of human insulin.

Several strategies have been developed to produce recombinant insulin. In the original process, as described by Genentech Inc., the A and B chains are expressed separately in *E. coli* as proteins that are fused with either tryptophan synthetase or β-galactosidase. This allows the A and B chains to be readily identified and recovered from

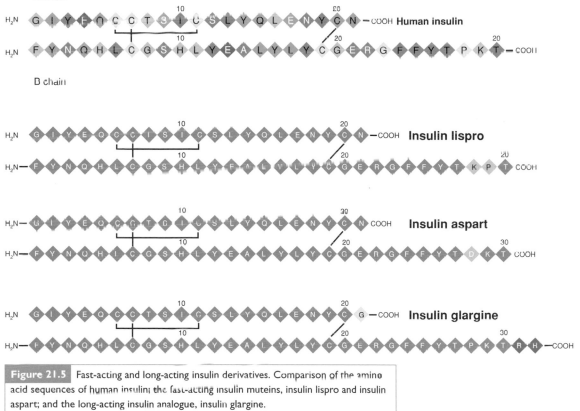

Figure 21.5 Fast-acting and long-acting insulin derivatives. Comparison of the amino acid sequences of human insulin; the fast-acting insulin muteins, insulin lispro and insulin aspart; and the long-acting insulin analogue, insulin glargine.

the two separate cultures. Then, after processing by cleavage with cyanogen bromide, the two chains are finally connected by chemical re-oxidation. In alternative processes, the physiological biosynthetic intermediate, proinsulin, or its analogues with shortened connecting peptide sequences, are expressed in *E. coli* or yeast (*Saccharomyces cerevisiae*), and the connecting peptide is then removed by proteolytic excision.

After an insulin injection into a diabetic patient, the plasma concentration of insulin rises slowly so that the injection should be done at least 15 minutes before a meal. Similarly, the plasma level of insulin also decreases more slowly than physiologically required, so there is the danger of hyper-insulinaemia. The slower increase in concentration is due to the time needed for dissociation of insulin hexamer to the pharmacologically active dimers and monomers. To accelerate this process, a large number of insulin muteins have been constructed that still are biologically active but show faster dissociation of hexamers in solution. Among these fast-acting insulin analogues (Fig. 21.5) are: *insulin lispro*, where, in analogy to the naturally occurring insulin homologue insulin-like growth factor-I (IGF-I), the order of the amino acid residues B28 and B29 was changed; and *insulin aspart*, which has an Asn(B28) instead of Pro. Both these changes lead to diminished self-association. Therefore, insulin lispro and insulin aspart reach pharmacologically efficient levels faster and, therefore, can be injected immediately before a meal. On the other hand, *insulin glargine* (an insulin mutein where Asn(A21) is replaced by glycine, and two additional Arg residues have been added to the C-terminus of the B chain) has been developed as a long-acting insulin analogue: it is formulated as a solution at pH 4.0, and, when injected sub-cutaneously, precipitates due to the pH change and forms a slowly dissolving precipitate. This results in a relatively constant rate of absorption of the insulin over 24 hours.

Interferons

Interferons, the first class of cytokines to be discovered, are a group of proteins that show a wide range of biological effects, including interference with viral replication, regulation of immune function, and regulation of growth and differentiation. In humans, three families (interferon-α, -β and -γ) are distinguished.

INTERFERON-α

In humans, at least 24 related *interferon-α* (IFN-α) genes or pseudogenes are known. The recombinant commercial versions include IFN-α2a and IFN-α2b, which both contain 165 amino acid residues, as well as a 'consensus interferon' (IFN alfacon-1), which is a synthetic version (166 amino acid residues) whose amino acid sequence was derived by comparison of the sequences of several naturally occurring interferon-α sub-types, and assigning the most frequently occurring residue to each position in the chain. Interferons-α have antiviral, antiproliferative and immunomodulatory properties and, therefore, are used for treatment of viral diseases (e.g. hepatitis C), as well as several types of cancer (e.g. hairy cell leukemia) and AIDS-associated Kaposi sarcoma. Pegylated versions (PEG-IFN α) have also recently been introduced.

INTERFERON-β

Normally produced by fibroblasts, displays significant sequence homology to IFN-α and also comprises 166 amino acid residues. It also shows both antiviral and immunomodulatory effects, and has shown activity in the treatment of relapsing–remitting multiple sclerosis (MS). Among the three IFN-β products presently approved, two are produced in CHO cell lines, and one in recombinant *E. coli* cells; the latter differs from the human protein because Cys-17 is replaced by Ser. The exact mechanism of IFN-β activity in the treatment of MS is unknown.

INTERFERON-γ

Often referred to as 'immune interferon', is produced by human T-cells that have been stimulated by an antigen. IFN-γ exhibits little evolutionary homology to IFN-α and -β. The mature polypeptide contains 143 amino acid residues and can be differentially glycosylated. Its antiviral properties are less than with IFN-α, but it promotes activation, growth and differentiation of a wide variety of cells involved in the immune and inflammatory response. A recombinant version of IFN-γ (140 amino acid residues) has been approved for use in chronic granulomatous disease (CGD), a rare genetic condition characterised by a deficiency in phagocytic oxidative metabolism.

Erythropoietin

Erythropoietin (Epoetin-α and -β, EPO) is a glycoprotein of 165 amino acid residues. It is formed in the foetal liver and in the kidneys of adults. The EPO hormone belongs to the haematopoietic growth factors and induces the formation of erythrocytes from precursor cells (termed BFU-E and CFU-E) in the bone marrow. Recombinant erythropoietin is produced in mammalian cell systems (Chinese hamster ovary (CHO) cells are used in the commercial processes – see also Chapter 22) due to the necessity of glycosylation: the EPO molecule contains one O- and three N-linked carbohydrate chains, and the latter are essential for bioactivity. Erythropoietin is used therapeutically mainly in renal anaemia, but also in other indications, e.g. in tumour anaemia; it was the first recombinant therapeutic protein whose global annual sales value reached US$1 billion.

Recently, an EPO mutein (*Darbepoetin*) has been approved, which contains five N-linked oligosaccharide chains resulting from amino acid substitutions in the erythropoietin peptide backbone. This increases the serum half-life and allows less frequent dosing.

Granulocyte colony stimulating factor

Granulocyte colony stimulating factor (G-CSF) also belongs to the class of haematopoietic growth factors: it stimulates proliferation and differentiation of neutrophil precursor cells to mature granulocytes. It is therefore used as an adjunct in chemotherapy of cancer to treat neutropenia caused by the destruction of white blood cells by the cytotoxic agent. Furthermore, G-CSF is also used in the treatment of myelosuppression after bone marrow transplantation, chronic neutropenia, acute leukaemia, aplastic anaemia, as well as to mobilise haematopoietic precursor cells from peripheral blood. Granulocyte colony simulating factor is a glycoprotein containing 174 amino acid residues. Products have been launched that contain either the glycosylated molecule produced from recombinant CHO cells (*Lenograstim*) or alternatively an unglycosylated, but therapeutically equally effective, form produced from recombinant *E. coli* (*Filgrastim*), which additionally possesses an N-terminal methionine residue. In order to prolong the half-life and reduce dosing frequency, a pegylated form of G-CSF (*Pegfilgrastim*) has been developed, where poly(ethylene glycol) residues are covalently attached to the G-CSF molecule.

Tissue plasminogen activators

Acute myocardial infarction (AMI) is the principal cause of deaths in most Western hemisphere countries. One approach to improve treatment of AMI is the use of thrombolytic enzymes. Plasminogen

Figure 21.6 General scheme of fibrinolysis. Thick arrows ($\downarrow$) designate catalytic activation by proteolysis, which is under control of plasma inhibitors ($\perp$).

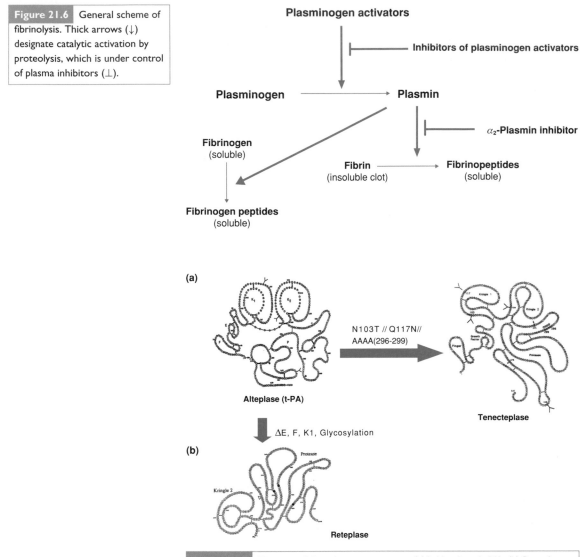

Figure 21.7 Diagram of the primary structures of (a) Alteplase (t-PA), (b) Reteplase, (c) Tenecteplase. The protein domains are: F, finger domain; E, epidermal growth factor-like domain; K1, kringle-1; K2, kringle-2; P, protease domain. Reteplase comprises only the K2 and P domains. Glycosylation is present in Alteplase at the positions marked **Y**, but absent in Reteplase. In Tenecteplase, two additional glycosylation sites have been introduced, and the stretch of amino acid residues 296–299 is replaced by AAAA.

activators catalyse the proteolytic processing of the inactive proenzyme plasminogen, which circulates in the bloodstream, into the active protease plasmin. Plasmin is able to cleave the insoluble fibrin of blood clots into soluble fibrin fragment peptides so that the clot is dissolved and the blood vessel is opened. The reaction scheme is outlined in Fig. 21.6.

Tissue plasminogen activator (*Alteplase*, Fig. 21.7), as well as muteins with an increased serum half-life, are used as thrombolytic agents in the treatment of AMI, and are also under study in related diseases such as stroke or deep-vein thrombosis. The latter proteins include: *Reteplase*, which is a mutein where the 'finger', 'EGF-like', and 'kringle-1' domains of the t-PA molecule are removed and which is not glycosylated due to its production by *E. coli*, and *Tenecteplase*, where six amino acid residues have been replaced by other amino acids to improve its efficacy.

Monoclonal antibodies

The largest proportion of therapeutic proteins now in clinical development are monoclonal antibodies. A number of them have already been approved for marketing (Table 21.4). Due to their immunogenicity, mouse monoclonal antibodies can only be used therapeutically in exceptional cases and, usually, chimeric or humanized antibodies (where rodent variable-region sequences are combined with a human constant-region framework) are used instead. Meanwhile, it has also become possible to provide fully human antibodies (e.g. Humira), either using phage display techniques, or generating them in transgenic mice that carry the human immunoglobulin gene repertoire. Monoclonal antibodies have proven successful especially in the treatment of cancer (such as Herceptin and Rituximab), rheumatoid arthritis (Remicade) and transplant rejection (e.g. Simulect, Zenapax).

Fusion proteins

By fusion of originally unrelated protein sequences, advantageous properties can be combined in a single molecule. Examples in this respect are recombinant immunotoxins used in experimental treatment of various cancers. These are chemical conjugates or recombinant fusion proteins constructed from a cell-binding part (mostly the antigen-binding parts of an antibody), a translocation domain that mediates transfer of the entire protein through the cell membrane, and a cytotoxic portion, e.g. protein domains taken from bacterial toxins (such as diphtheria toxin or pseudomonas exotoxin) or a chemical cytotoxic agent. The idea is that the toxic agent should be targeted to the selected cancer cell population by the antibody domain directed against specific surface antigens of these cells, which then should be killed after the uptake of the toxin part of the protein into the cancer cell. This has been done successfully in *Denileukin Diftitox*, which is a fusion construct consisting of the receptor-binding domain of the cytokine, Interleukin-2 and diphtheria toxin. This compound will bind specifically to the IL-2 receptor, which is overexpressed on the surface of tumor cells. It then induces cell death. Denileukin Diftitox was approved in 1999 for treatment of cutaneous T-cell lymphoma.

Another fusion protein that has been approved for marketing is *Etanercept* (Fig. 21.8), which comprises the extracellular domain of human p75 TNF receptor and the Fc part of human IgG1. Etanercept will neutralise the pro-inflammatoric mediator, tumor necrosis factor and is used in treatment of rheumatoid arthritis. The Fc part of the molecule serves to increase the half-life of the protein in the plasma of the patient.

Table 21.4 Monoclonal antibodies licensed as medicinal products

	Product name	Generic name	Indication	Originator/partner	Approval
Murine	OrthoClone OKT3	Muromomab-CD3l	Transplant rejection	Johnson & Johnson	1986
	Panorex	Edrecolomab	Colon cancer	Centocor/GSK	1995
	Antilfa	Odulimomab	Transplant rejection	Immunotech/ SangStat	1997
	Zevalin	Ibritumomab tiuxetan	Non-Hodgkin lymphoma	IDEC/Schering AG	2002
	Bexxar	Tositumomab and iodine-131	Non-Hodgkin lymphoma	Corixa/GSK	2003
Chimeric	Remicade	Infliximab	Rheumatoid arthritis	Centocor/Schering-Plough	1996
	Simulect	Basiliximab	Transplant rejection	Novartis	1996
	MabThera/Rituxan	Rituximab	Non-Hodgkin lymphoma	IDEC/Genentech/Roche	1997
	Erbitux	Cetuximab	Colorectal cancer	Imclone/Merck KGaA	2003
Chimeric Fab fragment	ReoPro	Abciximab	Cardiovascular prophylaxis	Centocor/Eli Lilly	1995
Humanised	Synagis	Palivizumab	Respiratory syncytial virus infection	MedImmune/Abbott	1996
	Zenapax	Daclizumab	Transplant rejection	PDL/Roche	1997
	Herceptin	Trastuzumab	Breast cancer	Genentech/Roche	1998
	Mylotarg	Gemtuzumab ozogamicin	Acute myeloic leukemia	Celltech/Wyeth	2000
	Campath	Alemtuzumab	Chronic lymphatic leukemia	ILEX/Schering AG	2001
	Xolair	Omalizumab	Allergic asthma	Genentech/Novartis	2002
	Raptiva	Efalizumab	Psoriasis	Xoma/Genentech	2003
	Avastin	Bevacizumab	Metastatic colorectal cancer	Genentech/Roche	2004
Human	Humira	Adalimumab	Rheumatoid arthritis	CAT/Abbott	2002

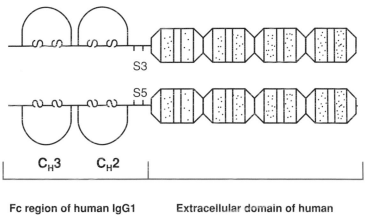

Fc region of human IgG1   **Extracellular domain of human p75 TNF receptor**

Figure 21.8 Domain structure of Etanercept.

Others

Among the first generation of recombinant therapeutic proteins, there are also enzymes such as glucocerebrosidase, used for treatment of glucocerebrosidase deficiency (Gaucher's disease), coagulation factors (Factor VIIa, Factor VIII and Factor IX) used for substitution therapy of haemophilia, hormones such as human growth hormone or follitropin. Additional examples of first- and second-generation biopharmaceuticals are listed in Table 21.3.

21.4 | Regulatory aspects of therapeutic proteins

21.4.1 Development and approval risk

Compound-related toxicity is not usually an issue with proteins in contrast to substances that have been chemically synthesised; they also have fewer undesirable side-effects associated with them, unless these are related to the biological target to which the protein is addressed. As natural substances, proteins are neither carcinogenic nor teratogenic. If the principle of action has been identified, and has proven to be valid as a target for therapeutic intervention, the development of recombinant human proteins into therapeutic agents thus generally carries less risk than the development of new low-molecular weight drugs. Indeed, it has turned out that the attrition rate (i.e. the percentage of projects which have to be terminated) in the later clinical development phases, where the main part of development costs arises, is significantly lower for biopharmaceuticals than for small molecule drugs. Furthermore, after completion of clinical development, innovative protein therapeutics will usually be approved faster for market launch due internationally to agreed common quality standards.

In the USA, approval of recombinant protein drugs (except vaccines) is regulated by the Center for Drug Evaluation and Research (CDER) of the Federal Drug Administration (FDA); in Europe, via a centralised procedure by the European Agency for the Evaluation of Medical Products (EMEA). These regulatory bodies have defined guidelines for approval of therapeutic proteins.

21.4.2 Safety

In contrast to proteins isolated from humans or animals, including transgenic sources, or from pathogenic organisms, e.g. vaccines obtained from bacteria or viruses (even if these are highly purified and carefully analysed), recombinant proteins do not bear the risk of contamination with allergenic substances, pathogenic viruses, e.g. HIV, or prions, e.g. from cattle or humans causing new variant Creutzfeldt–Jakob disease. For this reason, products such as coagulation factors (formerly produced from human blood or plasma), human growth hormone (in the past obtained from adenohypophysis extracts), or hepatitis B vaccines are today manufactured from recombinant systems.

Recombinant human proteins are not expected to be immunogenic. Depending on the expression system used, however, proteins may differ from original human proteins in their post-translational modification (e.g. glycosylation, processing of N-terminus, etc.), and modifications of the amino acid sequence (as in muteins) may lead to the emergence of neoepitopes. Furthermore, even recombinant human proteins may be immunogenic depending on the manufacturing process, especially if the downstream and formulation conditions do not preclude the presence of protein aggregates. Depending on the mode of action, this may lead to inactivation of the drug, allergic reactions or (in the worst case) to breaking self-tolerance and neutralisation of the body's naturally-occurring proteins. At present, in-vitro analytical tools and animal models to predict immunogenicity in patients are lacking. Therefore, immunogenicity of protein drugs has to be evaluated carefully during clinical development as well as after launch.

21.5 | Outlook to the future of protein therapies

Protein therapeutics are not equally attractive in all therapeutic areas and indications, when compared with competing approaches such as low-molecular weight chemical substances. Protein drugs would be especially useful in the following cases:

- In indications where no alternative therapy is available, particularly for potentially *life-threatening diseases* such as cancer, inflammation or viral infections.
- For *substitution therapy* if essential human proteins are missing or inactive, e.g. in ADA deficiency or in coagulation factor deficiencies.

- To modulate the *regulation of biological processes* such as metabolism, cell growth, wound healing, etc., or to influence the *immune system* by proteins acting as hormones, growth factors or cytokines (e.g. insulin, erythropoietin, G-CSF (granulocyte colony stimulating factor), somatotropin, interferons or interleukins). In these cases, protein–protein interactions have to be modulated. This may be more effective with therapeutic proteins as 'Nature's own ligands' optimised in the course of evolution, than with small chemical substances.

- As *vaccines,* especially against viral infectious diseases.

Human proteins identical to the body's own substances have become available through the advent of gene technology. Besides the first-generation biotherapeutics, an increasing number of redesigned, second-generation protein muteins with improved properties are being introduced to the marketplace, especially humanised or fully human antibodies. Once the problems of low transfection and expression efficiency have been solved, it may be possible in future to substitute defect genes, or add therapeutic genes, to human cells in vivo so that the patient's body itself will act as the manufacturing facility where the synthesis of therapeutic proteins occurs. In this sense, *gene therapy* may represent the future third-generation of therapeutic proteins, and may help to approach the final goal to cure, rather than treat, disease.

21.6 | Further reading

- Bergmeyer, H. U., Grassl, M. and Bergmeyer, J. (eds.) *Methods of Enzymatic Analysis,* Vols. 1–12. Weinheim: VCH, 1983–1986.

Crommelin, D. J. A. and Sindelar, R. D. *Pharmaceutical Biotechnology,* second edition. London: Taylor & Francis, 2002.

Dembowski, K. and Stadler, P. *Novel Therapeutic Proteins.* Weinheim. Wiley-VCH, 2001.

Ibelgaufts, H. *Cytokines Online Pathfinder Encyclopedia.* http://www.copewithcytokines.de/, 2003.

Kopetzki, E., Lehnert, K. and Buckel, P. (1994). Enzymes in diagnostics: achievements and possibilities of recombinant DNA technology. *Clinical Chemistry* **40**: 688–704, 1994.

Kresse, G.-B. Analytical uses of enzymes. In *Biotechnology,* second edition, Vol 9, eds. H.-J. Rehm and G. Reed. Weinheim: Verlag Chemie, pp. 138–163 (1995).

Lauwers, A. and Scharpé, S. *Pharmaceutical Enzymes.* New York: Marcel Dekker, 1997.

Rudolph, R. and Lilie, H. In vitro folding of inclusion body proteins. *Federation of American Societies for Experimental Biology* **10**: 49–56, 1996.

Walsh, G. *Biopharmaceuticals: Biochemistry and Biotechnology,* second edition. Chichester: John Wiley & Sons, 2003.

Walsh, G. and Headon, D. R. *Protein Biotechnology.* Chichester: John Wiley & Sons, 1994.

Chapter 22

Insect and mammalian cell culture

C. J. Hewitt
The University of Birmingham, UK

B. Isailovic
The University of Birmingham, UK

N. T. Mukwena
The University of Birmingham, UK

A. W. Nienow
The University of Birmingham, UK

22.1 | Introduction

Bacteria and yeasts have been the organisms of choice for the industrial production of heterologous recombinant proteins for many years. The ability to cultivate bacterial strains to high cell density at large scale has become an increasingly important technique throughout the field of biotechnology, from basic research programmes (structural or kinetic studies) to large-scale pharmaceutical production processes. *Escherichia coli* remains one of the most attractive organisms for the production of recombinant proteins (see Chapters 4, 5, and 21 for

Basic Biotechnology, third edition, eds. Colin Ratledge and Bjørn Kristiansen.
Published by Cambridge University Press. © Cambridge University Press 2006.

examples) where no complex post-translational modifications (e.g. glycosylation or disulphide bond formation) are required for biological activity and because its genetics and physiology are well understood. However, there are important drawbacks associated with the use of prokaryotic organisms. The low percentage of GC nucleotides in their genomes, when compared to mammalian genes, and the existence of rare codons that often result in low expression levels or inactive truncated forms and, in many cases, proteins are expressed as insoluble inclusion bodies in the bacterial periplasmic space. Bacteria are also incapable of carrying out any post-translational modifications, which strongly influences protein stability, folding, solubility and, hence, its biological activity. Yeasts (e.g. *Saccaromyces cerevisiae* or *Pichia pastoris*), though, can perform some post-translational modifications similar to those of the more complex eukaryotic cells (see Chapter 5). However N-glycosylation of mammalian proteins in yeast seems to be very inefficient. Additionally, both bacteria and yeast cells are surrounded by a mechanically strong cell wall that may hinder recovery of any non-secreted proteins. Therefore, since neither insect nor mammalian cells have a cell wall, they have been developed for the production of a wide range of heterologous recombinant proteins otherwise difficult to recover and purify.

22.2 | Mammalian cells

The first demonstration that mammalian cells could be cultured in vitro for biotechnology purposes was in 1949 when J. F. Enders showed that polio virus could be produced from cultured cells derived from primate neural and kidney tissue. In the 1950s, polio viral vaccines were produced in the laboratory from cultures of monkey kidney and testicular cells. This was closely followed by the production of other viral vaccines – mumps (1951), measles (1958) and adenovirus (1958), all produced by cultured cells from various animal species. It was only in the 1970s that modern mammalian cell culture truly emerged with the development of the hybridoma cell lines and the emergence of recombinant DNA technologies. A *cell line* is a population of genetically identical cells (clones) derived from a single parent cell. Although the production of biological material for vaccines is still important today, mammalian cells are also cultured for use in pharmaceutical testing and toxicological research and are being used for the in vitro synthesis of skin and cartilage tissues for surgical purposes.

In vivo mammalian cells (see Fig. 22.1) do not exist in isolation, like a microbial cell, but are organised within a whole animal into functioning organs (e.g. kidney, liver, etc.) with a specific purpose, e.g. to ensure the reproductive success of that entire animal. When specific cells are isolated from an animal and placed under appropriate culture conditions (see Section 22.6), some cell lines will divide, others will maintain their viability without dividing

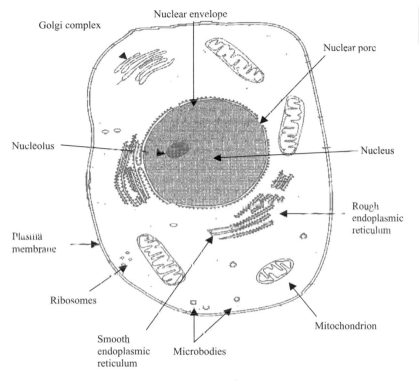

Golgi complex

Nuclear envelope

Nuclear pore

Nucleolus

Nucleus

Plasma membrane

Rough endoplasmic reticulum

Ribosomes

Smooth endoplasmic reticulum

Microbodies

Mitochondrion

Figure 22.1 Schematic diagram of a generalised eukaryotic cell.

and a few will die almost immediately. Epithelial (skin), myeloma (cancerous) and fibroblast (connective tissue) cells that are always growing and dividing in the parent organism are those best suited to growth in pure cell culture. The isolation of mouse *monoclonal antibodies* (mAbs) by Köhler and Milstein in 1975 revolutionised the use of mammalian cells in biotechnology, unearthing the profound medical and commercial potential of mammalian cells (see Chapter 25). Köhler and Milstein achieved this by fusing specifically immunised B-lymphocytes (white blood cells that secrete antibodies) from mice with myeloma cells (bone marrow cancer cells) to create the first hybridoma cell. In so doing, the capacity for specific antibody production of B-lymphocytes and the limitless growth capacity of myeloma cells were harnessed within a single entity. This means that such cells have the ability to grow and divide continuously provided the environmental conditions are correct. Other advantages of such cells include a reduced dependency on growth factors, increased growth rates and ease of cultivation despite a fluctuating microenvironment, particularly in suspension culture. However, such cells often have increased metabolic rates resulting in a concomitant increase in inhibitory by-product formation. Significantly, these developments have allowed the production (and, in some instances, secretion) of proteins bearing the correct post-translational modifications, in particular glycosylation and hence the required biological activity. The value of these first mouse monoclonal antibodies as human therapeutics was, however, restricted due to their rapid inactivation by the human immune system and patient allergic responses to them. In 1986, G. Winter and

Table 22.1 Monoclonal antibodies produced by animal cells that have been approved for various purposes

Category	Product	Application
Therapeutic	Rituxan	Non-Hodgkins lymphoma
	Centoxin	Sepsis
	Panorex	Colorectal cancer
In vivo diagnostic	Prosta Scint	Prostate cancer
	Myscint	Cardiac muscle necrosis
Preparative	Roferon A	Purification of IFNα2A from cell lysates
	MonoNine	Purification of the blood clotting agent Factor VIII from plasma
	Kogenate	Purification of the blood clotting agent Factor VIII from animal cell culture medium

colleagues pioneered techniques to 'humanise' mouse antibodies such that they closely resembled human antibodies thereby augmenting the suitability and efficacy of using 'artificially' produced monoclonal antibodies in human medicine (see Table 22.1).

22.2.1 Genetic modification of mammalian cell lines

The first recombinant DNA (rDNA) or genetic manipulation experiments were reported in 1973 by Walter Gilbert and colleagues who developed protocols to construct artificial functional pieces of DNA or genes by first cutting out (restricting) and then combining fragments of DNA (splicing) from different species. These pieces of recombinant DNA are then inserted into a host cell by attaching them to a vector, which is often a bacterial plasmid. Such constructed vectors are first amplified by insertion into a fast-growing bacterium, typically *Escherichia coli*, before being spliced into the genome (DNA) of a host (mammalian) cell (see Chapter 4). Such technology was used to produce tissue plasminogen activator (tPA), which is used for preventing blood clots in heart attack patients. It was first marketed by Genentech, Inc. (USA) and licensed in 1987. Tissue plasminogen activator (tPA) was cloned into and expressed by genetically modified mammalian Chinese hamster ovary (CHO) cells.

Hybridoma cells are not the only mammalian source of commercially viable biotechnology products. The exploitation of recombinant DNA technology has led to the development of a myriad of cloned mammalian cells (cell lines) from the organs (e.g. lungs, ovaries, liver and kidneys) of many mammals including humans, hamsters, rats, sheep and horses (see Table 22.2). This development was achieved by differential mutation or transfection with a cancerous gene (oncogene), while other cell lines are derived from cancerous tissue by viral infection. Genetic manipulation techniques have also been exploited for the production of recombinant antibodies using myelomas as host cells. Chinese hamster ovary (CHO) cells are presently the preferred choice for production of recombinant proteins because of their ease of growth in suspension culture, while baby hamster kidney (BHK)

Table 22.2 The most commonly used cell lines in biotechnology

Cell line	Mammalian source
CHO	Chinese hamster ovary
MDCK	Dog cocker spaniel kidney
HeLa	Human cervix carcinoma
NS0	Myeloma
BHK21	Syrian hamster kidney fibroblast
HEK293	Human embryonic kidney
Vero	Monkey kidney cells
GH3	Rat pituitary tumour
WI-38	Human foetal lung cells
J558L	Mouse myeloma
HepZ	Rat liver cells

Table 22.3 Pharmaceutical therapeutic agents produced by mammalian cells that have been approved for clinical purposes

Product	Protein	Cell line
Epogen, Eprex	Erythropoietin (anti-anaemia agent)	CHO
Saizen	Human growth hormone	CHO
Recombinate	Factor VIII (blood anticlotting agent)	CHO
Gonal	Follicle stimulating hormone (infertility treatment)	CHO
Avonex	Interferon-β (anticancer drug)	CHO
Novo Seven	Factor VIIa (blood anticlotting agent)	BHK

cells are used for production of vaccines because their infection with a virus does not affect growth (see Table 22.3). These landmark events paved the way for the large-scale manufacture of proteins in what has become a multi-billion dollar 'biotech' industry.

22.2.2 Commercial products from mammalian cell lines

Most proteins that are secreted by a mammalian cell, or are transported to other organelles within the cell, are glycoproteins. Glycoproteins are proteins where a sugar group has been added after (post) translation via a process called glycosylation in the endoplasmic reticulum (ER) and Golgi apparatus of a eukaryotic cell (see Fig. 22.1). Soluble proteins retained within the cytosol of a cell are rarely glycosylated. Since glycoproteins have specific sites of activity within the entire organism, they have become the most common products from mammalian cell culture because they have the potential to be high value therapeutic agents. Glycosylation follows no blueprint like protein sythesis (no DNA or RNA template). Therefore, a wide range of oligosaccharide structures of glycoproteins exists. This results in a range of glycoforms, i.e. glycoproteins with the same amino acid sequence but different oligosaccharide structures. There are two types of glycosylation, N-linked and O-linked, of which the former is the most common. In N-linked glycosylation, one species of oligosaccharide, made up of N-acetylglucosamine, mannose and glucose, is linked to the NH_2 group on the side chain of an asparagine residue of the protein in the ER of the cell. Subsequent modification of this asparagine-linked oligosaccharide in the Golgi apparatus gives rise to a whole range of mature glycoproteins. In the less common O-linked glycosylation, oligosaccharides are linked to the OH group on the side chain of a serine, threonine or hydroxylysine residue. The presence and composition of the correct oligosaccharide is often essential for full biological activity and directs the glycoprotein to its site of activity. If glycosylation is a requirement for biological activity, then the protein is usually produced in mammalian cell culture since bacteria have neither the correct enzymes nor organelles to do this. Yeast, fungi and insect cells may be used since they can carry out some types of glycosylation (see Chapter 5 and Section 22.3), but the extent and type of this is different to that of mammalian cells, so the choice of expression system becomes very important. Those proteins (e.g. insulin, human serum albumin, human growth hormone and haemoglobin) that do not require glycosylation for full biological activity can be more cheaply produced by bacterial expression systems.

Monoclonal antibodies (mAbs) remain the most renowned mammalian cell culture glycoprotein products comprising one-quarter of therapeutic developments in the biotechnology industry and valued at US\$ 2.7 billion in 2001 (see Table 22.1). The majority of these have applications in the treatment of cancer and infectious diseases. Tumour or infected cell-specific antibodies coupled to a cytotoxic compound (e.g. ricin) can be used to target and kill cancerous or diseased cells without causing damage to surrounding healthy tissues. Monoclonal antibodies can also be used to prevent transplant rejection. The superior and highly specific binding capability of mAbs also means they are invaluable as medical diagnostic tools (e.g. pregnancy testing) and probes for analytical molecular biology techniques, for example in *Western blotting*. Western blotting is a technique for measuring protein expression in cell or tissue extracts using the antibody/antigen interaction. Monoclonal antibodies can also be used as components of chromatographic apparatus for protein purification in downstream processing. Monoclonal antibodies for the specific product to be purified are immobilised onto an inert support held in a flow-through column. The supernatant containing the required protein is passed through the column where the protein binds to the immobilised antibody and the supernatant containing the waste products discarded. The protein can then be eluted via a variety of methods from the column in purified form.

Today's humanised antibodies (that is antibodies raised to human proteins) are manufactured by mammalian cell lines rather than

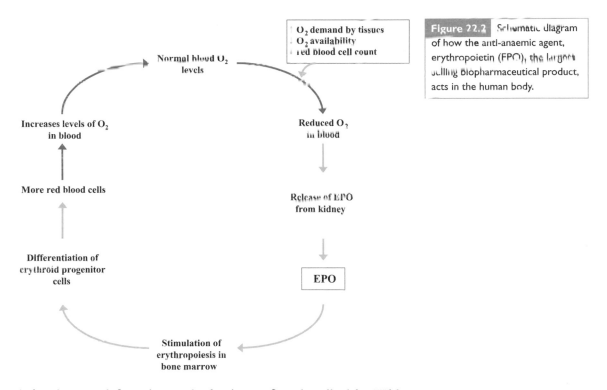

Normal blood O₂ levels

O₂ demand by tissues
O₂ availability
red blood cell count

Figure 22.2 Schematic diagram of how the anti-anaemic agent, erythropoietin (EPO), the largest selling biopharmaceutical product, acts in the human body.

Increases levels of O₂ in blood

Reduced O₂ in blood

More red blood cells

Release of EPO from kidney

Differentiation of erythroid progenitor cells

EPO

Stimulation of erythropoiesis in bone marrow

being harvested from immunised mice as first described by Köhler and Milstein. This results in an antibody containing more human amino acids than before (only the epitopes are derived from mice), therefore immunogenic responses have all but been eliminated and they can now be given to human patients in multiple doses. A therapeutic monoclonal antibody that is now on the market is Abciximab (ReoPro), a mouse/human antibody that inhibits platelet aggregation. It is licensed as an adjunct to aspirin and heparin in patients undergoing high-risk coronary angioplasty to prevent recurrent coronary obstruction. Currently (2005), there are no licensed therapeutic mAbs for cancer treatment, although a large number are in late-stage development and clinical trials.

With sales of US$ 7 billion, the anti-anaemic agent erythropoietin, (EPO), is the largest selling biopharmaceutical product (see Fig. 22.2). Erythropoietin is a recombinant protein marketed under various names and derived from various sources. Erythropoietin marketed by Amgen Co. Ltd. (Epogen) in 1989 is produced by CHO cells that have been genetically engineered to produce human EPO by insertion of DNA encoding human urinary EPO.

22.3 | Insect cells

Historically, the study of insect morphology and physiology was initially motivated by the need to broaden the knowledge of animal and plant infectious diseases caused by viruses transmitted by insects.

Some of the well-known examples are: Japanese encephalitis and St Louis encephalitis caused by arboviruses carried by mosquitoes and widespread filarial disease caused by the *Simulium* fly species. In the 1970s, special attention was drawn to agricultural problems such as uncontrolled insect pest propagation. A potential solution appeared in the form of baculoviruses, a group of viruses that proved to be pathogenic only for insects and not for the allied crops or vertebrates. Soon after, the first baculovirus products were authorised by the regulatory authorities to be marketed for pest control. In 1983, insect cells (see Fig. 22.1), in conjunction *with baculovirus expression vector systems* (BEVS), were recognised as alternative and powerful protein expression vehicles for large-scale production. Since then, numerous examples of the expression of functional mammalian proteins, such as receptors, channel proteins, viral antigens, enzymes, antibodies and biologically active peptides from cDNA libraries, have been reported. In addition, BEVS form the basis of many present biotechnological ventures aimed at the production of therapeutic pharmaceuticals, vaccines and diagnostic reagents.

The major advantage of the BEVS lies in their ability to produce large quantities of a heterologous recombinant protein and to provide the necessary eukaryotic modifications of the protein, such as phosphorylation, fatty acid acylation and O-glycosylation, for optimal biological activity. The only exception is N-glycosylation, which seems to be incomplete in insect cells due, in part, to the absence of functional levels of appropriate glycotransferase enzymes. For example, mosquito glycoproteins are terminated in a mannose residue and, thus, may be immunogenic when compared to the native mammalian glycoprotein that is terminated in sialic acid. The glycans (sugar compounds) linked to recombinant proteins produced by BEVS typically differ from those found on native mammalian products and importantly can influence their functions in many different ways.

The question therefore remains: if post-translational modification (e.g. N-glycosylation) in insect cells is insufficient, why is there the need to substitute already developed mammalian expression systems by BEVS? The answer is that insect cells have several advantages when compared to mammalian cells: ease of culture, genetic manipulation, higher tolerance to osmolarity (i.e. salt solutions), lower by-product concentrations and higher levels of DNA expression when they are infected with a recombinant baculovirus. Additionally, the baculovirus, which is used to infect particular insect cells is relatively large when compared to plasmid expression vectors used with bacteria (see Chapter 4). Consequently, baculoviruses can accommodate large DNA inserts without detriment to their ability to infect the insect cells. These inserts of DNA can therefore be sufficiently large to include several new genes coding for a series of proteins that can carry out several related functions. Other advantages of BEVS include the ability of insect cells to grow well in suspension (see Section 22.6.1), which, in turn, enables easy scale-up for the production of recombinant proteins in large-scale bioreactors. Baculoviruses are essentially

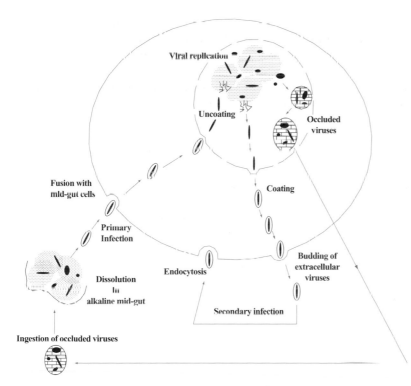

Viral replication

Uncoating

Occluded viruses

Fusion with mid-gut cells

Coating

Primary Infection

Endocytosis

Budding of extracellular viruses

Dissolution in alkaline mid-gut

Secondary infection

Ingestion of occluded viruses

Figure 22.3 In vivo baculovirus infection cycle. The main difference between the *in-vitro* and *in-vivo* infection processes, is that the polyhedrin gene has been removed and replaced with the recombinant gene or cDNA fragment of choice. Therefore occlusion bodies are not formed so no insect gut is required.

non-pathogenic to mammals or plants and have a restricted host range, being mainly limited to specific invertebrate species. Therefore such infected cell lines can be handled under minimal laboratory containment conditions, as they pose no danger to the operators at any stage of the production process.

These expression systems, however, are not perfect and have certain drawbacks aside from their post-translational modification deficiencies. One major problem appears to be the high level of breakdown of the expressed proteins due to the lytic nature of the BEVS. Promoters are regions of DNA that control whether the next sequence of DNA encoding for the required protein is expressed and at what levels. The polyhedrosis and p10 promoters (most commonly used in BEVS) are very strong. These promoters are also induced rather late on in the post-infection period. Hence, the recombinant protein expression peak may easily appear after the lytic phase has started, which involves the presence of cell or baculovirus proteases as the main factors in degradation events (see Fig. 22.3).

22.3.1 In vivo baculovirus infection

Baculoviruses are the most widespread viruses that infect insects. They are double stranded, supercoiled, circular molecules of ~120–150 kb DNA encased in a rod-shaped protein outer shell (nucleocapsid). They are isolated from infected insects and currently more than 500 baculoviruses have been identified. The most abundant group of these viruses comprises nuclear polyhedrosis viruses, where viral nucleocapsids are embedded in polyhedrin protein occlusion bodies.

Two of the most commonly used baculoviruses for foreign gene expression are *Autographa californica* multiple nuclear polyhedrosis virus (AcMNPV) and *Bombyx mori* (silkworm) nuclear polyhedrosis virus (BmNPV).

In such viruses, the promoter to instigate gene expression is very strong. Hence polyhedrin protein is produced at very high levels in wild-type strains (up to 20% of the total protein synthesised). Initial interest in polyhedra occlusion bodies arose when it was discovered that polyhedra made their way first into the insect mid-gut after infecting the insect larva (see Fig. 22.3). There, under alkaline conditions, they dissolve and release individual viruses that then fuse with mid-gut cell membranes and release nucleocapsids into the cytoplasm. After the viruses have been transported to the nucleus, they begin to replicate. Around 8 h later, budded viruses are released into the haemolymph, where they may infect other cells, or they are occluded into the polyhedra. Seven to 14 days later, cells lyse and the larva dies. Subsequently, polyhedra are released from the dead insect onto the plant surface and the cycle repeats.

22.3.2   In vitro baculovirus infection

The salient feature of the in vitro infection process, when compared to the natural in vivo infection, is that the polyhedrin gene in the wild-type baculovirus genome, which is not essential for viral propagation, is removed and replaced with the recombinant gene or cDNA fragment of choice. The two major techniques for recombinant baculovirus generation are homologous recombination and site-specific transposition. Homologous recombination is the substitution of a segment of DNA by another that is identical (homologous) or nearly so. The process occurs naturally during meiotic recombination and division. Site-specific transposition involves the use of restriction enzymes to cut out a known piece of the native DNA marked by specific nucleotide sequences. A new piece of DNA or a gene that has identical terminal nucleotide sequences to that previously removed can now be spliced in its place by use of a specific ligase enzyme.

The recombinant gene is most commonly placed under the transcriptional control of the very strong polyhedrin and p10 promoters. This ensures that the recombinant product (i.e. heterologous protein) is expressed in large quantities instead of the naturally occurring polyhedrin protein. In the very late phase of the recombinant baculovirus–infection cycle, within 20 to 36 hours post-infection, cells cease to produce budded viruses and begin assembly, production and expression of the recombinant gene product.

Both the polyhedrin and p10 promoters are termed 'late promoters' because they only switch on recombinant protein expression about 24 hours after the original infection. Consequently, the desired protein is only produced in large amounts 48–72 hours post-infection. This late production can lead to low recombinant protein yields because the viral cycle is lytic (cells break down to release viruses). Thus, the recombinant protein being produced can be rapidly degraded by the cells own proteases, which are synthesised before the peak protein production rate is reached. This sequence of events may also result in incomplete post-translational modification because there is too little time to modify the protein fully before cell lysis and proteolysis occurs. Therefore, a quantity of the produced heterologous protein may be biologically inactive.

The most common in vitro insect cell culture process is carried out batchwise in bioreactors (see Section 22.6). Generally three stages can be identified as occurring within the bioreactor of whatever type,

- *Growth phase*: Cells are inoculated into fresh culture medium in the bioreactor within the range 2 to 4×10^5 cells ml^{-1} and are grown to mid-exponential or late-exponential phase (2 to 3×10^6 cells ml^{-1}) and then infected with the appropriate baculovirus expression vector system (BEVS).
- *Infection phase*: The mid- or late-exponential (log) culture is infected at a certain multiplicity of infection (MOI), which may vary from values as low as 0.05 p.f.u. $cell^{-1}$ (p.f.u. = plaque-forming units, i.e. the number of viruses that have infected one cell) to values as high as 10 p.f.u. $cell^{-1}$. Multiplicity of infection (MOI) is the term used to quantify culture infection and is quoted as p.f.u. $cell^{-1}$: MOI can be calculated from the following formula:

$$MOI\ (p.f.u.\ cell^{-1}) = virus\ titre\ (p.f.u.\ ml^{-1})$$
$$\times\ ml\ of\ virus\ inoculum/total\ number\ of\ cells$$

Protein yields at lower MOI values are comparable to, or even better than those at a high MOI, provided lower cell concentrations and longer infection times are employed. However, a longer infection time means increased process cost as well as the problem of proteolysis and the presence of a significant quantity of cell debris, which complicates downstream processing. Therefore many large-scale processes operate at high MOI (5–10 p.f.u. $cell^{-1}$). This mode of operation, however, requires larger amounts of viral stock. Therefore, a thorough economic analysis of the process is required to determine the optimum MOI.

- *Protein expression phase*: This phase is started when 'late promoters' are switched on 24 hours after infection and the recombinant gene is then expressed. Protein expression is affected by many factors, such as MOI, dissolved O_2 concentration and temperature. The maximum cell density is also an important factor and for Sf-9 and Sf-21 cells (see Section 22.3.3) this is usually around 10^7 cells ml^{-1}, although it is possible to support higher cell densities by using optimised fed-batch strategies. Peak expression is reached at about 48–72 hours post-infection (lytic phase), so a thorough process analysis is required to determine the optimum harvest point in order for the best balance between protein synthesis and proteolysis to be reached. The rate of infection of Sf-9 insect cells is controlled by the rate of diffusion and transport of the virus to the cell by Brownian

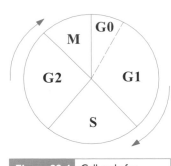

Figure 22.4 Cell cycle for eukaryotic cells. The interval between two mitotic divisions, i.e. that of a parent and a daughter cell, is called the cell cycle. The cell cycle consists of four major phases: G1 (gap 1), protein synthesis; S, DNA synthesis; G2 (gap 2), post-synthetic or pre-mitotic; M, mitosis.

Table 22.4 | The most commonly used insect cell lines used in biotechnology

Cell line	Insect source
Sf-9, Sf-21	Ovarian tissue of *Spodoptera frugiperda*
Tn-365	*Trichoplusia ni*
High-Five BTI-TN-5B1-4	*Trichoplusia ni*
SL-2, SL-3	*Drosophila melanogaster*

motion. As a result, the rate of infection is roughly proportional to the multiplicity of infection (MOI).

22.3.3 Commercial products from insect cell lines

Insect cell/baculovirus technology for the large-scale commercial production of recombinant protein is relatively new compared to mammalian cell technology. Therefore there is very little published work on industrial-scale processes involving baculovirus expression vector systems. However, the most common cells used for BEVS applications are known as Sf-9 and Sf-21, which were both isolated from the ovarian tissue of *Spodoptera frugiperda* (the fall armyworm from the Lepidoptera family), and Tn-368 and High-Five BTI-TN-5B1-4, which were isolated from *Trichoplusia ni*. Other insect cell lines, such as SL-2 and SL-3 (isolated from *Drosophila melanogaster*, see Table 22.4) have also been successfully utilised for recombinant protein production, e.g. β-galactosidase. The latter cell lines are frequently used to model large-scale recombinant protein expression in insect cells.

22.4 | Mammalian and insect cell cycles

The interval between two mitotic divisions, i.e. that of a parent and a daughter cell, is called *the cell cycle* (see Fig. 22.4). The cell cycle consists of four major phases: G1 (gap 1), protein synthesis; S, DNA synthesis; G2 (gap 2), post-synthetic or pre-mitotic; and M, mitosis. The time taken to complete the cell cycle is about 24 hours, but this depends on which cell line is being used. Some mammalian cell lines (e.g. hepatocytes, etc.) may leave the cell cycle in G1, where they enter G0 or the 'dormant' phase. This phenomenon is generally regarded as a result of an active repression of the genes needed for mitosis. Some G0 cells are terminally differentiated, i.e. they will never re-enter the cell cycle but will perform their specific function until they die. Other cells in G0 (e.g. human blood lymphocytes) may re-enter the cycle if the appropriate stimulus (i.e. an antigen) is encountered.

G1 corresponds to the stationary phase and S-G2 corresponds to the actively growing/dividing phase (exponential phase) in animal cell culture; whereas for insect cells (e.g. Sf-9), the resting phase is in G2. During insect cell growth, initially the proportion of cells in S and G1

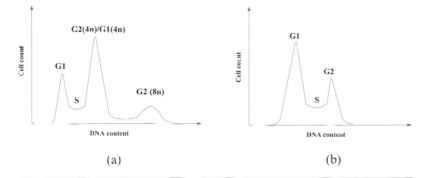

Figure 22.5 A typical cell cycle analysis for an insect cell (a) and a mammalian cell (b) population by flow cytometry based on DNA content of individual cells. For mammalian cells, the first peak represents G1 (2n-diploid), then S; the second peak G2 (4n-tetraploid). For insect cells, the first peak is G1 (2n-diploid), then S; and the second peak is an overlapping of G2 (4n-tetraploid) from the diploid cell cycle and G1 (4n-tetraploid) from the tetraploid cell cycle. The third peak is G2 (8n-octaploid) from the tetraploid cell cycle

increase and those in G2 decrease. During the mid-exponential phase, those in G2 increase and G1 and S decrease. The opposite behaviour is observed for all mammalian cell lines studied so far. The insect cell cycle (particularly for Sf-9 and Sf-21) is more complex than the mammalian cell cycle in that two separate cell cycles can be identified. First, there is the normal diploid cell cycle, G1 (2n–diploid), S and G2 (4n-tetraploid); but, second, there is also a tetraploid cell cycle, G1 (4n-tetraploid), S and G2 (8n-octaploid). This is because Sf-9 and Sf-21 cell lines are cytologically unstable: their chromosomes are susceptible to fusion and fragmentation during growth in vitro leading to the appearance of polyploidy or the second (tetraploid) cell cycle. A thorough understanding of the position of a cell or populations of cells in the cell cycle is an important part of any research and development programme leading to the optimal production of recombinant proteins at large scale and such measurements can be made by flow cytometry, an analytical technique discussed later (see Section 22.5 and Fig. 22.5).

In their natural environment, when they form part of an organism or when they have not been adapted to continuous cell division, mammalian cells exist in the G1 phase where normal metabolic activity and protein synthesis occur. Mammalian cells used in most biotechnological processes are adapted to continuous proliferation and have lost the ability to withdraw from the replication cycle. Therefore, if the environment becomes unsuitable for continued growth these cells may die via a mechanism called *apoptosis* or programmed cell death (PCD). There has been a lot of work done on the characteristics of mammalian cell death, especially on the active process of cell death, apoptosis. However, there is little information on death mechanisms in insect cell lines, although it has been shown that both Sf-9 and hybridoma cells share some of the typical features of apoptosis, which include cell shrinkage, loss of their spherical shape, swollen endoplasmic reticulum/golgi bodies, chromatin condensation and specific DNA degradation. On the other hand, distinctive morphological and kinetic differences between both cultures revealed that Sf-9 cells died by an atypical PCD process characterised by the absence of nuclear fragmentation, little association of condensed chromatin to the nuclear envelope, swollen mitochondria and high non-specific DNA degradation. These features, distinctive of necrosis (passive death process), were not observed in the normal apoptotic process of hybridomas. Cell death via apoptosis in animal cell culture is a particular problem often leading to truncated bioprocesses and poor product yields. Such programmed cell death is often associated with serum/nutrient limitation, fluid mechanical stress or the absence of a particular growth factor. Much research is being done to find out what controls apoptosis so that its effects during cultivation can be avoided.

22.5 | Flow cytometry

Figure 22.6 Schematic diagram of standard flow cytometry equipment. Cells pass individually through the centre of a laser beam and scattered light is detected at two angles. Forward angle light scatter (FALS) is measured in the plane of the beam and right angle light scatter (RALS) is measured at 90° to the beam. Emitted light from fluorescent stains that have a specific intracellular binding site is also measured at the 90° angle by photo multiplier tubes (PMT).

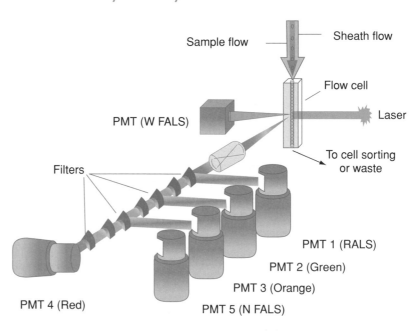

Flow cytometry is an analytical technique that has been used extensively for studying animal cell culture, where it is a powerful technique for the rapid characterisation of cell populations using scattered light (see Fig. 22.6). Cells pass individually through a laser beam and scattered light is detected in two planes. Forward angle light scatter (FALS) is measured in the plane of the beam and may give relative information on particle (cell) size. Right angle light scatter (RALS) is measured at 90° to the beam and provides information on cell granularity or the refractive properties of a cell. Emitted light from

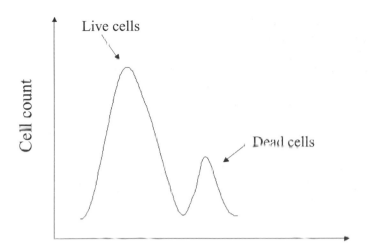

Live cells

Dead cells

Cell count

Propidium iodide fluorescence
(log scale)

Figure 22.7 Typical viability analysis of a eukaryotic cell culture by flow cytometry. All cells are bounded by the cytoplasmic membrane. A cell cannot exist without an intact fully functional cytoplasmic membrane. Therefore fluorescent stains that have specific intracellular binding sites, but cannot cross an intact cytoplasmic membrane (e.g. propidium iodide), can be used as a measure of a cell's viability, i.e. positive staining by propidium iodide indicates irreversible cell death.

fluorescent stains, which have specific intracellular or extracellular binding sites, is also measured at the 90° angle. This information coupled with the rapid throughput of thousands of cells per second provides real-time, statistically reliable information on cell cycle (see Fig. 22.5), cell physiology and cell viability (see Fig. 22.7) at the individual cell level. Importantly, cells can be sorted immediately post-analysis, such that sub-populations or even individual cells can be isolated for further analysis and investigation. If fluorescent substrates or products for the recombinant protein of choice are used, then highly producing cells can be selected for, greatly enhancing the efficiency of any cell line developmental programme. Many flow cytometric methods have been used for cell cycle analysis. Commonly, DNA-specific fluorescent stains (Hoechst 33342, 4,6-diamidino-2-phenylindole (DAPI), etc.) are used with permeablised cells to measure the specific DNA content of individual cells and the phase of the cell cycle identified. Similar information can also be obtained with nucleic acid specific stains (e.g. propidium iodide) after treatment with RNAse (see Fig. 22.5).

All eukaryotic cells are bounded by the cytoplasmic membrane, allowing the cell to communicate selectively with its immediate environment. A cell cannot exist without an intact, fully functional cytoplasmic membrane. Fluorescent stains that have specific intracellular binding sites, but cannot cross an intact cytoplasmic membrane (e.g. propidium iodide), can therefore be used as a measure of a cell's viability, i.e. positive staining by propidium iodide can indicate irreversible cell death (see Fig. 22.7). Other stains, e.g. Rhodamine 123 and Mitotraker Green, can be used to measure mitochondria (metabolic) activity, while Acridine Orange can be used to follow cell death by either apoptosis or necrosis.

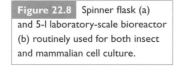

Figure 22.8 Spinner flask (a) and 5-l laboratory-scale bioreactor (b) routinely used for both insect and mammalian cell culture.

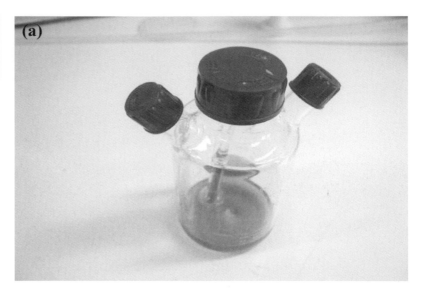

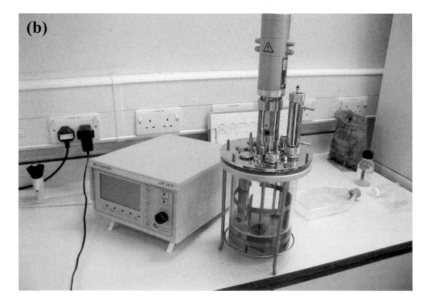

22.6 | Bioprocess engineering considerations

22.6.1 Cell culture techniques

Both insect cells and mammalian cells can be grown in free suspension culture (roller bottles, T-flasks, spinner flasks, continuously stirred tank or airlift bioreactors, see Figs. 22.8 and 22.9). Like microbial cells, both types of cells can be grown in batch (see Fig. 22.10), fed-batch or continuous culture and many of the same principles apply (Chapter 6). In free suspension, both insect cells and mammalian cells assume a spherical shape of between 5 and 20 μm, with insect

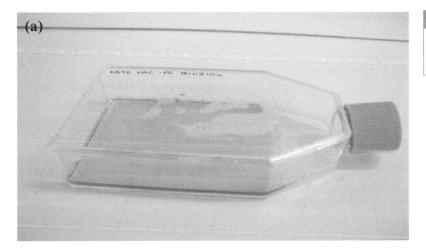

(a)

(b)

Figure 22.9 T-flask (a) and roller bottle (b) routinely used for both insect and mammalian cell culture.

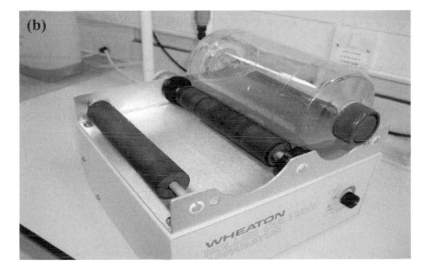

cells being nearer the higher end of that scale. Some cell lines are anchorage dependent; that is they need a surface on which to grow, which may be plastic or glass. The surface may be the wall of the bio-reactor, e.g. roller bottles, T-flasks (see Fig. 22.8), or suspended micro-carriers (see Table 22.5 and Section 22.6.6). Microcarriers provide a much greater area for growth per unit volume of medium than the original cell growth system. However, in all cases, the engineer needs to provide a closed sterile system for the cells to proliferate and syn-thesise the product of choice. Cells are maintained by diluting (pas-saging) them in fresh medium to $\sim 4 \times 10^5 \, \text{cells}^{-1} \, \text{ml}^{-1}$ (dependent on cell line), approximately every three days. Anchorage-dependent cells will adhere quite strongly to the microcarriers or to the base sur-face of the bottle/flask via a secreted protein-based, gelatinous matrix. Thus, for a successful passage, trypsin, a proteolytic enzyme, is added

Figure 22.10 Generalised growth curve for eukaryotic cell batch cultures.

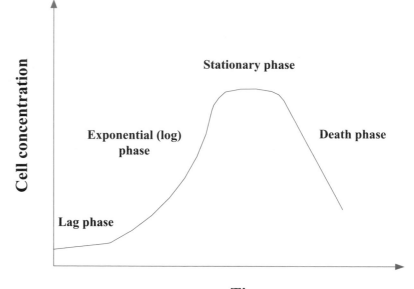

to aid cell detachment from the surface. Cells growing in suspension may also attach to the vessel walls, but in this case they can be removed quite easily by agitation. With sequential passaging, cell lines can retain the desired biological activity for up to three months. When such cells are present in the insect or animal of origin, they receive nutrients from the organism's circulatory system. Therefore, when cultivating these cells in vitro, the growth environment must provide similar nutrients and physical conditions (temperature, osmolarity, pH, O_2 and CO_2 concentration) as the parent organism.

The precise composition of growth media for the cultivation of such cells is often a closely guarded secret; the recipes are known only to, and sometimes patented by, companies specialising in growth media production. Such media, though, are commercially available. However, almost all growth media are based on a salt buffer, with the correct osmolarity and pH, containing various quantities of glucose, amino acids, vitamins and other growth factors. Each growth medium is optimised and is often specific for a particular cell line. Glutamine is often included, particularly for mammalian cells. It is often added in greater quantities than other amino acids because it can be used not only as a nitrogen source but also as an energy source and as an anabolic precursor (see Chapter 2). Therefore, its absence can lead to nitrogen limitation and rapid amino acid depletion in the culture medium. This possibility is less so for insect cells since it is known that the consumption rate of glutamine in Sf-9 cells is one-tenth that of hybridoma cell lines.

Frequently, particularly when the exact growth factors are not known, a quantity of blood serum (often from foetal calves) is added to the culture medium. This serum supplies trace elements, miscellaneous growth factors and lipids to the medium and also increases its

Table 22.5 Physical properties of some of the microcarriers commonly used for culture of mammalian and insect cells

Microcarrier	Cell line	Average particle size (μm)	Pore size (μm)	Particle density (g ml⁻¹)	Material	Use
Cytopore 1[a] (Amersham Biosciences)	Cells that require high recirculation rates and high nutrient availability, eg. CHO	230, diameter	30	1.03	Cross-linked cotton cellulose with a DEAE[b] coat	Stirred tank, perfusion cultures
Cytopore 2[a] (Amersham Biosciences)	Truly anchorage-dependent cells, e.g. BHK	230, diameter	30	1.03	Cross-linked cotton cellulose with a DEAE[b] coat	Stirred tank, perfusion cultures
Cytoline 1 (Amersham Biosciences)	Cells that attach well, are less sensitive to shear and require high recirculation rates, e.g. CHO	500–1000, thick; 1700–2500, length	10–400	1.32	Polyethylene and silica	Fluidised bed reactors
Cytoline 2 (Amersham Biosciences)	Cells that attach less well, are more sensitive to shear and require lower recirculation rates, e.g. hybridomas	500–1000, thick; 1700–2500, length	10–400	1.03	Polyethylene and silica	Varied
Cytodex 1 (Amersham Biosciences)	Truly anchorage-dependent cells, e.g. BHK	190, diameter	N/A	1.03	Cross-linked dextran with DEAE functional groups	Stirred tank cultures
Cytodex 3 (Amersham Biosciences)	Truly anchorage-dependent cells, e.g. BHK	170, diameter	N/A	1.04	Cross-linked dextran with a gelatin coat	Stirred tank cultures
Cultispher-G[c] (Percell via Sigma)	Majority of cell lines	130–380, diameter	20	1.04	Cross-linked porcine gelatin	Varied
Cultispher-S[c] (Percell via Sigma)	Majority of cell lines	130–380, diameter	20	1.04	Cross-linked porcine gelatin	Varied

[a] The major difference between Cytopore 1 and Cytopore 2 is the charge density, which is 1.0 meq g⁻¹ and 1.8 meq g⁻¹ respectively.

[b] Diethylaminoethyl.

[c] The major difference between Cultispher-G and Cultispher-S is the use of a different cross-linking procedure for Cultispher-S, which therefore has a higher thermal and mechanical stability. They may also be used for tissue engineering purposes as a support for transplanted material since the matrix can be fully dissolved by proteolytic enzymes.

buffering capacity, while also solubilising otherwise insoluble essential metals such as iron.

Due to the perceived problems associated with viruses (e.g. human immunodeficiency virus, HIV) and prions (the causative agent of bovine spongiform encephalopathy, BSE) from animal origin that can infect the human end user, the use of blood serum in growth media for therapeutic purposes is slowly being phased out and serum-free media are rapidly being developed. Other disadvantages of using serum additions are similar to those when using complex undefined growth media for prokaryotic expression systems in that performance, because of batch variation, becomes difficult to predict, and downstream processing for product recovery and purification becomes more involved. Additionally, the controlling factors are often not known to the experimenter.

There are also reports that foetal calf serum protects the cells from so called 'shear' forces and bubble coalescence in aerated, agitated bioreactors. Such issues are discussed separately later (see Sections 22.6.4 and 22.6.5). In most applications, a pH range of between 6.0 to 6.4 is satisfactory for insect (lepidopteran) cell lines, whereas the optimal pH range for mammalian cell lines is between 6.7 and 7.9. The optimal temperature range is again cell-line specific, but for mammalian cells varies between 36 and 38 °C, while for insect cells it lies between 25 and 30 °C. A typical batch process can last up to 5 days when a final cell concentration approaching $\sim 5 \times 10^6$ cells ml^{-1} is reached (see Fig. 22.10).

The main metabolic difference between insect and mammalian cells is in the accumulation of lactate in the growth medium. Unlike mammalian cells, which have a low glucose/lactate ratio in batch culture, insect cells accumulate lactate at low concentrations and only a small amount of glucose is oxidised to CO_2. Sf-9 cells do not produce lactate in the medium, even with a relatively high initial glucose content (40–50 mm). Metabolic flux analysis for the Sf-9 cell line showed that these cells possess a fully functional tricarboxylic acid (TCA) cycle (see Chapter 2), except under conditions of anoxic stress. Glucose is converted to pyruvate through glycolysis, which then enters the TCA cycle (to produce higher quantities of ATP) rather than the anaerobic pathway to produce lactate. This pathway explains why glucose consumption by hybridoma cell lines is 6 to 8 times higher than for Sf-9 cell lines with a concomitant 2 to 3 times higher O_2 demand for hybridoma cells. Conversely, however, High-Five cells accumulate lactate from 7 to 16 mm in suspension culture. Therefore, for both mammalian and insect cells, the inhibitory effect of lactate may be case specific.

Another important catabolic product in animal cell culture is ammonia. Insect cells are not as sensitive as mammalian cells to the presence of ammonia. Sf-9 cells do not usually accumulate ammonia during growth, whereas High-Five cells do so at concentrations dependent on the initial glutamine and asparagine content of the culture medium.

22.6.2 Large-scale protein production

Until recently bioreactors of up to 8000 litres were sufficient to satisfy the demand for high-value therapeutic proteins from mammalian cells. However, now that some products have reached the market and others are in late-stage clinical trials, such sizes are inadequate and commercial bioreactors of up to 20 000 litres are being commissioned. Insect cell technology for large-scale recombinant protein production is relatively new when compared to mammalian cell technology. Therefore bioreactors used in the laboratory are rarely larger than 5–10 litres, whereas volumes of 60 litres or more are used in industry. However, there is no reason to believe that, in the future, the demand for the products of insect cell culture will be any less than for those from mammalian cell culture today.

Scale-up is usually the last stage in a research and development programme, leading to the large-scale synthesis of recombinant products from mammalian or insect cells. Unlike microbial systems, the scale-up of both insect and mammalian cell processes involves a number of intermediate steps. Initially, cells are transferred from a stationary culture to shake flasks or spinner flasks (see Fig. 22.8). The latter were originally designed for the gentle agitation of microcarrier cultures, but are now routinely used in all cultures. They are equipped with a top-mounted magnetically driven stirrer that is suspended above the bottom of the flask. Sometimes cells are transferred along with a little 'spent medium' that may contain secreted growth factors essential for the stimulation of fresh growth. Conversely, however, 'spent medium' may also contain cytotoxic or cytostatic by-products, which must be removed by centrifugation before inoculation. Such cultures are then used to inoculate a bioreactor (see Fig. 22.8). Since the scale-up factor from flask or bottle (where pH is uncontrolled) to the fermenter is no more than 1 : 5, i.e. using a 20% (v/v) inoculum, a number of scale-up steps may be needed to obtain the required production volume. Pulsed-batch culture, where quantities of fresh medium are added periodically, and fed-batch culture, where fresh medium is added continuously at a pre-determined rate, both to a closed system, have been used. In this way, problems associated with catabolic repression or O_2 limitation can be overcome and by the continuous feeding of the correct balance of nutrients, higher cell densities ($\sim 10^7$ cells ml^{-1}) and product titres have been reported when compared to an equivalent batch process.

The use of continuous culture has been reported mainly for physiological studies since such processes are not favoured by industry because of the long culture duration time (up to five weeks). This long time scale can lead to cell-line instability and an increase in the risk of contamination or mechanical breakdown. A modification of the continuous process is perfusion culture. As cells grow and divide, they are retained within the bioreactor mechanically (spin-filter, hollow fibres, centrifugation) or ultrasonically. Fresh medium is added, while spent medium (and hence any secreted product or toxic by-products) is removed. Cell densities of $\sim 3 \times 10^7$ ml^{-1} and product titres x10 higher than that achieved in batch processes have been reported. However, problems can occur when spin-filters or hollow fibres become fouled or blocked.

22.6.3 Mass transfer and O_2 demand

Oxygen, an essential requirement for all aerobically respiring organisms, is sparingly soluble in weak salt solutions like growth media (~1.1 mmol l^{-1} or 33 mg l^{-1} at 35 °C) and therefore needs to be added on a continuous basis. Both insect and mammalian cells have somewhat similar O_2 demands in the range 1×10^{-17} to 1×10^{-16} mol s^{-1} $cell^{-1}$, with insect cells commonly being on the lower side. On the other hand, post-infection, insect cells generally double their O_2 demand. Maximum cell densities at the commercial scale tend to be similar at ~5×10^6 cells ml^{-1}, but the use of fed-batch techniques at the smaller scale has increased this to ~10^7 cells ml^{-1}. The level of dissolved O_2 over which the cultivation of mammalian cells can be undertaken satisfactorily is generally quite broad, ranging from 5 to 100% of air saturation. Insect cells have a narrower operating range of 40 to 60%, otherwise they are similar to mammalian cells. The overall O_2 demand of the cells throughout the cultivation (including post-infection) must be met by the O_2 transfer rate, which in turn depends on the mass transfer coefficient, $k_l a$, and the driving force for mass transfer.

The $k_l a$ is only dependent on the mean specific energy dissipation rate, $\bar{\varepsilon}_T$, imposed on the system by the impeller on the one hand, and the superficial air velocity in the bioreactor [$v_s = (vvm/60)$ (volume of broth/cross-sectional area of the bioreactor)] on the other. Thus, $\bar{\varepsilon}_T$ and v_s must together be sufficient to provide the necessary $k_l a$. Equations for determining the value of these parameters are available elsewhere in the literature, but two further comments are worth making here. First, up to the cell densities obtainable so far at the commercial scale, the O_2 demand and hence the $k_l a$ are very low compared to microbial fermentations. Second, the choice of agitator (see Chapter 7) does not alter the relationship between $k_l a$ and $\bar{\varepsilon}_T$ and v_s. Clearly, this level of agitation and aeration intensity must not significantly alter the cells' ability to grow and generate the desired product.

22.6.4 The impact of mechanical stress arising from agitation

Due to the lack of a cell wall, mammalian and insect cells are vulnerable to changes in osmolarity (insect cells less so) and have long been perceived to be 'shear' sensitive, i.e. they are physically damaged by the rotating impeller used in bioreactors. As a result, historically, the use of very low agitation intensities (expressed as mean specific energy dissipation rate, $\bar{\varepsilon}_T$ W kg^{-1} culture medium) has been recommended (~0.01 W kg^{-1}) for stirred bioreactors. In turn, these agitation conditions lead to heterogeneities in dissolved O_2 and CO_2 concentration and especially in pH at large scales of operation. For these reasons, during the 1980s, many attempts were made to introduce other systems, such as air-lift (see Chapter 7), hollow-fibre and circulating fluidised beds (for anchorage dependent cells). It is now recognised that this concern for 'shear' sensitivity was excessive and the majority of industrial processes use free-suspension, stirred tank bioreactors especially on the large scale. If anchorage-dependent cells are to be utilised, then agitated bioreactors containing microcarriers are employed. However, given that animal cells are potentially more sensitive to agitation and aeration in stirred tank bioreactors compared to microbial cells, much effort has gone into the proper design and operation of bioreactors in relation to agitation and aeration.

Typical bacterial fermentations operate with $\bar{\varepsilon}_T$ values of 1 to 2 W kg^{-1} while the early stirred mammalian cell bioreactors used $\bar{\varepsilon}_T$ values of the order of 0.01 W kg^{-1}. Yet, even at $\bar{\varepsilon}_T$ of 0.2 W kg^{-1}, a wide range of mammalian (e.g. hybridomas, myelomas, CHO) cells will grow and produce their product quite satisfactorily under unsparged conditions. Such an increase in agitation intensity, from 0.01 to 0.2 W kg^{-1}, would enable the $k_{L}a$ to be increased four- to five-fold. Sf9 insect cells have also been grown at $\bar{\varepsilon}_T$ values up to 0.25 W kg^{-1}. However, studies in spinner flasks (see Fig. 22.8) with insect cells indicate that damage can occur due to abrasion between the spinner and the base. With levels of agitation up to 0.2 W kg^{-1}, it is possible at the bench scale to get sufficient O_2 transfer through the top surface of the media without bubbling in air, i.e. without sparging, and by using O_2-enriched air, higher cell densities can be achieved.

Cell strength can be measured using micromanipulation. This technique confirmed that cells can withstand significantly more severe agitation than was initially thought. These agitation studies were initially conducted with radial flow Rushton turbines (often misleadingly called high-shear impellers, see Chapter 7) but the results were the same when axial flow propellers (so called low-shear impellers, see Chapter 7) were used. Many vendors, especially of bench-scale bioreactors specifically for use with mammalian or insect cells, still purport to equip them with special low-shear impellers. However, there is no evidence to suggest that such impellers actually enhance performance when a comparison is made on the basis of $\bar{\varepsilon}_T$.

22.6.5 The impact of sparging and the use of Pluronic F68

As the scale of cultivation increases, it becomes necessary to sparge air directly into the medium (especially for insect cells post-infection) in order to keep the desired level of dissolved O_2 concentration. Any mechanical damage to freely suspended cells is due to bubbles bursting at the medium surface. Fluid dynamic modelling of bursting bubbles has shown that there are huge local specific energy dissipation rates (10^4 to 10^5 W kg^{-1}) associated with it. This is many orders of magnitude greater than those due to agitation. Modelling also shows that smaller bubbles give locally higher $\bar{\varepsilon}_T$ and hence very high stresses are experienced by cells if attached to them. However, as first shown in 1968, the use of the surfactant Pluronic F68 essentially eliminates damage and it does so by preventing bubble/cell attachment and reduces medium surface tension so that the cells do not experience such high local stresses. Additionally, Pluronic F68 can render a protective effect biologically by incorporation into and strengthening the cytoplasmic membranes of insect cells, which grow and produce better in the presence of Pluronic F68 even when sparging is not required.

The realisation that bursting bubbles are the major cause of cell damage came too late to prevent airlift and bubble column bioreactors being used because they were considered to have 'low-shear' environments. Also, because of the perceived problem of agitation-induced 'shear', unbaffled stirred bioreactors are often used. However, under such conditions, even at low values of $\bar{\varepsilon}_T$, bubbles are easily sucked into the medium due to vortexing; and such bubbles, when they burst, are also damaging, so the addition of Pluronic F68 is still needed. Therefore, operating without baffles is of no advantage and indeed may cause difficulties.

22.6.6 The use of microcarriers

Many animal cell lines cannot be adapted to suspension culture and such adherent cells are often grown on microcarriers (see Table 22.5). Microcarriers are particles of various shapes and sizes (ranging from 100 μm to 2 mm) that can support high cell densities by providing a large surface area for anchorage-dependent growth. Microcarriers are also able to maintain a homogenous physical environment and provide relatively easy separation of cells from the growth medium at the end of the process. However, a major problem is that cells can be removed from the microcarrier surfaces relatively easily by agitation. This removal is accompanied by a loss of viable cells and, hence, productivity. Macroporous microcarriers provide some protection to the cells since cells can penetrate and grow in the internal spaces. However, in order to maximise this advantage, the internal space must be of the correct size and allow the transfer of O_2 to the cells and CO_2 away. Thus, the main goal of microcarrier cultivation is to maximise cell density without the detrimental effects of agitation. Adequate O_2 transfer and adequate suspension of the microcarriers must be provided.

Agitation intensities sufficient for microcarrier suspension may be kept to values of $\bar{\varepsilon}_T$ below those at which damage occurs by the choice of a down-pumping hydrofoil (see Chapter 7) coupled with a contoured bioreactor base. Also, by selecting a suitable medium feeding strategy, a well-mixed bioreactor environment may be achieved. However, higher levels of agitation, which can damage the cells, may be required if oxygenation is via surface aeration alone especially at large scales of operation or if high cell densities are required.

22.6.7 Physical and chemical environment

If mammalian and insect cells are cultivated with a low agitation speed then it becomes difficult to keep the medium homogeneous in a large-scale bioreactor. In turn, this lack of homogeneity means poor mixing and pH control can be very inaccurate. The pH probe is often situated close to the impeller and, on demand, 3 M Na_2CO_3 is often added on to the top surface of the medium. As a result, the upper regions of the bioreactor are badly mixed, yielding a significantly higher pH just below the liquid surface than in the main body of the medium. Scale-down studies, where myeloma cells and medium were circulated between two sparged bench-scale bioreactors, one held at pH 7.3 and one at pH 8 or 9, showed that when cells experience regular cyclic movement through regions of high pH, there is a significant increase in cell death (~30%). Feeding the pH controlling agent near to the impeller can essentially eliminate such changes in pH with obvious advantages for bioreactor operation; but, practically, this rarely occurs.

One consequence of using low aeration rates to prevent bubble-associated cell damage is the possible accumulation of dissolved CO_2 with increasing hydrostatic pressure (which occurs in large fermenters due to the depth of liquid medium) to toxic concentrations. Chinese hamster ovary (CHO) cells cultivated in laboratory-scale bioreactors are moderately tolerant to dissolved CO_2 (up to 18% saturation dissolved CO_2), while an inhibitory effect at 14% saturation dissolved CO_2 has been found in large-scale fermenters. The CO_2 ventilation rate is affected by the strategy used to determine the dissolved O_2 concentration (surface aeration, air sparging and partial pressure of oxygen in the inlet gas) and, therefore, a balance between oxygenation, CO_2 ventilation and pH control needs to be made.

22.7 | Further reading

Alberts, B., Johnson, A., Lewis, J., et al. *Molecular Biology of the Cell*, fourth edition. New York: Garland Science, 2002.

Bailey, J. E. and Ollis, D. F. (eds.) *Biochemical Engineering Fundamentals*, second edition. New York: McGraw-Hill, 1986.

Maramorosch, K. and McIntosh, A. H. *Insect Cell Biotechnology*. Boca Raton, FL: CRC Press, 1994.

Old, R. W. and Primrose, S. B. *Principles of Gene Manipulation: An Introduction to Genetic Engineering*, fifth edition. Oxford: Blackwell Science, 1994.

Shapiro, H. M. (ed.) *Practical Flow Cytometry*, third edition. New York: Alan R. Liss, 2003.

Spier, R. E. (ed.) *The Encyclopaedia of Cell Technology*. New York: John Wiley & Sons, 2000.

Chapter 23

Plant cell biotechnology

Robert Verpoorte
Leiden University, The Netherlands

Hens J. G. ten Hoopen
Delft University of Technology, The Netherlands

23.1 | Introduction

Plants are the basis of all human activities: they serve us as foods and medicines; as a source of building materials, of fibres for clothes, of bulk chemicals (such as cellulose, amylose and rubber) and of fine chemicals (such as flavours, fragrances, insecticides and dyes). Consequently, since ancient times, people have been searching for new applications of plants and plant-derived products and have tried to improve the production of known products.

At the advent of biotechnology also, plants became an important target for biotechnological research.

The basis of all plant biotechnology applications is the *totipotency* principle. Totipotency means that every individual plant cell carries all the genetic information needed for all the functions of the plant and, in principle, should be able to grow out to a complete plant again.

Agrobiotechnology concerns the growth of plants as crops and aims at improving yields or changing traits connected with the quality of the plant. This can be done via the classical breeding approach,

Basic Biotechnology, third edition, eds. Colin Ratledge and Bjørn Kristiansen.
Published by Cambridge University Press. © Cambridge University Press 2006.

in which plant tissue culture has become a major tool that reduces the time of developing a new cultivar considerably, enabling the production of many identical plants in a short time. Molecular biology is the other major tool employed for improving plants. In this case, genes are overexpressed, giving a plant improved or new (and desirable) traits. For improving yields, the first generation of transgenic plants (genetically modified, GM) developed, overexpressed a gene that either made the plant herbicide-resistant or resistant against pests or disease. By introducing into a plant, for example, a gene that encodes for BT-toxin, a toxic protein found in *Bacillus thuringiensis*, which is lethal for insects, the plant then became resistant against insect attack. These applications have raised many questions. As there were no obvious advantages for consumers to use or consume these GM plants, they were not accepted by the public in many countries, causing a major setback in the development of such crop plants.

Changing quality traits that do have extra, clear value for the consumer will be a more difficult task; although generating new flower colours for ornamental plants or cut flowers has been successfully achieved, these changes do not pose any perceived threat to the public. Genes for producing various health-promoting compounds in plants are presently a major target. The 'golden' rice, in which vitamin A biosynthesis is introduced, is a very promising proof-of-principle for this approach, as the rice now produces increased amounts of vitamin A, which then prevents the development of blindness in children who have a diet based almost exclusively on rice alone.

For industrially used plants, other traits are being addressed: e.g. the changing ratios of amylose and amylopectin, the major types of starch, in potatoes will make industrial processing easier. Lowering lignin levels in wood for cellulose and paper production is another example of GM plants for the production of bulk chemicals. For the production of fine chemicals, efforts are now being aimed at compounds to be used as medicines.

Plant cell biotechnology aims at the production of fine chemicals by means of biotechnological methods. This can involve the growth of plant cell or organ cultures in bioreactors. Genetic engineering is also used in this field to improve yields of required products.

In this chapter we will focus on plant cell biotechnology as a production method for fine chemicals. For agrobiotechnology, the reader is referred to the further reading list at the end of this chapter.

23.2 | Plant cell biotechnology

Plants are a source of a large number of highly valuable compounds (see Table 23.1 for some examples). Several different reasons have stimulated interest in the biotechnological production of such compounds:

Table 23.1 Some examples of important plant secondary metabolites

Medicines	Applications
Vinblastine	Antitumour
Vincristine	Antitumour
Camptothecin	Antitumour
Podophyllotoxin	Antitumour
Taxol (paclitaxel)	Antitumour
Quinine	Antimalaria
Artimisinin	Antimalaria
Quinidine	Antiarhythmic
Digoxin	Cardiotonic
Morphine	Relief of pain
Codeine	Relief of pain
Δ^9-Tetrahydrocannabinol	Relief of pain
Galanthamine	Alzheimer's disease
Colchicine	Gout
Hyoscyamine	Anticholinergic (parasymphatolytic)
Scopolamine	Anticholinergic (parasymphatolytic)
Caffeine	Tonic
Flavours and fragrances	
Vanillin	E.g. in ice cream, cola drinks
Hop bitter acids	Beer
Capsaicin	Chili pepper
Essential oils	Complex mixtures of terpenoids applied in food and cosmetics
Menthol	Candies
Glucosinolates	Mustard
Insecticides	
Azadirachtin	
Pyrethrins	
Dyes	
Anthraquinones	
Naphthoquinones (shikonin)	
Anthocyanins	
Indigo	
Miscellaneous	
Cocaine	
Nicotine	
Shikonin	

- only small volumes are required (kilograms to a few tonnes);
- source plants only grow in the wild and are being overcollected, leading to their possible extinction;
- source plants grow in areas with very unstable climatic or political conditions, causing supply problems;

- compounds are only produced in a certain phase of the plant development;
- plants grow very slowly and it takes many years before they are ready for harvesting;
- development of a high-quality product requires strict control of the production process (good manufacturing practice, GMP).

The products of interest are usually derived from plant *secondary metabolism*. Plant secondary metabolism is defined as those metabolic pathways specific for the plant species that are connected with the interaction of the plant with its environment rather than in the process of providing key precursors for the synthesis of major cell components (see also Chapter 2).

23.2.1 Plant cell and tissue culture

More than 100 years ago the first efforts were made for the culture of plant cells and tissues in vitro (meaning 'in glass', i.e. growing in laboratory glassware). The discovery of some plant hormones some 50 years ago enabled the first successful growth of plant tissues to occur. The potential of plant tissue cultures for the production of fine chemicals was then realised and the first efforts with cultures of plant roots were described in 1954. Plant tissue culture then developed into a major method for large-scale micropropagation of many ornamental plants and cut flowers, guaranteeing a constant quality of disease-free, genetically identical plants. This is presently the most important commercial industrial application of plant biotechnology, with hundreds of millions of plants being produced in this way every year.

23.2.2 Plant secondary metabolism

Each plant species has its own set of secondary metabolites that helps it to survive in its environment. These compounds are very varied and include, among many others, metabolites that are involved in the attraction of pollinators (flower colours and fragrance) and defence against insects and microorganisms. Some of the secondary metabolites (such as the phytoanticipins) are produced constitutively, i.e. all the time, while others (such as the phytoalexins) are only produced after induction following wounding or infection with a microorganism. By now, some 150 000 natural products are known, of which some 80% originate from plants. The majority of these compounds are derived from a few building blocks: the isoprenoid (C_5) unit, the phenylpropanoid (C_9) unit, the acetate (C_2) unit and amino acids. The *phenylpropanoid pathway* (Fig. 23.1) is well developed in plants, with 20–30% of the total carbon flux going through this pathway. This leads to various products ranging from lignin and lignans to flavonoids and anthocyanins (plant pigments).

Terpenoids are built up from C_5 units (Fig. 23.1). Monoterpenes ($2 \times C_5$), sesquiterpenes ($3 \times C_5$), diterpenes ($4 \times C_5$), steroids and

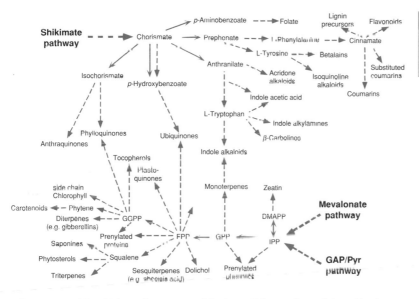

Figure 23.1 Two major secondary metabolite pathways in plants, the shikimate and the terpenoid pathway.

triterpenes ($6 \times C_5$) and carotenoids ($8 \times C_5$) are found in all plants and quite a few of these have great economic value.

The *acetate pathway* leads to the synthesis of a variety of polyketides. In combination with the phenylpropanoid pathway, this leads, for example, to the formation of the flavonoids (one C_9 unit + $3C_2$ units), which are plant colour compounds.

Amino acids are precursors of alkaloids, an important class of plant products, characterised by the occurrence of a heterocyclic nitrogen.

Usually, plants contain different types of secondary metabolites; several closely related compounds of each type are often present. Sometimes complex mixtures are found, e.g. essential oils containing hundreds of different monoterpenes. Each plant part has its own specific secondary metabolites, sometimes these compounds are stored at high concentrations in specialised cells such as glandular hairs.

Only about 15% of all plant species have been studied to some extent for their secondary metabolites. The biosynthetic pathways involved are not well known and only a few have been studied down to the level of determining what intermediates are involved, and which enzymes and genes.

23.3 | Plant cell-culture techniques

23.3.1 Initiating a cell culture

Plant cell cultures are obtained by cutting a small piece of any part of the plant after thorough sterilisation, but without killing the plant cells. This plant material, the explant, is placed on a solid medium. A callus, or lump, of undifferentiated cells usually develops out of the explant. After some weeks, this callus is cut from the explant and is put on an appropriate solid growth medium. By cutting the callus into smaller pieces and by finally sub-culturing into a liquid medium in Erlenmeyer (conical) flasks with continuous shaking, a suspension of growing cells can be obtained. Such cell suspensions can be cultured in bioreactors. By choosing a special combination of plant growth hormones, either root or shoot cultures can be produced. In principle, cell cultures from any plant can be obtained; in practice, it appears that some plants are much easier to develop into cell cultures than others. Because of the totipotency principle, it does not make any difference from which part of the plant a culture is initiated: in all cases, in principle, genetically the same, undifferentiated cells will be obtained. Sometimes products that occur in the plant can be found in the cultures in the first months after initiation but, later on, after stabilisation of the culture, they are not present anymore. Because of such 'memory' effects, product formation in cell cultures should only be assessed after stable cultures are obtained, which may take up to 6–9 months.

23.3.2 Media

Plant cell and tissue culture media were developed in the 1950s and 1960s. Most of the media presently used are based on these original formulations. The most often used are: *Murashige and Skoog* (MS), *Gamborg B5* (B5), (see Table 23.2), *Linsmaier and Skoog* (LS) and *Schenk and Hildebrand* (SH) media. In particular, the MS medium is used with many minor modifications.

Culture media consist of so-called micro- and macro-elements (micro and macro refer to the quantities), which are inorganic salts necessary to support growth. Moreover, the media contain various organic constituents such as vitamins. The difference between the media mentioned above is the ratio between the various constituents. Besides these three groups of compounds, the media contain a carbon source in the form of a sugar (usually glucose or sucrose), which is used as an energy source by the cells, as they have no photosynthetic capacity, and for building up the biomass. Finally, different growth hormones are added: the most important ones being the *auxins* (particularly useful for stimulating root formation in plants) and *cytokinins* (particularly useful for stimulating shoot formation), see Table 23.3. Both together stimulate callus formation and rapid cell proliferation.

Cell cultures of each plant species have their own specific requirements for optimum growth. Moreover, for the production of certain compounds, media conditions might be different from those for optimum growth. Consequently, both growth and production media have been described in which biomass is grown in the growth medium and then secondary metabolites are produced in a production medium.

23.3.3 Characteristics of plant cells

Plant cells differ from mammalian cells and microorganisms. The most obvious difference is the presence of a large central vacuole in

Table 23.2 Two examples of the plant cell growth media. The plant growth hormones vary for each individual culture

	Medium (mg l^{-1})	
Constituents	Murashige and Skoog	Gamborg B5
Macronutrients		
NH_4NO_3	1 650	
$(NH_4)_2SO_4$		134
KNO_3	1 900	2 500
$CaCl_2.H_2O$	440	150
$MgSO_4./H_2O$	370	250
KH_2PO_4	170	
$NaH_2PO_4.H_2O$		150
Micronutrients		
KI	0.83	0.75
H_3BO_3	6.2	3
$MnSO_4.4H_2O$	22.3	
$MnSO_4.H_2O$		10
$ZnSO_4.7H_2O$	8.6	2
$Na_2MoSO_4.2H_2O$	0.25	0.25
$CuSO_4.5H_2O$	0.025	0.025
$CoCl_2.6H_2O$	0.025	0.025
$FeSO_4.7H_2O$	27.8	27.8
$Na_2EDTA.2H_2O$	37.3	37.3
Organic supplements		
Myo-inositol	100	100
Nicotinic acid	0.5	100
Pyridoxine.HCl	0.5	1
Thiamine.HCl	0.5	1
Glycine	2	
Carbon source		
Sucrose	30 000	20 000

Table 23.3 Some commonly used growth hormones

Auxins
   Indole-3-acetic acid (IAA)
   Indole-3-butyric acid (IBA)
   Naphthalene-acetic acid (NAA)
   2,4-dichlorophenoxy-acetic acid (2,4D)
Cytokinins
   Benzylaminopurine (BAP)
   Cytokinin
   Zeatine

Table 23.4 Basic characteristics of plant cells and bacteria

	Bacteria	Plant cells
Size		
Diameter, μm	1–10	40–200
Surface, μm^2	3–300	5000–125000
Volume, μm^3	0.5–500	30000–4000000
Growth		
Doubling time, h	0.33–3	15–75
Specific growth rate, h^{-1}	0.2–2	0.01–0.05
O_2 uptake rate, mmol C-mol $^{-1}$ h^{-1}	700	15
Aeration rate required	High	Low
Yield		
C-mol biomass/C-mol C-source	0.50	0.65
Maintenance, h^{-1}	0.015	0.0075
Other characteristics		
Shear sensitivity	Low	Low to intermediate
Variability	Medium to high	High
Product localisation	Mostly extracellular	Mostly intracellular
Morphology	Single cells	Aggregates

plant cells. These vacuoles often are the site of accumulation of secondary metabolites. In Table 23.4 some basic characteristics of plant cells and bacteria are summarised.

The growth rate of plant cell cultures is not very high. The fastest doubling times are less than 24 h, but 48–72 h is not uncommon. The growth curves are similar to those for microorganisms, consisting of a lag phase, perhaps a short logarithmic phase, followed by a linear growth rate and, finally, a stationary phase. Growth usually lasts 1–2 weeks, but can be up to 4 or 6 weeks. Though ideally a plant suspension culture should consist of single cells, in reality most cultures contain small aggregates (up to 20 cells). Sometimes the aggregates can become much larger (0.5–1 cm diameter or even more) and may show clear differentiation in different types of cells. Cell suspension cultures can reach 10–20 g dry wt l^{-1} but, under special conditions, this may be higher: 120 g DW l^{-1} is the highest ever reported. At such densities there is only a little free medium (5–10%) left in the culture.

Plant cells are usually grown at 25 °C, in the light or in the dark, but this may result in differences in metabolic profiles. For large-scale culture in bioreactors, the use of light is not practical. Photoautotrophic cell cultures can be obtained, but are only used as an experimental system for studying photosynthesis.

The variability of plant cell cultures is high, which means that cells producing high amounts of a product may rapidly lose this trait. Cryopreservation of plant cells is applied to keep a stock of high-producing cell lines.

Table 23.5 Some examples of high producing plant cell suspension cultures

Plant species		Biomass production (g DW l^{-1})	Yield of product (% DW)	Yield (g l^{-1})	Productivity (g l^{-1}day^{-1})
Coleus blumei	Rosmarinic acid	25,7	21.4	5.5	0.91
Anchusa officinalis	Rosmarinic acid	35	11.4	4	0.16
Coptis japonica	Berberine	70	5	3.5	0.6
Perilla fructens	Anthocyanins	13.5	8.9	1.2	0.17
Papaver somniferum	Sanguinarine	12.1	2.5	0.3	0.025
Taxus chinensis	Taxuyunnanine C			0.89	0.025
Taxus canadensis	Paclitaxel			0.12	0.01
Catharanthus roseus	Ajmalicine + serpentine		1	0.23	0.008
Atropa belladonna	Hyoscyamine		0.95		0.0002
Morinda citrifolia	Anthraquinones		27	3	0.4

23.3.4 Production of secondary metabolites

Many plant cell and organ cultures have been studied for production of pharmaceuticals, flavours, fragrances, insecticides and dyes. The results vary from no production at all, to very high levels of secondary metabolites (Table 23.5).

Unfortunately, some of the most interesting pharmaceuticals are either not produced at all or are only produced in trace amounts in cell suspension cultures. On the other hand, the alkaloid, berberine, is produced at 7 g l^{-1}. In terms of commercial industrial production, the successful examples are shikonin, ginseng roots and paclitaxel (Taxol). The last is particularly important as it shows that it is feasible to develop a commercially viable process for expensive specialty chemicals.

Cell cultures can also be used for conversions of cheap precursors into more valuable products, as evident from the conversion of digitoxin into digoxin, which requires a single stereospecific hydroxylation. This was developed to a large-scale, commercially feasible process, though the patent was never implemented. Many other potential commercial examples have been reported, but none has yet been developed into a commercial process.

23.4 Optimisation of productivity

Because of the low productivity in most plant cell-culture systems, different strategies are being followed to increase production of the compounds of interest. These are described below; in general, they are similar to those used for the improvement of production when microorganisms are being used. However, one has to keep in mind that, in the case of plant cells, there is always the alternative option of the plant itself being grown in the field for production of a metabolite.

Price, flexibility of the production system and GMP are the elements that will play a major role in choosing the final production system.

23.4.1 Screening and selection; medium optimisation

The most common approach for obtaining high-producing cell lines is by screening and selection followed by optimisation of the growth and production media. *Screening* involves the selection of plants from which callus cultures and subsequently cell suspension cultures are initiated. On each level, the productivity is measured and high-producing strains are used for further development. The aim is to find a high volumetric production per time unit (g l^{-1} day^{-1}) in cell suspension cultures. Unfortunately, there is not always a direct relation between high-producing plants and the derived cell cultures. A better correlation seems to exist between callus cultures and cell suspension cultures.

In the case of *selection*, the approach is different; an external condition is created that favours the survival of potentially high-producing cells. This is done, for example, by adding a toxic compound to the medium, which is detoxified by an enzyme involved in the pathway, leading to the product of interest. Fluorophenylalanine has, for example, been used to select tobacco cells that are able to convert this compound rapidly; the enzyme phenylalanine lyase (PAL), which is capable of acting on this compound, is the rate-limiting step for the synthesis of caffeoyl putrescine. Consequently, the cells that survive exposure to fluorophenylalanine do so because they have an increased activity of PAL. This increased enzyme activity then removes the bottleneck and leads to overproduction of the final product (1.5 g l^{-1}, 6–10 times higher than original cell line).

A major problem with the screening and selection procedures is that a stable strain is not always obtained. In general, in about 50% of cases, stable cell lines are obtained.

Medium optimisation is a complex procedure, not only because of the large number of components that are involved, but also because the plant cell needs several sub-cultures (perhaps as many as 10) before the final result is observed of a change in medium composition. Experimental set-ups in which several parameters can be changed at the same time, enabling multi-variate analysis of the results, is preferred to experiments that optimise one component at a time. The most important components that appear to effect growth and secondary metabolite production are the growth hormones, carbohydrates, nitrogen source and phosphate. Other growth conditions, such as the composition of the gas phase, light and temperature, are further important parameters to be considered.

As rapid growth and secondary metabolism are mutually exclusive, two-stage procedures are often used. In the first stage, the biomass is produced, so it is necessary to select media that specifically promote rapid growth. In the second stage (the production phase), the cells are transferred into a medium which stimulates synthesis of the

Table 23.6 Examples of the effects of various treatments on the production of paclitaxel in cell cultures of *Taxus* species

Taxus species	Treatment	Paclitaxel level (mg l^{-1})	
		Untreated	Treated
T. cuspidata	Ethylene	0.02	2
	MeJ[a]		2.7
	Ethylene + MeJ		3.8
	Optimised oxygen, carbon dioxide and ethylene	0.5	6.5
	Light	7[b]	14[d]
T. chinensis	Ethylene	1.1	0.3
	Ag$^+$ (ethylene inhibitors) and fungal elicitor		10.8
	Fungal elicitor		5.2
	Abscisic acid	0.2	1.1
	Abscisic acid + MeJ		18
	McJ		10.6
	Ethylene + MeJ + sucrose	1.1	20.2
(Taxuyunanine)			
	MeJ + sucrose		18.6
	Lanthanum ions	1.1	4.7
	Osmotic pressure (sucrose + mannitol)	2.1	78.5
	Brassinolide	0.28[c]	0.6[e]
	Ag$^+$ + MeJ + chitosan	0.9	25
	2-phase system		5.20
	Elicitation + 2-phase system		48
	2-phase system	3.4	12
	2-phase system, extra sugar, precursor feeding		16.7
	Temperature	16.4	62.3
	Intermittent maltose feeding	3.8	67
	Ag$^+$ + temperature shift	30.9	137.5
T. media	MeJ	28.2	110

[a] MeJ: methyl jasmonate.
[b] 7 mg g^{-1} (light).
[c] 0.28 mg g^{-1}.
[d] 14 mg g^{-1} (dark).
[e] 0.6 mg g^{-1}.

secondary metabolite. Optimisation of a production medium is easier than for a growth medium as only one sub-culture is needed.

Although this approach requires a lot of effort, it may improve productivity by a factor of 20–30. Table 23.6 gives some examples of the effects of various treatments on the production of paclictaxel in *Taxus* cell cultures.

23.4.2 Culture of differentiated cells
Secondary metabolites are, by definition, a product of differentiation; however, in cell suspension cultures such differentiation does not

Table 23.7 Various compounds and solvents used to improve permeability of plant cell membranes

Dimethyl sulphoxide
Phenylethyl alcohol
Chloroform
Triton X-100
Cetrimide
Tween 20
Tween 40
Tween 80

always occur. For this reason a lot of research has been done on the in vitro culture of differentiated cells, e.g. of roots, shoots and embryos. This is achieved by using different combinations of growth hormones. Such organ cultures have similar patterns of secondary metabolite formation as the original plant. For example, the tropane alkaloids, hyoscyamine and scopolamine, are produced in root cultures. By transformation of the plant cell with *Agrobacterium rhizogenes*, so called 'hairy roots' (see p. 563) can be obtained that can grow without plant growth hormones. They have a growth rate somewhat less than that of cell suspension cultures (minimum doubling times of about 35 h), but they are good producers of the typical root secondary metabolites. The major problem of the organ is their large-scale culture. Although all types of bioreactors have been described for the culture of roots and/or shoots, commercial large-scale production using these systems remains expensive (see also Section 23.5.3).

Immobilisation of plant cells improves interactions between adjacent cells and may result in some differentiation and thus improved productivity. Immobilisation can, for example, be achieved by inclusion of cells in natural gels, such as calcium alginate, or in polyurethane foam cubes. However, as with organ cultures, the costs of scaling up to industrial production is the major constraint (see also Section 23.5.3)

23.4.3 Secretion of product

As most products are stored intracellularly, methods have been developed to induce secretion of the products. An advantage of excretion is that lowering the internal concentration of a product might increase its production. A common approach is to add permeabilising agents such as an organic solvent like dimethylsulphoxide or detergents (Table 23.7). Ultrasonic treatment can also be applied. Addition of a second phase to the culture (a solid adsorbent or a non-miscible liquid, Table 23.8) to create a 'sink' for the product(s) improves the productivity in certain cases, as this then physically removes the product

Table 23.8 Some solvents and adsorbents used for two-phase plant cell culture systems

Solvents
  Myglyol
  Paraffin
  Dibutylphthalate
  Decane
  Hexadecane
  Dioctylphthalate
Solid phases
  XAD4
  XAD7
  RP
  Ion exchangers

from the production system, thereby preventing it from interacting with the cells.

23.4.4 Elicitation

In plants, certain secondary metabolic pathways are induced by infection with microorganisms. The compounds formed are *phytoalexins*: low molecular weight compounds with antimicrobial activity. Each plant species has its own specific set of phytoalexins. They include terpenoids, phenylpropanoids, alkaloids; in fact, almost any class of natural product. They are formed by degradation of the plant cell wall or from the microbial cell wall during infection. They may be peptides or oligosaccharides, or a hybrid of both. These molecules can also be obtained from extracts of phytopathogenic microorganisms or common organisms, such as yeast. Also, some small molecules are capable of inducing phytoalexin biosynthesis. Jasmonic acid (and its methylester) is one such universal elicitor. It is involved as a signal in the response of the plant to defend itself against microbial infections and this involves the synthesis of the phytoalexins.

Besides these so-called biotic elicitors, *abiotic elicitors* are also known. These include heavy metal ions and inorganic salts (e.g. vanadate). Stress factors, such as osmotic shock or ultraviolet radiation, also can act as elicitors.

Elicitors, besides being active in a plant, are also active in plant cell cultures. Elicitation increases, for example, the production of paclitaxel (Table 23.6). Unfortunately, most of the plant secondary metabolites of interest are not phytoalexins.

The disadvantages and advantages of the various approaches for increasing production are summarised in Table 23.9.

23.4.5 Metabolic engineering

With the presently available tools of molecular biology, new possibilities are constantly arising for improving the productivity of the plant

Table 23.9 Methods for improving productivity in plant cell cultures

Method	Experiments	Advantage	Problems
Screening	Analyse large numbers of cell lines	Many-fold increase possible	Stability, laborious method
Selection	Create special selective condition for cells	Easy way to increase productivity	Improves one step, not always whole pathway
Medium optimisation	Test different media compositions	Many-fold increase possible, production medium might be successful	Laborious, for growth medium a series of sub-cultures is needed
Immobilised cells	Chose immobilisation system	Sometimes increased productivity, continuous process	Costly procedure on industrial scale, nutrient limitation
Elicitation	Select optimal elicitor	Very high production can be achieved on selected point in time	Phytoalexins are not necessarily the products of interest
Differentiated cells	Find media for root or shoot culture	Similar production as in plants can be obtained	Large-scale culture is difficult
Metabolic engineering	Overexpression of biosynthetic genes	Targeted approach	Biosynthetic pathways not well known, no genes cloned

cell factory for known compounds or, even, for producing completely novel compounds. However, this requires a thorough knowledge of the secondary metabolite pathway(s), including the identification of the intermediates in the pathway as well as knowing the enzymes involved and the genes that encode them. This then allows the dedicated researcher to develop a strategy for increasing the flux of carbon directly towards the product of interest. Unfortunately, for most pathways this knowledge is very limited.

Biosynthetic pathway mapping

Most of the pathways of plant products are often only based on a hypothesis. Though reasonable, often they lack rigorous proof for the involvement of all proposed intermediates. This hampers further studies on the enzymes and genes involved in these pathways. Consequently, extensive mapping of the pathways is required. Basically, two approaches can be used. One starts from the metabolite side and the other from the side of the genes.

For the first approach, putative intermediates are fed to the plant or plant cell cultures and in vitro enzyme reactions are performed to confirm their involvement in the pathway. For each individual step, this is followed by isolating and purifying the enzyme. Amino acid sequence information from the enzyme can subsequently be used to clone the gene. A novel approach to establish possible intermediates in a pathway uses precursors, such as a ^{13}C-labelled glucose, followed by analysis of the final product using ^{13}C-NMR to show in which position(s) the ^{13}C has been incorporated in the molecule of interest. Based on this information, a possible pathway can be proposed and likely intermediates can be predicted. This so-called *retro-biosynthetic* approach has been shown to be very successful in mapping complex biosynthetic pathways.

In the gene-based approach, different strategies are used. A well-known strategy is the induction of mutants. Instead of the at-random production of mutants (e.g. by radiation or mutagenic chemicals), molecular biology tools are nowadays available to knock out genes in a more selective way (e.g. transposon tagging, antisense genes, RNAi; see Chapter 5). The mutant and knock-out approaches require the analysis of the metabolites in the plant to determine what step(s) in the pathway is (are) affected. When the intermediates are not known, this approach will be difficult. For the time being, the classical approach of identifying each individual step in a biosynthetic pathway and, subsequently, isolating the enzymes and cloning of the encoding gene, is still the most certain way to unravel a biosynthetic pathway.

Techniques for plant transformation

Two methods are the most common for introducing new genes into plants. These are the *Agrobacterium-mediated gene transfer* and *direct gene transfer by particle bombardment*.

Agrobacterium tumefaciens is a soil-dwelling, Gram-negative bacterium that causes crown gall disease of plants. The bacterium can infect a plant at a wound site. After infection it transfers some genes from a tumour-inducing (Ti) plasmid into the genome of plant cells, causing an increase in the production of *auxins* and *cytokinins*. This makes the cells proliferate rapidly, resulting in the formation of a gall. This natural transformation system has been modified in such a way that the tumour-inducing genes are replaced by other genes and are introduced into plant cells destined to laboratory cultivation.

The binary *A. tumefaciens* vector system is now widely used for the transformation of isolated plant cells. In this system, an *A. tumefaciens* strain that contains two plasmids is used. One is a vector plasmid, containing non-oncogenic (non-cancer forming) T-DNA, which carries the expressible foreign gene(s) to be introduced, together with suitable selection and reporter genes. The second, the 'helper' plasmid, harbours virulence genes that effect transfer of the non-oncogenic T-DNA. Unfortunately, most monocotyledonous plants (e.g. cereals and grasses, including rice and corn) are not amenable to transformation with *Agrobacterium*. A related species, *Agrobacterium rhizogenes*, causes the tumourous growth of roots, the so-called *hairy roots*. This system is used for inducing hairy root cultures for the production of secondary metabolites.

Direct gene transfer applicable to all plants can be achieved, literally, by shooting small tungsten or gold particles (∼0.4–1.2 μm diameter) coated with the DNA to be delivered into the plant cells (e.g. in a plant leaf or plant cell suspension). The particle-gun (microprojectile bombardment or biolistics) approach is widely used nowadays.

Irrespective of the means used to introduce foreign DNA into a plant cell, besides the gene(s) of interest, the piece of DNA that is being transferred also contains a selectable marker gene and a suitable promoter (see Chapter 4). This selection marker gene introduces resistance against a toxic compound: in plants this is usually resistance against an antibiotic, such as kanamycin and hygromycin, or a herbicide, such as glyphosate. By growing the cells on a medium containing such a toxic compound, only those cells that have received and incorporated the transgene, which codes for resistance to the compound, will be able to survive. Cells not expressing this *resistance* gene will die. A promoter is required to achieve constitutive or a localised expression of genes of interest in the plant cells. The cauliflower mosaic virus 35S (CaMV 35S) promoter is widely used for a constitutive expression in all parts of the plant. A variety of constitutive, tissue-specific and inducible (e.g. by ultraviolet light, glucocorticoids or tetracycline) promoters are available for more specific expression in the plant or plant tissues.

To confirm that cells are transformed, *reporter genes* are also usually incorporated into the DNA that is transferred to the plant cells (see p. 109). Such genes are, for example, the GUS gene that encodes a β-glucuronidase and genes encoding fluorescent proteins, such as the green fluorescent protein (GFP). The fluorescent proteins enable direct confirmation of transformed cells using microscopy, which means that it is not necessary to sacrifice the cells as in the GUS-colouration reaction (see p. 110).

In general, any plant species can be transformed genetically. Problems in genetic modification of plants are low transformation rates, i.e. only a few cells receive the desired gene(s), and even when the DNA has been incorporated it may not result in the production of a functional protein. In case of overexpression of an endogenous gene, the transformation may result in the opposite effect: the silencing of the gene. The major problem, however, is generation of viable healthy plants from the transformed cells.

Targets for metabolic engineering

The goals one can envisage for metabolic engineering are many and may include:

- improving the production of a desired compound/protein for subsequent extraction and isolation;
- improving resistance against pests and diseases;
- lowering level of undesired compounds in food plants;
- increasing the level of a desired compound in food (e.g. vitamins);
- giving a new trait (colour, taste, smell) to food, flowers or ornamental plants.

For improving the productivity in a plant or plant cell culture, one can envisage several approaches: overexpression of genes encoding rate-limiting enzymes; blocking competitive pathways or blocking catabolic pathways of the product of interest. In the first-mentioned

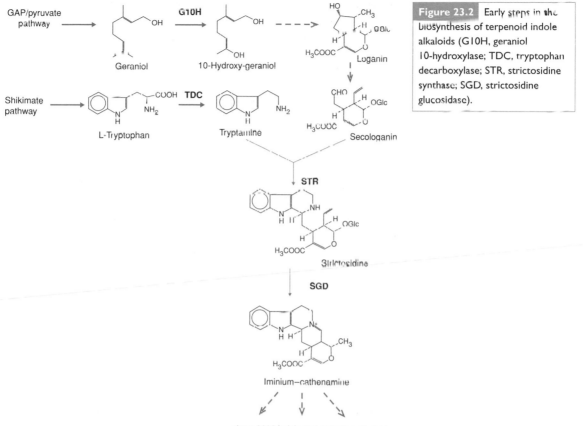

Figure 23.2 Early steps in the biosynthesis of terpenoid indole alkaloids (G10H, geraniol 10-hydroxylase; TDC, tryptophan decarboxylase; STR, strictosidine synthase; SGD, strictosidine glucosidase).

about 3000 indole and quinoline alkaloids

approach, genes are required that result in the overexpression of an active enzyme. The last two approaches can be achieved by introducing an antisense gene (see p. 138) or using the RNAi approach. In both cases, a step in a pathway is blocked at the level of messenger RNA, by interacting of the transgenic RNA with the native RNA resulting in a lowered level of activity of the encoded enzyme.

An example of metabolic engineering is the improved production of terpenoid indole alkaloids in *Catharanthus roseus* cells. This plant is an important source of pharmaceuticals such as ajmalicine (from roots), vinblastine and vincristine (from leaves). All these products are derived from two precursors, tryptophan and geraniol (see Fig. 23.2). Several genes of the pathway have been cloned. Over-expression of the gene encoding tryptophan decarboxylase (TDC) in *C. roseus* cell cultures, resulted in higher tryptamine production only, showing that secologanin availability is a limiting factor for the biosynthesis of the alkaloids. Whereas, unexpectedly, over-expressing strictosidine synthase (STR) resulted in a higher production of alkaloids.

Studies on metabolic engineering using a single structural gene from a pathway in plants show, in general, that the increase in the production of the desired compounds is not very large. Several reasons for this can be advanced: several limiting steps may occur in a pathway, or intra- and intercellular transport may play an important role. To overcome these problems, regulatory genes that control the expression of the genes of all, or most, of the pathway are of great interest. Overexpression of such genes may result in the permanent up-regulation of a series of enzymes in a pathway.

Production of secondary metabolites in other plants
To obtain a better source for the production of a compound, one may consider the overexpression of (a part of) the biosynthetic pathway in another plant species, rather than the original producing plant species. For example, the secologanin biosynthetic pathway involved in the biosynthesis of terpenoid indole alkaloids (Fig. 23.2) occurs in many plants that do not produce these alkaloids. By overexpressing the *Tdc*- and *Str*-genes from the alkaloid pathway (Fig. 23.2) in a plant cell culture of *Weigelia* 'Styriaca', the cells start to produce indole alkaloids (tryptamine, ajmalicine and serpentine; Fig. 23.2).

Production of proteins
Any protein can, in principle, be overexpressed in plants or plant cell cultures. As plants are cheap to grow, this has raised much interest in using plants for the production of various pharmaceutical proteins, vaccines and antibodies. The fact that plant cells are capable of protein glycosylation gives them a further advantage and some cell lines have been used to produce proteins such as insulin and human serum albumin (HSA). However, plants and plant cells are not generally recognised as safe (GRAS) organisms for the production of therapeutic proteins. To register any product from a non-GRAS organism as a drug is a major effort requiring extensive studies on safety. This will be far more expensive than the cost of developing the plant or plant cell culture for overexpressing the protein. So, only in case of non-medical applications, one may expect some commercial applications in the near future. Other applications will first require the production system to be recognised as safe.

23.5 | Large-scale production

23.5.1 Introduction
The ultimate goal of plant cell biotechnology is the development of large-scale processes for the production of secondary metabolites of commercial interest. The development of a large-scale production process is one with many interrelated steps, as shown in Scheme 1 (Fig. 23.3). In the next sections, these various steps will be discussed in more detail.

23.5.2 Process options
In the design of a production process with plant cells or tissue, three points are very important in the choice of the process type: the culture type (free cells, immobilised cells or organ cultures), the localisation of the product (inside the cell or released) and the

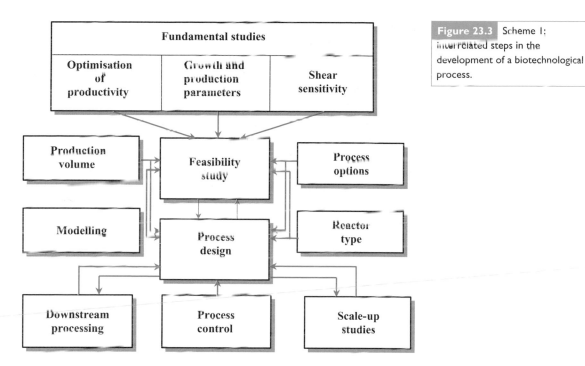

Figure 23.3 Scheme 1: interrelated steps in the development of a biotechnological process.

production period (during the growth phase or during the stationary phase). For production, different systems can be considered:

- cell suspension cultures,
- immobilised cells,
  - surface immobilisation (biofilms),
  - gel-entrapped cells,
- organ cultures,
  - roots,
  - shoots,
  - hairy roots.

A characteristic of many plant cell cultures is that growth and production phases are separated in time. This requires two-stage processes in which the conditions for growth and production are optimised separately.

Fermentation processes can be carried out as a batch, fed-batch, or continuous process (see Chapter 6). In plant cell biotechnology, batch and fed-batch technology are usually preferable. The fed-batch culture system provides the advantage of gradually changing the conditions in the reactor from growth medium into production medium without there being a sharp transition phase. Furthermore, plant cell cultures have to be inoculated with relatively large quantities of biomass to obtain fast-growing cultures (10–20% of the final biomass concentration). This causes the necessity of a long fermentation sequence, starting with a laboratory culture and then using stepwise volume increases by a factor of 5–10 from one fermenter to the next. By using a fed-batch operation, the fermenter train can be shortened (volume steps of 1 to 15–30), because the next larger fermenter is filled by about 30% with inoculum and fresh medium and, when growth is started, is then gradually filled up to 100% of the working volume.

Plant cell suspension cultures have some characteristics that complicate the application of a continuous culture. The low specific growth rate means that a long time is required to reach a steady state and then this has to be maintained for several months if the economics of using this technique are to be attained. The risk of a calamity happening (contamination, equipment failure) during this extended cultivation period is considerable and thus there is a reluctance on behalf of companies to consider this as a valid means of achieving production.

23.5.3 Bioreactors

Plant cells and hydrodynamic stress

When compared to microorganisms, plant cells are much bigger, mainly due to the presence of large vacuoles, which may form up to 95% of the total cellular volume. Originally, it was thought that stirring plant cells, being essentially a bag of water with a thin cell wall, in a bioreactor would cause them to collapse due to the shear forces produced (shear effects on microorganisms are discussed in Chapter 7). The common opinion was that the airlift bioreactor (see Chapter 7) would be the preferred reactor type, but other specially designed low-shear bioreactors were also developed to avoid exposing plant cells to high shear forces. However, recent research has shown that most plant cell cultures are robust enough to be cultured in a conventional stirred tank bioreactor. This is confirmed by the commercial production of plant products using this type of bioreactor.

Bioreactors for cell suspensions

Plant cells and small aggregates can successfully be cultured in stirred tank reactors, airlift systems, bubble columns and fluidised bed reactors (for details see Chapter 7). Stirred tank reactors are the preferred systems for several reasons. They are the standard equipment in the fermentation industry and stirred tank reactors can handle the highest concentrations of plant cells, maintaining good mixing and oxygen transfer characteristics.

Much of the available knowledge for microorganisms is directly applicable on plant cells. However, there are also some differences, which cannot be neglected (see Table 23.4).

Plant cell suspensions at low concentrations behave as Newtonian fluids; however, at higher concentrations they often become pseudo-plastic fluids. This can cause the formation of packages of biomass far from the stirrer, which are not then optimally mixed and also suffer from oxygen depletion. Several studies have been made on the implementation of alternative agitator designs for plant cells (low-shear, good-mixing characteristics for pseudoplastic fluids, adequate bubble dispersion and low foam formation). An upward-pumping axial-flow turbine offers important advantages for gas handling and mixing at restricted power input to avoid shear problems.

Bioreactors for artificially immobilised systems

Immobilised plant cells are protected against hydrodynamic stress and cell-to-cell contact might stimulate production. Moreover, they are easily separated from the medium, so high dilution rates can be employed without washout of the biomass and repeated use of the biomass becomes possible.

The bioreactors that are used for growing plant cells embedded in gel beads or in foam cubes are stirred vessels, packed columns, airlift systems or fluidised bed reactors. Because of optimal gas exchange, the stirred vessel is the first choice.

Bioreactors for natural immobilised systems

Organ cultures differ from the other immobilised systems in being highly organised structures, but they are relatively vulnerable to damage in stirred bioreactors.

Most research has been done on transformed root cultures. Although the cells in these *hairy roots* are protected against shear stress, the roots themselves may be damaged by the agitator, causing the development of undifferentiated callus-like tissue. A specific problem of hairy roots is the need for attachment onto a fixed point for good growth. For optimal use of a large bioreactor, it is essential to have many attachment points for the roots. The inoculation itself needs a dedicated design to achieve transfer of the roots from one vessel into the next. After attachment, the roots start growing and may form dense clumps.

The possibility of growing hairy roots in a moist environment has been achieved using mist (droplet size, 0.01–10 μm), spray (droplet size, 10–100 μM) or drip (droplet size 1–5 mm) reactors. The advantage of the mist or spray systems is a thinner fluid film on the roots, thereby providing better gas exchange between the cells and the cultivation medium. However, the drip technology offers better prospects for large-scale development.

Studies have also been carried out on the culture of *shoots* and the development of somatic embryos in bioreactors. Shoots are sensitive to physical stress: if they are wounded, they may excrete undesirable products; inoculation is also difficult. Shoots need light for photosynthesis. They do not need continuous agitation because the exchange rates between shoots and medium are low. A successful approach for the large-scale production of shoots was inoculation with primordial cells (the earliest stage of development of a leaf in a bud which is relatively robust) in a 500-l stirred and aerated vessel equipped with interior fluorescent lamps to provide a light–dark cycle.

The development of *somatic embryos* (small organised structures of cells capable of developing in plant-like seeds) as the basis for the large-scale propagation of plants is another interesting process. It requires easy change of medium composition to support the embryo development, and a stirring system avoiding shear damage. A spin-filter bioreactor was proposed for this purpose.

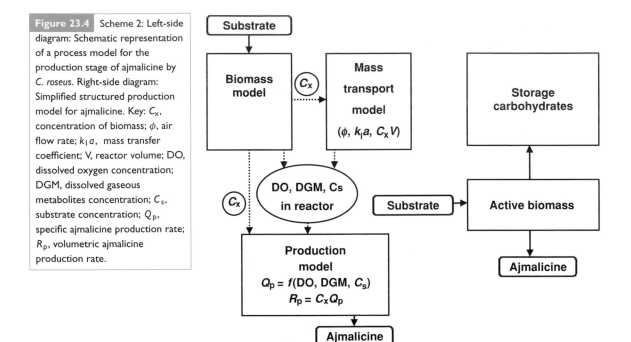

Figure 23.4 Scheme 2: Left-side diagram: Schematic representation of a process model for the production stage of ajmalicine by *C. roseus*. Right-side diagram: Simplified structured production model for ajmalicine. Key: C_x, concentration of biomass; ϕ, air flow rate; $k_l a$, mass transfer coefficient; V, reactor volume; DO, dissolved oxygen concentration; DGM, dissolved gaseous metabolites concentration; C_s, substrate concentration; Q_p, specific ajmalicine production rate; R_p, volumetric ajmalicine production rate.

23.5.4 Mathematical modelling

General aspects of setting up macroscopic models for fermentation processes are discussed in Chapters 3 and 6. The same approach can be applied to plant cells. Some particular characteristics, typical for growing or producing plant cells, have to be taken into account because they can cause complications. Plant cells change their composition considerably during batch growth because the cells possess the capacity to store the carbon source as starch-like products. Storage products are consumed by the cells when the external carbon source is exhausted.

For most applications, growth and production have to be described by structured models in which the biomass is divided in two compartments: the active biomass compartment (where the biochemical transformation processes take place) and the storage compartment (containing starch-like products).

Two-stage batch fermentation appears, in many cases, to be the optimal process operation for the production of secondary metabolites. Both growth and production stages require their specific model (see Scheme 2, Fig. 23.4, for an example of a structured model).

A quite different situation appears in the case of mathematical modelling of hairy root cultures. Three types of cells are present in hairy roots: cells dividing at their tips, cells in the state of cell elongation and non-dividing differentiated cells. They all have typical growth characteristics and have to be dealt with as different populations, coupled by rate equations for the transfer of cells from one population to another. This results in a segregated model instead of

Table 23.10 Examples of oxygen and carbon dioxide percentages in the gaseous phase of a well-mixed and ventilated bioreactor and a shake flask

	Bioreactor		Shake flask	
	O_2 (% v/v)	CO_2 (% v/v)	O_2 (% v/v)	CO_2 (% v/v)
After inoculation	21	0.03	21	0.03
At the end of the exponential growth phase	20.3	0.7	13	11

a continuous model, as is usually applied to suspension cultures of microbial and plant cells.

23.5.5 Process control

Process control of plant cell production follows the general principles described in Chapter 10.

Essential, of course, is to find out which parameter has to be optimised and which parameter is critical. To achieve maximal productivity during the first stage of a two-stage process, a high biomass concentration is aimed at. Here, O_2 transfer is most probably the critical factor. Possibilities for maximising the O_2 transfer are: intensive agitation, high sparging rate or O_2-enriched ventilation gas. Process control has to take into account the maximum acceptable stirrer speed, sparge rate and maximum allowable oxygen concentration in the ventilation gas.

The critical parameter during the production stage of the required compound is more difficult to establish. Many factors may play a part in the stimulation of the production, such as the O_2 and the CO_2 concentrations; the concentration of other, sometimes unknown, gaseous metabolites; the glucose concentration; or the concentration of plant hormones and elicitors.

23.5.6 Scale-up

From a technological point of view, a suspended cell system in a bioreactor is the preferred production system because it is relatively homogeneous and, therefore, easy to mix, aerate and control. The commonly used 'bioreactor' in plant cell research is the shake flask. However, it differs from a stirred vessel in almost every aspect: such as geometry, mixing and ventilation. This causes large differences in the conditions for growth and product formation. The composition of the gaseous phase, especially, is different (Table 23.10) and, in the case of shake-flasks, is also very dependent on the type of flask closure being used. Therefore, experiments on a plant cell production system at the laboratory scale should be performed as early as possible in a small-scale reactor of the type intended for commercial production.

There are no straightforward guidelines to solve the scale-up problem because there is an interaction of the various mechanisms involved; for example, the stirring speed will increase the oxygen

Table 23.11	Scale-up methods
1. Trial and error	
2. Rules of thumb	
3. Scale down approach/regime analysis	
4. Dimensional analysis/regime analysis	
5. Semifundamental methods	
6. Fundamental methods	

transfer rate, but might have a negative shear effect on plant cells. Consequently, compromises have to be made. Different approaches to solve this problem are summarised in Table 23.11.

The objective of scale-up methodology is to avoid trial and error because it implies that trials and errors will still be needed at full scale, which will be quite expensive. Methods 4, 5 and 6 in Table 23.11 are based on having more quantitative knowledge of the involved mechanisms than presently available in most plant biotechnological processes. Therefore, a combination of rules of thumb and regime analysis/scale-down is most appropriate. The regime analysis/scale-down approach implies that the rate-limiting mechanism at the large scale is determined on theoretical grounds or through experience in a running process.

This rate-limiting step can be studied in detail in a small-scale set-up. From such a study, improvements at the large scale can be developed.

23.5.7 Feasibility

Plant cell biotechnology aims at the commercial production of economically important secondary metabolites. Here we describe an evaluation of the costs of such a commercial production. The general approach of a feasibility study is comprehensively dealt with in Chapter 11.

The most frequently proposed process design in industrial plant biotechnology is the two-stage (growth and production) approach as described above.

A different approach involves the re-use of the biomass. This can be achieved by naturally or artificially induced product release from the cells. The production strategies discussed here are:

• the batch process, with a single use of biomass,
• continuous or semicontinuous processes with
  – repeated use of biomass with spontaneous release of product,
  – repeated use of biomass with forced release of product through permeabilisation,
  – repeated use of immobilised biomass.

It must be stressed here that downstream processing, wastewater treatment and manpower are not included in this cost calculation.

Estimation of costs

Two products have been selected as examples of cost analysis: ajmalicine and berberine.

Ajmalicine has been the subject of several feasibility studies, and a considerable amount of data on the growth of *Catharanthus roseus* cell cultures and production of ajmalicine by these cultures have been published.

Berberine is selected as the second target for this work. High productivity of cell cultures for the production of this compound has been achieved.

The cost price estimations are made for a production of 3000 kg product during a production period of 300 days per year. The product loss during recovery and purification is assumed to be 20%.

Growth and production media

The total costs of a standard medium with 3% (w/v) glucose is about 50 € m^{-3}, the price of a concentrated fed batch medium works out at about 800 € m^{-3}. These data should be considered as very rough estimates because the prices of the individual chemicals are very much dependent on the purity, the quantity and the supplier. Furthermore, the market price of the most cost-determining compound (sugar) varies considerably (the carbon source represents about 30% of the medium costs).

In many production media, only the concentration of the carbon source is increased compared to growth medium; such a medium with 8% glucose will cost 75 € m^{-3}. Most media contain balanced quantities of nitrate and ammonium, as nitrogen sources, to avoid unacceptable pH shifts. In bioreactors with pH control, this restriction does not apply, and the choice of the nitrogen source is rather free.

Biomass concentration

Biomass concentration in shake flasks usually reaches 15–20 kg m^{-3} dry weight. However, cell densities up to 120 kg m^{-3} have been reported in other reactor systems. At biomass concentrations over 40 kg m^{-3}, mixing and aeration problems start to occur.

Ajmalicine or berberine production in cell cultures

GROWTH AND PRODUCTION PARAMETERS

The size of the equipment and the final price of the product are determined by four important process parameters: annual production, maximum specific growth rate, specific product formation rate and the maximum biomass concentration. The commercially interesting ajmalicine, which is produced in *Catharanthus roseus* cell cultures, and berberine, which so far is the compound with the highest reported production at 7 g l^{-1} in *Coptis japonica* cell cultures, were selected for these calculations. *Thalictrum minus* also produces berberine, though not at as high levels, but it is an example of a cell culture that excretes the product. A selection from cell-culture parameters in the literature has been made for use in the cost calculations (Table 23.12).

PRODUCTION PROCESS BASED ON SINGLE USE OF BIOMASS

Biomass is grown in a fermentation train consisting of a series of reactors of increasing size, and serves as an inoculum for the ajmalicine production stage. After a production reactor is inoculated, the biomass concentration further increases. When growth of the culture begins to decline, production will start; in the case of *C. roseus* this results in a maximum ajmalicine concentration after 21 days. In the case of berberine, *Coptis japonica* is the preferred culture for a fed-batch procedure. The residence time in the reactor is 14 days. Assuming one day for cleaning, sterilisation and refilling, the run time will be 15 days, resulting in 20 runs per year.

PRODUCTION IN A CELL RETENTION SYSTEM WITH SPONTANEOUS PRODUCT RELEASE

The first phase of the process is comparable with the single-use set-up. The biomass of *Thalictrum minus* in the last reactor serves to inoculate one of the production bioreactors. The production medium is fed continuously into the production vessel. At the same time, spent medium and biomass are withdrawn. The extraction of the product from spent medium can be done either by extraction with an organic solvent (or combination of solvents) or adsorption by a polymeric adsorbent in an adsorption column. In a semi-continuous mode, the greater part of the cell mass is harvested from the bioreactor at once, leaving sufficient biomass to serve as the inoculum for the next run.

PRODUCTION IN A CELL RETENTION SYSTEM WITH PRODUCT RELEASE BY PERMEABILISATION

In contrast to the *Th. minus* cells that excrete berberine, ajmalicine release from *C. roseus* cells may have to be forced by permeabilisation of the cells using dimethylsulphoxide (DMSO).

The first phase of the process is the same as that for spontaneous release of the product. The last phase of the process is the permeabilisation phase. The plant cells are allowed to settle for two hours, half of the medium is then withdrawn and replaced by 10% (v/v) DMSO in water, resulting in DMSO at 5% (v/v) in the medium. After agitation for 20 minutes, release of ajmalicine is assumed to be complete, biomass is allowed to settle, and half of the medium is withdrawn and replaced by an 8% (w/v) glucose solution. To remove the ajmalicine completely, this washing step must be repeated three times. After the washing phase, new production medium is fed into the production fermenter and the whole procedure can start again. For the purposes of the calculation, it is assumed that the plant cells can be permeabilised and recycled six times.

Table 23.12 Process parameters used in the cost calculations

Process type	Design parameters		Production costs (€ kg^{-1})
Ajmalicine			
Single use of biomass	Productivity: 9 g kg^{-1} DW after 21 days production period Final dry wt: 40 kg m^{-3}	Spec. growth rate: 0.029 h^{-1} Inoculation ratio 1 : 7 (v/v) Initial dry wt: 2.5 kg m^{-3}	1500
Spontaneous release of product	Productivity: 24 mg kg^{-1} h^{-1} Final dry wt: 20 kg m^{-3}	Dry wt. yield on glucose: 0.65 C-mol/C-mol^{-1} Maintenance on glucose: 0.0083 C-mol/C-mol h$^-$	3300
Forced release by permeabilisation	Productivity: 9 g kg^{-1} DW after 21 days production period Final dry wt: 20 kg m^{-3}	Max C_2 uptake: 0.0154 kmol m^{-3} h^{-1} at 20 kg m^{-3}	4300
Berberine			
Single use of biomass	Initial dry wt: 8 kg m^{-3} Final dry wt: 55 kg m^{-3} Final berberine: 0.07 kg kg^{-1} DW Total growth and production time: 14 days		320
Spontaneous product release, discontinuous	Biomass growth reactor Initial dry wt: 1.25 kg m^{-3} Final dry wt: 40 kg m^{-3}		670
Spontaneous product release, continuous	Berberine production reactor Initial dry wt: 2.5 kg m^{-3} Final dry wt: 20 kg m^{-3} Final berberine: 0.07 kg kg^{-1} DW Total growth and production time: 18 days		750
Immobilised cells	Initial dry wt: 10 kg m^{-3} in 0.5 m^3 Ca alginate beads m^{-3} Final berberine: 20 kg m^{-3} after 100 days Medium renewal every 10 days		535

REPEATED USE OF IMMOBILISED BIOMASS

The necessary bioreactor volume to achieve a given amount of product will be larger when using immobilised cells than when using free cells because of the space taken up by the matrix – always assuming that the rates of production are approximately the same in the two systems. The cost of the matrix must also be taken in consideration. However, the downstream process time could be shortened because of the ease in separating the biomass and medium. The ajmalicine production processes that could be developed using this technique would give a price comparable with that for the production process with spontaneous release from free cells.

RESULTS OF THE COST ESTIMATES

Comparing the various process options (Table 23.12), it is obvious that single use of biomass in a batch process is the most economic approach. The continuous processes are more expensive than batch processes in our analysis. This is caused by the lower biomass concentration assumed for the continuous processes, which is necessary to enable the separation of the product-containing liquid phase from the broth. The negative effect of the lower biomass concentration is not compensated by the multiple use of the biomass, because the biomass costs have only a limited contribution to the total costs in the analysed processes.

In fact, at the core of the economic problem are the costs of the investment in equipment. The return on investment is determined by the productivity of the system, which is the amount of product produced per time and volume (kg m^{-3} day^{-1}). Alternative process options become interesting only if the productivity can be improved to make the process competitive. A comparison between the ajmalicine and the berberine data clearly shows that the use of traditional methods to enhance media and process conditions can already give significant improvement in the productivity and process costs.

23.5.8 Conclusions

Plant cell cultures on a large scale are feasible for industrial production processes. However, for the presently commercially interesting phytochemicals, only a few processes have been successfully developed. For the others, the productivity is too low to compete with existing production methods. As the markets for most of the products are well established, and the profits small, little money is available to invest in a new biotechnological production system.

In the coming years, new plant products will certainly come out of the high-throughput screening programmes now being used to find new biologically active compounds (see Chapter 12). This will eventually result in new plant-derived drugs. Plant cell cultures offer the possibility of producing materials at least during the first phases of drug development, after which other production methods can then be considered and eventually may be the method of choice for production. This would avoid problems such as have been encountered with achieving an adequate supply of paclitaxel in recent years.

Metabolic engineering is, in this context, an important tool to improve the plant cell factory for production of desired phytochemicals. It can be used both for plants and plant cell cultures, and even short pathways (bioconversions) can be introduced into microorganisms. However, more basic knowledge about the pathways involved in their biosynthesis and in their regulation is still needed.

23.6 | Further reading

Alfermann, A. W. and Petersen, M. Natural product formation by plant cell biotechnology: results and perspectives. *Plant Cell Tissue and Organ Culture* **43**: 199–205, 1995.

DiCosmo, F. and Misawa, M. (Eds.) *Plant Cell Culture Secondary Metabolism. Toward Industrial Application.* Boca Raton, Fl., CRC Press, 1996.

Doran, P. M. (Ed.) *Hairy Roots: Culture and Applications.* Amsterdam: Harwood Academic, 1997.

Giri, A. and Narasu, M. L. Transgenic hairy roots: recent trends and applications. *Biotechnology Advances* **18**: 1–22, 2000.

Oksman-Caldentey, K.-M. and Barz, W. H. *Plant Biotechnology and Transgenic Plants.* New York: Marcel Dekker, 2002.

Schlatmann, J. E., ten Hoopen, H. J. G. and Heijnen, J. J. A simple structured model for maintenance, biomass formation, and ajmalicine production by nondividing *Catharanthus roseus* cells. *Biotechnology and Bioengineering* **66**: 147–157, 1999.

Spier, R. E. (Ed.) *Encyclopedia of Cell Technology.* New York: John Wiley & Sons, 2000.

Su, W. W. Bioprocessing technology for plant cell suspension cultures. *Applied Biochemistry and Biotechnology* **50**: 189–230, 1995.

Verpoorte, R. and Alfermann, A. W. (Eds.) *Metabolic Engineering of Plant Secondary Metabolism.* Dordrecht: Kluwer Academic, 2000.

Verpoorte, R., Contin, A. and Memelink, J. Biotechnology for the production of plant secondary metabolites. *Phytochemistry Reviews* **1**: 13–25, 2002.

Verpoorte, R., van der Heijden, R., van Gulik, W. M. and ten Hoopen, H. J. G. Plant biotechnology for the production of alkaloids: present status and prospects. In *The Alkaloids*, Vol. 40, ed. A. Brossi. San Diego, CA: Academic Press, pp. 1–187, 1991.

Verpoorte, R., van der Heijden, R., ten Hoopen, H. J. G. and Memelink, J. Metabolic engineering of plant secondary metabolite pathways for the production of fine chemicals. *Biotechnology Letters* **21**: 467–479, 1999.

Chapter 24

Biotransformations

Pedro Fernandes
Instituto Superior Técnico, Lisbon

Joaquim M. S. Cabral
Instituto Superior Técnico, Lisbon

24.1 | Introduction

Biotransformation deals with the use of biological catalysts to convert a substrate into a product in a limited number of enzymatic steps. The establishment of an efficient biotransformation process requires the extensive examination of factors affecting the development of optimal biocatalysts, reaction media and bioreactors (Fig. 24.1).

The chemical industry currently takes advantage of enzyme technology in various sectors, namely in the food, pharmaceutical and detergents sectors. An on-going trend towards the implementation of commercial processes based on the use of biocatalysts in other areas (e.g. polymers, fine and agricultural chemicals, and miscellaneous chemicals) is noticeable. It is foreseeable that in the near future the use of biocatalysts in these fields will be enhanced which, coupled to the already established bioprocesses, will further broaden the overall impact of biocatalysis in the chemical industry. When compared to equivalent chemical processes, bioprocesses are simpler,

Basic Biotechnology, third edition, eds. Colin Ratledge and Bjørn Kristiansen.
Published by Cambridge University Press. © Cambridge University Press 2006.

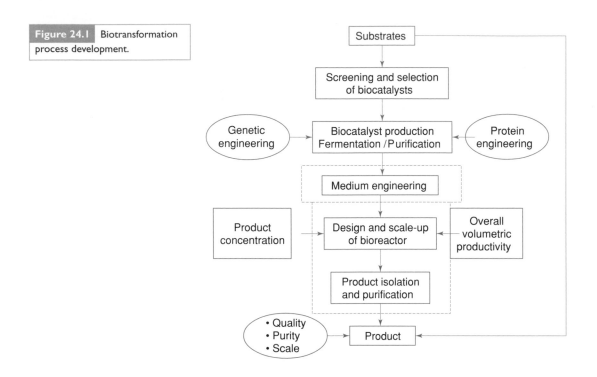

Figure 24.1 Biotransformation process development.

less demanding in raw materials and in energy, lead to higher quality products (i.e. with fewer impurities) and produce higher yields, lower the involvement of toxic wastes and decrease the emission of wastewater. Such features decrease production costs and, since bioprocesses easily comply with the stringent environmental legislation in highly regulated countries, these processes are given a competitive edge when matched up to conventional (chemical) methods. In many cases, near-term benefits will increase as the market penetration of the product and process continues to grow, leading to further cost reduction and performance improvements relative to competing products and processes. Some representative examples of successful applications of biocatalysts in industry are given in Table 24.1.

Biological catalysts when compared with chemical catalysts have the advantages of their regioselectivity and stereospecificity, which lead to single enantiomeric products with regulatory requisites for pharmaceutical, food and agricultural use. They are also energy effective catalysts working at moderate temperatures, pressures and pH values.

Biotransformations have been performed by a variety of biological catalysts, such as isolated enzymes, immobilised enzymes and cells. The developments of recombinant DNA technology have led to improvements in the enzyme production in different host organisms giving the bioprocess engineer a greater choice of biocatalyst option.

The optimal biocatalyst must be selective, active and stable under operational conditions in the bioreactor, which may not be necessarily conventional in terms of composition, concentration, pressure and

Table 24.1 | Examples of commercial-scale bioprocesses

Class	Product	Substrate	Biocatalyst	Company	Scale (tons a^{-1})
Alcohols, amides and amines	Acrylamide	Acrylonitrile	*Rhodococcus rhodochrous* J1 cells entrapped in polyacrylamide	Mitsubishi Rayon Co., Ltd	20 000
	Enantiomerically pure alcohols	Racemic primary aminoalcohols	Immobilised lipases	BASF	1 000
	Chiral amines	Racemic amines	Immobilised lipases	BASF	>2 000
Amino acids	L-Methionine, L-Tryptophan, L-Phenylalanine, L-Valine	Acyl-D,L-amino acids	Aminoacylase ionic binding to DEAE-Sephadex	Tanabe	6–21[a]
	L-Alanine	Fumaric acid and ammonia	*E. coli* and *Pseudomonas dacunhae* cells entrapped in κ-carrageenan	Tanabe	100[b]
	L-Aspartic acid	Fumaric acid and ammonia	*E. coli* cells entrapped in κ-carrageenan. Immobilised ammonia lyase	Tanabe DSM	100[b] 1 000
Antibiotics	7-Aminocephalosporanic acid	Cephalosporin C	D-amino acid oxidase	Biochemie (Novartis)	~2 000
	6-Aminopenicillanic acid	Penicillin G/V	Immobilised penicillin acylase	DSM	6 000
Lactams	(−)-Lactam, intermediate for the production of carbovir™ and abacavir™	Racemic lactam	Recombinant γ-lactamase	ChiroTech (Dow Chemicals)	10s

(cont.)

Table 24.1 (cont.)

Class	Product	Substrate	Biocatalyst	Company	Scale (tons a⁻¹)
N-Heterocyclic chemicals	cis-3R-(acetyloxy)-4-phenyl-2-azetidinone acetate (intermediate in the synthesis of paclitaxel, Taxol)	Racemic acetate cis-3-(acetyloxy)-4-phenyl-2-azetidinone	Immobilised lipase	Bristol–Myers–Squibb	–[c]
	6-Hydroxynicotinic acid	3-Cyanopyridine	Mutants of *Agrobacterium* sp. DSM 6336	Lonza	N.a.
	Niacinamide	3-Cyanopyridine	*Rhodococcus rhodochrous* J1 cells	Guangzhou Fine Chemicals/Lonza	3 000
	Nicotinamide	3-Cyanopyridine	*Rhodococcus rhodochrous* J1 cells entrapped in polyacrylamide	Lonza	4 000
Polymers	Cyclodextrins	Starch	Enzymatic conversion	Wacker Specialties	3 000
	Polyurethane	Residues of an aliphatic hydroxy carboxylic acid	Lipase bound to a macroporous acrylic resin	Baxenden	2
	Polylactic acid	Unrefined dextrose		Cargill Dow LLC	140 000
Sweeteners	Aspartame	N-Protected L-aspartic acid, D/L-phenylalanine methyl ester	Immobilised thermolysine	Holland Sweetener Company	1 000
	High-fructose syrups	Maize	α-Amylase, amyloglucosidase, pullulanase, immobilised glucose isomerase	A. E. Staley, ADM, Cargill	23 000 000
Vitamins	Riboflavin (Vitamin B2)	Glucose	*Bacillus subtilis* (mutant)	Hoffman La-Roche	2 000

Miscellaneous compounds in agriculture and health

Product	Substrate	Biocatalyst	Company	Production (tonnes)
Androstenedione	Sitosterol	Mycobacterium spp. mutants	Schering	1 000
L-Carnitine	4-Butyrobetaine	Rhyzobia spp. mutants	Lonza	
S-2 Chlorpropionic acid (CPA) (agricultural intermediate)	Racemic CPA	Recombinant Pseudomonas spp	Avecia	2 000
5-Cyanovaleramide, intermediate for the production of the herbicide Milestone™	Adiponitrile	Pseudomonas chlororaphis B23 entrapped in calcium alginate beads	Commercial–DuPont	130
5-Hydroxypyrazinecarboxylic acid	2-Cyanopyrazine	Whole cells of Agrobacterium DSM 6336	Lonza	
S-Ibuprofen (non-steroidal anti-inflammatory drug)	Racemic ibuprofen	Immobilised lipase (hollow fiber membrane)	Sepracor	–[c]
S-Naproxen (non-steroidal anti-inflammatory drug)	Racemic naproxen methyl ester	Esterase	Chiroscience	–[d]
(+)-(2S,3R)-trans-3-(4-methoxy-phenyl)-glycidic acid methylester (Diltiazem precursor)	Racemic mixture	Immobilised lipase	Tanabe BASF	–[e]

(cont.)

Table 24.1 | (*cont.*)

Class	Product	Substrate	Biocatalyst	Company	Scale (tons a^{-1})
Miscellaneous uses in environment, food and pulp and paper areas	Pulp bleaching	Hydrolyse the xylan polymer	Xylanase	Domtar; Oji Paper and other paper mills	
	Vegetable oil degumming Water and oxygen	Seed oils Hydrogen peroxide	Phospholipase A2 Catalase	Cereol/Lurgi Windel Textil GmbH and Co.	
	ZnS (solid)	ZnSO$_4$ (aqueous)	Sulphate-reducing bacteria	Budel Zink	8.5 daily of ZnS

[a] Tons per month in continuous process.
[b] Ton per month.
[c] Multi-kelogramme scale.
[d] Tons per year.
[e] Several 100 tons per year.

temperature. In particular, it is necessary to evaluate the biocatalyst performance in non-conventional media (e.g. organic solvents and super-critical fluids).

A key issue is the availability of suitable biocatalysts. More rational screening and selection techniques are required to: (a) isolate biocatalysts, e.g. enzymes and cells, able to catalyse novel reactions of industrial interest; and (b) select and design catalysts suitable for industrial use with improved operational stabilities and kinetic properties. This requires a much greater understanding of the mechanisms of protein denaturation and decay of catalytic activities under process conditions and an evaluation of methods to maintain and improve biocatalyst stability, e.g. chemical modification, immobilisation and protein engineering.

In the optimisation of the overall process, it is also important to enhance the predictability and performance of the biocatalyst in the reaction media, in particular in multi-phasic media involving a solid phase, e.g. an immobilised biocatalyst, and one (aqueous) or two (aqueous and organic) liquid phases. It is very important to obtain reliable data and models on physical/chemical transport and interfacial phenomena. Medium engineering plays an important role in the definition of the optimal biocatalyst operation and to evaluate the effect of medium composition on the biocatalyst.

The optimal bioreactor should be simple, safe, well controlled, easy to design and flexible. The design of bioreactors requires knowledge of reaction kinetics as well as fluid dynamics, substrate dispersion and mass transfer. In addition, for multi-phase bioreactions, interfacial phenomena, substrate and product partitioning, and separation of two liquid phases should also be taken into account.

24.2 | Biocatalyst selection

A better and deeper understanding of fundamental biology and enzymology, coupled to the development of bioinformatics and of high-throughput methods, are broadening the field of biocatalysis, besides enhancing the impact of enzyme technology in industry. Comprehensive databases assembling data on enzymes, such as BRENDA (http://www.brenda.uni-koeln.de), are being rapidly developed. This trend is expected to be further enhanced since fully automated high-throughput crystallography systems have been put into use, enabling a faster (less than 100 hours) determination of protein structure. Besides, databases dedicated to the determination of the three-dimensional structure of proteins have been developed (e.g. http://www.structuralgenomics.org). The development of robotics and software, together with improved and fully automated analytical tools improved the methodologies for biocatalyst screening and improvement (see also Chapter 12).

After selecting an appropriate starting material to be converted into the product, it is necessary to select the appropriate biocatalyst with suitable activity, selectivity and stability to work under the required operational conditions (temperature, salt concentration, pH, organic solvents, substrate and product concentrations). Several strategies can be followed to obtain the biocatalyst for the pertinent biotransformation: (a) screening for novel biocatalysts, (b) use of existing biocatalysts and (c) genetic modification of existing biocatalysts.

24.2.1 Screening for novel biocatalysts

Selection of new micro-organisms with novel activities is still worthwhile taking into account the overwhelming biochemical diversity present in nature. The screening of large numbers of organisms requires that cheap, simple, rapid and selective detection methods, preferably capable of some automation, should be available to facilitate this usually tedious process.

Selective selection methods for colonies on plates can be very useful, as shown for the isolation of micro-organisms able to hydroxylate L-tyrosine to L-DOPA, a drug used in the treatment of Parkinson's disease. The colonies that produce L-DOPA turn violet–black as a result of the reaction of L-DOPA with ferrous ions added to the agar plates.

Microbial selection has also been performed in the presence of high concentrations of the target compound. This approach was used to isolate benzoic-acid-assimilating strains for the production of *cis,cis*-muconic acid from benzoic acid. Similar approaches have been followed to isolate nitrile-hydrolysing enzymes, such as nitrile hydratase, nitrilase and amidase, which have great potential as catalysts for producing high-value amides and acids from the corresponding nitriles.

The resistance to organic solvents is often an important criterion in the selection of a suitable biocatalyst. *Pseudomonas* strains have been isolated with the ability to grow in the presence of toluene and aromatic and aliphatic hydrocarbons and long chain alcohols. These strains and their enzymatic activities are therefore important biocatalytic sources for the degradation of harmful compounds as well as for the synthesis of important chiral compounds. Extremophiles have been receiving a great deal of attention. These microorganisms that thrive in extreme environments are likely to provide biocatalysts able to cope with the often harsh industrial reaction conditions. Different types of extremophiles have been identified, namely thermophiles, hyper-thermophiles, psychrophiles, halophiles, alkaliphiles, acidophiles and piezophiles.

24.2.2 Use of existing biocatalysts

A well-known way to accomplish a desired biotransformation is the use of existing biocatalysts (e.g. commercial enzymes) on natural and unnatural substrates. The substrate specificities of lipases and proteases are currently under intense investigations. The hydrolytic capacity of lipases is not restricted only to triacylglycerols. This type of enzyme is also able to hydrolyse mono-, di- and tri-acyl esters with different chain lengths of the various acyl groups.

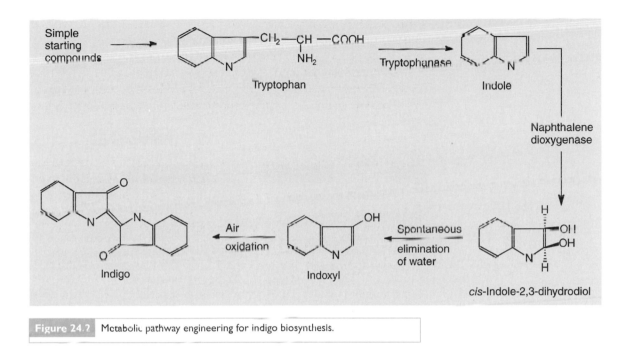

Figure 24.2 Metabolic pathway engineering for indigo biosynthesis.

The exploitation of existing enzymes under different reaction conditions could lead to the finding of a biocatalyst for the desired biotransformation. For example, lipases have been used to perform synthetic reactions in media under controlled water activity, e.g. esterification, inter-esterification and trans-esterification reactions. Methods to optimise the enantioselectivity of lipases have been reported, namely the non-covalent modification of lipase and the control of the surface tension of an emulsion.

24.2.3 Genetic modification of existing biocatalysts

A distinct way to obtain a biocatalyst is by in vivo (*metabolic pathway engineering*) and in vitro (*protein engineering*) construction of a novel biocatalyst. In vivo genetic engineering has been applied in large scale to obtain a recombinant organism with the desired enzymatic activity. Mutational events leading to the novel enzyme activities include transfer of genes, gene duplication, gene fusion, recombination between genes, deletion or insertion of gene segments, and one or more single-site mutations, or combination of these activities. An example of this metabolic pathway engineering is the production of dyes, such as the indigo biosynthesis in *E. coli* (Fig. 24.2). By assembling, on a single operon genes encoding for tryptophan formation, the gene specifying tryptophanase and a fragment of the NAH plasmid of a *Pseudomonas* encoding the naphthalene dioxygenase, a recombinant *E. coli* was obtained that was able to synthesise indigo from simple starting compounds.

Another example is the production of cortisol from glucose, using genetically engineered *Saccharomyces cerevisiae* cells. An artificial

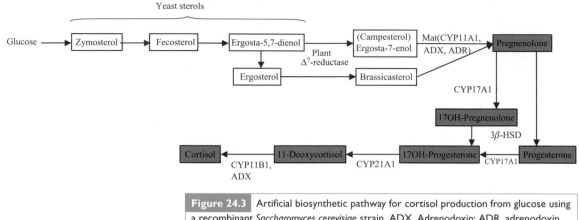

Figure 24.3 Artificial biosynthetic pathway for cortisol production from glucose using a recombinant *Saccharomyces cerevisiae* strain. ADX, Adrenodoxin; ADR, adrenodoxin reductase; β-HSD, 3-β-hydroxysteroid dehydrogenase (adapted from Szczebara, F. N., Chandelier, C., Villeret, C., *et al.*, 2003. Total biosynthesis of hydrocortisone from a single carbon source in yeast. *Nature Biotechnology* **21**: 143–149).

biosynthetic pathway involving 13 engineered genes was expressed in a single *S. cerevisiae* strain. The total biosynthetic pathway for cortisol production involved the natural endogenous yeast biosynthetic pathway, the re-route of the pathway using plant Δ^7-reductase and additional enzymatic steps catalysed by eight mammalian proteins, which mimic the adrenal synthesis of cortisol. The exogenous mammalian enzymes included mature and mitochondrial adrenodoxin, mitochondrial CYP11B1, mature adrenodoxin reductase and CYP11A11, 3-β-hydroxysteroid dehydrogenase, CYP17A1 and CYP21A1. CYP enzymes belong to the P450 superfamily of monooxygenases (for details on P450 check http://www.icgeb.org./~p450srv/). Adrenodoxin and adrenodoxin reductase are electron carriers. The further modulation of the two mitochondrial systems, the metabolic flux equilibration and the disruption of the unwanted side reaction related to three gene products, enabled the production of cortisol from a simple carbon source (e.g. glucose; Fig. 24.3).

Another approach is the use of protein engineering to modify an existing protein/enzyme or create *de novo* a protein of pre-specified properties. The protein engineering process can be viewed as an interactive cycle of several interconnected steps (protein engineering cycle). The aim of protein engineering has been to elucidate the structure–function relationship of proteins and to use this information to develop novel/modified proteins (enzymes) with improved characteristics for process applications. An elucidative example is the design of subtilisin mutants with altered properties (substrate specificity and pH activity profile) and improved thermal and oxidative stabilities. For example, in subtilisin BPN′, two methionines, Met[124] and Met[222], are especially susceptible to oxidation. To prevent the negative influence caused by the formation of methionine sulphoxide, Met can be replaced, using site-directed mutagenesis, by a non-oxidative amino acid, such as Ala, Ser or Leu, without losing more than 12–53% of the initial activity. The mutant Met^{222}– Ala^{222} is currently in use as a commercial detergent enzyme: Durazyme.

Biocatalyst engineering and biosynthetic pathway engineering gained considerably from directed evolution technology, since this provides an effective tool to optimise enzymatic activity rapidly and without need for structural or mechanistic information. In an iterative Darwinian optimisation algorithm, molecular diversity is created by random mutagenesis and/or recombination of target gene or family of related genes. Genes encoding for improved variants are identified by high-throughput screening methods (see Chapter 13) and used as parents for a further round of evolution. This tool has been used to develop biocatalysts with enhanced stability, such as N-carbamyl-D-amino-acid amidohydrolase from *Agrobacterium tumefaciens*, an enzyme currently used in the industrial production of D-amino-acids, or horseradish peroxidase; to enhance stability and activity, characteristic of variants of mesophilic subtilisin E, psychrophilic subtilisin S41, and mesophilic p-nitrobenzyl esterase. Catalytic activity can also be improved, as observed in variants of benzoylformate decarboxylase from *Pseudomonas putida*, which have a five-fold greater carboligase activity than the wild-type enzyme. An increase in the oxidation activity of toluene *ortho*-monooxygenase of *Burkholderia cepacia* G4 for both chlorinated ethenes and naphthalene was also achieved. Altered substrate specificity, allowing galactose oxidase to use glucose as substrate could also be accomplished. Other goals that were attained through this approach include increased specificity, as observed with D-selective hydantoinase mutants (90% *ee*) obtained from a wild type with D selectivity of 40% *ee*; to change stereoselectivity, as shown by a variant of D-hydantoinase from *Arthrobacter* sp. DSM 9771 towards L-5-(2-methylthioethyl)hydantoin; novel specificity and activity, as displayed by triazine hydrolase variants that were able to hydrolyse triazines that were not substrates for the original enzyme, or by a mutant toluene dioxygenase able to accept 4-picoline as substrate for its conversion to its 3-hydroxy derivative. Directed evolution of pathways has been used to increase two-fold carotenoid production in *E. coli*; to create novel carotenoid compounds; to evolve *Rhodobacter sphaeroides* phytoene desaturase, a neurosporene-producing enzyme; to produce lycopene; or to increase the yield of *cis*-(1S,2R)-indandiol, a precursor in an engineered biosynthetic pathway for the production of Crixivan, a pharmaceutical product, by a toluene dioxygenase variant from *P. putida*.

The development of large libraries of mutant biocatalysts, created by directed evolution demands experimental power to access activity, which is basically done by measuring the conversion of substrate to product by some means. Such high-throughput experiments, where several hundreds or thousands of samples must be analysed each day, involve such an enormous task that the analyses can only be effectively dealt with by the development of simple chromogenic or fluorogenic tests, since high-pressure liquid chromatography (HPLC), gas chromatography (GC) and nuclear magnetic resonance (NMR) are often impractical for they are too slow and too expensive. (These aspects of high-throughput screening are covered in detail in Chapter 12.)

24.3 | Biocatalyst immobilisation and performance

24.3.1 Biocatalyst immobilisation

The immobilisation of biocatalysts for laboratory studies, analytical and medical applications and large-scale industrial processes is presently a widespread technique. Immobilisation can be defined as the confinement of a biocatalyst inside a bioreaction system, with retention of its catalytic activity and stability, and which can be used repeatedly and continuously. Table 24.2 lists some advantages and limitations that can arise from the use of immobilised biocatalysts.

The biocatalysts that can be immobilised range from purified enzymes to viable microbial cells, animal and plant tissues. Isolated enzymes can give high activities per unit mass or mole, high specificity and minimum side reactions. They are, however, often difficult and costly to prepare. In addition, they are frequently unstable and, in many cases, require parallel co-factor regenerating systems. Due to their relatively simple chemical nature, as compared to organelles or whole cells, isolated or partially purified enzymes are the biocatalysts most extensively studied in relation to immobilisation. Immobilised, purified enzymes find suitable applications in developing biosensors and preparing high added-value substances, such as chiral compounds. In more crude forms, immobilised enzymes are also used in large-scale applications in the carbohydrate, food and pharmaceutical industries.

Multi-enzyme systems, such as organelles, whole cells or cell tissues, have some clear advantages for immobilisation over isolated enzymes. They can be efficiently retained by mild, physical means, preserving, in adequate conditions, the enzyme-synthesising and co-factor regenerating capabilities and producing a suitable microenvironment for single and multiple enzymatic activities. However, the efficient use of immobilised cells relies on the control of metabolic and physiological alterations throughout the retention procedure and the subsquent catalytic process. The major large-scale utilisations of immobilised cell systems take advantage of the natural tendency of many microbial species to flocculate or to adhere to solid surfaces. Other applications are restricted to single-enzyme transformations with non-growing cells in the manufacture of pharmaceuticals and amino acids.

24.3.2 Methods for biocatalyst immobilisation

A wide range of basic immobilisation procedures with their specific variations has been described in a large number of reviews. Several classification schemes have also been proposed, one of which is given in Fig. 24.4.

Table 24.2 Advantages and limitations of the use of immobilised biocatalysts

General aspects		Specific aspects
Advantages		
Retention of the biocatalyst in the bioreactor		Possible biocatalyst re-use
		Product contamination avoided
		High dilution rates allowed without biocatalyst wash-out
High biocatalyst concentration		Increased volumetric productivity
		Rapid conversion of unstable substrates
		Minimised side reactions
Control of biocatalyst microenvironment		Manipulation of biocatalyst activity and specificity
		Stabilisation of biocatalyst activity
		Protection of shear-sensitive biocatalysts
Facilitated separation of the biocatalyst from the product		Precise control of bioreaction time
		Minimisation of further product transformation
Limitations		
Increased costs of biocatalyst production		Increased requirements of materials and equipment
		Need for specific reactor configurations
Loss of biocatalyst activity during immobilisation	Biocatayst-related	Exposure to pH and temperature extremes
		Exposure to toxic reactants
		Exposure to high shear or mechanical strain
	Microenvironment related	Exclusion of macromolecular substrates
		Blocking of the enzymatic active site
		Local pH shifts
		Mass transfer limitations
Loss of biocatalyst activity during bioreactor operation	Leakage of biocatalyst	Matrix erosion or solubilisation
		Small support particles carried in the outflow
		Cell growth inside the matrix
		Broad pore-size range
	Matrix poisoning or fouling	Build-up of inhibitors in the microenvironment
		Retention of suspended solids
		Growth of contaminating species (biofilms)
		Need for a stricter control of feed composition
Empiricism		Need for case specific, multi-parameter optimisation
		Difficult process modelling and control

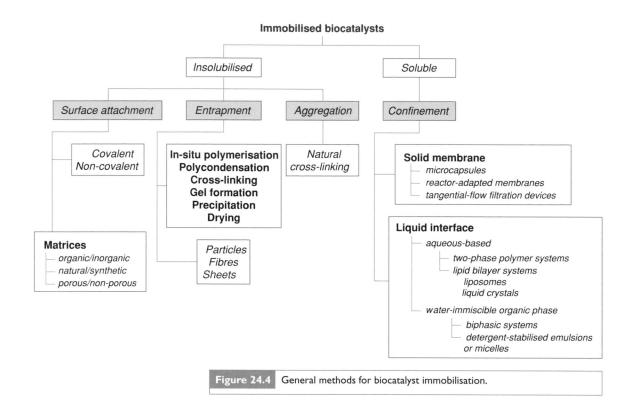

Figure 24.4 General methods for biocatalyst immobilisation.

Cross-linking with bifunctional reagents

Both cells and enzymes can be covalently cross-linked with bi- or multi-functional reagents, such as aldehydes or amines. However, the toxicity of these reagents limits their applicability to the immobilisation of non-viable cells and enzymes. This method produces three-dimensional, cross-linked enzyme aggregates, which are then insoluble in water. Glutaraldehyde has been the most extensively used cross-linking reagent, which reacts with the lysyl residues of the enzyme forming a Schiff's base:

$$\text{Enzyme-NH}_2 + \text{OHC(CH}_2)_3\,\text{CHO} + \text{H}_2\text{N-Enzyme} \rightarrow$$
$$\text{Enzyme-N}\!=\!\text{CH(CH}_2)_3\text{CH}\!=\!\text{N-Enzyme}$$

The linkages formed between enzyme and glutaraldehyde are irreversible and survive extreme values of pH and temperature, which suggests that the aldimine bond is stabilised.

Biocatalyst cross-linking with glutaraldehyde is critically dependent on a delicate balance of factors such as the concentration of the biocatalyst and cross-linking reagent, pH and ionic strength of the aqueous solution, temperature and time of reaction. The most important advantage of this method is that only a single reagent is required and the reaction is easy to carry out. Furthermore, biocatalyst immobilisation on a carrier often leads to a loss of native activity. Besides, a large mass fraction, roughly 90 to 99.9%, of the solid support used as carrier is free of biocatalytic activity. This leads to lower space-time yields and lower productivity. The use of carrier-free immobilised enzymes provides an approach to overcome such drawbacks, while maintaining the advantages of biocatalyst immobilisation. They are prepared by direct cross-linking of enzyme preparations. These may be in the form of aggregates, crystalline enzymes, dissolved enzymes or spray-dried enzymes. The various cross-linking methods therefore give rise to: *cross-linked enzyme aggregates* (CLEAs), *cross-linked enzyme crystals* (CLECs), *cross-linked enzymes* (CLEs) and *cross-linked spray-dried enzymes* (CSDEs).

Carrier-free immobilised enzymes generally display specific volumetric activities that are 10–1000 times greater than the corresponding carrier-bound immobilised enzymes. They are also highly stabilised against unnatural conditions, such as heating and organic solvents. Application of this approach includes immobilisation of penicillin G amidase, thermolysin, elastase, asparaginase, lipase, lysozyme, glucoamylase and urease as CLECs, trypsin and papain as CLEs, and penicillin acylase as CLEA.

Supported immobilisation methods

The available methods for biocatalyst immobilisation, involving solid supports, fall into two general categories: *surface attachment* and *lattice entrapment*. By surface attachment, the enzyme, organelle or cell is bound to a solid interface through interactions that range from weak van der Waals forces essentially to irreversible, covalent bonding. The milder interactions can result from direct contact, in suitable conditions, between the biocatalyst and a natural, unmodified surface. However, the versatility and effectiveness of surface immobilisation have been greatly increased by introducing synthetic carriers and chemical modifications to natural and fabricated matrices. In lattice entrapment, a chemical or physical solidification process is induced in a solution containing the biocatalyst, ideally resulting in a water-insoluble lattice retaining the biocatalyst in its active or viable form. Mechanisms like polymerisation, thermal gelation or precipitation can be employed in this type of procedure. Figures 24.5 and 24.6 give a general overview of biocatalysts, supports and retention methods used in surface attachment and entrapment

Supports for biocatalyst immobilisation

The development of a useful, support-immobilised biocatalyst necessarily involves a choice of a solid support. Ideally, this selection step should be based on established structural and activity data for the biocatalyst and the general immobilisation method to be used, and process conditions. The important factors for examining a broad range of possible supports are summarised in Tables 24.3 and 24.4. Because several factors have usually to be considered when integrating biocatalyst immobilisation in a process, the optimal solution is frequently a compromise. In view of this, a support with a more flexible character is most often used. For example, a porous support can immobilise large biocatalyst loads; however, to avoid diffusional limitations, this same

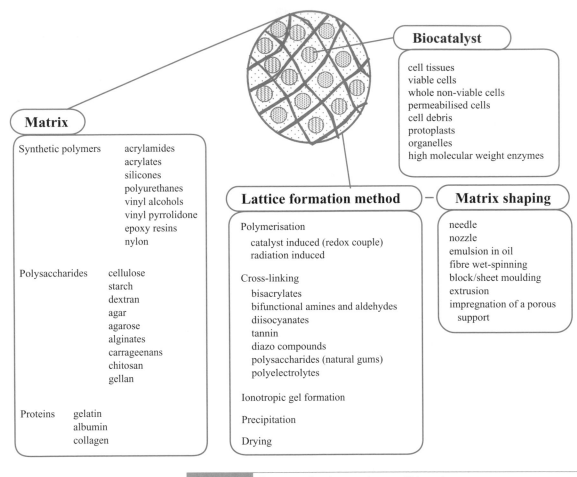

Biocatalyst

cell tissues
viable cells
whole non-viable cells
permeabilised cells
cell debris
protoplasts
organelles
high molecular weight enzymes

Matrix

Synthetic polymers   acrylamides
                     acrylates
                     silicones
                     polyurethanes
                     vinyl alcohols
                     vinyl pyrrolidone
                     epoxy resins
                     nylon

Polysaccharides   cellulose
                     starch
                     dextran
                     agar
                     agarose
                     alginates
                     carrageenans
                     chitosan
                     gellan

Proteins   gelatin
              albumin
              collagen

Lattice formation method – **Matrix shaping**

Polymerisation
    catalyst induced (redox couple)
    radiation induced

Cross-linking
    bisacrylates
    bifunctional amines and aldehydes
    diisocyanates
    tannin
    diazo compounds
    polysaccharides (natural gums)
    polyelectrolytes

Ionotropic gel formation

Precipitation

Drying

needle
nozzle
emulsion in oil
fibre wet-spinning
block/sheet moulding
extrusion
impregnation of a porous
    support

Figure 24.5   Overview of surface attachment of biocatalysts.

support should be used as very small particles (see Section 24.3.3). In other cases, a single or a few factors determine the choice of the support. Such is the case of systems where the aim is to preserve biocatalytic activity in the presence of aggressive components in the reaction medium, such as toxic species, organic solvents or strong inhibitors. With these systems, a porous matrix entrapping the bio-catalyst and excluding the inhibitor is often the only efficient choice, regardless of the diffusional hindrances slowing down the reaction. Here, the possibility of changing the shape, porosity or hydrophobi-city of the support can be advantageous in fine-tuning substrate or non-substrate size exclusion and external and internal mass transfer rates.

Organic polymers are the most widely employed supports for bio-catalyst immobilisation (for examples, see Figs. 24.5 and 24.6). This preference derives from the adaptability of these supports to nearly all kinds of surface-binding or entrapment techniques and to the broad variety of their chemical and physical characteristics. Their

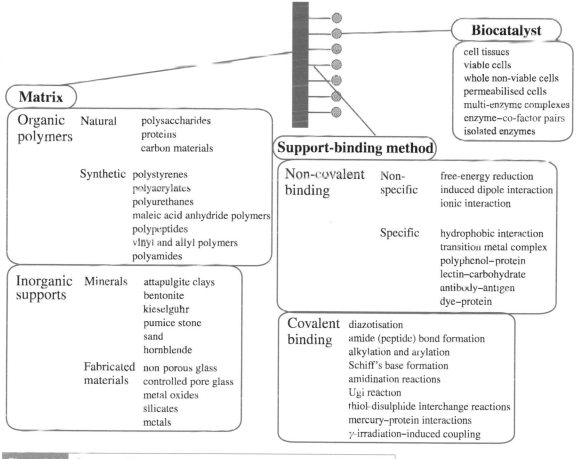

Figure 24.6 Overview of lattice entrapment of biocatalysts.

major drawbacks come from insufficient mechanical and chemical resistances, which limit both their use under harsher conditions and their regenerability.

Adsorption and ionic binding

Adsorption on a support is the oldest and simplest retention method for biocatalysts, involving no previous modification of the solid surface and relying on weak interactions of van der Waals, electrostatic, hydrophobic or hydrogen-bond types. This is a low-cost procedure largely retaining the native conformation of an immobilised enzyme and its intrinsic catalytic activity. The general application of physical adsorption methods is, however, severely limited by the reversible nature of the biocatalyst-support bond, which is critically dependent on process conditions, such as temperature, pH, ionic strength and dielectric constant. This factor makes it difficult to operate large-scale bioreactors without significant biocatalyst leakage, which then result in loss of productivity and product contamination. On the other hand, reversible adsorption methods allow straightforward regeneration of

Table 24.3 Important aspects in the chemical nature of potential supports for biocatalyst immobilisation

| | Chemical nature/Origin[a] | | | |
| | Organic | | Inorganic | |
	Natural	Synthetic	Mineral	Fabricated
Availability of reactive functional groups				
Usable with large variety of biocatalysts	++	+++	+	+
Wide range of techniques for surface activation	++	+++	+	+
Commercially available pre-activated supports	+++	++	−	+
Usable with lattice formation techniques	+++	+++	−	−
Possibility of adjusting hydrophilic/hydrophobic character	+	+++	+	+
Sensitivity to physical, chemical and microbial agents				
Resistance to changes in reaction medium composition (pH, ionic strength, organic media)	+	++	+++	+++
Resistance to high temperatures	−	+	+++	+++
Resistance to large hydrostatic or hydrodynamic pressures	−	++	+++	+++
Regenerability	−	+	+++	++
Low cost/availability	+++	+	+++	+
Obtainable support morphology				
Usable diameter or thickness ranges	++	+++	+	+++
Available porosity ranges	+	++	++	++
Obtainable shapes				
Sphere	++	++	−	+++
Fibre	++	+++	−	+++
Sheet/membrane	++	+++	−	+++

[a] −, Inadequate; +, poor; ++, fair; +++, good.

the supports. After adsorption, the enzyme may be cross-linked; however, this limits the possibility of reusing the support.

A growing field for applying physically adsorbed enzymes is non-aqueous biocatalysis. By using an organic solvent in which the protein is insoluble, an enzyme bound to a carrier by simple adsorption undergoes virtually no desorption in prolonged processes. A lipase from *Rhizomucor miehei* was adsorbed on a polyacrylate support with a very high activity retention (90%) and used in hydrolytic and synthetic reactions. An industrial example is the use of a *Rhizopus* lipase adsorbed onto Celite for the continuous production of cocoa butter-like fats in organic media. Other applications include the immobilisation of xylanase on Eudragit L-100 for the degradation of xylan or the immobilisation of catalase on poly(2-hydroxyethylmethacrylate) (pHEMA) based flat sheet membranes, the adsorption of lipases to Sepabeads to be used in hydrolytic reactions, the oxidation of resveratrol catalysed by a laccase adsorbed onto glass beads, or the adsorption of subtilisin and α-chymotrypsin on standard silica chromatography

Table 24.4 Important aspects of the morphology of potential supports for biocatalyst immobilisation

Characteristics	Morphology[a]	
	Porous	Non-porous
Total surface area available per unit weight	+++	+
Low incidence of diffusional limitations	+	+++
Attainable biocatalyst load	+++	+
Biocatalyst protection from external aggressions	++	+
Usable with macromolecular substrates	+	+++

	Fabricated			
	Mineral	Inorganic	Gel	
Pore size uniformity	+	+++	++	Na.
Pore size stability	++	+++	+	Na.
Low cost	+++	−	++	+++

[a] −, inadequate; +, poor; ++, fair; +++, good.

gel leading to a 1000-fold enhancement in catalytic activity in aceto-nitrile and tetrahydrofuran as compared to the respective freeze-dried enzyme powders.

A slightly stronger biocatalyst–support linkage can be achieved by the use of ionic supports. Their advantages and limitations are mostly the same as those of physical adsorption. The stability of the established ionic bonds is particularly sensitive to pH and ionic strength. Glucose isomerase from *Streptomyces rubiginous* was adsorbed onto an anion-exchange resin consisting of DEAE-cellulose agglomerated with polystyrene and TiO_2. This process was industrially implemented for the isomerisation of glucose into fructose. Other examples are the immobilisation of β-galactosidase on to an anionic exchanger resin, which was based on coating the internal surfaces of commercial beads (Sepabeads) with polyethylenimine (PEI). The preparation was then used for the hydrolysis of lactose. Similarly, keratinase has been immobilised on Dowex and DEAE-cellulose for the hydrolysis of different proteinaceous substrates.

Covalent coupling of enzymes
Probably the most thoroughly investigated approach to enzyme immobilisation involves covalent binding of amino acid residues in the protein to reactive groups in the support. In principle, the wide variety of surface activation and coupling reactions available makes it a generally applicable method. However, the high cost of materials, the often complicated procedures and the almost unavoidable loss of part of the catalytic activity, restrict practical applications of covalent surface immobilisation to specific cases with outstanding advantages.

Covalent coupling of enzymes to supports produces highly stable conjugates with no protein leakage over a wide range of operational conditions. Trypsin, penicillin acylase and lipases immobilised by multi-point covalent attachment onto CNBr-activated agarose yielded derivatives much more stable (300- to 50 000-fold) than their free counterparts. A 1000-fold stability enhancement was the outcome of the multi-point attachment of carboxypeptidase A to aldehyde-agarose gels. Ideally, the binding reaction should not interfere with the amino acids residues at the active site of the enzyme and should not significantly distort the native protein conformation nor alter its flexibility, either as a result of single or multi-point linkages. To meet these requirements, methods include multi-stage activation steps. Although ten different amino acid residues from enzymes can, in principle, be used for covalent coupling, most procedures are targeted at amino, thiol, phenolic and hydroxyl groups. Some of the basic coupling reactions are presented in Fig. 24.7.

Recently, multi-point covalent attachment of penicillin G acylase to organically modified xerogels yielded a biocatalyst with high specific activity and thermal stability. These *xerogels* are prepared by co-hydrolysis and co-condensation of alkoxydes functionalised with a selected organic group to match enzyme requirements. *Sepabeads*, epoxy-based supports, have also been used for multi-point attachment of β-galactosidase (see above). Covalent coupling of enzymes (e.g. β-fructosidase, GL-7-ACA acylase and lactate dehydrogenase) to supports modified by silanisation with (3-aminopropyl)triethoxysilane and activated with glutaraldehyde has been performed as a tool for the development of lactate and sucrose biosensors or for the production of 7-aminocephalosporanic acid. Penicillin G acylase was covalently immobilised on organically modified xerogels, yielding biocatalysts with high specific activity and thermal stability. Eupergit C, a carrier composed of macroporous beads with a diameter of 100–250 μm and made by co-polymerisation of N, N-methylene-bis-methacrylamide, glycidyl methacrylate, allyl glycidyl ether and methacrylamide, has been extensively used for covalent immobilisation of enzymes, namely pepsin, trypsin, phosphodiesterase, lipase, glucoseoxidase, glycolate oxidase, cytidine deaminase and penicillin acylase. Glucose oxidase has also been covalently bonded to a carbon sol-gel composite to develop a glucose sensor. Gold nanoparticles bound with a high surface coverage on 3-aminopropyltrimethoxysilane (APTS)-functionalised zeolites have been used for the covalent immobilisation of pepsin. This procedure has yielded a biocatalyst with high specific activity and enhanced pH and thermal stability compared to the free form.

Lattice entrapment

The immobilisation of biocatalysts within the lattices of solid matrices aims to take advantage of the size difference between the substrates, or products, and the biocatalyst so as to achieve total retention of the latter while the former move freely between the bulk medium

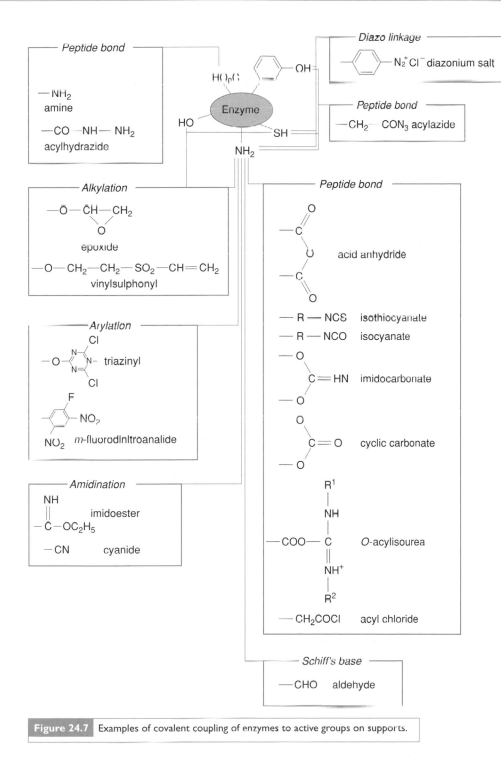

Figure 24.7 Examples of covalent coupling of enzymes to active groups on supports.

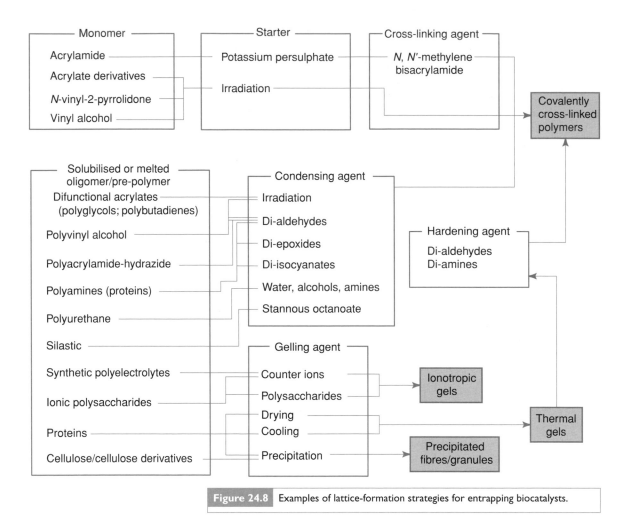

Figure 24.8   Examples of lattice-formation strategies for entrapping biocatalysts.

and the catalytic site. In lattice entrapment, the biocatalyst is not generally subject to strong binding forces; no structure distortion or active site blocking take place. Some deactivation can, nevertheless, occur during the immobilisation process due to pH and temperature changes and contact with aggressive monomers or solvents. Matrices are formed in the presence of the biocatalyst by *in situ* polymerisation, starting from the appropriate monomers, or by solidifying polymer solutions through ionic (alginates) or covalent (chitosan, polivinyl alcohol, polyurethanes) cross-linking, cooling (agarose, gelatin), drying or induced (carrageenan) precipitation (Fig. 24.8). Critical parameters in such processes are always related to optimising pore size and its influence on support rigidity and substrate diffusion within the lattice.

Several attempts have been made to entrap isolated enzymes; however, due to enzyme leakage, this immobilisation method is mainly used for whole-cell immobilisation. Several industrial examples include the use of entrapped cells for the production of amino acids (L-aspartic acid, L-isoleucine), L-malic acid, hydroquinone and acrylamide. Other examples of enzyme entrapment include: porcine liver esterase entrapped in calcium alginate and polyacrylamide gel for the enantioselective cleavage of ofloxacin butyl ester to levofloxacin, and glucoamylase and pullulanase being entrapped in alginate beads for starch hydrolysis. Cross-linking the enzyme with glutaraldehyde prior to entrapment is carried out to diminish enzyme leakage. Beads can be reinforced by treatment with glutaraldehyde and, although this may decrease the activity, it ensures a longer active life for the catalyst.

A more radical approach to produce effective entrapped biocatalysts is based on the use of sol-gel composites. These are oxide glasses that can be produced under mild polymerisation conditions and with controlled hydrophilicity, and lead to particles that can be fabricated in a variety of shapes, with high biocatalytic activity and high chemical and mechanical stability. Furthermore, the biocatalyst is physically entrapped in a rigid glass framework that provides a matrix of stabilising interactions and virtually abolishes enzyme leaching. The high degree of biomolecule rigidity also reduces biocatalyst deactivation. This approach has been used in a wide variety of systems, namely esterification and synthesis with lipases or sulphoidations by horseradish peroxidase and in the development of biosensors.

Biosilica has also been assessed as an effective tool for butyrylcholinesterase immobilisation. Silica bioactive nanoparticles are obtained by the precipitation of silica catalysed by a silica-condensing peptide added to a solution of silicic acid. Higher activity retention and storage stability were observed when compared to a sol-gel-based approach.

Immobilised soluble enzyme and suspended cell methods

All the methods of biocatalyst immobilisation described so far involve the modification of the biocatalyst (enzyme) or its microenvironment, with subsequent alteration of its kinetics and catalytic properties. In order to use a biocatalyst in its native state continuously over a long period of time, biocatalysts have been confined within semipermeable membranes in the form of hollow fibres or flat sheet ultrafiltration membrane reactors (Fig. 24.9). The membrane retains the biocatalyst but is permeable to the products and sometimes to the substrates. This method offers several advantages relative to other immobilisation methods. Chemical modification of the biocatalyst is not necessary and the biocatalyst retains its kinetic properties.

This method is particularly suited for conversion of high molecular weight or insoluble substrates, such as starch, cellulose and proteins, as it allows the intimate contact of the biocatalyst with the substrate achieving an efficient conversion of the substrates. However, some disadvantages are inherent in the method: the possible decrease in the reaction rate as a result of the permeability resistance of the membrane; and the adsorption of the biocatalyst and/or substrates and products on the membrane surface. This

Figure 24.9 Enzyme membrane reactors: (a) continuous stirred tank reactor with recirculation, (b) dead-end cell and (c) tubular.

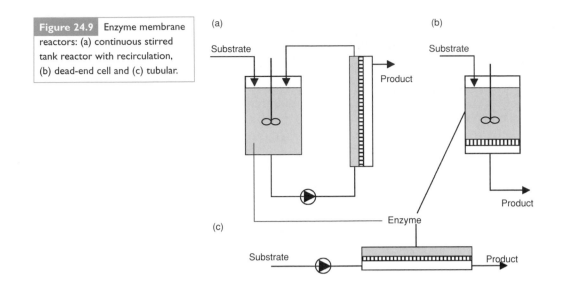

type of immobilisation has found applications on the modification of fats and oils (e.g. olive oil, palm oil) by lipases and dipeptide synthesis (acetylphenylalanine-leucinamide) by proteases in organic media. Other recent examples include: the continuous production of R-(–)-phenylacetylcarbinol, which is a key intermediate in the synthesis of ephedrine using pyruvate decarboxylase; penicillin G hydrolysis using penicillin acylase; conversion of fumaric acid into L-malic acid by fumarase; and xylan hydrolysis catalysed by xylanases.

Immobilisation of multi-enzyme systems and cells

One of the strong disadvantages of single-enzyme systems, free or immobilised, is their limitation to single-step transformations. This limitation is particularly acute with thermodynamically unfavourable conversions and those requiring the regeneration of enzyme co-factors, such as redox reactions or phosphorylations. Among the possible solutions is coupling the intended enzymatic reaction to a chemical one or to a second enzymatic reaction. The latter alternative has been investigated for several NAD(P)- or ATP-dependent systems, using a pair of enzymes and two substrates with the co-factor shuttling between them. When two or more biotransformations are carried out simultaneously in the same vessel – to regenerate co-factors, to shift thermodynamic equilibria, or to favour process economics – the intermediate products should be rapidly converted. In this context, co-immobilisation of the involved enzymes is likely to minimise the diffusion paths of the intermediates between active sites, thus accelerating the potential rate-limiting steps. However, such systems suffer from severe problems related to the correct relative positioning of the immobilised enzymes and co-factor, which are extremely difficult to achieve in practice. An example of this type of immobilisation method is the synthesis of L-tertiary leucine (Fig. 24.10), a chiral intermediate for chemicals.

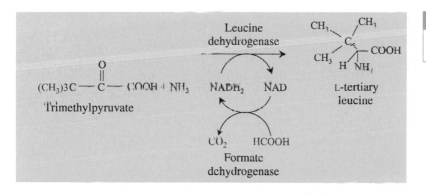

Figure 24.10 Synthesis of L-tertiary leucine from trimethylpyruvate and ammonia.

The immobilisation of the multi-enzyme systems contained in whole cells or cell particles can lead to marked improvements in a process when compared to using free cells or immobilised single or multiple enzymes. However, a clear distinction should be made between the cases in which cell viability is indispensable and those employing whole cells or cell parts as non-viable, crude preparations of single-activity biocatalysts.

In the first situation, one deals with sensitive catalytic forms that require very mild immobilisation and close control of operating conditions in order that cell viability is preserved. This situation corresponds, for example, to the immobilised cell fermentations and the culture of anchorage-dependent mammalian cells.

Immobilised, non-viable cell systems are sometimes preferred to immobilised single enzymes to avoid costly purification processes, or to increase catalytic stability and to retain lattice-entrapped enzymes more efficiently without the need for light control of matrix porosities. With this type of biocatalyst, entrapment or attachment procedures designed for enzymes can be safely used, though lower productivities per unit weight of biocatalyst are to be expected. In addition, diffusional resistances are enhanced by the cell membrane, and permeabilising treatments with heat, surfactants or solvents are often required. Such treatments can also be required to inactivate contaminating enzyme activities in the cells. On the whole, single-activity, immobilised cell preparations are convenient for industrial applications, where cost reduction is necessary and process control as well as sanitisation procedures are feasible.

One important and industrial example is the immobilisation of glucose isomerase; being an expensive intracellular enzyme, the producing cells were successfully immobilised and used continuously at industrial scale in packed bed reactors. A heat treatment was included that degraded other enzymes and thus avoided substrate (glucose) and product (fructose) degradation. Other examples are listed in Table 24.5.

24.3.3 Effect of immobilisation on enzyme kinetics and properties

Although enzyme immobilisation can be very useful, immobilisation may also change the kinetics and other properties of the enzyme,

Table 24.5 Examples of immobilised whole cells for single- or two-enzyme conversions of industrial interest

Microbial biocatalyst	Immobilisation method	Application
Escherichia coli	Entrapment	L-Tryptophan production from indole and DL-serine, L-Aspartic acid production from fumaric acid and ammonia
Escherichia coli, Pseudomonas putida	Entrapment	Production of cis-dihydrodiols from aromatics
Pseudomonas chlororaphis	Entrapment	Hydration of adiponitrile to 5-cyanovaleramide
Saccharomyces cerevisiae	Surface attachment	Sucrose hydrolysis
Rhodococcus rhodochrous JI	Entrapment	Acrylamide from acrylonitrile
Rhodococcus rhodochrous JI	Entrapment	Hydrolysis of 3-cyanopiridine to nicotinamide
Solanum aviculare and Dioscorea deltoidea	Entrapment	S-(-)-Limonene into cis and transcarveol and carvone
Mycobacterium sp. NRRL B-3805	Surface attachment	Sitosterol to androstenedione
Zymomonas mobilis	Entrapment	Sorbitol and gluconic acid production from glucose and fructose
Pseudomonas AMI	Entrapment	L-Serine production from glycine and methanol
Arthrobacter simplex and Bacillus sphaericus	Entrapment	Chlormadinone acetate to delmadinone acetate, prednisolone production from cortisol
Saccharomyces cerevisiae	Entrapment	Alcohols to aldehydes

usually with a decrease of enzyme-specific activity. This may be ascribed to several factors: (i) conformational and steric effects, (ii) partitioning effects and (iii) mass transfer or diffusional effects.

Conformational and steric effects

The decrease of specific activity of enzymes, which occurs on their binding either to solid supports or upon intermolecular cross-linking, is usually attributed to conformational changes in the tertiary structure of the enzymes. For instance, covalent bonds between the enzyme and the matrix can stretch the enzyme molecule and thus the three-dimensional structure at the active site. Denaturation of the enzyme can arise by the action of reagents used in entrapment methods.

The specific activity decrease may also be attributed to steric hindrance resulting in limits on the accessibility of the substrate. In these two cases, the decrease in enzyme activity can be minimised, or prevented, by choosing suitable conditions for immobilisation. Thus the active centre of the enzyme can be protected with a specific inhibitor, substrate or product, and the shielding effect of the support that causes steric hindrances can be reduced by the introduction of *spacers* that keep the enzyme at a definite and certain distance from the support. By introducing bifunctional compounds, such as

1,6 diaminohexane, as *spacers*, the specific activity of covalent coupled glucoamylase on porous silica was increased ten-fold.

In addition to their influence on the enzyme activity, any physical or chemical matrix–enzyme interactions may additionally modify the selectivity and stability of the bound enzyme from that which it normally possesses in free solution.

Partition effects

In the support-binding method, when the support is charged or has a hydrophobic character, the kinetic behaviour of the immobilised enzyme may differ from that of the free enzyme even in the absence of mass transfer effects. This difference is commonly attributed to partition effects that cause different concentrations of charge species, substrates, products, hydrogen ions, hydroxyl ions and so on, in the microenvironment of the immobilised enzyme and in the domain of the bulk solution, owing to electrostatic with fixed charges on the support.

The main consequences of these partition effects is a shift in the optimum pH, with a displacement of the pH–activity profile of the immobilised enzyme towards more alkaline or acidic pH values for negatively or positively charged carriers, respectively. For example, chymotrypsin immobilised on a polyanionic support – ethylene/maleic anhydride co-polymer – shifted 1 pH unit to the alkaline side; while immobilised on a polycationic support, polyornithine, a shift of 1.5 pH units to the acid side occurred.

By similar considerations, the partitioning of charged compounds, substrate or product, between a charged enzyme particle and the bulk solution can also be evaluated. For a positively charged substrate, when using a negatively charged immobilised enzyme, a higher concentration of substrate is obtained in the local environment or microenvironment than in the bulk solution, and a higher value of relative activity is obtained than with a neutrally charged matrix. However, when effects other than partitioning are present, it is possible to have no shift of the enzyme's pH optimum on charged supports.

Mass transfer effects

When an enzyme is immobilised on or within a solid matrix, mass transfer effects may exist because the substrate must diffuse from the bulk solution to the active site of the immobilised enzyme. If the enzyme is attached to non-porous supports, there are only external mass transfer effects on the catalytically active outer surface; in the reaction solution, being surrounded by a stagnant film, substrate and product are transported across the Nernst layer by diffusion. The driving force for this diffusion is the concentration difference between the surface and the bulk concentration of substrate and product.

When an enzyme is immobilised within a porous support, in addition to possible external mass transfer effects, there could also be resistance to the internal diffusion of the substrate (as it must diffuse through the pores in order to reach the enzyme) and resistance of product for its diffusion into the bulk solution. Consequently, a substrate concentration gradient is established within the pores, resulting in a concentration decreasing with increased distance (in depth) from the surface of immobilised enzyme preparation. A corresponding product concentration gradient is obtained in the opposite direction.

Unlike external diffusion, internal mass transfer proceeds in parallel with the enzyme reaction and takes into account the depletion of substrate within the pores with increasing distance from the surface of the enzyme support. The rate of reaction will also decrease, for the same reason. The overall reaction is dependent on the substrate concentration and the distance from the outside support surface.

Miscellaneous effects

Other properties of the enzyme can change upon immobilisation. The substrate specificity alters, particularly when using a substrate of high molecular weight, by the effect of steric hindrance and diffusional resistances. The kinetics constants K_m and V_m (i.e. the standard Michaelis–Menten constant for the concentration of substrate needed for the enzyme to proceed at half its maximum velocity) of the immobilised enzyme are different from the free enzyme as a consequence of conformational changes of the immobilised form, which affect the affinity between enzyme and substrate. The increase of activity energy for some immobilised enzymes may be attributed to diffusional resistances, mainly in porous supports.

24.4 | Synthesis of chemicals

24.4.1 Synthesis of oligosaccharides

Oligosaccharides are a complex class of compounds widely used in glycobiology which have numerous medical applications. Chemical synthesis is a laborious multi-step task, making biological synthesis an attractive approach.

Glycosyltransferases promote the transfer of a monosaccharide to saccharide acceptors. Examples are the production of acetyllactosamine using β-1,4-glycosyltransferase. This enzyme has also been used for solid-phase synthesis of tetrasaccharides on a Sepharose matrix. Glycosyltransferases are also used to promote chemically difficult glycosidic linkages, such as those involved in the formation of α-sialosides and β-mannosides, synthesised with β-1,4-manosyltransferase. Recently, β-1,3-N-acetylglucosaminyltranserases have been used for polylactosamine synthesis. Glycosyltransferases, however, are scarce and the relative cost of the substrates is high.

Glycosidases have been used for reverse hydrolysis (equilibrium-controlled synthesis) or transglycosylation (kinetically controlled reactions). These ubiquitous enzymes are robust and generally tolerant to organic solvents. Recent screenings have identified fucosidase for the synthesis of α-1,3-linked fucosides and β-galactosidase for

β-1,3-, β-1,4-, β-1,6- and α-1,6-galactoside synthesis. The use of whole cells has also been considered for oligosaccharide synthesis allowing biotransformation from inexpensive precursors. Genetically engineered *E. coli* cells have been effectively used for the synthesis of chitooligosaccharides and O-acetylated and sulphate analogues. However, only modest product yields (hardly over 40%) are usually obtained, thus making the use of this approach for large-scale synthesis economically unfeasible.

A third, more recent option for the enzymatic synthesis of oligosaccharides lies in the use of glycosynthases. Glycosynthases are glycosidases specifically mutated in given residues in order to synthesise oligosaccharides but preclude product hydrolysis. Since the unwanted hydrolysis in avoided, high product yields are obtained. Pioneering work led to a limited number of glycosynthases able to produce a range of oligosaccharides from commonly available glycosyl donors. In order to widen the application of this approach, several glycoside hydrolases have been mutated to yield glycosynthases for the synthesis of oligosaccharides such as β-1,4-linked cellooligosaccharides, 4-nitrophenyl-β-acetyllactosamine, β-1,3- or β-1,6-linked tetrasaccharides, β-1,3- or β-1,4-linked mannosides or glycans. Product yields exceeding 60% are obtained.

Further residue mutation has been performed in order to improve the characteristics of glycosynthases, namely leading to increased glycosylation activity, higher product yields, lower reaction times and a wider array of products.

Mutant glycosidases able to produce thioglycosides have recently been obtained. These biocatalysts, termed thioglycoligases use SH-sugars as acceptors, which are more nucleophilic than OH-sugars.

24.4.2 Synthesis of C–C bonds in biotransformations

The biosynthesis of C–C bonds is a crucial matter of organic synthetic chemistry. Biosynthesis of C–C bonds is naturally performed by ligases which require expensive ATP as a co-factor. Thus other enzymes such as (trans)aldolases and (trans)ketolases, which do not require ATP, are preferably used for such goals. Most aldolases, however, require phosphorylated precursors, but 2-deoxyribose-5-phosphate aldolase can be used in the production of epothilones, a class of compounds with possible anticancer properties, without using a phosphorylated substrate. Pyruvate decarboxylase, a ketolase that normally breaks a C–C bond, is currently used to synthesise phenylacetylcarbinol, an intermediate in the production of ephedrine, from pyruvate or acetaldehyde and benzaldehyde. This enzyme also promotes the production of pyruvic acid from acetaldehyde and carbon dioxide, with a product yield in excess of 80%. Benzoylformate decarboxylase catalyses the carboligation of a wide array of cyclic aldehydes and conjugated unsaturated aldehydes to acetaldehyde. The genes for these enzymes, originally isolated from plants, have been successfully cloned and overexpressed in *Escherichia coli*, *Saccharomyces cerevisiae* and *Pichia pastoris*, thus providing useful biocatalysts for the synthesis of *S*- and

Table 24.6 Biocatalytic synthesis of some enantiomers

Biocatalyst	Substrate	Product	Yield[a]	Ee (%)
Sphingomonas paucimobilis	4-benzyloxy-3-methanesulfonylamino-2'-bromoacetophenone	(R)-Alcohol	>85	>98
Mycobacterium neoaurum	Racemic methyl-phenylalanine amide	(S)-Amino acid	48[a]	98
Pig liver esterase	Methyl-(4-methoxyphenyl)-propanedioic acid, ethyl diester	(S)-Monoester	96.7	96
Rhodococcus MB 5655	Indene	*Cis*-(1S, 2R)-indandiol	–	99
Rhodococcus MA 7205	Indene	*Trans*-(1R, 2R)-indandiol	–	98
Aspergillus niger, Rhodotorula glutinis	Racemic 1-{2',3'-dihydro-benzo[β]furan-4'-yl}-1,2-oxirane	(R)-Diol	45[a]	95
Immobilised lipase	(3R)-*cis*-3-acetyloxy-4-(1,1-dimethylethyl)-2-azetidinone	(S)-Alcohol	>48	>99

[a] 50% theoretical maximum.

R-cyanohydrins. These provide building blocks for the synthesis of α-hydroxycarboxylic acids, α-amino acids, 1,2-aminoalcohols or 1,2-diamines.

24.4.3 Synthesis of chiral intermediates

The efficiency of many drugs depends on chirality, since often only one enantiomer of a racemic mixture has the required activity. Enzyme-catalysed reactions are often highly enantio- and regio-selective making this approach an effective tool for the production of chiral intermediates and fine chemicals. Table 24.6 gives some examples of the use of biocatalysts for the synthesis of single enantiomers for key chiral compounds.

Other applications include enzymatic synthesis of chiral synthons for the production of hyper-tensive drugs, such as Omapatrilat, in a multi-enzyme process that requires regeneration of the co-factor (NAD/NADH); of antiviral drugs, such as Crixivan, a leading HIV protease inhibitor, or Abacavir, a selective reverse transcriptase inhibitor, used for treatment of HIV and hepatitis B, or Lobucavir, used for the treatment of herpes; anticholesterol drugs; anticancer drugs, such as paclitaxel, an inhibitor of the depolymerisation process of micro-tubulin, or (−)-15-deoxyspergualin, an immunosuppressive agent and antitumour agent.

Acyloin condensation can be achieved using either pyruvate decarboxylase from a yeast, a bacterial benzoylformate decarboxylase, or phenylpyruvate decarboxylase. Acyloins (α-hydroxyketones) are relevant in organic synthesis owing to their bifunctional nature, mainly due to one chiral centre which is amenable to further modification.

Between 87 and 98% of the final product is in one chiral form, indicating that the enzymes carry out a highly selective reaction.

24.4.4   Redox biocatalysis

Redox reactions are relevant for the regio-, stereo-, or enantio-selective production of chemicals that are important in the agrochemical, food and pharmaceutical industries. Oxido-reductases catalyse redox reactions. They, therefore, act on a substrate through electron transfer. These enzymes are mostly co-factor dependent, therefore, commercial bioconversion systems are limited by the development of a process for the efficient recycling of the expensive co-factors. The most commonly needed co-factors are $NADH/NAD^+$, $NADPH/NADP^+$, $FADH/FAD^+$ and ATP/ADP. The use of whole cells is often a viable alternative to using enzymes, provided that the presence of other enzymes within the cells has no negative impact on product purity and yield. Co-factor regeneration is assured, costly enzyme recovery and purification is avoided, and a more stable microenvironment is given.

Oxidative biocatalysts

Oxidative reactions can be performed by a wide variety of oxidising enzymes: monooxygenases, dioxygenases, oxidases and peroxidases. Current applications of these monooxygenases include the oxidation of ketones to esters or lactones through Bayer–Villiger-type reaction, the production of (R)-epoxides from terminal alkenes, the conversion of arenes to aldehydes and the production of hydroxybenzaldehydes from substituted phenols. Dioxygenases are used to hydroxylate cyclohexene and to hydroxylate arenes to diols. Oxidases can be used in regio-specific oxidation at nucleosides and in the selective oxidation of pyranoses. Laccases, in particular, have a wide array of substrates, namely alkenes, aryl amines, phenol derivatives and polyphenols and polyamines. They also recognise lignin (in wood) as a substrate. When substrates with a high redox potential are used, a mediator (e.g. 1-hydroxybenzotriazole) is required. This acts as an intermediate substrate for the enzyme: the oxidised form of the mediator then oxidises the real substrate. Peroxidases are used to oxidise aromatic hydrocarbons to aldehydes, to convert sulphide to chiral sulphoxides, and to introduce the oxo-functionality into cyclic conjugated dienes.

Reductions

The asymmetric reduction of ketones to yield non-racemic chiral alcohols can be performed by different biocatalysts including baker's yeast and various dehydrogenases, including alcohol dehydrogenases from baker's yeast, *Thermoanaerobium brockii* and *Pseudomonas* sp.; horse liver and hydroxysteroid dehydrogenase from *Pseudomonas testosteroni* and *Bacillus sphaerisus*; or glycerol dehydrogenase from *Geotrichum candidum*. Reductants (hydrogen sources) are necessary to perform these reactions. For biocatalytic reduction, alcohols such as ethanol and 2-propanol, glucose and formic acid, among others, can be used.

Table 24.7 Methods for co-factor regeneration

Cofactor	Regeneration method	Reaction
ATP	Acetate kinase and acetyl phosphate	Phosphoryl transfer
NAD^+	Glutamate dehydrogenase with α-ketoglutarate	Removal of hydrogen
NADH	Formate dehydrogenase with formate	Addition of hydrogen
$NADP^+$	Glutamate dehydrogenase with α-ketoglutarate	Removal of hydrogen
NADPH	Glucose dehydrogenase with glucose	Addition of hydrogen
Flavins	Self-regeneration	Oxygenation

Regeneration of co-factors

Due to the high cost of co-factors (NADH/NAD$^+$ or NADPH/NADP$^+$), they cannot be used as stoichiometric agents in preparative biocatalysis, thus *in situ* regeneration is required. An efficient co-factor regeneration system has to fulfil several requirements, but, above all, the *total turnover number* (TTN) of the co-factor must be high. TTN is defined as the total number of moles of product formed per mole of co-factor during the course of a complete reaction. As a rule of thumb a TTN between 10^3 and 10^5 can assure a feasible reaction system. Chemical, electrochemical and enzymatic methods have been assayed as effective approaches for co-factor regeneration. However, since the former two lack the adequate selectivity required to obtain high TTN, the enzymatic approach is currently favoured. Examples of enzymatic methods for co-factor regeneration are given in Table 24.7.

Recent developments on the enzymatic regeneration of pyridine nucleotide co-factors include the discovery of phosphite dehydrogenase, a promising enzyme for NADH regeneration. Another approach for NADH regeneration involved the use of cross-linked enzyme crystals for the production of cinnamaldehyde, where the co-factor was present during crystallisation and involved NADH-alcohol dehydrogenase and cross-linked enzyme crystals.

A recent development for the regeneration of NADPH involves the use of soluble pyridine nucleotide transhydrogenase that promotes the transfer of reducing equivalents between NAD(P) and NAD(P)H.

An NADH oxidase from *Lactobacillus brevis*, which generates water as product from NADH oxidation, provides a potential alternative for the conventional enzymatic method of NAD$^+$ regeneration where toxic H_2O_2 is produced.

Two novel genes from *L. sanfranciscensis* and *Borrelia burgdorferi* expressing NADH oxidases were recently cloned and heterologously overexpressed in *E. coli*. The novel oxidases accept both NADH and NADPH and may, therefore, be used for regeneration of NAD(P)$^+$.

The development of preparative electrochemical reactors for co-factor regeneration has been challenging both due to scale-up costs and the need for large electrode surface areas. In spite of these difficulties, an ultrafiltration membrane reactor has proved a promising tool for the electrochemical regeneration of NADH coupled to the synthesis of cyclohexanol from cyclohexanone.

Many applications of dehydrogenases or monooxygenases involve the use of whole cells. The natural NAD(P)H regeneration rate should not limit oxygenase/dehydrogenase activities of about 100 µg dry wt^{-1}, but may become limiting at higher activities or if resting cells are used. To deal with these situations, simultaneous overexpression of production and regeneration enzymes has been performed. Alternatively, purified co-factor regeneration enzymes can be added to whole-cell preparations. A different, more radical approach has involved directed evolution of a cytochrome P450 variant in which a peroxide-mediated electron donor activity replaces the requirement for NADPH.

24.4.5 Combinatorial biocatalysis

Combinatorial biocatalysis is another field of knowledge that takes advantage of high-throughput methods (see also Chapter 12). It focuses on the generation of libraries through the iterative conversion of lead compounds catalysed by enzymes or whole cells. Large arrays of derivatives are generated in successive rounds of biocatalytic steps including acylation, glycosylation, halogenation, oxidation and reduction, creating a large pool of potentially useful building blocks for the construction of new molecules or for the modification of complex natural compounds. Combinatorial biocatalysis is, therefore, a useful tool in drug discovery for the pharmaceutical industry. For example, lipases were used to prepare a combinatorial library of 24 esters starting from four aromatic alcohols and six vinyl esters as acyl donors. Similarly, a range of peptides have been produced using combinations of peptide synthetases with various amino acid substrates.

24.5 | Immobilised enzyme reactors

24.5.1 Classification of enzyme reactors

Among the applications of immobilised enzymes, their utilisation in industry is perhaps the most important and consequently the most frequently discussed. The use of immobilised enzymes in industrial processes is performed in basic chemical reactors. A classification of enzyme reactors based on the mode of operation and the flow characteristics of substrate and product is presented in Table 24.8. The configurations of the different reactor types are shown in Fig. 24.11.

24.5.2 Batch reactors

Batch reactors are most commonly used when soluble enzymes are used as catalysts. The soluble enzymes are not generally separated from the products and consequently are not recovered for re-use.

Table 24.8 Classification of enzyme reactors

Mode of operation	Flow pattern	Type of reactor
Batch	Well mixed	Batch stirred tank reactor (BSTR)
	Plug flow	Total recycle reactor
Continuous	Well mixed	Continuous stirred tank reactor (CSTR)
		CSTR with ultrafiltration membrane
	Plug flow	Packed bed reactor (PBR)
		Fluidised bed reactor (FBR)
		Tubular reactor (other)
		Hollow fibre reactor

Since one of the main goals of immobilising an enzyme is to permit its re-use, the application of immobilised enzymes in batch reactors requires a separation (or an additional separation) to recover the enzyme preparation. During this recovery process, appreciable loss of immobilised enzyme material may occur as well as loss of enzyme activity. Traditionally, the stirred tank reactor has been used for batchwise work. Composed of a reactor and a stirrer, it is the simplest type of reactor that allows good mixing and relative ease of temperature and pH control. However, some matrices, such as inorganic supports, are broken by shearing in such vessels, and alternative designs have therefore been attempted. A possible laboratory alternative is the *basket reactor*, in which the catalyst is retained within a *basket* either forming the impeller *blades* or the baffles of the tank reactor.

Another alternative is to change the flow pattern, using a plug flow type of reactor: the total recycle reactor or batch recirculation reactor, which may be a packed bed or fluidised bed reactor, or even a coated tubular reactor. This type of reactor may be useful where a single pass gives inadequate conversions. However, it has found greatest application in the laboratory for the acquisition of kinetic data, when the recycle rate is adjusted so that the conversion in the reactor is low and it can be considered as a differential reactor. One advantage of this type of reactor is that the external mass transfer effects can be reduced by the operational high fluid velocities.

24.5.3 Continuous reactors

The continuous operation of immobilised enzymes has some advantages when compared with batch processes, such as ease of automatic control, ease of operation and quality control of products. Continuous reactors can be divided into two basic types: the *continuous feed, stirred tank reactor* (CSTR) and the *plug flow reactor* (PFR).

In the ideal CSTR, the degree of conversion is independent of the position in the vessel, as a complete mixing is obtained with stirring and the conditions within the CSTR are the same as the outlet stream, that is, low substrate and high product concentrations. With the ideal PFR, the conversion degree is dependent on the length of the reactor,

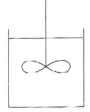

Batch stirred tank reactor

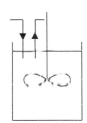

Continuous stirred tank reactor

Figure 24.11 Examples of immobilised biocatalyst reactors.

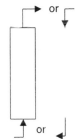

Packed bed reactor

Fluidised bed reactor

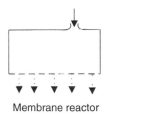

Membrane reactor

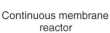

Continuous membrane reactor

as no mixing device at all exists and the conditions within the reactor are never uniform.

While a nearly ideal CSTR is readily obtained (since it is only necessary to have good stirring to obtain complete mixing), an ideal PFR is very difficult to achieve. Several adverse factors to obtaining an ideal PFR often occur, such as temperature and velocity gradients normal to the flow direction and axial dispersion of substrate.

Several considerations influence the type of continuous reactor to be chosen for a particular application. One of the most important criteria is based on kinetic considerations. For Michaelis Menten kinetics, the PFR is preferable to the CSTR, as the CSTR requires more enzyme to obtain the same degree of conversion as a PFR. If product inhibition occurs, this problem is accentuated, as in a CSTR high product concentration is always in direct contact with all of the catalyst. There is only one situation where a CSTR may be kinetically more favourable than a PFR, namely, when substrate inhibition occurs.

The form and characteristics of the immobilised enzyme preparations also influence the choice of reactor type, and operational requirements are still another factor to be taken into account. Thus, when pH control is necessary, for instance with penicillin acylase, the CSTR or batch stirred tank reactor is more suitable than PFR reactors. Due to possible disintegration of support through mechanical shearing, only durable preparations of immobilised enzyme should be used in a CSTR. With very small immobilised enzyme particles, problems such as high pressure drop and plugging arise from the utilisation of this catalyst in packed bed reactors (the most used type of PFR). To overcome these problems, a fluidised bed reactor, which provides a degree of mixing intermediate to the CSTR and the ideal PFR, can be used with low pressure drop.

Reactant characteristics can also influence the choice of reactor. Insoluble substrates and products and highly viscous fluids are preferably processed in fluidised bed reactors or CSTR, where no plugging of the reactor is likely to occur, as would be the case in a packed bed reactor.

As can be deduced from this outline, there are no simple rules for choosing reactor type and the different factors mentioned must be analysed individually for a specific case.

24.6 | Biocatalysis in non-conventional media

Water as an essential reaction medium for biocatalysts has been advocated for many years as one of the major advantages of biotransformations. However, this so-called advantage has proved to be one of the severest limitations for broadening the scope of applications of biocatalysts, especially when the reactants are poorly soluble in water. Non-conventional media that have been used include organic solvents, some gases and super-critical fluids. The scopes and limitations of these different systems are described below.

24.6.1 Biocatalysis in organic media

The first examples of biocatalyst/enzyme use in organic solvents for the conversion of hydrophobic compounds were presented over 20 years ago. Several examples show the synthesis of peptides (e.g. AcPheAlaNH$_2$) from amino acids catalysed by proteases, the production of the sweetener, Aspartame (L-aspartyl-L–phenylalanine methyl ester), catalysed by thermolysin using ethyl acetate as solvent, and the use of lipases on esterification, transesterification and interesterification reactions and the resolution of enantiomers.

The introduction of an organic solvent in the reaction system has several advantages (Table 24.9). The organic solvent increases the solubility of the poorly water-soluble or insoluble compounds, thereby increasing the volumetric productivity of the reaction system. Another important advantage is that the equilibrium of a hydrolytic reaction can be shifted in favour of the product, this being extracted

Table 24.9	Characteristics of two-liquid-phase bioconversion

Potential advantages
    High substrate and product solubilities
    Reduction in substrate and product inhibition
    Facilitated recovery of product and biocatalyst
    High gas solubility in organic solvents
    Shift of reaction equilibrium
Potential disadvantages
    Biocatalyst denaturation and/or inhibition by organic solvent
    Increasing complexity of the reaction

into the organic phase, therefore biocatalyst and product recovery will be facilitated (extractive bioconversions). High product yields may also be achieved by decreasing possible substrate or product inhibition and prevention of unwanted side reactions. In spite of these advantages of using organic solvents, limitations also exist. The biocatalyst may be denaturated or inhibited by the solvent and, in addition, the introduction of an organic solvent leads to an increased complexity of the reaction process system.

These reaction systems were first applied to enzymatic conversions before their use was extended to whole-cell systems. Recently, the discovery of bacterial strains that are able to grow in the presence of organic solvents has made this field even more promising, opening further possibilities for the understanding of the mechanisms underlying the tolerance or toxicity responses of microorganisms to organic solvents.

Selection of solvent

Two of the most important technical criteria for solvent selection are high product recovery and biocompatibility; although other characteristics, like chemical and thermal stability, low tendency to form emulsions with water media, non-biodegradability, non-hazardous nature and low market price, are desirable.

Whereas the other desirable solvent attributes are relatively mild conditions, the requirement of biocompatibility is a particularly restrictive criterion. Several attempts have been made to associate the toxicity of different solvents to some of their physico-chemical properties. The parameters used to classify solvents in terms of biocompatibility have been related to the polarity of the solvent. Laane and co-workers from Wageningen Agriculture University have described a correlation between bioactivity and the logarithm of the partition coefficient of the solvent in the octanol/water two-phase system (log P_{oct}), known as the *Hansch parameter*. Log P_{oct} denotes hydrophobicity, which is not exactly the same as polarity, but it shows a much better correlation with the biocatalytic rates than other models based on solvent polarity. The Hansch parameter has currently been used in the pharmaceutical and medical fields as a part of drug activity

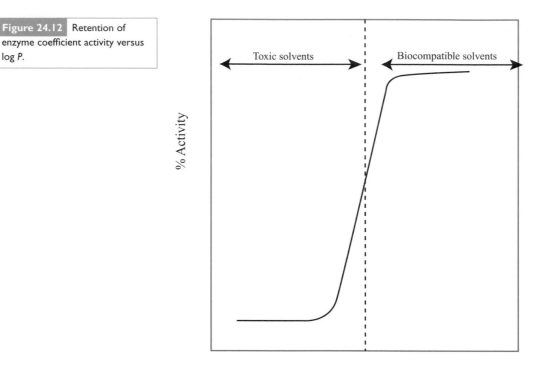

Figure 24.12 Retention of enzyme coefficient activity versus log P.

$\log P$

studies and can be determined experimentally or calculated by Rekker's hydrophobic fragmental constant approach. Many attempts have been made to explain the empirical correlation between log P_{oct} and the activity retention of cellular-biocatalysts, but so far the mechanisms of solvent-caused toxicity are poorly understood.

Laane and co-workers observed that a correlation exists between log P_{oct} and the epoxidising reaction activity of immobilised cells and the gas-producing activity of anaerobic cells in various water-saturated organic solvents. When plotting the cellular activity retention against log P_{oct}, sigmoidal curves are obtained (Fig. 24.12). A solvent with a log P_{oct} value lower than the inflection point is usually toxic and one with a log P_{oct} value higher than the inflection point is biocompatible. The inflection point of these curves depends on the microorganism studied. In general, solvents having a log P_{oct} lower than 2 are relatively polar solvents not suitable for biocatalytic systems, and biological activities vary in solvents having a log P_{oct} between 2 and 4, being high in apolar solvents having log P_{oct} values above 4 (Table 24.10).

Similar sigmoidal shapes were observed for the effect of solvents on microorganisms; however, different inflection points were obtained for different microorganisms, which could be due to differences in the characteristics of their cellular membranes. It has also been observed that increasing the agitation rate caused the log P_{oct} curve to shift to the right. A good correlation between the metabolic

Table 24.10 Biocompatible organic solvents

Solvents	Hansch parameter (log P)
Alcohols	
Decanol	4.0
Undecanol	4.5
Dodecanol	5.0
Oleyl alcohol	7.0
Ethers	
Diphenyl ether	4.3
Carboxylic acids	
Oleic acid	7.9
Esters	
Pentyl benzoate	4.2
Ethyl decanoate	4.9
Butyl oleate	9.8
Dibutylphthalate	5.4
Dipentylphthalate	6.5
Dihexylphthalate	7.5
Dioctylphthalate	9.6
Didecylphthalate	11.7
Hydrocarbons	
Heptane	4.0
Octane	4.5
Nonane	5.1
Decane	5.6
Undecane	6.1
Dodecane	6.6
Tetradecane	8.8
Hexadecane	9.6

activity of *Arthrobacter, Acinetobacter, Nocardia* and *Pseudomonas* and the log P_{oct} of the solvent was found; however, the transition between toxic and non-toxic solvents was observed in the log P_{oct} range from 3 to 5. Tramper and co-workers have investigated the relationship between the metabolic activity of cells exposed to organic solvents at 10% (v/v) concentrations and their log P_{oct} values for different homologous series of solvents. They found that the log P_{oct} value, above which all solvents are non-toxic, is different for different homologous series: e.g. *Arthrobacter* and *Nocardia* tolerate alkanols with log P_{oct} above 4, but are only able to tolerate phthalates having a log P_{oct} value higher than 5.

The influence of the characteristics of the cell membrane on the solvent tolerance of the micro-organisms has been evaluated for Gram-negative and Gram-positive bacteria. Gram-negative bacteria, and particularly *Pseudomonas*, are in general more tolerant than Gram-positive bacteria. The difference in solvent tolerance is probably due to the presence of the outer membrane of Gram-negative

Figure 24.13 Classification of biocatalysis in organic media systems. (a) Water-in-oil biphasic emulsion; (b) oil-in-water biphasic emulsion; (c) enzyme immobilised in a porous support in a biphasic system; (d) enzyme in a reversed micelle; (e) enzyme modified with polyethylene glycol and solubilised in organic media; (f) immobilised enzyme suspended in organic media; and (g) enzyme powder suspended in organic media.

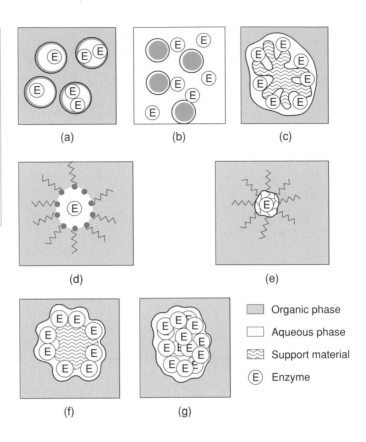

bacteria. This membrane contains major structural proteins, lipoproteins and lipopolysaccharides. A percentage of the total lipoproteins of the outer membrane is bound covalently to the peptidoglycan layer. This linkage might be expected to protect cells from environmental stress. Plant cells appear to be even more sensitive to the presence of organic solvents, as shown for cell suspensions of *Morinda citrifolia*, which had a biocompatibility limiting log P_{oct} value of 5. Thus the transition range from toxic to non-toxic clearly depends on the type of cellular biocatalyst.

Other criteria for correlation with solvent biocompatibility have recently been described, especially for the effect of solvents on enzyme stability. These are the *three-dimensional solubility parameter* or the *denaturing capacity* used to predict, for example, the concentration of the organic solvent at which half-inactivation is observed.

Classification of organic reaction systems

Biocatalysts can be used in different ways in combination with organic solvents: (a) homogeneous mixture of water and water-miscible solvent; (b) aqueous/organic two-liquid-phase systems; (c) microheterogeneous systems (microemulsions and reversed micelles); (d) enzyme powder and immobilised biocatalysts suspended in solvent without aqueous phase; and (e) covalently modified enzymes dissolved in organic solvent (Fig. 24.13a–g).

Homogeneous mixture of water and water-miscible solvent

An easy way to increase the solubility of a hydrophobic substrate is to add a water-miscible organic solvent, such as methanol, acetone, ethyl acetate, dimethyl formamide, dimethylsulphoxide, etc., to the reaction medium. These systems have the advantages of generally not presenting mass transfer limitations as they are homogeneous systems. However, the biocatalyst in the presence of these systems usually has poor operational stability, particularly if a high concentration of solvent is needed. This results from the fact that water-miscible solvents are polar compounds with log P values lower than 2, being considered as toxic solvents. For example, ribonuclease dissolved in increasing concentrations of 2-chloroethanol undergoes a transition from the native state to an unfolded form.

Aqueous/organic two-phase systems

Two-liquid-phase (aqueous/organic) systems are useful when reactants of poor water solubility have to be employed. The organic solvent may be the substrate itself (e.g. olive oil) to be converted or may serve as a reservoir (a hydrocarbon) for substrate(s) and/or product(s), (Figs. 24.13a,b,c and 24.14). These systems can also be used to confine (immobilise) the biocatalyst physically in the aqueous phase while the organic phase is being renewed. In these systems, it is important that the interfacial area is large enough to improve mass transfer. The partitioning of the substrate(s) and product(s) in the two liquid phases can be controlled by choosing a suitable solvent and, in certain cases, such as those involving ionic species (e.g. organic acids), the pH (which should be lower than the pK_a of those ionic species in order to get the unprotonated compound, which is the one readily to be extracted) of the water phase. In the latter case, the pH selected should also be compatible with the enzymatic activity. The partitioning of substrate(s) and product(s) is particularly suited when one or both of these compounds is an inhibitor of the enzymatic activity. Its accumulation in the organic phase will alleviate this inhibition. The overall displacement of reaction equilibrium by extraction of the products is also an advantage of this type of system. The phase ratio can be varied over a wide range, leading to an optimisation of reactor capacity. Application of two-liquid-phase systems include: epoxide production [e.g. (S)-styrene oxide], steroid transformation (phyosterols side-chain cleavage, Δ^1-dehydrogenation of cortisol and cortisol derivatives), catechol production, generation of (2R,3S)-3-(p-methoxyphenyl)glycidylmethylester (an intermediate for the synthesis of Diltiazem) peptide synthesis, carvone production, olive oil hydrolysis, kinetic resolution of Ibuprofen ester and of racemic Naproxen, production of flavour ketones, oxidation of n-alkanes, reduction of aldehydes to alcohols or oxidation of alcohols to aldehydes.

Microheterogeneous systems

Microemulsions and *reversed micelles* represent a special case of two-liquid-phase systems in which the aqueous phase is no longer

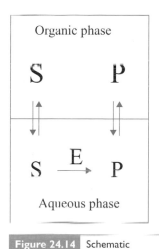

Figure 24.14 Schematic presentation of an enzymatic conversion in a two-phase system. S, substrate; P, product; E, enzyme.

Table 24.11 Example of surfactant-forming reversed micelles

Surfactant	Solvent
Sodium dioctyl sulphosuccinate (AOT)	n-Hydrocarbon (C_6–C_{10})
	Isooctane
	Cyclohexane
	Carbon tetrachloride
	Benzene
Cetyltrimethylammonium bromide (CTAB)	Hexanol/isooctane
	Hexanol/octane
	Chloroform/octane
Methyltrioctylammonium chloride (TOMAC)	Cyclohexane
Brij 60	Octane
Triton X	Hexanol/cyclohexane
Phosphatidylcholine	Benzene
	Heptane
Phosphatidylethanolamine	Benzene
	Heptane

macroscopically distinguishable from the continuous organic phase. These systems usually contain surfactants to stabilise the distribution of water and its contents in the continuous organic phase.

Reversed micelles are aggregates formed by surfactants in apolar solvents. Surfactants are amphipathic molecules that possess both a hydrophilic and a hydrophobic part (Fig. 24.13d). The hydrophobic tails of the surfactant molecules are in contact with the apolar bulk solution; the polar head groups are turned towards the interior of the aggregate, forming a polar core. This core can solubilise water (water pool) and host macromolecules such as proteins. The group of amphipathic molecules used in the formation of reversed micelles in hydrocarbon solvents include both natural membrane lipids and artificial surfactants (Table 24.11).

The amount of water solubilised in the reversed micellar systems is commonly referred to as w_0, the molar ratio of surfactant to water ($w_0 = H_2O$/surfactant). This is an extremely important parameter, since it will determine the number of surfactant molecules per micelle, the availability of water molecules for protein hydration and biocatalysis, and is the main factor affecting the micelle size.

The formation of reversed micelles depends largely on the energy change due to dipole–dipole interactions between the polar head groups of the surfactant molecules. The solubilisation properties of surfactants are often expressed by a three- or four-component phase diagram, the reversed micelles being identified by the regions of optical transparency. Most of the work performed with reversed micelles in biological systems uses sodium dioctyl sulphosuccinate (AOT), an anionic surfactant. AOT forms stable micellar aggregates in organic solvents, the most used being isooctane. The maximum amount of solubilised water for an AOT/isooctane/H₂O system is around $w_0 = 60$. Above this value, the transparent reversed micelle solution becomes a turbid emulsion and phase separation occurs.

Biocatalysis in reversed micelles was first reported in 1978, since when several major studies and biocatalytic applications have been described in the literature. Examples include the controlled hydrolysis of lipids and vegetable oils, peptide synthesis by proteases, degradation of pesticides catalysed by organophosphorus hydrolase, stereospecific reduction of progesterone and reduction of 2-heptanone by alcohol dehydrogenases, penthylferulate synthesis catalysed by feruloyl esterase, chiral epoxidation catalysed by *Mycobacterium* whole cells solubilised in microemulsions, and synthesis of galactooligosaccharides and alkyl glycosides catalysed by glycosidases. The optimum water level can be controlled by the w_0 value, this value being greater than 10 for synthesis reactions. Currently important aspects of research on these systems include the stabilisation of biocatalysts and the development of appropriate reactors to accomplish enzyme retention, product separation and avoid product contamination with the surfactant molecules.

Very low water systems

For many biotransformations it is advantageous to decrease the amount of water in the reaction medium considerably. The first studies in this area were performed in 1966 and since then extensive research has been carried out. It is believed that retention of enzyme activity is due to the minimum essential water necessary to maintain the protein structure and the enzymatic function. The selection of the organic solvent is critical as hydrophilic solvents strip the essential hydration shell from the enzyme molecule. The amount of water bound to the enzyme decreases dramatically with the increasing hydrophilicity of the solvent. For example, the reactivity of α-chymotrypsin in octane is 10 000-fold higher than that in pyridine.

The amount of water in the reaction medium can be measured in several ways. The most common way is to measure the water concentration (in % v/v or mol 1^{-1}). This parameter, however, does not describe the reaction conditions for the enzyme. A better way to characterise the degree of hydration of the reaction medium is to use the thermodynamic water activity, a_w, as a parameter. This parameter, which is a measure of the amount of water in the system, directly determines the effects of water on the chemical equilibrium. During the reaction the water activity may change, especially if water is formed (esterification reactions) or consumed (hydrolysis). Therefore it is important to keep the water activity constant by controlling its concentration during the reaction, for example by adding salt hydrates directly to the reaction medium, which give a constant water activity suitable for the enzymatic conversion. The salt hydrates act as a *buffer* of the water activity.

Very low water systems involve the use of enzymes as solid suspension powders immobilised onto a support, in organic solvents

(Fig. 24.13g) or immobilised in the form of CLECs or CLEAs; and covalently modified enzymes soluble in organic media (Fig. 24.13e).

When enzyme powders are used as biocatalysts, problems can occur due to aggregation of the enzyme molecules. A solution to solve these problems is the immobilisation of the enzyme onto an appropriate solid support. The support should be judiciously selected taking into account its surface properties, namely its capacity to attract water (*aquaphilicity*), as the water in the reaction medium will partition between the enzyme, the support and the reaction medium affecting the enzyme microenvironment.

A very interesting feature of enzyme suspensions in organic media is the phenomenon of *pH memory*. It has been observed that lyophilised lipases and proteases and several oxido-reductases display pH optima in organic media identical to optima in aqueous solutions. This phenomenon is attributed to the right ionisation state of the enzyme for catalysis. Enzymes suspended in organic solvents have been observed to exhibit altered substrate specificity compared with those in aqueous media. This has been attributed to steric hindrance caused by the lack of conformational mobility of the enzyme (lipases and proteases) in organic solvents and to the substrate's inability to displace water from the hydrophobic binding pockets of the enzyme molecules in organic media.

Since dehydration drastically decreases the conformational mobility of enzymes, it has been observed, as expected, that the thermal denaturation process is slowed down considerably for enzymes suspended in organic solvents.

An approach to improve the activity of enzymes in organic solvents is the use of either excipients or salts, added to the aqueous enzyme solution prior to lyophilisation. These additives can improve the activity by different mechanisms. Additives, such as competitive inhibitors or substrate analogues that are removed after lyophilisation by anhydrous extraction, induce desirable conformational changes of the enzyme active site. These are then retained in organic solvents because of the enhanced enzyme rigidity. A lyoprotective effect can also result from the addition of sucrose or sorbitol, poly(ethylene glycol) or crown ethers. These chemicals tend to prevent conformational changes of the protein during the lyophilisation process.

Suspensions of solid enzymes in organic solvents have been used for a number of biotechnological applications, namely the transesterification of fats and oils by lipases, which is an industrial process for upgrading triacylglycerols. Other examples of biocatalysis in low water media include enzymatic oxido-reductions, such as the asymmetric sulphoxidation of organic sulphides catalysed by peroxidase; asymmetric reduction of racemic aldehydes and ketones and oxidations of racemic secondary alcohols catalysed by horse liver alcohol dehydrogenase; or the regio-selective hydroxylation of phenols with O_2 to catechols and subsequent dehydrogenation to orthoquinones, promoted by polyphenol oxidase.

In spite of the advantages of solid enzyme suspensions in organic solvents, these systems are limited by mass tranfer. To overcome these diffusional limitations, enzymes have been covalently modified, namely using polyethylene glycol for this purpose, to make them soluble in organic solvents. As the enzyme becomes soluble in the reaction, there are no diffusional limitations; however, in order to re-use the enzyme, it has to be recovered by precipitation from the reaction mixture with a non-polar solvent such as hexane. Other drawbacks of this type of enzyme are inactivation of the enzyme that may occur during the derivatisation procedure and that the enzyme preparations are soluble only in a limited number of solvents, like aromatic and chlorinated hydrocarbons.

24.6.2 Gas-phase reaction media

Solid–gas-phase systems present several advantages when compared to other systems, namely enhanced solubility of substrates and products. Enzymes and co-factors are more stable and the recovery of the biocatalyst from the conversion medium is simpler. Furthermore, mass transfer is usually not an overall rate-limiting step since diffusion in the gas phase is more efficient than in liquid solution. Since relatively high temperatures are used (e.g. from 45 to 85 °C), microbial contamination of the bioreactor can be avoided.

Enzymes, such as alcohol dehydrogenase, alcohol oxidase and lipases, have been mostly used in solid–gas biocatalysis. Such enzymes are involved in the production of volatile compounds, such as aldehydes, esters and ketones, through transesterification (alcoholysis) and redox reactions, mainly for the food and fragrance industries. Enzymes involved in redox reactions are co-factor dependent and, since these are expensive and have to be regenerated, the use of whole cells is an attractive approach since it allows co-factor regeneration. Besides, pure enzymes are often less stable than in their natural cell environment and their recovery and purification is frequently expensive. Dried cells of *Saccharomyces cerevisiae* have thus been used for the reduction of aldehydes and ketones in continuous solid–gas bioreactors. Similarly, lyophilised cells of *Rhodococcus erythropolis* have been used to hydrolyse 1-chlorobutane to 1-butanol in a solid–gas bioreactor, in an example of the validity of this approach for the bioremediation of volatile organic compounds.

24.6.3 Super-critical fluids as bioreaction media

Enzymatic reactions in super-critical and near-critical fluids require pressurised systems. Such systems permit high mass transfer rates and easy separation of reaction products. Due to its non-toxic character and its relatively low critical temperature (31 °C), super-critical CO_2 is the most frequently used fluid. Several bioconversions have been effectively performed in super-critical CO_2, namely the oxidation of cholesterol by cholesterol oxidase, the stereo-selective hydrolysis of racemic glycidyl butyrate by immobilised *Rhizomucor miehei* lipase yielding the homochiral R(-)glycidyl butyrate, the lipase-catalysed synthesis of aliphatic polyesters by ring-opening polymerisation of lactones and by polycondensation of divinyl esters and glycols, lipase-catalysed degradation of polyesters yielding oligomers, esterification between n-butyric acid and ethanol using free lipases, esterification of oleic acid with oleyl alcohol using immobilised lipase, lipase-catalysed synthesis of triolein-based sunscreens, transesterification between triolein and ethyl behenate by immobilised lipase, dipeptide synthesis by surfactant-coated α-chymotrypsin complexes, and sunflower oil hydrolysis by a lipase in a continuous membrane reactor. The non-polarity of CO_2, which preferentially dissolves only hydrophobic compounds, proves to be a limitation for its applications although the development of novel surfactants that allow dissolution of both hydrophilic and hydrophobic materials in CO_2 can overcome this constraint. The solubility of some compounds may also be improved by the addition of small amounts of co-solvents, known as entrainers. For example, methanol (3.5% mol mol^{-1}) was used as an entrainer to enhance the solubility of cholesterol in super-critical CO_2. Furthermore, super-critical CO_2 can occasionally strip essential water from an enzyme's surface leading to its deactivation. Thus, near-critical propane was used to overcome such drawbacks, in lipase-catalysed esterification between n-butyric acid and ethanol. Subtilisin CLECs, suspended in super-critical ethane, were also used for transesterification and hydrolysis and several other compressed gases (Freon R23, butane, dimethyl ether and sulphur hexafluoride) have been evaluated. The major drawback of these reaction systems is the high energy requirement and equipment costs due to the use of high pressure.

24.6.4 Biocatalysis in ionic liquids

Ionic liquids are salts that do not crystallise at room temperature. They are mainly composed of either a 1,3-dialkylimidazolium cation or an N-alkylpyridinium cation and a non-coordinating anion, e.g. BF_4^-, BF_6^- or NO^-_3. These chemicals are envisaged as possible *green* replacements for organic solvents. Ionic liquids have no vapour pressure, are thermally stable, and their polarity, hydrophobicity and solvent miscibility can be adequately tuned by adequate modifications of the cation or the anion. Enzymes tend to remain active in the presence of ionic liquids provided that they do not dissolve but, instead, remain suspended as a powder. A considerable array of enzyme types, but particularly lipases, are catalytically active in the presence of ionic liquids. The ability to use these solvents in bioconversion media enables high concentrations of polar substrates (e.g. sugars and vitamins) to be used. This, in turn, leads to fast reactions and high product yields.

The thermal stability of enzymes, such as lipases, can be enhanced when they are in ionic liquids, possibly because a more active conformation of the enzyme is induced. (Enantio)selectivity is also enhanced as compared to traditional media. Although biocatalysis in ionic media has focused mainly on the use of enzymes, whole cells of *Rhodococcus* B312, baker's yeast and *E. coli* also retain catalytic activity in such media probably because ionic liquids are less deleterious to cell membranes than organic solvents.

Table 24.12 Some examples of biocatalysts retaining activity in ionic liquids

Biocatalyst	Reaction
Esterases	Transesterification
Glycosidases hydratases	Carbohydrate synthesis
Rhodococcus B312	Hydration of 1,3-dicyanobenzene
Lipases	Alcoholysis
	Amide synthesis
	Esterification
	Perhydrolysis
	Polyester synthesis
	Transesterification
Proteases	
Thermolysin	Peptide synthesis
α-Chymotrypsin	Transesterification
Subtilisin	Enantio-selective hydrolysis
Redox systems	
Baker's yeast	Ketone reduction
Formate dehydrogenase	NADH regeneration
Laccase	Syrringaldazine oxydation
Peroxidases	Guaiacol oxidation

Examples of biocatalysts that are active in ionic liquids are given in Table 24.12. Despite their many advantages, these solvents present some drawbacks, among them their high viscosity, complex recovery and purification procedures. Also, the control of water activity and pH in these liquids is difficult.

24.7 | Concluding remarks

This chapter described the use and performance of biocatalysts in biotransformations relevant to industrial, analytical and biomedical applications and environment bioremediation.

From a process point of view, there are advantages and limitations for both chemical and biochemical routes. Part of the limitations of the biocatalytic route has been solved through new developments in the areas of biology, chemistry and process engineering. The recent advances in recombinant DNA technology, metabolic engineering, fermentation and biocatalysis in non-conventional media have also broadened the applications of biocatalysts to synthetic and oxidative/reductive biotransformations. It is also important to emphasise the integration of both processes and disciplines (engineering, biology and chemistry), which is a key feature for the development of competitive biocatalytic routes. New applications of biocatalysts (native or modified) in the fields of chemical synthesis, biomedical (biosensors), and environment analyses are foreseen.

24.8 | Further reading

van Beilen, J. B., Funhoff, E. G. Expanding the alkane oxygenase toolbox: new enzymes and applications. *Current Opinions in Biotechnology* **16**: 308–314, 2005.

Breuer, M. and Hauer, B. Carbon–carbon coupling in biotransformation. *Current Opinions in Biotechnology* **14**: 570–576, 2003.

Burton, S. G. Oxidizing enzymes as biocatalysts. *Trends in Biotechnology* **21**: 543–549, 2003.

Burton, S. G., Cowan, D. A. and Woodley, J. M. The search for the ideal biocatalyst. *Nature Biotechnology* **20**: 37–45, 2002.

Cao, L. Immobilised enzymes: science or art? *Current Opinions in Chemical Biology* **9**: 217–226, 2005.

Cao, L., van Langeny, L. and Sheldon, R. A. Immobilised enzymes: carrier-bound or carrier-free? *Current Opinions in Biotechnology* **14**: 387–394, 2003.

Gavrilescu, M., Chisti, Y. Biotechnology–a sustainable alternative for chemical industry. *Biotechnology Advances* **23**: 471–499, 2005.

Gill, I. and Ballesteros, A. *Bioencapsulation within synthetic polymers. 1: Sol-gel encapsulated biologicals. Trends in Biotechnology* **18**: 282–296, 2000.

Ishige, T., Honda, K., Shimizu S. Whole organism biocatalysis. *Current Opinions in Chemical Biology* **9**: 174–180, 2005.

Krishna, S. H. Developments and trends in enzyme catalysis I in non-conventional media. *Biotechnology Advances* **20**: 239–266, 2002.

Müller, M. Chemical diversity through biotransformations. *Current Opinions in Biotechnology* **15**: 591–598, 2004.

OECD. *The Application of Biotechnology to Industrial Sustainability.* Paris: OECD Publications, 2001.

Schmid, A., Dordick, J. S., Hauer, B., *et al.* Industrial biocatalysis: today and tomorrow. *Nature* **409**: 258–268, 2001.

Schmid, A., Hollmann, F., Park, J. B. and Bühler, B. The use of enzymes in the chemical industry in Europe. *Current Opinions in Biotechnology* **13**: 359–366, 2002.

Straathof, A. J. J. and Adlercreutz, P. (eds.) *Applied Biocatalysis*, second edition. Switzerland: Harwood Academic, 2000.

Szczebara F. N., Chandelier, C., Villeret, C., *et al.* Total biosynthesis of hydrocortisone from a single carbon source in yeast. *Nature Biotechnology* **21**: 143–149, 2003.

Turner, N. J. Directed evolution of enzymes for applied biocatalysis. *Trends in Biotechnology* **21**: 474–478, 2003.

Van Beilen, J. B. and Li, Z. Enzyme technology: an overview. *Current Opinions in Biotechnology* **13**: 338–344, 2002.

van der Donk, W. A. and Zhao, H. Recent developments in pyridine nucleotide regeneration. *Current Opinions in Biotechnology* **14**: 421–426, 2003.

Zhao, H., Chockalingam, K. and Chen, Z. Directed evolution of enzymes and pathways for industrial biocatalysis. *Current Opinions in Biotechnology* **13**: 104–110, 2002.

Chapter 25

Immunochemical applications

Mike Clark

University of Cambridge, UK

Glossary

Adjuvants Substances that when mixed with an antigen will make them more immunogenic, i.e. they enhance the immune response. Adjuvants cause inflammation and irritation and help to activate cells of the immune system.

Affinity The measured binding constant of an antibody for its antigen at equilibrium.

Alloimmunisation Immunisation of an animal with cells or tissues derived from another animal of the same species where there are allelic differences in their genes.

Antibody Adaptive proteins in the plasma of an immune individual with binding specificity for antigens (cf immunoglobulin).

Antigen A molecule, or complex of molecules, that is recognised by an antibody (immunoglobulin) by binding to the antibody's variable or V-regions.

Basic Biotechnology, third edition, eds. Colin Ratledge and Bjørn Kristiansen.
Published by Cambridge University Press. © Cambridge University Press 2006.

Antigen-presenting cells (APCs) An antigen-presenting cell is a specialised cell (dendritic cells and macrophages) that can ingest, degrade and then present on its cell surface, fragments of pathogens and other antigens, to other cells of the immune system (e.g. B-cells and T-cells).

Autoimmune Immunity to molecules (antigens) within an animal's own body that can lead to a disease, e.g. rheumatoid arthritis, or some forms of diabetes.

Avidity Antibodies frequently interact with antigen using multiple antigen-binding sites and thus they have a functional affinity termed avidity which is a complex function of the individual binding affinities.

B-cells A sub-set of white cells (lymphocytes) in the blood which produce antibodies.

CDR (1, 2 and 3) The three complementarity determining regions of the immunoglobulin variable-region domains that form the major interaction with antigen. Structurally, the complementarity determining regions form the loops at one end of the globular domain.

Chimaeric antibody Recombinant DNA technology allows artificial antibodies to be prepared in which domains from one antibody are substituted by domains from another antibody or protein.

Class The major type or classification of an immunoglobulin, e.g. IgM, IgG, IgA or IgE.

Complement An autocatalytic enzyme cascade found in the plasma that can be triggered by antibody–antigen complexes and that can lead to antigen destruction and removal.

D-segment The diversity segment, a gene segment found in immunoglobulin heavy chains that is re-arranged between the V-segment and the J-segment.

Effector functions Immune functions triggered through specific binding of antibody to antigen. These include complement in the plasma and Fc receptors on many different cell types.

Epitope The epitope is a single antibody-binding site on an antigen. Any given antigen may bind different antibodies through different epitopes.

ELISA An enzyme-linked, immunoadsorbent assay is a commonly used assay system in which an antibody is covalently linked to an enzyme so that conversion of a substrate can be used to quantify the amount of antibody bound.

Fab The antigen-binding proteolytic fragment of an immunoglobulin.

F(ab')$_2$ A proteolytic fragment of an immunoglobulin in which the two antigen-binding 'Fab' fragments are still attached at the hinge.

Fc The crystallisable proteolytic fragment of an immunoglobulin. This fragment also contains the sequences needed for interacting with and triggering effector functions.

Fc receptor A protein molecular complex expressed on a cell that is able to bind specifically to and recognise sequences within the Fc fragment of an immunoglobulin.

FR (1, 2, 3 and 4) The framework regions are four partially conserved (less variable) regions of sequence within the immunoglobulin variable-region domains. Structurally, the framework regions form the conserved antiparallel βstrands of the protein domains.

Fv fragments The minimal component of an immunoglobulin still capable of binding to antigen. It consists of the heavy- and light-chain variable domains.

Hapten A hapten is a small molecule that can be recognised by antibodies but which is not immunogenic in itself. They thus must be coupled covalently to carrier proteins in order to use them for immunisation.

Humanised antibodies In order to reduce the immunogenicity of monoclonal antibodies in human patients many of the rodent-derived sequences are substituted with homologous human sequences. This can also be done for the framework regions within the variable-region domains to give a 'fully humanised' or 're-shaped' antibody.

Hybridoma cells In order to produce long-term cell lines secreting a single specific antibody, B-cells from the spleens of immunised animals are fused with myeloma cells adapted to growth in cell culture. These hybrid cell lines made with myeloma cells are called hybridomas.

Immunoadhesins Fusion proteins, generated using recombinant DNA technology, in which cellular adhesion molecules are made as a chimaeric hybrid molecule with an immunoglobulin Fc region.

Immune complex A complex of antibodies bound to their antigens.

Immunogenic A form of an antigen that is capable of generating an immune response when injected or administered to an animal.

Immunoglobulin A globulin fraction of plasma that contains the specific immune proteins termed antibodies.

Immunoprecipitation The use of antibodies to remove an antigen from solution through the formation of an insoluble or immobilised immune complex.

Immunosuppress To lower, or suppress, the ability of an animal to make an active immune response. This may be desired, and can be achieved using drugs, or antibodies, specific for regulatory cells of the immune system. It can also occur as an unwanted effect in some diseases such as in AIDS resulting from HIV infection.

J-chain Is a 'joining' protein sub-unit that is found covalently associated, through disulphide bonds, with multi-meric immunoglobulins such as IgA dimers and IgM pentamers. The J-chain should not be confused with the similar sounding 'J-segment' (see below).

J-segment Is the junctional or joining DNA segment that is rearranged with the V-segment for immunoglobulin light chains, or the V-and D-segments for immunoglobulin heavy chains, to give a fully formed immunoglobulin variable (V-) region.

MHC class I and class II Major histocompatibility locus class-I and class-II molecules are the molecules on a cell surface used to present peptide fragments of an antigen to the T-cell receptor.

Monoclonal antibody This term is applied to an antibody produced from a clonal cell line in tissue culture. It is a well-defined antibody of predictable characteristics, unlike the complex mixtures of antibodies found in an animal's plasma.

Polyclonal antisera This term is used to distinguish the inherently heterogeneous mixture of antibodies found in the sera derived from an immunised animal, from the laboratory prepared monoclonal antibodies.

Sub-class A sub-classification of an immunoglobulin within a given class, e.g. IgG1, IgG2, IgG3 and IgG4 are all IgG sub-class antibodies.

ScFv A single chain Fv fragment is an artificial genetic construct in which a polypeptide linker has been inserted between the N-terminus of one variable-region domain and the C-terminus of the other variable-region domain.

Specificity The specificity of an antibody is the ability to show a level of discrimination in binding avidities between different antigens. It is thus in a sense a relative term, i.e. the antibody is specific for 'antigen A' but not for 'antigen B'. This would then be termed an *anti-A antibody*.

T-cells A sub-set of white cells (lymphocytes) in the blood that either directly kill infected cells or help other cells, such as B-cells, to respond to an antigen.

V-region Variable region of an immunoglobulin.

V_H The variable region domain of the immunoglobulin heavy chain.

V_L The variable region domain of the immunoglobulin light chain.

V-segment A gene segment that is re-arranged to give a functional immunoglobulin variable region.

Xenoimmunisation Immunisation of one species with cells or tissues of a different species.

25.1 | Introduction

This chapter will discuss immunochemical applications in basic biotechnology and thus will mainly concentrate on the derivation and applications of **antibodies** otherwise known as **immunoglobulins** (Ig). These proteins are so named because of the way in which they were first discovered. They were first identified as a particular globulin protein fraction of the blood, which was called the gammaglobulin and, because it was then recognised that this protein fraction was a major specific component of the immune response made to infection, they were also called immunoglobulins. The term 'antibody' refers to the fact that they recognise or are specific ('anti-') for 'foreign bodies'. Antibodies are important within biotechnology because of the ease with which it is possible to exploit the immune system's ability to generate a diverse population of immunoglobulins with specificity for binding to a huge range of different molecular structures, the 'foreign bodies' recognised by antibodies, which we call **antigens**.

In order to describe these applications it is necessary that the reader has some basic knowledge of the immunobiology of antibody production and of immunoglobulin structure and function. A very brief and simplified overview will be given here but it should be noted that the immune system has evolved of necessity to be highly complex in organisation and the interested reader is recommended to look at more detailed and fuller explanations given in the many widely available immunology textbooks (see the Further reading list).

25.2 | Antibody structure and functions

Antibodies are proteins made as part of the humoral immune response to immunogenic substances and infectious agents. They serve as key adapter molecules within the immune system, enabling the host's inherited **effector functions** to recognise the many unpredictable, diverse and varied antigen structures that might be encountered during an animal's lifetime. These **effector functions** are inherited mechanisms for inactivating or killing infectious pathogens and then causing their breakdown and removal from the body. However, these **effector systems** do not have the ability to recognise the infectious agents easily in all of their many diverse forms. This recognition, or targeting, of the effector systems is, in part, dependent upon the antibody's ability to interface between antigens on the infectious agent and also the body's effector systems. The effector systems are inherited within the germ-line genes of an individual, but the antibody specificities are derived by complex somatic re-arrangements of the genes encoding immunoglobulins within the so-called B-cells (a sub-population of the white blood cells or lymphocytes). This means that even two identical twins, or two mice from the same laboratory strain, will have different immunoglobulin sequences expressed at any one time.

The basic schematic representation of an antibody is the familiar Y-shaped structure of an IgG with two identical **Fab** (antigen binding) arms and a single **Fc** (crystallisable) region joined by a more flexible **hinge region** (see Fig. 25.1). Again, these terms come about from the original protein chemistry in which the whole molecule was fragmented by cleavage with proteolytic enzymes and different properties were then assigned to the different isolated fragments. This basic molecular structure (or sub-unit) is made up of two identical heavy (**H**) chains and two identical light (**L**) chains, based upon their molecular size, and each chain contains repeated immunoglobulin-type globular domains with a conserved structure. In protein structural terms, the domains have antiparallel strands that loop back on themselves to form β-sheets and these sheets are then rolled up into a barrel-like structure (see Fig. 25.2). Light chains have two of these globular domains, whereas heavy chains have four or more (depending upon their **class**, see below). The heavy and light chains come in several different forms, which give rise to the concept of immunoglobulin classes and sub-classes, and, for example in man (and most other mammals), we have heavy-chain types μ, γ, ε and α giving, respectively, the classes of antibody IgM, IgG, IgE and IgA. Each of these classes can have light-chains of either the κ or the λ type. The proportion of immunoglobulins in the plasma with each light-chain type varies between species with humans having a $\kappa : \lambda$ ratio of approximately 60 : 40, whereas mice have a ratio of about 90 : 10. In humans, the IgG class has four sub-classes called IgG1, IgG2, IgG3 and IgG4, using $\gamma 1$, $\gamma 2$, $\gamma 3$ and $\gamma 4$ chains; whilst the IgA class has two sub-classes IgA1 and IgA2, using $\alpha 1$ and $\alpha 2$ chains. Some of these classes of immunoglobulin are secreted into plasma in the form of more complex oligomerised structures of sub-units often associated with a molecule called a J-chain. Thus IgM is a pentamer of five identical

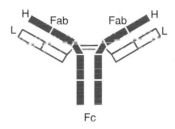

Figure 25.1 The basic IgG immunoglobulin structure of two heavy chains (black) and two light chains (white). The two heavy chains are disulphide bonded together and each light chain is disulphide bonded to a heavy chain. The antibody also has two antigen-binding Fab regions and a single Fc region.

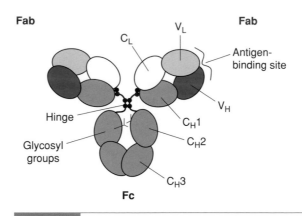

Figure 25.2 An alternative schematic of an IgG structure. Each globular domain of the molecule is illustrated as an ellipse. The heavy-chain domains are shown in darker shades and the light-chain domains in lighter shades. The heavy- and light-chain variable domains V_H and V_L are also indicated along with the position of the antigen-binding site at the extremities of each Fab. Each C_H2 domain is glycosylated and the carbohydrate sits in the space between the two heavy chains. Disulphide bridges between the chains are indicated as black dots within the flexible hinge region.

protein sub-units, and IgA is frequently found as dimers and trimers of identical protein sub-units, again associated with a J-chain (see Fig. 25.3).

It is the heavy chain that is largely responsible for the 'effector functions' (antigen destruction and removal) triggered through interactions with cells of the immune system by *ligation* (binding to and cross-linking) of cell surface receptors (called **Fc receptors** because they require the Fc fragment of the antibody) or, alternatively, through activation of the **complement cascade** and the binding to **complement receptors**. *Complement* is another family of proteins found in the blood and are involved in immune reactions. The components of complement are mainly specific proteolytic enzymes whose substrates are themselves other complement components that are activated by proteolysis. This gives rise to a classical biochemical amplification of an initial small activation step. Once activated, some of these complement components also rapidly form covalent chemical bonds with antigen, thus marking them for clearance by complement receptors of the immune system, whilst others are able to create pores in cell or viral membranes of infectious organisms and thus kill the cells or viruses.

Each of the different immunoglobulin (antibody) classes, and also sub-classes, exhibit a different pattern of effector functions, some of which may be more appropriate in dealing with certain types of antigens or infectious agents. Each of the different classes of immunoglobulin has their own class of Fc effector functions. Thus there are well-characterised Fc receptors for the IgG class (FcγRI, FcγRII, FcγRIII), the IgA class (FcαR) and the IgE class (FcϵRI and FcϵRII) that have different cellular distributions, affinities for Fc type and sub-class, and

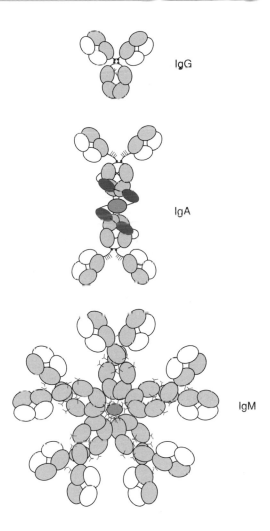

IgG

IgA

IgM

Figure 25.3 The origins of immunoglobulins. Different classes of immunoglobulin are built up from the same basic structure. The top shows IgG, which can be compared with Fig. 25.2. In secretory IgA, two sub-units of IgA, each of which is similar to IgG, are joined together by covalent disulphide bridges and through a sub-unit known as a J-chain (dark grey). During transport and secretion of IgA across the gut lining, a second set of sub-units, which are derived from the transport receptor, also become associated. These extra sub-units found only on secreted IgA are known as 'secretory components' (black). IgM has a pentameric structure of five sub-units covalently bonded together by disulphide bonds and associated like IgA, with a single sub-unit of J chain (dark grey).

that also mediate different signals and thus trigger different effector functions. In addition, for some of these classes, there are **transport receptors** that enable, for example, IgA to be secreted into the gut, the urinary tract, the respiratory tract, into tears and saliva, and also into milk and colostrum.

The receptor for transport of IgA is the poly Ig receptor and, during the transport of the IgA, the receptor is cleaved leaving a fragment of the receptor, termed secretory component (because it was initially characterised on secreted, but not plasma, IgA), associated with secreted IgA (see Fig. 25.3). In humans, IgG is actively transported across the placenta during the late stages of pregnancy to provide the neonate with a primary immune defence; whilst in other animals, such as rodents, the IgG is transported across the gut from colostrum during the first few hours after birth. The receptor that transports IgG, is called FcRn (the neonatal Fc receptor). FcRn is also responsible for protecting IgG from catabolism and is thus responsible for extending the plasma half-life of IgG from days to weeks. FcRn achieves this by binding at low pH to the Fc region of IgG, which is within intracellular endosomal vesicles containing proteins destined for degradation. The bound IgG is then recycled back to the plasma before it is degraded, whereupon it is released under the neutral pH conditions encountered at the plasma membrane. This has considerable importance and consequences with regard to pharmaceutical applications of IgG antibodies in vivo. A long antibody half-life in the plasma means that a smaller amount of antibody is needed at less frequent intervals to maintain a required plasma concentration. The extent of the half-life is a function of the specific binding of receptor FcRn to the Fc region of IgG and is thus lost in fragments of antibodies such as Fab fragments. Obviously, because FcRn is an IgG-specific receptor, these properties of placental transfer and extended half-life are unique to this class of immunoglobulins. The name FcRn had originally been applied to just the form of receptor found in the gut of neonatal rats, but in a much earlier series of papers, published by Professor Brambell in the mid 1960s, the existence of both forms of receptor had been predicted, and thus some now refer to both functions of the receptor under the unified name of FcRB.

As already mentioned, the antigen specificity of the antibody is a property of the Fab fragment of the molecule. Specificity is the result of variation in parts of the sequences of the Fab. The N-terminal domain of both the heavy and light chain is called the variable region (V_H and V_L domains). Sequence analysis of amino acids of large numbers of variable regions for both V_H and V_L has allowed three small regions of hyper-variability to be defined within four more conserved framework regions (FR1, FR2, FR3 and FR4). In the three-dimensional structures, the hyper-variable regions form loops that combine together to form the principal antigen-binding surfaces and thus these sequences have also been named the **complementarity determining regions** or CDRs (CDR1, CDR2 and CDR3; see Fig. 25.4).

In terms of the genetics of immunoglobulin expression, the unique sequences of each different antibody are the direct result of somatic re-arrangements of different gene segments during B-cell development (see Fig. 25.5). In the case of the heavy chain, three segments, V, D and J, are re-arranged, and in the case of light chains, two segments, V and J, are re-arranged. These gene re-arrangements lead to expression of a surface immunoglobulin receptor and this is followed by selection of individual B-cell clones based on their binding to antigen. Further differentiation can result in somatic mutations of the V-region sequences and/or further somatic cell re-arrangements to bring the constant region segments for different heavy-chain subclasses adjacent to the variable-domain-encoding gene segments.

25.3 | Antibody protein fragments

Various protein fragments of antibodies can be produced individually and separately from the other protein components, which may be of practical use in different circumstances (see Fig. 25.6). These

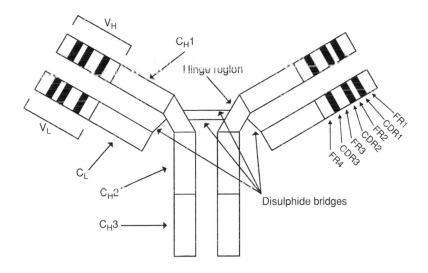

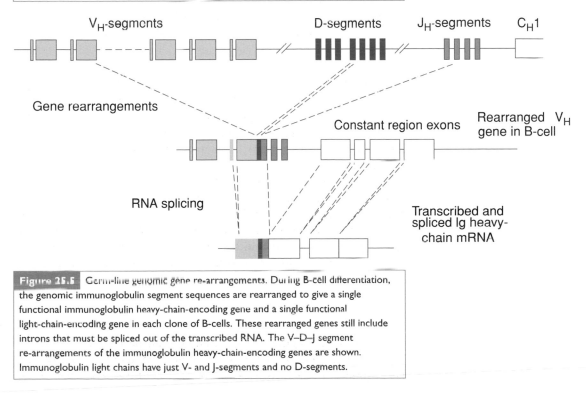

Figure 25.4 Regions of the variable domains of IgG. The sequences of these domains are classified as either framework region sequences (FR1, FR2, FR3 and FR4) or complementarity determining regions (CDR1, CDR2 and CDR3). Framework region sequences are sequences that go to make up the conserved β-pleated strands, which form the globular barrel shape of the domain structure. The complementarity determining regions form the variable loop structures that make the antigen-binding sites. There are three CDR loops from each heavy chain and three CDR loops from each light chain. These six loops act together to form the antigen-binding site of the antibody.

Figure 25.5 Germ-line genomic gene re-arrangements. During B-cell differentiation, the genomic immunoglobulin segment sequences are rearranged to give a single functional immunoglobulin heavy-chain-encoding gene and a single functional light-chain-encoding gene in each clone of B-cells. These rearranged genes still include introns that must be spliced out of the transcribed RNA. The V–D–J segment re-arrangements of the immunoglobulin heavy-chain-encoding genes are shown. Immunoglobulin light chains have just V- and J-segments and no D-segments.

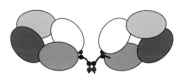

F(ab')$_2$ fragment

Fab fragment

F$_v$ fragment

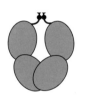

Fc fragment

Figure 25.6 Functional sub-fragments of IgG molecule. These can be generated either through limited proteolysis or through expression of recombinant genes.

fragments can conveniently be derived by enzyme proteolysis. In general, the Fab region is relatively resistant to proteolysis; whereas the Fc region and, particularly, the hinge region are comparatively susceptible. Depending upon which protease is used and the particular antibody isotype under examination (and the animal species from which the antibody is derived), the proteolytic cleavage may occur at the hinge region. If it does, and the cleavage site is on the C-terminal side of the inter-chain disulphide bridges, then F(ab')$_2$ fragments are generated; if cleavage is on the N-terminal side, Fab fragments are generated. Alternatively, mildly reducing conditions can be used to separate the F(ab')$_2$ fragment into two F(ab') fragments.

Protein fragments can also be expressed using recombinant DNA techniques. Other recombinant products, such as the so-called **Fv fragments**, contain only the V-region domains, which are not covalently associated and could be considered as the smallest unit of antibody that should still be capable of antigen binding with the original single-site affinity. In order to stabilise this association of the V-regions of the recombinant heavy and light chains, a gene segment encoding an artificial linker from the C-terminus of one domain to the N-terminus of the other can be introduced and the whole fusion protein expressed, by a suitable cell, as a single-chain Fv (**ScFv**).

All the small fragments of antibodies may be of use, both in vitro and *in vivo*, because they are still capable of binding to an antigen but have lost the ability to bind to Fc receptors and to activate the complement cascade. Their smaller size can in certain situations improve their diffusion and penetration properties; particularly, for example, when they are used, for staining of tissue sections in vitro, or for targeting of cellular antigens in vivo. However, for IgG, the loss of the Fc in addition to the smaller size of the fragments will, of course, result in a considerable decrease in the plasma half-life as discussed above.

It should also be noted that post-translational modifications of an antibody may be critical for its functions. Antibodies of different classes and sub-classes show conserved sites for both N- and O-linked sugars. In IgG, the conserved N-linked glycosylation of the C_H2 region is essential for many of the molecule's effector functions (i.e. binding to some Fc receptors and also activation of complement is dependent upon the correct glycosylation). Similarly, the intra- and interchain disulphide bridges are important for the overall structure and function of the antibody. Thus the manner in which antibodies are produced, as well as the particular methods of purification, are important issues to consider. This is the case particularly with recombinantly produced immunoglobulins, for example where the inability of bacteria to glycosylate or reliably assemble, and disulphide bond complex proteins must be taken into account.

25.4 | Antibody affinity

The concept of the **affinity**, or more correctly the **avidity**, of an antibody for antigen is important. For many uses, both in vivo and in vitro, the affinity of the antibody for antigen is an important factor in determining not only the utility but also the commercial success of a product. Strictly, the affinity of an antibody for its antigen (association constant or K_a expressed in units of m^{-1}) is a measure of the ratio of the concentrations of bound antibody–antigen complex to free antibody and free antigen at a thermodynamic equilibrium. It assumes that the interaction with bound antigen is of single valency, which is more likely to be the case only for very simple antigens or for antibody Fab or Fv fragments. In the past, antibody affinities were often determined by equilibrium dialysis or by measuring radiolabelled antibody binding to antigens under conditions near to equilibrium. It is quite common today, however, to carry out direct determination of percentage of antibody association and disassociation using techniques such as plasma resonance. However, it is worth remembering that a good approximation to the affinity of an antibody for an antigen can be estimated by measuring the concentration of antibody needed to give half maximal binding to the antigen. This gives the dissociation constant, K_d, expressed in units of m, which is, in fact, the reciprocal of the association constant K_a (i.e. $K_d = 1/K_a$).

It must be remembered that antibodies usually have two or more identical binding sites for an antigen. Often the interaction of a bivalent (e.g. whole IgG with two Fab regions) or multi-valent (e.g. IgM with ten Fab regions) antibody with multivalent antigen (e.g. a cell surface or antigen immobilised on a solid surface) is the critical parameter in determining the strength of interaction between antibody and antigen. This functional affinity of an antibody is referred to as its **avidity**. The affinity or avidity of an antibody (Ab) for an antigen (Ag) is related to the ratio of the rates of the forward reaction for formation of the complex to back reaction for decay of the complex:

$$[Ab] + [Ag] \underset{k_{backward}}{\overset{k_{forward}}{\rightleftharpoons}} [AbAg] \tag{25.1}$$

$$K_a = \frac{1}{K_d} = \frac{[AbAg]}{[Ab] \cdot [Ag]}$$

Two antibodies can have a similar affinity for antigen measured at equilibrium, but one may have a much slower on-rate ($k_{forward}$) and, of course, a proportionally slower off-rate ($k_{backward}$). In many instances, the antibody will not be used under conditions of thermodynamic equilibrium: for example, when using an antibody to affinity purify an antigen or when using antibodies in immunometric assays. In such situations, the antibody is usually in excess and a faster rate of the forward reaction ($k_{forward}$) may then be desirable. In a different example, such as the use of radiolabelled antibodies for the radioimaging of tumours in vivo, the antibody needs first to circulate through the body and then to diffuse and penetrate through the tissues before it even has a chance to interact with the antigen. The stability of antibody on the tumour once it is bound (affinity and off-rate) as well as the diffusion rates of the antibody in tissues (a product of the antibody or fragment size) are both factors that determine the suitability of one antibody versus another.

25.5 | Antibody specificity

The **specificity** of an antibody is another important concept and one that is often highly confused with the concept of affinity. In a practical sense, the specificity of an antibody for its antigen is only, in part, related to its affinity or avidity. It is highly likely that an antibody will have a spectrum of affinities for a range of different antigens. Sometimes these antigens may be completely unrelated whilst more often they may share related structural features (for example many different complex carbohydrate structures share features in common). Different antibodies to the same antigen may therefore show different functional cross-reactions on other antigens. Clearly, if the intended use of the antibody is to discriminate between different antigens in a complex mixture then the cross-reactions of the antibody are as critical as the avidity for the correct antigen. For an antibody that is to be used in a situation where the 'alternative' antigens are not likely to be encountered, for example in the affinity purification of an antigen product from a batch culture process, any cross-reactions may be considered as irrelevant. In the use of antibodies for in vivo therapy or diagnostics, there are so many different tissue antigens that unexpected cross-reactions of the antibody on tissues other than the intended target may frequently be a complicating factor in the development of an antibody-based product. The observation of the cross-reaction of an antibody on a second antigen is, of course, related to the avidity of the antibody for that antigen and the sensitivity of the assay being used to measure the interaction. This can lead to the situation where an apparent improvement in the sensitivity of an assay leads to a deterioration in the specificity of the assay.

25.6 | Immunisation and production of polyclonal antisera

The earliest, but still a widely used, way to exploit the immune system is to immunise an animal with an **immunogenic** form of the substance or a pathogen of interest (perhaps repeatedly over several months) and then, some weeks after the final immunisation, to collect the blood plasma or serum and use it whole or fractionated. It is necessary to understand some of the complexity of the immune response in order to appreciate some of the problems associated with derivation of antisera to different types of antigen. Figures 25.7 and 25.8 show a highly schematic and simplified view of two different types of B-cell response to antigen, T-cell-independent (Fig. 25.7) and T-cell-dependent (Fig. 25.8) responses to antigen. The T-cell-independent, B-cell response is largely the result of triggering the surface immunoglobulin on the B-cells by cross-linking

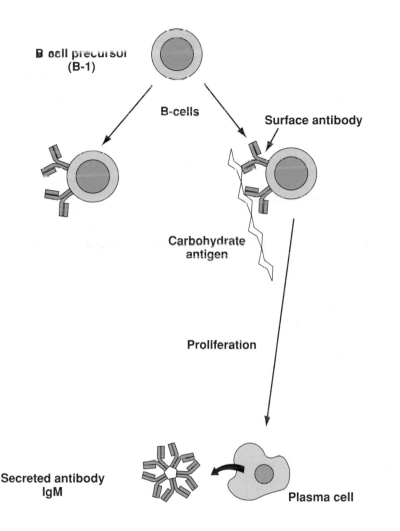

**B cell precursor
(B-1)**

B-cells

Surface antibody

**Carbohydrate
antigen**

Proliferation

**Secreted antibody
IgM**

Plasma cell

Figure 26.7 The T-cell-independent, B-cell response. Some key steps in the production of secreted IgM by a so-called T-cell-independent, B-cell response are illustrated. The critical feature is that the antigen is usually a multi-meric repeating structure (e.g. bacterial carbohydrate) and is capable of cross-linking the surface antibody on the B-cells which have specificity for this antigen. These B-cells are then activated by this event and go on to differentiate into plasma cells secreting the IgM.

with an antigen of a highly repetitive structure. Such antigens include carbohydrates, glycolipids, phospholipids and nucleic acids. The B-cells are driven into proliferation and differentiate into plasma cells that secrete large amounts of immunoglobulin (mainly of the IgM class). Immune responses of this type include the human antiblood group A and antiblood group B responses that are thought to be triggered by exposure to bacterial carbohydrates and that then cross-react with the blood group antigens from other individuals. This is an excellent example of natural cross-reactions of antibodies because, except for individuals who have been transfused with mismatched blood or women following pregnancy, a majority of individuals with such antibodies are unlikely to have encountered blood cells of these other blood groups. Antiblood group A and B antibodies, as well as being principally of the IgM class, are also generally of low affinity but, because of the valency of IgM (five sub-units and thus ten possible binding sites per molecule) and the repetitive structures within the antigen, they may interact with a high avidity.

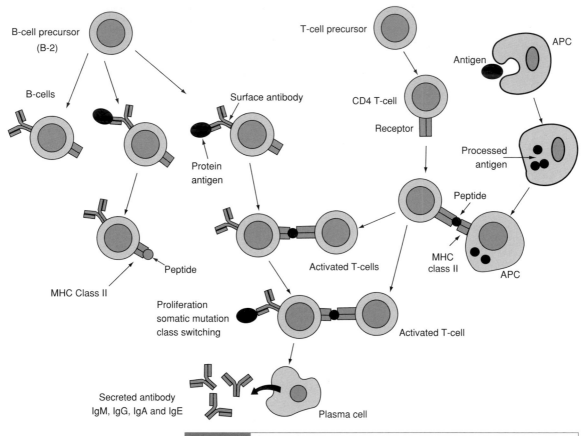

Figure 25.8 The T-cell-dependent, B-cell response. Antibody production resulting from the T-cell-dependent, B-cell response involves antigen recognition and cooperation between a number of different cell types including T-helper cells (which express the CD4 molecule, a co-receptor for MHC Class II) and so-called antigen-presenting cells or APCs (macrophages and dendritic cells). Antigen-presenting cells are called this because they present on their cell surface a complex of the MHC Class II molecule containing, within a binding groove, peptides from the antigen. These peptides are derived through proteolysis from antigen molecules that have been endocytosed. Before these antigen-specific B-cells can differentiate antibody secreting plasma cells they must be helped by an activated, CD4-positive, T-helper cell. For this activation, the CD4-positive T-helper cells must first see 'processed' antigen presented by macrophages or dendritic cells (APC).

In contrast, immune responses to T-cell-dependent antigens seem more complex and involve several steps whereby different cell types are required to interact in an antigen specific way thus allowing for complex regulation (see Fig. 25.5). Proteins are taken up by specialist **antigen-presenting cells** (APCs) and are broken down into peptides. Some of these peptides are capable of binding to MHC Class II molecules and are presented as a complex on the surface of the APC. CD4-positive, Class II restricted T-cells are able to bind the MHC peptide complex and can be activated by the APCs. B-cells are also capable of taking up antigen through their specific receptor, which is the membrane-bound surface immunoglobulin, and as a consequence they too can present peptides in the context of MHC Class II. If an activated CD4 T-cell interacts with such an antigen-presenting B-cell, it is able to help the B-cell by providing signals that activate the B-cell to divide, differentiate and secrete its antibody. During several such rounds of specific T- and B-cell cooperation, the B-cell may switch to produce other antibodies such as IgG, IgA and IgE and it may also undergo somatic mutation and be selected for higher-affinity binding to the antigen. Thus, in general, T-cell-dependent, B-cell antigens should be proteins or protein associated.

There is an important feature that is common to both T-cell-independent and T-cell-dependent B-cells and that is the concept of self-tolerance. In general, the immune system has checks and controls that act to minimise the chances of an immunoglobulin recognising a self-antigen being made in quantity. Such autoreactive B-cells are generally eliminated. In extreme situations, a breakdown of tolerance can occur and, in such cases, pathology can result from this so-called **autoimmune response**.

Self-tolerance means that it is again, in general, easier to generate antibody responses to antigens that are unrelated to any self-antigens within the animal being immunised. For example, there are more likely to be many differences if human-derived proteins are used to immunise a mouse (**xenoimmunisation**) than if mouse-derived proteins are used to immunise a different strain of mouse (**alloimmunisation**). The different regions on the antigen recognised by antibodies are called **antigenic epitopes** and thus a xenoimmunisation is likely to raise antibodies to more epitopes of an antigen than an alloimmunisation. This may be important and will be discussed later because simultaneous recognition of an antigen by several antibodies to different epitopes may result in apparently improved affinity (avidity) and specificity of reaction.

Another important factor of immunisation is that some antigens are more immunogenic than others. Partly this may relate to self-tolerance, but it is also now thought that an important component of an immune response is the activation of the immune system by danger signals. Thus an antigen can be combined with other substances, such as mineral oils and components derived from micro-organisms, that can act as **adjuvants** and activate the immune system and improve antigen processing and presentation by the APCs.

Following production, the antisera can be used in very many systems as a specific tool for detection of antigen. The immunoglobulin fraction of the antisera can be purified and then used in several assay and detection systems. For example, it can be labelled by covalent conjugation with fluorescent dyes and used in microscopy or flow cytometry for detecting antigen binding on or in cells. Equally, the antibody could be labelled with an enzyme and used in histology or in

Figure 25.9 Production of monoclonal antibodies. This involves fusion of spleen cells, from immunised rodents, with myeloma cells adapted to cell culture. The resulting hybridoma cells are selected for growth in media that is toxic to the parental myeloma cells and they are then cloned. Each clone produces a single monoclonal antibody.

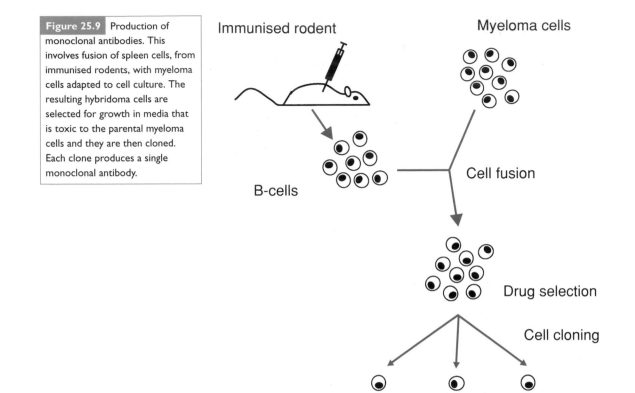

an enzyme-linked, immunosorbent assay (ELISA; see Section 25.10.2) again for detection of the specific antigen.

25.7 | Monoclonal antibodies

Conventionally, cell lines secreting monoclonal antibodies have been derived by taking immune B-cells, which have a limited capacity to proliferate in vitro, and then immortalising them by somatic cell fusion with a suitable tissue culture cell line (see Fig. 25.9). For reasons that are most likely to be related to the complex interactions of regulatory genes (e.g. transcription factors) encoded on different chromosomes in different species, this technique has proved to be most successful for a limited range of species, particularly for monoclonal antibodies of the IgM and IgG classes derived from rat and mice, although other species such as sheep, hamsters and humans have been used.

In the methods used for cell fusion and subsequent selection of hybridomas, a large number of variations exist. These are well documented in text books and reviews devoted to the methodology. Although Kohler and Milstein used the *Sendai* virus to induce cell fusion in their earlier experiments, this virus has been replaced almost universally with polyethylene glycol (PEG) or electrofusion techniques. For mouse and rat hybridomas, the efficiencies of these procedures are all high and typically several hundreds to thousands of individual hybridoma clones can be obtained from one animal spleen.

Using somatic cell fusion or cell transformation, either alone or in combination, it has proved very difficult to make human monoclonal antibodies. The time and effort expended is far greater than that needed to produce the equivalent mouse or rat monoclonal antibodies. It is this difficulty in production of human monoclonal antibodies that has driven the strategies for the rescue of human antibodies by phage display or alternatively to 'humanise' or 're-shape' rodent antibodies using recombinant DNA technology for so-called 'antibody engineering'.

25.8 | Antibody engineering

It is now possible to engineer genetically and express a whole range of differing novel antibody constructs thus freeing biotechnologists from the constraints imposed by the natural biology of the immune system. It is the modular structure of antibody molecules, which are composed of a collection of discrete globular domains, encoded by genes with a similar modular structure whereby each domain is coded in a separate exon, that makes the manipulation of immunoglobulin genes a relatively straightforward proposition (see Fig. 25.5). There are several obvious advantages of recombinant antibodies over conventionally derived monoclonal antibodies.

It is technically feasible, through the use of appropriate cloning strategies, to isolate the genes encoding any antibody made from any immunised species; and, so, future applications need not be restricted to the derivation of the mouse, rat and human antibody classes.

Often monoclonal antibodies can be derived with the correct specificity, but they may exhibit the wrong effector functions because they are not of the desired species, class or sub-class of immunoglobulin. Obviously, using recombinant DNA technology, any V-regions can be expressed in combination with any constant regions selected for desirable properties. These antibodies are called **chimaeric antibodies** (see Fig. 25.10). Thus variable regions from rodent antibodies specific for chosen antigens can be combined with constant regions encoding human immunoglobulin classes/sub-classes, the final product having potential in vivo therapeutic uses in humans. It is also possible to introduce further mutations into the Fc regions to modify the properties to suit the proposed applications of the antibody, for example to remove the ability to bind to some Fc receptors or to activate complement.

Where in vivo therapeutic applications are concerned, rodent antibodies often are limited because they provoke an immune response in the patient to the antibody usually within a week of their first use. This precludes any further treatment beyond this time. As described above, useful rodent monoclonal antibodies can be partially

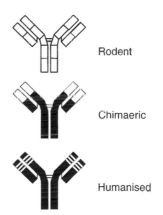

Rodent

Chimaeric

Humanised

Figure 25.10 Chimaeric antibodies. Through the use of recombinant DNA technology it is possible to engineer antibodies with novel properties. One simple step is to make chimaeric antibodies in which the variable regions from a rodent antibody (white) are combined with the constant regions of a human antibody (black). A step further in the technology is to combine just the complementarity determining region (CDR) encoding DNA sequences of a rodent antibody with framework region (FR) encoding DNA sequences of a human antibody, to give a fully humanised antibody.

'humanised' by making chimaeric antibodies by combining the rodent variable regions with human constant regions, thus introducing the effector mechanisms of the human whilst at the same time minimising the number of potential immunogenic epitopes. For immunotherapy, there are several key features that an antibody should have if it is to be successfully used. Obviously, the antibody must possess a desired specificity to bind to a relevant antigen, such as an antigen expressed on a tumour cell surface, a viral antigen or perhaps a bacterial toxin. Once bound to that antigen, the antibody is then normally required to carry out a function. The antibody could be used for targeting of a radioimaging label or used for the destruction of a tumour cell or of a virus. Alternatively, the antibody might be used for neutralisation of a virus or toxin. The production of a chimaeric antibody and the selection of the most appropriate human immunoglobulin class/sub-class, allows for the retention or addition of desirable functions but, at the same time, reduces the 'foreignness' of the antibody to the patient (see Fig. 25.10).

As a further step in lessening the immunogenicity or 'foreignness', rodent monoclonal antibodies can also be fully 'humanised' or 're-shaped', to produce human antibodies that contain only those key residues from the rodent variable regions responsible for antigen binding combined with framework regions from human variable regions (see Fig. 25.10).

After manipulation of the antibody genes, they can be expressed in a number of different expression systems. Transfection of antibody genes cloned in suitable vectors into myeloma cells may result in expression of the antibody molecules which are processed and glycosylated in a manner that is characteristic of immunoglobulin produced by hybridoma cells and normal B-cells. It is also possible to express antibodies in other mammalian cell types such as Chinese hamster ovary (CHO) cells. Antibodies have also been expressed in a number of other eukaryotic and also prokaryotic expression systems including plant cells, yeast and bacteria. However, there are certain problems that are encountered in some of these different expression systems chiefly with regard to glycosylation and to disulphide bonding that preclude expression of complete molecules or complicate the purification of the antibody product. Natural antibodies have multiple domains per chain and multiple chains per molecule and these chains have intradomain disulphide bonds as well as interchain disulphide bonds. Thus the cells used for antibody expression must be capable of correctly assembling the molecule. In addition, for most of the IgG antibody effector functions, appropriate N-linked glycosylation is required. Bacteria are thus only really appropriate for the expression of smaller fragments from antibodies such as Fab or Fv fragments. At present, most commercial large-scale production of recombinant antibody molecules, particularly for therapeutic applications, is carried out using either B-lymphoid cell lines or CHO cells.

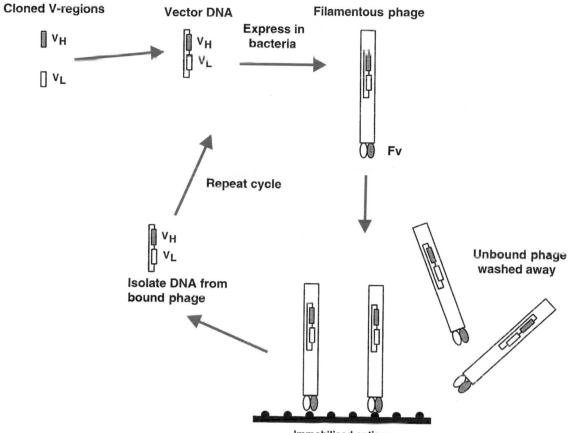

Figure 25.11 Making a phage display library. Antibody fragments can be expressed on the surface of a bacteriophage in which the antibody variable regions are encoded within the DNA which is packaged inside the phage. Thus by selecting for antigen-binding phage, it is possible to isolate the DNA, which in turn encodes the antigen-binding antibody V-regions. The cycle can be repeated to improve enrichment and to select for phage that bind with higher affinity.

25.9 | Combinatorial and phage display libraries

Recent advances in molecular biology mean that mammalian genes can be rapidly cloned and expressed in bacteria, usually using phage vector systems (see Chapter). In **phage display**, genes encoding variable regions of immunoglobulins are cloned into the phage vectors (see Fig. 25.11). These modified bacteriophage vectors are then used to transform bacteria and, during assembly of the phage particle, the immunoglobulin variable regions are expressed on the surface of the phage particles. Thus, if each bacterium is infected by only one phage type, all of the newly synthesised phage will carry the

DNA that encodes the same antibody Fv or Fab fragments on the surface of the phage. For the system to work, it is obvious that the phage that encodes the required antigen-specific Fv or Fab must be separated from other phage and then propagated further. This is conveniently achieved by affinity selection of the phage on antigen (see Fig. 25.11). During several rounds of selection, phage with higher affinity can be selected and propagated. Finally, it is possible to re-isolate the genes from the phage particles and to express them in other systems. For example, expression systems exist that produce soluble Fab or Fv fragments from the phage vector systems.

Antibody responses in a whole animal are transient, the antibodies appearing in reponse to immunisation or infection, and then disappearing over time once the antigen has been cleared from the body. Phage display provides the ability to rescue the antibody response from almost any immunised animal in the form of cloned genes encoding the individual heavy- and light-chain variable regions. Most strategies for cloning antibody genes in phage utilise random cloning of 'libraries' of the heavy- and light-chain sequences and then the expression of these libraries in randomised pairings of a single immunoglobulin heavy chain and a single immunoglobulin light chain in each individual phage. These **combinatorial libraries** are generated by cloning a repertoire of immunoglobulin heavy and light chains, usually by using the polymerase chain reaction, from mRNA isolated from tissue containing B-cells from an immune donor. It should be remembered, however, that the combinations rescued after screening such a library are not necessarily representative of the combinations present in the native B-cells. This last point may be of importance because, as described above, the B-cell repertoire found in vivo has been selected through a complex system of random gene re-arrangements followed by both positive and negative selection. The reason for this selection which involves T-cell antigen-specific recognition and T-cell help is to restrict the immune response to 'foreign' antigens and to prevent cross-reactions to self-antigens. Thus, certain combinations of heavy and light chains may be generated and selected for in combinatorial libraries that would be selected against in a normal immune response. Phage display can also be used to mimic the immune response by generating an artificial, randomised library of synthetic genes with random complementarity determining sequences (see Section 25.2; i.e. not derived by cloning genes from B-cells). Such libraries have been used successfully to screen for a number of different specificities.

A major disadvantage of phage display libraries is that the only antibody function being tested is antigen binding and this may not be the crucial function for the final application. Although the genes once isolated can be expressed along with any immunoglobulin constant regions, assays that are dependent upon the effector function cannot be used for the detection and isolation of the phage antibodies with appropriate specificity. Additionally, it is relatively easy to screen phage libraries on purified and homogeneous antigen preparations but it is very difficult to screen for specific binding to complex mixtures, such as cell surface antigens, where the required antigen may be a minor component of the mixture.

25.10 | In vitro uses of recombinant and monoclonal antibodies

25.10.1 Affinity purification

Major uses of antibodies include roles in the purification of other molecules using affinity binding procedures, often in single step. This relies on the ability to derive antibodies and, in particular, monoclonal or recombinant antibodies, that have a unique and discriminating specificity for the chosen antigen. To raise useful antisera for affinity purification of an antigen, it is usually necessary to have a highly purified antigen to start with. This is because the antisera will contain many different antibodies, i.e. it will be polyclonal, and thus the required antibodies must be affinity purified in some way. However, during the process of derivation of the monoclonal antibodies, it is possible to work with impure mixtures of antigens and yet still obtain a useful reagent for the affinity purification of the antigen. This is because when the animal is immunised with an impure antigen there will be antibodies made against all of the different antigens present, so the antisera from the animal will contain a complete mixture of antibodies. However, when the individual B-cell hybridomas are cloned in culture, all of these different antibody specificities are separated and the clones secreting antibody specific for a chosen antigen can be selected and large amounts of the antibody produced. Similarly, recombinant antibodies allow single, pure antibodies of defined specificity and affinity to be produced.

The affinity of an antibody for its antigen and its selectivity in binding can be exploited in techniques such as **immunoprecipitation**. The antibody is mixed with the antigen and it forms immune complexes. The basis for these immune complexes is that an antibody normally has at least two binding sites and so can, in theory, bind to at least two identical antigens. If the antigen, in turn, has more than one antigenic binding site (or epitopes), then the antigens and antibodies can form chains or higher-order aggregates (immune complexes). Sometimes, large immune complexes are formed and these then become insoluble and will form a precipitate. This insoluble immune precipitate can be separated away from the other antigens in solution by centrifugation and washing of the precipitate and, finally, it will contain a relatively pure mixture of the chosen antigen and its antibody.

There are several problems associated with immunoprecipitation reactions of this type. First, because they rely heavily on the valency of the antigen–antibody interactions in the immune complex, they do not work well using single monoclonal antibodies and they tend

Figure 25.12 Formation of immunoprecipitates. Antibodies and antigens can combine to form insoluble immune complexes. Thus the antigen is immunoprecipitated by the antibody. For this to occur, the antibody and antigen must be at appropriate concentrations otherwise small, soluble, immune complexes are formed.

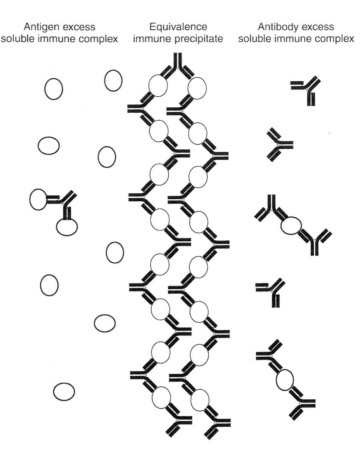

Antigen excess
soluble immune complex

Equivalence
immune precipitate

Antibody excess
soluble immune complex

to work better with mixtures of monoclonal antibodies or with polyclonal antisera. Also, the immunoprecipitation reaction works best over a narrow concentration range where the antibody and antigen are said to be at equivalence. Either side of this range, either the antigen or the antibody is in excess and only small soluble immune complexes are likely to be formed. This principle is exploited in immunodiffusion reactions where antibody and antigen are allowed to diffuse towards each other in a semi-solid agarose layer. Immunoprecipitation lines can be seen by eye where the points of equivalence have been reached (see Fig. 25.12). With appropriate standards and controls it is possible to adapt this technique to estimate the concentrations of antigen or antibody in mixtures and even to assess the purity of them.

An alternative strategy is to immobilise the antibody onto a solid matrix support, such as on Sepharose beads, using a covalent chemical reaction. The beads can then be packed into a column and solutions containing the antigen passed through (see Fig. 25.13). The antibody will remove the antigen from the rest of the mixture by a process of affinity chromatography. This process can be of direct use, for example in the removal of a contaminant such as a toxin from another protein, when an antibody or antisera specific for the toxin exists. If the antigen that is adsorbed to the antibody on the matrix is required, it is necessary to find conditions that disrupt the affinity of binding. Several methods are appropriate under different conditions. For some low-affinity antibody–antigen interactions, adsorbtion may be achieved by competition with an alternative ligand. For higher-affinity interactions, it is usually necessary to use partially denaturing conditions and chaotropic agents or extremes of pH. There is often a compromise that has to be taken, between the ease of elution of the antigen and the long-term stability of the antibody on the column (if it is to be re-used) or of the antigen (if it is required intact and functional).

Immunoprecipitation reactions are often used in experimental situations where the antigen mixture is radiolabelled and then run in gel electrophoresis. Immunoprecipitating the antigen, or purifying it on an antibody-affinity column, allows the individual radiolabelled components to be separated and identified by their reactivity with the antibody. As described above, affinity purification on antibody columns can be used either to remove contaminants from a mixture, e.g. toxins, or alternatively to purify an antigen out of a mixture. These affinity columns tend to work best when its antibody is in excess over the antigen, whereas direct precipitation relies on antibody–antigen equivalence. If the column is to be recycled and re-used, or the antigen is to be recovered intact, then it is important that the antibody–antigen affinity is not too great. However, if it is important that, for example, all traces of an antigen, such as a toxin, are removed from a mixture, the antibody on the column must be in excess over antigen and not of too low an affinity.

It is possible to adapt the methods above to use indirect methods. Thus, molecules with an affinity for antibody such as Protein A or Protein G can be coupled to an affinity matrix and a mixture of antibody and antigen passed through. The binding of antibody to the column will indirectly adsorb the antigen. Similarly, antibodies can be chemically modified with chemical haptens (small molecules that can be recognised by antibodies but which must be coupled covalently to carrier proteins in order to make them immunogenic for use in immunisation), such as biotin, and then molecules, such as avidin or streptavidin, with affinity for biotin can be attached to the column matrix. Also anti-immunoglobulin antibodies (e.g. sheep antibodies specific for mouse IgG) can be used to affinity adsorb or immunoprecipitate soluble immune complexes.

25.10.2 Diagnostics

An important use of antibodies and, in particular, monoclonal antibodies is in diagnostic applications. The specificity of antibodies allows them to be used for the direct determination of the antigen even in complex mixtures. For example, they can be used to determine concentrations of a single hormone in samples of human blood. With appropriate standards and controls, the detection methods can quantify the chosen antigens in the system usually by labelling the antibody with a marker, which itself is quantitatively determined.

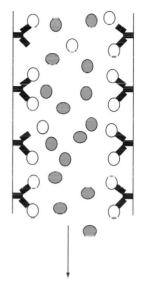

Unbound antigens

Figure 25.13 Affinity chromatography using an immobilised antibody. Purification based on the antibody's affinity for antigen can be easily carried out using antibody immobilised on a column matrix. In the schematic shown, the antibody is removing the white antigen from the blue antigen. Thus the fluid that flows through the column should be depleted of antigen to which the antibody is specific, whereas the fraction that is at first bound and then later eluted in a subsequent step will be enriched for antigen. The elution of bound antigen is usually carried out using mildly denaturing conditions, e.g. low pH buffers.

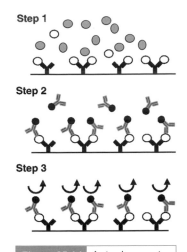

Step 1

Step 2

Step 3

Figure 25.14 A simple, two-site ELISA procedure. In the first step, antibody, which is immobilised onto a surface, is used to capture the antigen from solution. The excess and therefore unbound antigen is then washed away. In a second step, an enzyme-labelled antibody specific to a second site on the antigen is added. Again the excess-labelled antibody, which does not bind to the antigen, is then washed away. Finally, a substrate is added and the conversion of this by the enzyme is determined over a given time period. Usually a colour change resulting from formation of a coloured product is monitored using a spectrophotometer.

Commonly used labels are radioisotopes, enzymes or fluorochromes. Appropriate detection systems are then used to detect these.

The **enzyme-linked immunosorbent assay (ELISA)** is one of the most commonly used diagnostic techniques available today. The basic principle is simple. An enzyme is coupled directly to an antibody, usually using a chemical cross-linking procedure. The amount of antibody bound to an antigen can then be determined indirectly by measuring the conversion of a substrate to a product by the enzyme. This is stoichiometric; but also includes an amplification of the signal, because one molecule of enzyme can convert many molecules of substrate over a given time. If coloured substrates are used or coloured products are formed a simple photometric adsorbancy measurement will quantify the enzyme reaction. It is also possible to make this measurement as a real-time determination of the rate of the reaction.

There are many subtle variations on the basic ELISA system. In its simplest form, an antigen is adsorbed onto a solid surface, either non-specifically, or through an affinity ligand or covalent chemical bond. An enzyme-labelled antibody is then added in excess to the system and some of it binds to the immobilised antigen. Excess antibody is removed by washing and then substrate is added. The amount of enzyme, and hence amount of antibody–antigen complex in the system, is estimated from the amount of substrate it converts. More usually, ELISA involves a two-site recognition with two different antibodies or an indirect detection (see Fig. 25.14). For example, one antibody may be immobilised on a solid matrix and used to capture (affinity adsorb) the antigen. The amount of antigen captured can be determined by a second antibody coupled to an enzyme that recognises a different site on the antigen and so does not compete with the first antibody. Indirect detection systems can employ multiple layers of anti-antibodies or of biotin-avidin layers giving even greater amplification in the system. Alternatively, the systems can be designed to determine the quantity of unknown antigen in the system through competition with binding a known amount of a labelled and pure form of the same antigen (a method originally widely employed in radioimmunoassays). The maximum binding of labelled antigen is seen when there is no competitor antigen in the test sample and the minimum binding of labelled antigen is seen when there is a huge excess of competitor antigen in the test sample.

Enzyme-labelled antibodies are also employed in **immunocytochemistry**. Tissue sections or cell cytosmears are prepared on glass microscope slides. These are then incubated with antibodies specific for different tissue antigens and coupled with enzymes. After washing away excess antibody, the enzyme substrates are added. Substrates are chosen such that insoluble, coloured products are deposited in the section and these can be visualised in light microscopy and, along with suitable counter staining, may allow for very detailed classification of the cells stained. Using appropriate counter stains and, through co-localisation of test antibodies with known markers, it is possible to identify which parts of the cell, e.g. surface, cytoplasmic or nuclear staining, contain the antigen recognised by the antibody. Again, as described above for the ELISA system, the techniques can be modified to use multiple layers of antibody and anti-antibody in order to amplify the staining. As well as enzyme-labelled antibodies, it is possible to use antibodies coupled to fluorescent dyes (fluorophores) and to use them in fluorescent microscopy. Fluorescently conjugated antibodies can be used in the powerful technique of **confocal microscopy**, which allows the precise localisation of the fluorescence on, or in, the cell to be visualised in a time-dependent way. In confocal microscopy, images collected in a precise focal plane are digitised and then stored in a computer. These digitised images, which thus represent 'slices' through the cell, can then be built up into a three-dimensional representation of the intensity of fluorescence throughout the cell and a model can be displayed on a high-resolution graphics monitor. If images are collected at intervals over a given time, then the computer can also be used to generate a time-lapse movie of the movement of fluorescence within the cell.

Fluorescent antibody cell sorting and analysis have developed in parallel with monoclonal antibody technology. Again, the principles of the technique are simple. Monoclonal antibodies are labelled with a fluorochrome and used to stain cells. These cells are then passed at high velocity through a nozzle in a stream of liquid droplets such that the cells pass one at a time through a laser light beam that excites the fluorophore. Detectors then measure the fluorescence output from each cell on an individual basis. At the same time, other properties of the cells can be measured through their abilities to scatter the light beam (size and granularity of the cells). Also, different fluorophores with different emission spectra can be used to tag different antibodies. Thus, a very sophisticated analysis of cells even in a complex mixture can be carried out; for example, human blood cells can be separated into their various types and sub-types. The whole classification of human (and now other animal) cell surface antigens using the 'CD', which stands for cluster designation, nomenclature has relied very heavily on the use of fluorescent cell analysis. The results from the analysis, carried out in many laboratories, on panels of monclonal antibodies are used to cluster these antibodies into groups with similar reactivities, and provided this clustering seems to be statistically robust, an international committee authorises the designation of a cluster with a new sequential number in the CD series (e.g. CD1, CD2, CD3, etc.). Although many people now commonly refer to the antigens by the CD name, the original designation was of groups of antibodies. Thus 'anti-CD1 antibodies', for example, is nonsensical in the purest sense, since the cluster of antibodies is CD1, and the antigen is that which is recognised by the CD1 cluster of antibodies.

25.11 | In vivo uses of recombinant and monoclonal antibodies

Again, the uses of antibodies in vivo rely heavily on their great specificity for antigen. It is sometimes easy to forget when dealing with uses of monoclonal antibodies in vivo that our own antibodies play a major role in our natural immune system in protecting us from infection by killing pathogens and by removing harmful antigens from our system. However, despite this obvious role for antibodies, there are, in fact, only a few therapies currently in use that exploit monoclonal antibodies for these properties. This is largely due to the commercial, practical and also ethical considerations involved in developing antibody therapies. It is an enormously expensive and also a time-consuming undertaking to get even a single antibody through clinical trials and regulatory approval for widespread commercial sale and use. The situation is further complicated if accepted, existing treatments are already in use. Thus, polyclonal human IgG is manufactured and given (e.g. as a preparation called IVIG, i.e. intravenous IgG) for many disorders where passive immunity might be beneficial. Equally, polyclonal horse or sheep antisera against bacterial toxins (e.g. tetanus toxin), snake venoms or toxic drugs (e.g. digoxin) are a tried and tested treatment for acute poisoning. These antibody treatments work and could, in theory, be replaced with monoclonal antibodies, but this may not be economically and practically viable. Clearly, there is a potential role for monoclonal antibody-based therapies, wherever efficacy has already been demonstrated for polyclonal antisera. The obstacles are mainly commercial and regulatory issues. One example where these barriers might be overcome is the likely replacement of polyclonal human anti-RhD antibodies, used in the prevention of haemolytic disease of the newborn (HDN), with a monoclonal or mixture of monoclonal human antibodies specific for RhD antigen. The RhD antigen is not expressed on the red blood cells of a significant percentage of the population and, thus, mothers who are blood group RhD negative are able to make immune responses to their foetus's red blood cells if they are RhD positive as a result of inheriting this phenotype from their father. The mothers anti-RhD antibody can cross the placenta (if it is IgG) and cause red blood cell destruction in her unborn child. HDN does not affect the first born RhD-positive child because the mother's immune response takes time to develop IgG antibodies to the RhD antigen. However, during subsequent pregnancies with RhD antigen positive foetuses, the IgG antibodies develop more quickly (secondary immune response). It has been found that administering anti-RhD antibodies to the mother at the time of birth can suppress her immunisation by RhD antigens. In the example of RhD, concerns over the safe use (in the light of, for example, bovine spongiform encephalopathy, BSE, and new variant Creutzfeldt–Jakob disease, nvCJD) of pooled blood products, for treatment of young healthy women of child-bearing age, may play a significant role in pushing forward the switch to a monoclonal based product.

Thus, in contrast, many antibodies have been developed for use in vivo in situations where natural antibodies may not play any significant role, such as in attempts to eradicate tumour cells from the body. This is mainly because alternative treatments are not available making it logistically easier to try new antibody-based therapies. Requiring monoclonal antibodies to achieve what polyclonal antibodies are unable to do may be one reason for the large number of apparently unsuccessful antibody-based trials.

Imaging is an area where the combination of antibodies and modern computerised techniques can provide a detailed analytical tool for looking inside the human body in a non-invasive way. Thus, for example, radiolabelled antibodies that localise to a tumour can be detected with γ-cameras and, by using a series of moving detectors, a three-dimensional image can be built up as a computer model showing exactly where the labelled antibodies are sequestered. There are many problems with this technology: for example, for antibodies of moderate affinity, only a fraction will become localised to antigen, with the rest remaining unbound. Also, some antibody will be taken up non-specifically by some tissues or even specifically through Fc receptors and also receptors for carbohydrate. One way round this is to image two antibodies with different isotopes. One antibody will be chosen to be specific for antigen, for example a tumour-associated antigen, the other antibody will be a matched control, but with no specificity for the antigen. The two images can be subtracted one from the other leaving just the image of the specific binding. In this way, the antibody appears to be more specific than it really is, but it does provide a useful diagnostic tool in looking for tumour metastasis and similar malignancies.

Cancer therapy is one application where most people are familiar with the concept of antibodies as so-called 'magic bullets', a term used to describe them by the popular press and on broadcast news items. The idea is that the specificity of the antibody allows it to target tumour cells for destruction. The problems here are two-fold: first, it is necessary to identify a suitable specificity associated with the tumour; second, the antibody must be capable of delivering some kind of destructive effector mechanism to the tumour cells. Tumour-associated or tumour-specific antigens are not easy to identify and the examples where they can be found are usually such that a new antibody would have to be made for each patient. It is then often the case that tumour cells are resistant to killing by natural antibody-effector mechanisms, such as through complement or processes that are triggered by cross-linking of Fc receptors. There have been some examples where antibodies seem to be effective at least in a proportion of patients with some types of tumour, e.g. leukaemias and lymphomas, but there have been many failures in clinical trials.

As an alternative to natural effector mechanisms in tumour cell targeting and destruction, some scientists have tried coupling other toxic agents to antibodies. Obviously, radioisotopes may deliver a lethal radiation dose to the tumour tissue providing there is a high enough degree of specific localisation of the antibody (a function of the antibodies' affinity, half-life and ease of tissue penetration). Others have tried coupling highly active toxins to antibodies, such as the plant toxins ricin, abrin and gelonin. These work very well against some target antigens and for some cell types but there are still problems with non-specific toxicity to the patient versus the degree of tumour cell kill. The other aspect is that the toxins seem to be highly immunogenic and, in the medium to long term, provoke a strong antiglobulin response to the antibody–toxin conjugate. As another alternative approach, enzymes can be coupled to antibodies which will convert non-toxic, pro-drugs to highly toxic, but short-lived, active drugs at the site of tumour localisation. I would argue this is reminiscent of how the natural complement system works. One problem with all these strategies is that the degree of tumour localisation is critical. It is undesirable to have too much antibody circulating round the body and triggering non-specific toxicity in other tissues. Ironically, natural effector mechanisms have evolved to work under precisely these conditions, i.e. an antibody excess. They rely mainly on a succession of low affinity, but higher avidity, steps to distinguish immune complexes from free antibody.

One area where antibody-based therapies have had some success is in specifically targeting cells involved in immune functions and thus creating a state of **immunosuppression**. Antibodies have been targeted at whole populations of cells, such as all lymphocytes, at specific lineages, such as T-lymphocytes, or at activation-antigens expressed only by smaller sub-populations of cells, e.g. those expressing certain cytokine receptors. Earlier strategies were aimed at killing these cells either using natural antibody-effector mechanisms or through use of immunotoxins. More recently, there has been a shift in antibody therapy towards the use of non-depleting blocking antibodies. This comes from the realisation that cells respond to different signals and that the very nature of the signals, e.g. whether they are linked together or independent, can either result in cells that participate in an inflammatory reaction or, alternatively, regulatory cells that can attenuate a response. Through the use of antibodies that are able to block normal cellular processes, it is hoped that cells can be re-programmed in autoimmune reactions to stop reacting against self and, similarly, the immune system might be taught to accept foreign-grafted tissues.

These blocking functions of antibodies require that they still are able to bind to antigen, but that they should not activate complement or trigger Fc receptors on effector cells. Such properties can be achieved by modifying sequences within the constant regions of antibodies known to be critical for individual antibody functions. As an additional step on from these strategies, chimaeric molecules are being constructed in which the genes encoding Fc regions of antibodies are combined with genes encoding domains of cytokine receptors or adhesion molecules to create **immunoadhesins**. These domains replace the antibody variable region but still provide a highly specific recognition of a ligand The Fc region provides the whole molecule with a multiple valency and also a longer half-life.

As mentioned above the problems with use of antibodies in vivo is that the development time and clinical trials are procedures that last for many years. Thus, many of the antibodies in the final stages of clinical trials today are based on scientific ideas of perhaps ten or more years ago. Equally, it will be many years before some of the newest ideas in laboratory science today find their way into the next generation of clinical trials.

25.12 | Further reading

Antibody Engineering, Vol 65, *Chemical Immunology*. Capra, J. D. (ed.) Basel, London and New York: Karger, 1997.

Goldsby, R. A., Kindt, T. J., Osborne, B. A. and Kuby, J. *Immunology*, fifth edition. New York: W. H. Freeman & Company, 2003.

Harris, W. J. and Adair, J. R. (eds.) *Antibody Therapeutics*. New York and London: CRC Press, 1997.

Janeway, C. A., Travers, P., Walport, M. and Shlomchik, M. *Immunobiology: The Immune System in Health and Disease*, fifth edition. New York: Garland Science, 2001.

King, D. J. *Applications and Engineering of Monoclonal Antibodies*. London: Taylor & Francis, 1998.

Kontermann, R. and Dubel, S. (eds.) *Antibody Engineering*. Berlin: Springer-Verlag, 2001.

Parham, P. *The Immune System*, second edition. New York: Garland Science, 2004.

Index